Workbook for

Radiographic Positioning and Related Anatomy

Eleventh edition

John P. Lampignano, MEd, R.T.(R)(CT)(ARRT)

Leslie E. Kendrick, MS, R.T.(R)(CT)(MR)(ARRT)

ELSEVIER

Elsevier
3251 Riverport Lane
St. Louis, Missouri 63043

WORKBOOK FOR RADIOGRAPHIC POSITIONING
AND RELATED ANATOMY, ELEVENTH EDITION

ISBN: 978-0-323-93615-6

Previous editions copyrighted 2021, 2018, 2014, 2010, 2005, 2001, and 1997.

Content Strategist: Meg Benson
Senior Content Development Specialist: Tina Kaemmerer
Publishing Services Manager: Deepthi Unni
Project Manager: Thoufiq Mohammed
Cover Design: Amy Buxton

Printed in the United States of America

Last digit is the print number: 9 8 7 6 5 4 3 2

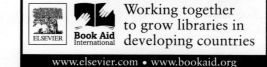

Acknowledgments

I am fortunate to have **Leslie E. Kendrick** as my friend and coauthor. Leslie is a dedicated educator, talented and professional writer who has brought a high degree of quality and currency to this edition. Leslie has the insights, skills, and dedication of a veteran educator and writer. She has made me a better writer, educator, and person. I am blessed to have her as a coauthor for this edition and other editions to follow.

Tina Kaemmerer, our editor, deserves praise for her dedication and vision in coordinating this project. She supported us tirelessly and professionally through every phase of this new edition. She has become a close friend to us, and we hope to work with her for many future editions. This workbook would not have been possible without her talents and dedication. Special thanks also to **Meg Benson**, Senior Content Strategist, for the leadership on the text and related ancillaries. **Dr. Chad Hensley, Professor, University of Nevada Las Vegas**, edited and validated each of the review exercises and assessments for this edition of the workbook. Chad has a keen eye for detail and ensured the accuracy of each exercise and assessment. Special thanks to **Thoufiq Mohammed**, the Production Project Manager, for his attention to detail and his professionalism during the editing phase of the workbook.

This edition is dedicated to the students who continue to provide us with valuable feedback on how we can improve the text and workbook materials.

Finally, my gratitude goes to the faculty who dedicated their careers to preparing future generations of health care professionals. The faculty at **Boise State University and GateWay Community College** have a special love for their profession and it is reflected daily in their dedication to quality instruction and mentoring of the next generation of technologists. Thank you.

John P. Lampignano

Thank you to my friend and coauthor, **John P. Lampignano** for collaborating with me on this project. It has truly been a life-changing experience. John's passion for the profession, true respect for others, and insatiable drive to provide a valuable, lasting resource for imaging technologists are admirable. It is truly an incredible honor to work with John and have such an amazing opportunity to contribute to the field of radiologic sciences. Thank you for your trust and friendship.

I wish to echo John's expression of appreciation to all the individuals at Elsevier who made this publication possible. Many thanks especially to **Tina Kaemmerer**, our editor. She truly is a master of her trade and a dear friend. It has been more than a pleasure to have Tina guiding us throughout the progression of this project. A special thank you to **Meg Benson**, our senior content strategist, for looking out for the best interest of the authors and the project. You are a gem and most appreciated for your attention to detail. A note of special recognition to **Chad Hensley** for his enthusiasm for the project, his eye for accuracy, and his talent for writing. Working with Chad is always a privilege.

A word of appreciation is also extended to all of the working technologists, physicians, faculty, and students who are so willing to provide us with feedback on methods for keeping these materials accurate, current, and useful. It is my hope that this workbook continues to be a valued teaching tool for the enhancement of student success.

Leslie E. Kendrick

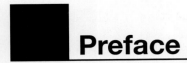

Preface

Because of the success of the first ten editions of this workbook and laboratory manual, as well as the accompanying textbook, along with the associated ancillary materials, many schools of radiologic technology throughout the United States and other countries have adopted and used all or parts of these instructional media for more than 40 years.

NEW TO THIS EDITION

The field of medical imaging is in constant evolution. It becomes a challenge to create a text and workbook that accurately reflect the technology and clinical practice of the profession. Through the diligence of the contributors and reviewers, we hope we have successfully made these learning tools as current as possible.

New illustrations, photographs, and expanded questions have been added to the eleventh edition of the *Textbook of Radiographic Positioning and Related Anatomy*. The use of visuals in these review exercises is aimed not only at increasing comprehension but also at increasing retention. *A team of educators has assessed every review question to ensure it as accurate as possible.*

The detailed laboratory activities have been updated, and the positioning question-and-answer exercises have been expanded, with less emphasis on rote memory recall. More situational questions involving clinical applications have been added. These questions assist in the application of positioning principles and the critical evaluation of images. The clinically situational questions require students to analyze and apply positioning criteria to specific clinical examples.

Pathology and clinical indication questions have been expanded to help students understand why they are performing specific exams and how exposure factors or positioning may be affected.

As in the textbook, updated information and concepts in digital imaging have been added in this edition.

HANDBOOK

The eleventh edition of the expanded *Handbook of Radiographic Positioning and Techniques* is now available from Elsevier as part of this comprehensive learning package on radiographic positioning and imaging. The 11th edition of this handbook includes the unique added feature of a printed radiographic image of the position being described along with a basic critique checklist alongside each image. These primary image evaluation criteria are grouped in a consistent manner for all projections and are listed in more detail in the positioning pages of the textbook in the *Evaluation Criteria* section.

This unique handbook provides a guide for students to carry with them in the clinical setting as they learn what to look for when they evaluate each radiograph after it has been taken and processed.

INFORMATION FOR FACULTY

Instructor Resources

Electronic resources are available on the Evolve website at http://evolve.elsevier.com/Lampignano/positioning/, and they consist of the following five components:

- **Radiographic Critique:** The textbook for Chapters 2–11 and 18 have been designed to provide students with a baseline, well-positioned image to compare and contrast with two or more images that reflect common technical and positioning errors. Our goal is to expand knowledge to distinguish between an excellent and a substandard image. The solutions for this exercise are found on the **Evolve website** under **Instructor Resources** so that educators may use these exercises for assessment.

- **Self-Test Answer Keys:** Each chapter in the workbook includes a self-test that appears after the review exercises, which the students can complete. Based on feedback in advance of the eighth edition from educators, the answer keys were removed from the student workbook and have been placed on the **Evolve website** under **Instructor Resources**.

- **Test Bank:** This test bank features more than 2000 questions divided into 20 chapters. It has been updated, expanded, and revised into more registry-level questions that can be used as final evaluation exams for each chapter. Each question and the answers have been verified by a team of educators and student reviewers. They can be used to produce paper-based exams, or they can be integrated into a Learning Management System such as Canvas. These questions can be downloaded to use for any assessment, and you will be able to delete or add questions to create your own personal test bank.

- **Electronic Image Collection:** Also available is an updated and expanded electronic collection of images from all 20 chapters of the eleventh edition of the textbook. These images can be used by faculty to create PowerPoint presentations or for other web-based applications.

- **Electronic Instructional Presentation in PowerPoint:** Now included is an updated and expanded electronic image PowerPoint program that is fully coordinated with all 20 chapters of the eleventh edition textbook and workbook. These electronic images include text slides, some of which contain embedded anatomy and radiographic images, resulting in a visually led instructional narrative. This can then be used as a complete chapter-by-chapter PowerPoint lecture guide. Sections from the more advanced chapters can also be used for in-service training or with postgraduate presentations. They may be downloaded to your desktop to personalize with your own content.

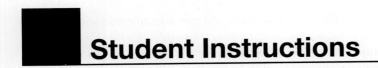

Student Instructions

The following information describes how to use this workbook and the accompanying textbook effectively to help you master radiographic anatomy and positioning.

Because this course becomes the core of all your studies and your work as a radiologic technologist, it is one that you must master. You cannot become a proficient technologist by marginally passing this course. Therefore please read these instructions carefully before beginning Chapter 1.

OBJECTIVES

Gain a clear understanding of the competencies by reviewing the list of objectives found at the beginning of each chapter.

TEXTBOOK AND WORKBOOK

Chapter 1 includes a comprehensive introduction that prepares you for the remaining chapters of this positioning course. This chapter contains basic positioning and technical principles that will apply to the remainder of the text and workbook exercises. Your instructor may assign all or specific sections of these chapters at various times during your study of radiographic positioning or procedures. There is an expanded section on digital imaging. The radiation protection section reflects the best practices to protect both patient and technologist.

Chapters 2–14 are specific positioning chapters that include the anatomy, positioning, and related procedures for most regions of the body.

Chapters 15–20 describe more specialized procedures and modalities that are commonly studied later in a medical radiography program.

LEARNING EXERCISES

These exercises are the focal point of this workbook. Using them correctly will help you learn and remember the important information presented in each chapter of the textbook. To maximize the benefits from each exercise, follow the correct six-step order of activities as outlined in the following.

ANATOMY ACTIVITIES

Step 1 (Textbook)

Carefully read and learn the radiographic anatomy section described in each of these chapters. Include the anatomic reviews on labeled radiographs provided in the textbook. Pay particular attention to those items in bold type and to the summary review boxes, where provided.

Step 2 (Workbook, Part I)

Complete Part I of the review exercises on radiographic anatomy. Do not look up the answers in the textbook or look at the answer key until you have completed the review exercises. Then refer to the textbook or the answer key and correct or complete those questions you answered incorrectly. Reread those sections of the textbook in which you could not answer questions.

POSITIONING ACTIVITIES

Step 3 (Textbook)

Carefully read and study Part II on all of the parts on radiographic positioning. Note the general positioning considerations, alternate modalities, and clinical indications for each chapter. Information from these sections will be seen on workbook review exercises and self-tests. Learn the specific positioning steps, the central ray location and angle, and the five-part radiographic criteria for each projection or position.

Step 4 (Workbook, Part II)

Complete Part II of the review exercises, which includes technical considerations and positioning. Also included is a section on problem-solving for technical and positioning errors. As before, complete as many of the questions as you can before looking up the answers in the textbook or checking the answers on the answer key.

The last review exercise in each positioning chapter covers radiographic critique questions in the workbook. These questions may involve radiographic evaluation of images from the textbook. These important exercises will help you make the transition from factual knowledge to application and will help you prepare for clinical experience. Compare each critique radiograph that demonstrates errors with the correctly positioned radiographs in that chapter of the textbook, and see if you can determine which radiographic criteria points could be improved and which are repeatable errors.

With digital imaging, you will learn that in some cases, postprocessing adjustments can be made to improve the exposures and the diagnostic value of the images rather than repeating the exam. Positioning errors, however, would still need to be repeated. Students who successfully complete these exercises will be ahead of those students who do not attempt them before coming to the classroom. The instructor will then explain and clarify the repeatable and nonrepeatable errors on each radiograph.

LABORATORY ACTIVITY

Step 5 (Workbook, Part III)

These exercises must be performed in a radiographic laboratory using a phantom or a student (without making exposure), an energized radiographic unit, and monitors for viewing digital images. Arrange for a time when you can use your radiographic laboratory or a diagnostic radiographic room in a clinic setting.

This is one of the most important aspects of this learning series and should not be neglected or underemphasized. Students frequently have difficulty transferring the information they have learned about positioning to effective use in a clinical setting. Therefore you must perform the laboratory activities as described in each chapter. Your instructors or lab assistants will assist you as needed in these exercises.

Each radiograph taken of the phantom or other radiographs provided by your instructor should be evaluated as described in your lab manual. Critique and evaluate each radiograph for errors of less-than-optimal positioning or exposure factors based on radiographic criteria provided in the textbook. Also, with the help of your instructor, learn how to discriminate between less-than-optimal but diagnostic radiographs, and those that need to be repeated. This generally requires additional experience and practice before you can make these judgments without assistance from a supervising technologist or radiologist.

SELF-TEST

Step 6

You should take the self-test only after you have completed all the preceding steps. Treat the self-test as if it is an actual exam. After completing the self-test, submit your test to your instructor. **The faculty possesses the self-test answer keys**. Please **DO NOT share the answer keys** with peers or share them online. It denies other students and faculty the ability to use them as authentic assessments. If your score is less than 90%–95%, you should go back and review the textbook again; pay special attention to the areas you missed before you take the final chapter evaluation exam provided by your instructor.

Note: Statistics prove that students who diligently complete all the exercises described in this section will invariably achieve higher grades in their positioning courses and will perform better in the clinical setting than those who do not. Avoid the temptation of taking shortcuts or looking for the answers online. If you bypass some of these exercises or just fill in the answers from the answer key or other resources, your instructors will know by your grade and by your clinical performance that you have taken these shortcuts. Most important, you will know that you are not doing your best and when you graduate you will have difficulty in competing with better prepared technologists in the workplace.

Go to it and enjoy the feeling of satisfaction and success that only comes when you know you're doing your best!

Contents

1 Terminology, Positioning, and Imaging Principles

CHAPTER OBJECTIVES

After you have successfully completed the activities in this chapter, you will be able to:

A. General, Systemic, and Skeletal Anatomy and Arthrology

_____ 1. List the four basic types of tissues.

_____ 2. List the 10 systems of the body.

_____ 3. Match specific bodily functions to their correct anatomic system.

_____ 4. List the four general classifications of bone.

_____ 5. Identify specific characteristics and aspects of bone.

_____ 6. Classify specific joints by their structure and function.

_____ 7. Classify specific synovial joints by their movement types.

B. Positioning Terminology

_____ 1. Define general radiographic and anatomic relational terminology.

_____ 2. Define the imaginary planes, sections, and surfaces of the body used to describe central ray (CR) angles or relationships among body parts.

_____ 3. Distinguish among a radiographic projection, position, and view.

_____ 4. Given various hypothetic situations, identify the correct radiographic projection.

_____ 5. Given various hypothetic situations, identify the correct radiographic position.

_____ 6. List the antonyms (terms with opposite meanings) of specific terms related to movement.

C. Positioning Principles

_____ 1. Given a hypothetic clinical situation, identify the response as required in the professional code of ethics.

_____ 2. Identify the correct sequence of steps taken to perform a routine radiographic procedure.

_____ 3. Given a set of circumstances, apply the three general rules of radiography concerning the minimal number of projections required for specific regions of the body.

_____ 4. Identify the correct way to view a conventional radiograph, computed tomography (CT) image, and magnetic resonance (MR) image.

_____ 5. List the three key elements of the American Society of Radiologic Technologists (ASRT) ACE campaign.

D. Imaging Principles

_____ 1. Describe the major exposure factors that influence the diagnostic quality of the radiograph.

_____ 2. List the four image quality factors and their impact on a radiograph.

_____ 3. Identify the exposure factors controlling receptor exposure and penetrability.

_____ 4. Explain SID and its impact on x-ray beam intensity.

_____ 5. Define the 15% rule.

_____ 6. Define grids and the factors for when they are used.

_____ 7. Explain the benefits of collimation.

_____ 8. Define Exposure Index (EI).

_____ 9. List the three critical concepts related to EI and radiation exposure to the IR.

_____ 10. Define spatial resolution and identify its controlling factors.

_____ 11. Define _blur_ and identify its controlling factors.

_____ 12. List the three geometric factors that influence image sharpness.

_____ 13. Identify the best ways of controlling voluntary and involuntary motion.

_____ 14. Given a hypothetic situation, select the correct factor to improve radiographic detail.

_____ 15. Define _radiographic distortion_ and identify its controlling factors.

_____ 16. Given a hypothetic situation, select the correct factor to minimize radiographic distortion.

E. Digital Imaging Characteristics

_____ 1. Define digital medical imaging.

_____ 2. Define _pixels_ and their impact on spatial resolution

_____ 3. Define _contrast resolution_ and identify its controlling factors in the digital image.

_____ 4. List the two types of pixel sizes.

_____ 5. Define _spatial resolution_ and identify its controlling factors in the digital image.

_____ 6. Define _detective quantum efficiency (DQE)._

_____ 7. List the three factors that influence scatter radiation.

_____ 8. Explain the concept of the signal-to-noise ratio (SNR).

_____ 9. Identify the dynamic range of digital imaging systems.

F. Digital Imaging Equipment

_____ 1. List the major components of a storage phosphor-based digital system (PSP).

_____ 2. Describe briefly how an image is recorded, processed, and viewed with a PSP system.

_____ 3. Explain the importance of correct centering, collimation, use of lead masking, and use of grids to the overall quality of the digital image.

_____ 4. Identify specific differences and similarities between PSP and digital radiography (DR).

_____ 5. Define the terms PACS, RIS, HIS, and DICOM.

_____ 6. Compare and contrast differently sized image receptors between metric and English units of measurement.

_____ 7. Define specific digital imaging terms and acronyms.

G. Radiation Protection

_____ 1. List the three methods to reduce exposure to patients and staff.

_____ 2. List and define the traditional units and International System of Units (SI units) of radiation measurement and the conversion factors used to convert between systems.

_____ 3. List the specific annual dose-limiting recommendations of whole-body effective dose for the general population and occupationally exposed workers.

_____ 4. Define ALARA.

_____ 5. Apply the principles of ALARA to a given hypothetic situation.

_____ 6. List the different types of personnel dosimeters.

_____ 7. Define and provide examples of effective dose (ED).

_____ 8. Identify specific methods to reduce exposure to the technologist during fluoroscopic and radiographic procedures.

_____ 9. Describe the seven methods to reduce exposure to the patient during radiographic procedures.

_____ 10. Identify the major types of specific area shields and how they should be applied during radiographic procedures.

_____ 11. Define patient dose terminology for specific regions of the body.

_____ 12. Identify methods to ensure a dose to the patient is minimized when using digital imaging systems.

_____ 13. Explain the Image Wisely and Image Gently initiative and its purpose.

The following review exercises should be completed only after careful study of the associated pages in the textbook as indicated by each exercise. Because certain topics may be too advanced for the entry-level student, the review exercises for Chapter 1 are divided into Sections A through C. You can complete specific sections of review exercises, as directed by your instructor, to best meet your learning needs.

After completing each of these individual exercises, check your answers with the answers provided at the end of the review exercises.

REVIEW EXERCISE A: General, Systemic, and Skeletal Anatomy and Arthrology (see textbook pp. 3–17)

1. The lowest level of the structural organization of the human body is the _____.

2. List the four basic types of tissues in the body.

   A. _____   C. _____

   B. _____   D. _____

3. List the 10 systems of the human body.

   A. _____   F. _____

   B. _____   G. _____

   C. _____   H. _____

   D. _____   I. _____

   E. _____   J. _____

4. Match the following functions to the correct body system.

   _____ 1. Eliminates solid waste from the body   A. Skeletal system

   _____ 2. Regulates fluid and electrolyte balance and volume   B. Circulatory system

   _____ 3. Maintains posture   C. Digestive system

   _____ 4. Regulates body activities with electrical impulses   D. Respiratory system

   _____ 5. Regulates bodily activities through various hormones E. Urinary system

   _____ 6. Eliminates carbon dioxide from blood   F. Reproductive system

   _____ 7. Receives stimuli, such as temperature, pressure, and pain   G. Nervous system

   _____ 8. Reproduces the organism   H. Muscular system

   _____ 9. Regulates body temperature   I. Endocrine system

   _____ 10. Supports and protects many soft tissues of the body   J. Integumentary system

5. True/False: One of the six functions of the circulatory system is to protect against disease.

6. Which of the following body systems synthesizes vitamin D and other biochemicals?

   A. Integumentary   C. Circulatory

   B. Digestive   D. Endocrine

7. What is the largest organ system in the body?

    A. Digestive

    B. Nervous

    C. Integumentary

    D. Respiratory

8. List the two divisions of the human skeletal system.

    A. _____

    B. _____

9. True/False: The adult skeleton system contains 256 separate bones.

10. True/False: The scapula is part of the axial skeleton.

11. True/False: The skull is part of the axial skeleton.

12. True/False: The pelvic girdle is part of the appendicular skeleton.

13. List the four classifications of bones.

    A. _____

    B. _____

    C. _____

    D. _____

14. The outer covering of a long bone, which is composed of a dense, fibrous membrane, is called what?

    A. Spongy or cancellous bone

    B. Compact bone

    C. Medullary aspect

    D. Periosteum

15. Which aspect of long bones is responsible for the production of red blood cells?

    A. Sesamoid bone

    B. Compact bone

    C. Medullary aspect

    D. Periosteum

16. Which aspect of the long bone is essential for bone growth, repair, and nutrition?

    A. Medullary aspect

    B. Compact bone

    C. Periosteum

    D. Articular cartilage

17. Identify the primary and secondary growth centers for long bones.

    A. Primary growth center: _____

    B. Secondary growth center: _____

18. True/False: Epiphyseal fusion of the long bones is complete by the age of 16 years.

19. The _____ is the wider portion of a long bone in which bone growth in length occurs.

    A. Diaphysis

    B. Epiphysis

    C. Metaphysis

    D. Epiphyseal plate

20. List the three *functional* classifications of joints.

    A. _____

    B. _____

    C. _____

21. List the three *structural* classifications of joints.

    A. _____

    B. _____

    C. _____

22. Match the following joints to the correct structural classification.

    _____ 1. First carpometacarpal of thumb   A. Fibrous joint

    _____ 2. Roots around teeth   B. Cartilaginous joint

    _____ 3. Proximal radioulnar joint   C. Synovial joint

    _____ 4. Skull sutures

    _____ 5. Epiphyses

    _____ 6. Interphalangeal joints

    _____ 7. Distal tibiofibular joint

    _____ 8. Intervertebral disk space

    _____ 9. Symphysis pubis

    _____ 10. Hip joint

23. List the seven types of movement for synovial joints. (List primary and secondary terms.)

    A. _____   E. _____

    B. _____   F. _____

    C. _____   G. _____

    D. _____

24. Match the following synovial joints to the correct type of movement.

  _____ 1. First carpometacarpal joint   A. Plane

  _____ 2. Elbow joint   B. Ginglymus

  _____ 3. Shoulder joint   C. Pivot

  _____ 4. Intercarpal joint   D. Ellipsoidal

  _____ 5. Wrist joint   E. Saddle

  _____ 6. Temporomandibular joint   F. Ball and socket

  _____ 7. First and second cervical vertebra joint   G. Bicondylar

  _____ 8. Second interphalangeal joint

  _____ 9. Distal radioulnar joint

  _____ 10. Ankle joint

  _____ 11. Knee joint

  _____ 12. Third metacarpophalangeal joint

25. The build, physique, and general shape of the body are defined as _____.

26. Which of the following body-type classifications makes up 50% of the population?
 A. Hypersthenic   C. Asthenic
 B. Sthenic   D. Hyposthenic

27. Which of the following body-type classifications makes up 35% of the population?
 A. Hypersthenic   C. Asthenic
 B. Sthenic   D. Hyposthenic

28. True/False: Approximately 5% of the population is classified as hypersthenic.

29. What is the specialty in medicine that deals with the study and treatment of obesity? _____

30. True/False: Body habitus has no impact on radiographic positioning.

REVIEW EXERCISE B: Positioning Terminology (see textbook pp. 18–32)

1. A(n) _____ is an image of a patient's anatomic part(s) as produced by the actions of x-rays on an image receptor.

2. The _____ is the aspect of an x-ray beam that has the least divergence (unless there is angulation).

3. An upright position with the arms abducted, palms forward, and head and feet together and directed straight ahead describes the _____ position.

4. The vertical plane that divides the body into equal right and left parts is the _____ plane.

5. The vertical plane that divides the body into equal anterior and posterior parts

   is the _____ plane.

6. A plane taken at right angles along any point of the longitudinal axis of the body

   is the _____ plane.

7. True/False: The *base plane of the skull* is a transverse plane located between the infraorbital margin of the orbits and the superior margin of the external auditory meatus (EAM).

8. The _____ refers to the back half of the patient and the _____ refers to the front half.

9. The direction or path of the central ray defines the following positioning term:

   A. Projection   C. Position

   B. View   D. Perspective

10. The positioning term that describes the general and specific body position is:

    A. Projection   C. Position

    B. View   D. Perspective

11. True/False: Oblique body and lateral positions are described according to the side of the body closest to the image receptor.

12. True/False: Decubitus positions always use a horizontal x-ray beam.

13. What is the name of the position in which the body is turned 90 degrees from a true anteroposterior (AP) or posteroanterior (PA) projection?

    _____

14. **Situation:** A patient is erect with the back to the image receptor. The left side of the body is turned 45 degrees toward the image receptor. What is this position?

    _____

15. **Situation:** A patient is recumbent facing the image receptor. The right side of the body is turned 15 degrees toward the image receptor. What is this position?

    _____

16. **Situation:** The patient is lying on his or her back. The x-ray beam is directed horizontally and enters the right side and exits the left side of the body. An image receptor is placed against the left side of the patient. Which specific position has been performed?

    _____

17. **Situation:** The patient is erect with the right side of the body against the image receptor. The x-ray beam enters the left side and exits the right side of the body. Which specific position has been performed?

    _____

18. **Situation:** A patient on a cart is lying on the left side. The x-ray beam is directed horizontally and enters the posterior surface and exits the anterior aspect of the body. The image receptor is against the anterior surface. Which specific position has been performed?

    _____

19. Match the following definitions to the correct term (using each term only once).

_____ 1. Palm of the hand	A. Posterior
_____ 2. Lying on the back facing upward	B. Anterior
_____ 3. An upright position	C. Plantar
_____ 4. Lying in any position	D. Dorsum pedis
_____ 5. Front half of the patient	E. Trendelenburg
_____ 6. Top or anterior surface of the foot	F. Erect
_____ 7. Position in which head is higher than the feet	G. Supine
_____ 8. Posterior aspect of foot	H. Palmar
_____ 9. Position in which head is lower than the feet	I. Recumbent
_____ 10. Back half of the patient	J. Fowler

20. What is the name of the projection in which the central ray enters the anterior surface and exits the posterior surface?

    _____

21. A projection using a Central Ray (CR) angle of ≥10 degrees directed parallel along the long axis of the body or body

    part is termed a(n) _____ projection.

22. The specific position that demonstrates the apices of the lungs, without superimposition of the clavicles, is termed

    a(n) _____ position.

23. What is the term that describes a decreasing of the angle between the top of the foot (dorsum) and the lower leg?

    _____

24. True/False: The term *varus* describes the bending of a part outward.

25. Match the following. (Indicate whether the following terms describe a position or projection.)

_____ 1. Anteroposterior	A. Position
_____ 2. Prone	B. Projection
_____ 3. Trendelenburg	
_____ 4. Left posterior oblique	
_____ 5. Left lateral chest	
_____ 6. Mediolateral ankle	
_____ 7. Tangential	
_____ 8. Lordotic	
_____ 9. Inferosuperior axial	
_____ 10. Left lateral decubitus	

26. For each of the following terms, list the word that has the **opposite** meaning.

   A. Flexion: _____

   B. Ulnar deviation: _____

   C. Dorsiflexion: _____

   D. Eversion: _____

   E. Lateral (external) rotation: _____

   F. Abduction: _____

   G. Supination: _____

   H. Retraction: _____

   I. Depression: _____

27. Match the following relationship terms to the correct definition (using each term only once):

   _____ 1. Near the source or beginning   A. Caudad or inferior

   _____ 2. On the opposite side   B. Deep

   _____ 3. Toward the center   C. Distal

   _____ 4. Toward the head end of the body   D. Contralateral

   _____ 5. Away from the source or beginning   E. Cephalad or superior

   _____ 6. Outside or outward   F. Proximal

   _____ 7. On the same side   G. Medial

   _____ 8. Near the skin surface   H. Superficial

   _____ 9. Away from the head end   I. Ipsilateral

   _____ 10. Farther from the skin surface   J. Exterior

28. Which two types of information should be imprinted on **every** radiographic image?

   A. _____   B. _____

29. True/False. It is acceptable to annotate an anatomic side marker on digital images.

30. Which of the following are additional markers that may be included on a radiograph?

   A. Time indicators   C. Inspiration or expiration

   B. Upright, erect, or arrows   D. Any of the above

REVIEW EXERCISE C: Positioning Principles (see textbook pp. 33–39)

1. The _____ describes the rules of acceptable conduct toward patients and other health care team members as well as personal actions and behaviors as defined within the profession.

2. True/False: A technologist is responsible for the professional decisions he or she makes during the care of a patient.

3. True/False: The technologist is responsible for communicating with the patient to obtain pertinent clinical information.

4. Which organization maintains the code of ethics for radiologic technologists?
   A. ASRT
   B. ARRT
   C. JRCERT
   D. OSHA

5. List the three recommendations stated in the ASRT ACE communication campaign.
   A. _____
   B. _____
   C. _____

6. List the two rules or principles for determining positioning routines as they relate to the maximum number of projections required in a basic routine.
   A. _____
   B. _____

7. Indicate the minimum number of projections (1, 2, or 3) required for each of the following anatomic regions.
   A. Foot _____
   B. Chest _____
   C. Wrist _____
   D. Tibia/fibula _____
   E. Humerus _____
   F. Fifth toe _____
   G. Postreduction of wrist (image of wrist in cast) _____
   H. Left hip _____
   I. Knee _____
   J. Pelvis (non hip injury) _____

8. **Situation:** A young child enters the emergency room with a fractured forearm. After one projection is completed that confirms a fracture, the child refuses to move the forearm for any additional projections.
   A. What is the *minimum* number of projections that must be taken for this forearm study?
      (a) One
      (b) Four
      (c) Three
      (d) Two

   B. If additional projections are required for a routine forearm series, what should the technologist do with the young patient described in this situation?
      (a) Because only one projection is required for a fractured forearm, the technologist is not required to take additional projections.
      (b) With the help of a parent or guardian, gently but firmly move the forearm for each additional projection required.
      (c) Rather than move the forearm for a second projection, place the IR and x-ray tube as needed for a second projection 90 degrees from the first projection.
      (d) Ask the emergency room physician to move the forearm for a second projection. This eliminates any liability for the technologist in case the patient is injured further.

9. What is the term for bony landmarks used for positioning that identify specific structures or organs?

   _____.

10. True/False. Patient consent should be obtained before palpating a topographic landmark.

11. True/False: In most cases, the long axis of the anatomic part is aligned to the longest dimension of the IR.

12. True/False: Most CT and MR images are viewed so that the patient's right side is to the viewer's left.

13. True/False: The technologist is expected to review the preliminary findings of the radiographic study with the patient.

14. True/False: Technologists are not allowed to ask female patients if they may be pregnant.

15. True/False: The technologist should verify that the correct patient is having the correct procedure by a minimum of two means.

REVIEW EXERCISE D: Imaging Principles (see textbook pp. 40–48)

1. What are the two terms that can be used for exposure factors?

    A. _____   B. _____

2. The degree to which an image receptor (IR) is exposed to ionizing radiation is known as _____.

3. Which of the following is the primary controller of receptor exposure?

    A. mAs   C. ALARA

    B. kVp   D. SID

4. Which specific exposure factor controls the energy or penetrating power of the x-ray beam?

    _____

5. Exposure time is usually expressed in units of _____.

6. True/False. The lowest kVp and highest mAs should be used to ensure the least exposure to the patient.

7. The distance from the x-ray source to the image receptor is known as _____.

8. If the SID is increased from 40 to 80 inches, what specific effect will it have on the intensity of the x-ray beam on the image receptor if other factors are not changed?

    A. Intensity will double.   C. Intensity will decrease by half.

    B. Intensity will increase by a factor of 4.   D. Intensity will decrease by a factor of 4.

9. What can be used to reduce the amount of scatter radiation reaching the image receptor? _____

10. Doubling the mAs will result in _____the image receptors radiation exposure.

11. Which percentage increase in kVp will result in an increase receptor exposure equivqlent to doubling the mAs?

    A. 5%   C. 15%

    B. 10%   D. 20%

12. If an anatomic part measures greater than _____ inches (cm), a grid should be used.

13. True/False. A physical grid is still needed if a virtual grid is used.

14. What are two benefits to collimation?

    A. _____   B. _____

15. Which of the following is a numeric value that represents the exposure to the image receptor?

    A. Exposure indicator (EI)   C. mAs

    B. Source to image distance (SID)   D. ALARA

16. What are the three critical concepts a technologist must understand when it comes to the relationship between EI and radiation exposure to the IR?

    1. _____

    2. _____

    3. _____

17. The recorded sharpness of structures or objects on the radiograph defines _____.

18. The lack of visible sharpness is called _____.

19. List the three geometric factors that control or influence image resolution.

    A. _____

    B. _____

    C. _____

20. The term that describes the unsharp edges of the projected image is _____.

21. What are four other terms can refer to spatial resolution?

    1. _____   3. _____

    2. _____   4. _____

22. The greatest deterrent to image unsharpness as related to positioning is _____.

23. Which of the following is not an example of involuntary motion?

    A. Peristaltic action   C. Tremors

    B. Breathing   D. Chills

24. Which of the following are methods to reduce blur due to voluntary motion?

    A. High mA with short exposure times   C. Clear communication from the technologist

    B. Immobilization devices   D. Any of the above

25. What is the area on the anode that is the actual source of x-rays? _____

26. The greatest deterrent to image unsharpness as related to positioning is _____.

27. Which of the following changes will improve image resolution?

    A. Decrease OID   C. Use a large focal spot

    B. Decrease source image receptor distance (SID)   D. Use a higher kilovoltage

28. **Situation:** The technologist is performing an elbow series on a pediatric patient. Because of the nature of the injury, the technologist has been asked to produce radiographs that have the highest degree of recorded resolution possible. Which of the following sets of factors will produce that level of detail?

   A. 0.3-mm focal spot and 30-inch (75 cm) SID

   B. 1.0-mm focal spot and 45-inch (115 cm) SID

   C. 0.5-mm focal spot and 40-inch (100 cm) SID

   D. 0.3-mm focal spot and 40-inch (100 cm) SID

29. The misrepresentation of an object size or shape projected onto a radiographic recording medium is called _____ _____.

30. True/False: Through careful selection and control of exposure and geometric factors, it is possible to eliminate penumbra completely.

31. List the four primary controlling factors for distortion.

   A. _____   C. _____

   B. _____   D. _____

32. True/False: A decrease in SID reduces distortion.

33. True/False: An increase in OID reduces distortion.

34. True/False: Distortion is reduced when the central ray (CR) is kept perpendicular to the plane of the image receptor.

35. The minimum SID for general radiographic procedures is:

   A. 40 inches (100 cm)   C. 36 inches (90 cm)

   B. 72 inches (180 cm)   D. 48 inches (120 cm)

36. **Situation:** A chest examination on a patient with an enlarged heart has been requested. Which SID is recommended for this study?

   A. 40 inches (100 cm)   C. 44 inches (110 cm)

   B. 72 inches (180 cm)   D. 48 inches (120 cm)

37. True/False: Every radiographic image reflects some degree of unsharpness, even if the smallest focal spot is used.

38. True/False: As the distance between the object and the image receptor is increased, magnification is reduced.

39. True/False: Image distortion increases as the angle of divergence increases from the center of the x-ray beam to the outer edges.

40. True/False: The greater the angle of inclination of the object or the IR, the greater the amount of distortion.

REVIEW EXERCISE E: Digital Imaging Characteristics (see textbook pp. 49–51)

1. True/False: Attenuation of the x-ray beam is different in a digital imaging compared to film-screen.

2. True/False: Digital images are a numeric representation of the x-ray intensities that are transmitted through the patient.

3. True/False: Digital radiographic images are two-dimensional.

4. The smallest unit in a digital image is a _____.

5. Columns and rows of pixels make up the _____.

6. What effect does an increase in pixels have on spatial resolution?

    A. Increase

    B. Decrease

    C. No change

7. In digital imaging, the term _____ is defined as the difference in brightness between light and dark areas of an image.

8. True/False. A high contrast image shows small differences between brightness (shades of gray).

9. True/False: Changes in mAs do not have a primary controlling effect on digital image brightness.

10. True/False: Brightness cannot be altered in the digital image after it has been processed.

11. A digital imaging system's ability to distinguish between similar tissues is termed:

    A. Brightness

    B. Image resolution

    C. Signal

    D. Contrast resolution

12. Radiographic contrast in the digital image is primarily affected by:

    A. kVp

    B. Signal-to-noise ratio

    C. Application of processing algorithms

    D. Matrix size

13. The greater the bit depth of a digital imaging system, the greater the:

    A. Size of the matrix

    B. Contrast resolution

    C. Brightness

    D. Pixel size

14. What describes how efficiently the digital image receptor detects and converts x-ray energy into an image signal?
    _____

15. Which of the following represents a perfect DQE?

    A. 0.25

    B. 0.50

    C. 0.75

    D. 1

16. What are the three factors that influence scatter?

    1. _____

    2. _____

    3. _____

17. True/False. Digital receptors are less sensitive to low-energy radiation; therefore controlling scatter is not important.

18. True/False. Digital imaging systems have a wide dynamic range.

19. What is the term that describes the acceptable level of exposure that produces the desired image quality?
    _____

20. True/False. In digital imaging, a patient may be overexposed but still result in a diagnostic image.

Chapter **1** **Terminology, Positioning, and Imaging Principles**

21. A random disturbance that obscures or reduces clarity is the definition for _____.

22. SNR is the acronym for the _____.

23. When insufficient mAs is applied in the production of a digital image, it produces a _____ (high- or low-) SNR image.

24. Another term for image noise is:

A. Variance

C. Mottle

B. Static

D. Digital spam

25. What is a secondary factor related to noise resulting from the electrical system, nonuniformity of the image receptor, or power fluctuations? _____

REVIEW EXERCISE F: Digital Imaging Components, Postprocessing Options, and Image Archiving (see textbook pp. 52–56)

1. What is photostimulable storage phosphor (PSP) technology most commonly called?

A. Digital radiography

C. Computed radiography

B. Analog film

D. Computed tomography

2. True/False: A PSP-based digital imaging system may be cassette based or cassetteless.

3. What is the device used to convert an analog electrical signal to a computer for digital processing?

A. Charged-coupled device (CCD)

C. Photostimulable storage phosphor (PSP)

B. Analog-to-digital converter (ADC)

D. Detective quantum efficiency (DQE)

4. Which of the following is produced when a PSP is exposed to radiation?

A. Protons

B. Neutrons

C. Electrons

5. True/False: After the PSP image plate has had an image recorded on it, it must be discarded.

6. True/False: A laser within the computed radiography reader scans the latent image on a PSP image plate.

7. True/False: The greater the exposure to the plate, the greater the intensity of the light emitted from the plate during the reading process.

8. Any residual latent image is erased on the PSP image plate by applying:

A. Bright light

C. Low-level radiation

B. Heat

D. Microwaves

9. The process of transferring the digital image to a storage device is termed _____.

10. What is the flat-panel detector with thin-film transistor (FPD-TFT) system commonly referred to as?

A. Digital radiography (DR)

C. Computed radiography (DR)

B. Analog film

D. Computed tomography (CT)

11. What two materials can digital radiography units be constructed with?

1. _____

2. _____

16

12. Which DR system requires the use of a scintillator to produce light when struck by x-ray photons?

   A. Direct
   B. Indirect

13. Which of the following imaging components is *not* required with direct digital radiography (FPD-TFT)?

   A. IP
   B. Image reader
   C. Technologist's workstation
   D. Both A and B

14. True/False: Patient dose may be lower with digital radiography (DR) as compared with analog radiography.

15. True/False: DR-based systems are capable of displaying the image faster than CR.

16. True/False: FPD-TFT and PSP-based systems do *not* provide the ability to preview an image to evaluate for positioning errors and to confirm the exposure indicator.

17. True/False: In both DR and CR systems, the technologist has the ability to post process and manipulate the image.

18. Match the following metric measurements for collimation field size to the nearest equivalent traditional size.

Metric		Traditional (English)
_____	1. 24 × 30 cm	14 × 17 inches
_____	2. 18 × 24 cm	7 × 17 inches
_____	3. 35 × 43 cm	11 × 14 inches
_____	4. 30 × 35 cm	10 × 12 inches
_____	5. 24 × 24 cm	8 × 10 inches
_____	6. 18 × 43 cm	9 × 9 inches

19. Digital imaging processing involves the systematic application of highly complex mathematical formulas called:

   A. Matrices
   B. PACS
   C. C, Analog-to-digital converters
   D. Algorithms

20. True/False. Collimation is not needed when using digital imaging.

21. Window _____ control contrast of the image and window _____ control brightness

22. Identify the type of postprocessing described by listing the correct term for the following definitions.

   A. Adding text to images: _____

   B. Increasing brightness along the margins of structures to increase the visibility of the edges: _____
   _____

   C. Reversing the dark and light pixel values of an image: _____

   D. Enlarging all or part of an image: _____

   E. The application of specific image processing to reduce the display of noise in an image: _____
   _____

   F. Removing background anatomy to allow visualization of contrast media–filled structures: _____
   _____

Chapter **1** Terminology, Positioning, and Imaging Principles

23. Define the acronym PACS.

P:_____   C:_____

A:_____   S:_____

24. What do the following acronyms represent? (Write the complete term.)

    A. DICOM: _____   C. HIS: _____

    B. RIS: _____   D. DR: _____

25. Provide the correct term for the following definitions.

_____ A. Series of "boxes" that give form to the image

_____ B. Range of exposure intensities that produce an acceptable image

_____ C. The user adjusting the window level and window width

_____ D. Unsharp edges of the projected image

_____ E. Numeric value that is representative of the exposure the image receptor received in digital radiography

_____ F. Representative of the number of shades of gray that can be demonstrated by each pixel

_____ G. Misrepresentation of object size or shape as projected onto radiographic recording media

_____ H. Controls the energy (penetrating power) of the x-ray beam

_____ I. Random disturbance that obscures or reduces clarity

_____ J. The recorded sharpness of structures on the image

_____ K. Changing or enhancing the electronic image to view it from a different perspective or to improve its diagnostic quality

26. List the complete term for the following acronyms.

    A. RIS: _____

    B. IR: _____

    C. OID: _____

    D. SID: _____

    E. AEC: _____

    F. HIS: _____

27. Match the following terms to the correct definition.

_____ A. Windowing

1. Term used by certain equipment manufacturers to imply exposure indicator

_____ B. Bit-depth

2. Range of exposure intensities that will produce an acceptable image

_____ C. Noise

3. Random disturbance that obscures or reduces clarity

_____ D. Exposure latitude

4. The point of least distortion of the projected image

_____ E. Exposure level

5. The user adjusting the window level and window width

_____ F. Central ray

6. Series of "boxes" that give form to the image

_____ G. Display matrix

7. Representative of the number of shades of gray that can be demonstrated by each pixel

REVIEW EXERCISE G: Radiation Protection (see textbook pp. 57–66)

1. List the three cardinal principles to protect patients and staff from excessive radiation exposure:

A. _____

B. _____

C. _____

2. Which radiation unit is used to measure the amount of ionizations created in air? (More than one answer is possible.)
_____

3. What is the preferred unit of radiation measurement for exposure? _____

4. Which unit of measurement is used to describe patient dose? (List both SI and traditional units.) _____

5. _____ dose allows comparisons of the relative risk from various imaging procedures.

6. In regard to equivalent dose, the radiation weighing factor for radiography is always a value of _____.

7. What is the whole-body effective dose limit per year for a technologist? _____

8. True/False. Higher dose limits are applied for partial body exposure.

9. For each of the following traditional units, list the equivalent SI unit of radiation measurement and its symbol.

Traditional Unit	SI Unit
A. Roentgen (R)	_____
B. Radiation absorbed dose (rad)	_____
C. Radiation equivalent man (rem)	_____

10. Convert the following doses, stated in traditional units, into the equivalent SI unit.

    A. 0.03 Grad = + 3 rad = _____ Gy   C. 38 rem = _____ Sv

    B. 448 mrad = _____ mGy   D. 15 rem = _____ mSv

11. What is the maximum dose limit for the embryo/fetus of a pregnant technologist?

    A. Per month: _____   B. For the entire gestational period: _____

12. The effective dose (ED) limit for minors under the age of 18 years is _____ per year.

13. Personnel monitoring devices must be worn if there is a possibility of acquiring _____% of the annual occupational effective dose limit.

    A. 1%   C. 15%

    B. 10%   D. 20%

14. Define the following personnel dosimetry devices.

    A. TLD: _____   B. OSL: _____

15. The acronym ALARA is _____.

16. **Situation:** A young child comes to the radiology department for a skull series. The child is combative and will not remain still for the procedure. Which of the following individuals should be asked to restrain the patient (if mechanical restraints are not available)?

    A. A family member (if not pregnant)   C. The oldest technologist

    B. A student technologist   D. A nuclear medicine technologist

17. True/False: Exposure to persons outside a shielded barrier is due primarily to scatter radiation from the patient.

18. True/False: Fluoroscopy procedures do not result in high exposures to the fetus of the pregnant technologist.

19. True/False: Exit dose is often a smaller percentage of the entrance dose.

20. True/False: Effective dose (ED) describes gonadal dose levels only for each radiographic procedure.

21. Which of the following projections provides the greatest amount of dose to the ovaries? (Review the patient dose chart in the text.)

    A. PA chest   C. AP abdomen

    B. Lateral skull   D. AP thoracic spine

22. Which of the following projections provides the greatest amount of bone marrow dose? (Review patient dose chart in text.)

    A. AP lumbar spine   C. Retrograde pyelogram

    B. PA chest   D. Lateral skull

23. What is one of the primary causes for repeat radiographs? (Select the *best* answer.)

    A. Excessive kilovoltage   C. Poor communication between technologist and patient

    B. Wrong IR selection

                                      D. Distortion caused by incorrect SID

24. In addition to the primary causes identified in the previous question, what two other factors often lead to repeat exposures?

    A. _____   B. _____

25. List the two major forms of filtration found in x-ray tubes that affect the quality of the primary x-ray beam.

    A. _____   B. _____

26. What are the two most common metals used for added filtration in diagnostic radiology equipment? _____
_____

27. What is the minimum total filtration for equipment operating at 70 kVp or higher?

    A. 0.5 mm aluminum   C. 2.5 mm aluminum

    B. 1.5 mm aluminum   D. 3.5 mm aluminum

28. True/False: Safety standards require that collimators be accurate to within 10% of the selected SID.

29. True/False: Positive beam limitation (PBL) collimators restrict the size of the exposure field to the size of the cassette in a Bucky tray.

30. True/False: PBL collimators became optional on new equipment manufactured after May 1993 because of a change in US Food and Drug Administration (FDA) regulations.

31. What are the two ways collimation will reduce patient dose?

    A. _____   B. _____

32. True/False: In general, collimation borders should be visible on the image receptor on all four sides.

33. True/False: A pregnant patient should never receive an x-ray.

34. Which of the following exams would deliver a dose less than 10 mGy (1 rad) to the fetus on a pregnant patient?

    A. Head CT   C. Scoliosis: full series

    B. Lumbar Spine series   D. CT pelvis

35. True/False: It is acceptable to process an image with a different algorithm to correct overexposure.

36. True/False: Current recommendations by the AAPM and NCRP are to discontinue the use of gonadal shielding.

37. A 1-mm lead equivalent shield can absorb _____ of the primary beam in the 50–100 kVp range.

    A. 70%–75%   C. 85%–90%

    B. 80%–85%   D. 95%–99%

38. Which of the following is true regarding specific area shielding?

    A. Follow local regulations and department policies.   C. Shielding is not a substitute for accurate beam collimation and careful positioning is essential.

    B. Gonadal shielding may be recommended if the organ of concern lies within 2 inches (5 cm) of the primary beam.   D. All of the above are true.

39. What is the federally set limit for exposure rates for intensified fluoroscopy units?

    A. 1 R/min

    B. 6–8 R/min

    C. 3–4 R/min

    D. 10 R/min

40. In high-level fluoroscopy (HLF) mode, the exposure rate measured at tabletop *cannot* exceed _____ _____.

41. With most modern fluoroscopy equipment, the average exposure rate is:

    A. 0.5 R/min

    B. 5–7 R/min

    C. 1–3 R/min

    D. 10 R/min

42. What are the two methods that monitor fluoroscopic radiation output?

    1. _____

    2. _____

43. Which method for monitoring fluoroscopic output indicates a combination of dose and the amount of tissue irradiated? _____

44. The minimum radiation dose that will produce temporary skin injury (epilation) is:

    A. 1 Gy (100 rad)

    B. 3 Gy (300 rad)

    C. 5 Gy (500 rad)

    D. 6 Gy (600 rad)

45. True/False: Pulsed fluoroscopy, when frames per minute are minimized, can produce a substantial dose reduction.

46. To reduce occupational exposure during fluoroscopy, which of the following is the best place for a technologist to stand?

    A. Head end of table

    B. Foot end of table

    C. Behind the radiologist (fluoroscopist)

    D. Next to the radiologist (fluoroscopist)

47. What is the best method of reducing scatter to a worker's eyes and neck during fluoroscopy? _____ _____.

48. What is the minimum lead equivalency recommended for a protective apron worn during fluoroscopy? _____.

49. True/False: Radiation-attenuating surgical gloves offer minimal protection of the interventionist's hands, provide a false sense of protection, and therefore are not recommended.

50. True/False: The ImageWisely initiative is intended to minimize radiation exposure to children.

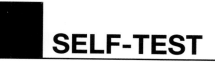

SELF-TEST

This series of self-tests should be taken only after completing all of the readings and review exercises for a particular section. This self-test is divided into seven sections. The purpose of this test is not only to provide a good learning exercise but also to serve as a strong indicator of what your chapter evaluation exam will cover. It is strongly suggested that if you do not achieve at least a 90%–95% grade on each self-test, you should review those areas in which you answered questions incorrectly before going to your instructor for the final evaluation exam.

Self-Test A: General, Systemic, and Skeletal Anatomy and Arthrology

1. Which of the following is (are) *not* one of the four basic types of tissue in the human body? (More than one answer is possible.)

   A. Integumentary

   B. Connective

   C. Nervous

   D. Osseous

   E. Muscular

   F. Epithelial

2. How many separate bones are found in the adult human body?

   A. 180

   B. 243

   C. 206

   D. 257

3. Which of the following systems distributes oxygen and nutrients to the cells of the body?

   A. Digestive

   B. Circulatory

   C. Skeletal

   D. Urinary

4. Which of the following systems maintains the acid-base balance in the body?

   A. Digestive

   B. Urinary

   C. Reproductive

   D. Circulatory

5. Which of the following systems is considered to be the largest organ system in the human body?

   A. Muscular

   B. Endocrine

   C. Skeletal

   D. Integumentary

6. The two divisions of the human skeleton are:

   A. Bony and cartilaginous

   B. Axial and appendicular

   C. Vertebral and extremities

   D. Integumentary and appendicular

7. Which portion of the long bones is responsible for the production of red blood cells?

   A. Spongy or cancellous

   B. Periosteum

   C. Hyaline

   D. Compact aspect

8. What type of tissue covers the ends of the long bones?

   A. Spongy or cancellous

   B. Periosteum

   C. Hyaline or articular cartilage

   D. Compact aspect

9. The narrow space between the inner and outer table of the flat bones in the cranium is called the:

   A. Calvarium   C. Medullary portion

   B. Periosteum   D. Diploe

10. What is the primary center for endochondral ossification in long bones?

    A. Diaphysis (body)   C. Epiphyses

    B. Epiphyseal plate   D. Medulla

11. What is the name of the secondary growth centers of endochondral ossification found in long bones?

    A. Diaphysis (shaft)   C. Epiphyses

    B. Epiphyseal plate   D. Metaphysis

12. The aspect of long bones where bone growth in length occurs is termed:

    A. Diaphysis (shaft)   C. Epiphyses

    B. Epiphyseal plate   D. Metaphysis

13. A skull suture has the structural classification of a _____ joint.

    A. Fibrous   C. Synovial

    B. Cartilaginous   D. Diarthrosis

14. The symphysis pubis has the structural classification of a _____ joint.

    A. Fibrous   C. Synovial

    B. Cartilaginous   D. Synarthrosis

15. Which specific joint(s) is (are) the only true syndesmosis, amphiarthrodial, fibrous joint(s)?

    A. Joints between the roots of teeth and adjoining bone   C. Distal tibiofibular joint

                                                                     D. Proximal and distal radioulnar joints
    B. First carpometacarpal joint

16. Match the following bones to their correct classification.

    _____   1. Sternum   A. Long bone

    _____   2. Femur   B. Short bone

    _____   3. Tarsal bones   C. Flat bone

    _____   4. Pelvic bones   D. Irregular bone

    _____   5. Scapulae

    _____   6. Humerus

    _____   7. Vertebrae

    _____   8. Calvarium

17. The three structural classifications of joints are synovial, cartilaginous, and:

   A. Amphiarthrodial   C. Diarthrodial

   B. Ellipsoidal   D. Fibrous

18. Classify the following synovial joints based on their type of movement.

   _____ 1.   First carpometacarpal joint   A. Plane (gliding)

   _____ 2.   Intercarpal joint   B. Ginglymus (hinge)

   _____ 3.   Hip joint   C. Pivot (trochoidal)

   _____ 4.   Proximal radioulnar joint   D. Ellipsoidal (condyloid)

   _____ 5.   Interphalangeal joint   E. Saddle (sellar)

   _____ 6.   Fourth metacarpophalangeal joint F. Ball and socket (spheroidal)

   _____ 7.   Knee joint   G. Bicondylar

   _____ 8.   Wrist joint

   _____ 9.   Joint between C1 and C2

   _____ 10.   Ankle joint

Self-Test B: Positioning Terminology

1. Which plane divides the body into equal anterior and posterior parts?

   A. Midsagittal   C. Midcoronal

   B. Transverse   D. Longitudinal

2. True/False: The terms *radiograph* and *image receptor* refer to the same thing.

3. A longitudinal plane that divides the body into right and left parts is the:

   A. Coronal plane   C. Sagittal plane

   B. Horizontal plane   D. Oblique plane

4. Match the following definitions to the correct term.

_____ 1. Near the source or beginning   A. Eversion

_____ 2. Away from head end of the body   B. Circumduction

_____ 3. Inside of something   C. Pronation

_____ 4. Increasing the angle of a joint   D. Contralateral

_____ 5. Outward stress of the foot   E. Proximal

_____ 6. Movement of an extremity away from the midline   F. Medial

_____ 7. Turning palm downward   G. Interior

_____ 8. A backward movement   H. Retraction

_____ 9. To move around in the form of a circle   I. Caudad

_____ 10. Toward the center   J. Extension

_____ 11. Away from the source or beginning   K. Abduction

_____ 12. On the opposite side of the body   L. Distal

5. Match the following definitions to the correct term.

_____ 1. Lying down in any position   A. Base plane of skull

_____ 2. Head lower than the feet position   B. Plantar

_____ 3. Upright position, palms forward   C. Palmar

_____ 4. Top of the foot   D. Reverse Trendelenburg position

_____ 5. Frankfort horizontal plane   E. Lithotomy position

_____ 6. A plane at right angle to the longitudinal plane   F. Anatomic position

_____ 7. Head higher than feet position   G. Trendelenburg position

_____ 8. Palm of hand   H. Horizontal plane

_____ 9. Sole of foot   I. Midcoronal plane

_____ 10. Front half of body   J. Dorsum pedis

_____ 11. A plane that divides body into anterior and posterior halves   K. Anterior

_____ 12. A recumbent position with knees and hips flexed   L. Recumbent with support for legs

6. The direction or path of the central ray of the x-ray beam defines the positioning term:

   A. Position

   B. View

   C. Perspective

   D. Projection

7. **Situation:** A patient is placed in a recumbent position facing downward. The left side of the body is turned 30 degrees toward the image receptor. Which specific position has been performed?

   A. LAO

   B. Left lateral decubitus

   C. LPO

   D. RAO

8. **Situation:** A patient is placed in a recumbent position facing downward. The x-ray tube is directed horizontally and enters the left side and exits the right side of the body. An image receptor is placed against the right side of the patient. Which position has been performed?

   A. Dorsal decubitus

   B. Left lateral decubitus

   C. Ventral decubitus

   D. Right lateral decubitus

9. **Situation:** A patient is erect with her back to the image receptor. The central ray enters the anterior aspect and exits the posterior aspect of the body. Which projection has been performed?

   A. Posteroanterior

   B. Tangential

   C. Ventral decubitus

   D. Anteroposterior

10. **Situation:** A patient is lying facing upward with the posterior surface of the body against the image receptor. The right side of the body is turned 45 degrees toward the image receptor. The x-ray tube is directed vertically and enters the anterior surface of the body. Which position has been performed?

    A. LPO

    B. RAO

    C. RPO

    D. LAO

11. **Situation:** An elbow projection is taken with the posterior surface placed against the image receptor. The elbow is rotated 20 degrees externally. Which specific projection has been performed?

    A. PA oblique with medial rotation

    B. PA oblique with lateral rotation

    C. AP oblique with medial rotation

    D. AP oblique with lateral rotation

12. **Situation:** A specific projection of the foot in which the central ray enters the anterior surface and exits the posterior surface is termed:

    A. Dorsoplantar

    B. Plantodorsal

    C. Axioplantar

    D. Posteroanterior

13. **Situation:** A patient is placed in a recumbent position with the body tilted so that the head is higher than the feet. The image receptor is under the patient and the x-ray tube is above the patient. Which is the general position of the patient?

    A. Trendelenburg

    B. Reid

    C. Sims

    D. Fowler

14. **Situation:** The anterior surface of the right knee of the patient is facing the image receptor. The anterior aspect of the knee and lower leg is rotated 15 degrees toward the midline. Which specific projection has been performed?

    A. AP oblique with medial rotation

    B. PA oblique with medial rotation

    C. PA oblique with lateral rotation

    D. AP oblique with lateral rotation

15. What is the name of the projection in which the central ray merely skims a body part?

    A. Tangential
    B. Decubitus
    C. Axial
    D. Trendelenburg

16. What is the name of the specific projection in which the central ray enters the left side of the chest and exits the opposite side?

    A. Parietoacanthial
    B. Axial
    C. Transthoracic
    D. Lordotic

17. What is the specific projection that enters the posterior aspect of the skull and exits the acanthion?

    A. Acanthioparietal
    B. Tangential
    C. Axial
    D. Parietoacanthial

18. Which of the following is an example of an axial projection?

    A. Transthoracic lateral
    B. Mediolateral ankle
    C. AP chest with 20-degree cephalic angle
    D. AP abdomen with 30-degree rotation to the left

19. Which of the following positioning terms is no longer considered valid in the United States?

    A. Radiographic view
    B. Radiographic position
    C. Radiographic projection
    D. Semiaxial projection

20. Match each of the following positioning terms to the term that is its direct opposite.

    _____ 1. Proximal   A. Kyphosis

    _____ 2. Cephalad   B. Inferior

    _____ 3. Ipsilateral   C. External

    _____ 4. Medial   D. Distal

    _____ 5. Superficial   E. Plantodorsal

    _____ 6. Internal   F. Lateral

    _____ 7. Lordosis   G. PA

    _____ 8. AP   H. Caudad

    _____ 9. Superior   I. Contralateral

    _____ 10. Dorsoplantar   J. Deep

Self-Test C: Positioning Principles

1. True/False: If a patient is younger than 18 years of age, any confidential information obtained during the procedure must be shared with the parent or guardian.

2. True/False: The technologist must provide a preliminary interpretation of any radiographs if requested by the referring physician.

3. True/False: Personal patient information can be shared with another technologist even if he or she has no role in that patient's procedure.

4. True/False: The technologist can explain a radiographic procedure to the patient without permission from the referring physician or radiologist.

5. List the three recommendations of the ASRT ACE initiative.

   A. _____

   B. _____

   C. _____

6. Indicate the minimum number of projections required for the following anatomic structures.

   _____ 1. Knee   A. Two

   _____ 2. Fourth finger   B. Three

   _____ 3. Humerus

   _____ 4. Sternum

   _____ 5. Ankle

   _____ 6. Tibia/fibula

   _____ 7. Chest

   _____ 8. Hand

   _____ 9. Hip (proximal femur)

   _____ 10. Forearm

7. Which of the following radiographic procedures requires that only a single AP projection be taken?

   A. Postreduction forearm   C. Hand on a pediatric patient

   B. Pelvis   D. Ribs

8. **Situation:** A patient enters the emergency room with a fractured forearm. The fracture is set, or reduced. The orthopedic physician orders a postreduction series. What is the minimum number of projections required?

   A. One   C. Two

   B. Three   D. Four

9. **Situation:** A patient enters the emergency room with a dislocated elbow. The patient is in extreme pain. What is the minimum number of projections that must be performed?

   A. One
   B. Three

   C. Two
   D. Four

10. **Situation:** A patient comes to radiology for a rib study. What is the minimum number of projections that must be performed?

    A. One
    B. Three

    C. Two
    D. Four

11. **Situation:** A patient enters the emergency room with a possible fractured ankle. She can move it but it is painful. What is the minimum number of projections that must be performed?

    A. One
    B. Three

    C. Two
    D. Four

12. **Situation:** A patient enters the emergency room with a small piece of wire embedded in the palm of the hand. What is the minimum number of projections required for this study?

    A. One
    B. Three

    C. Two
    D. Four

13. **Situation:** A patient has fallen on the ice and has a possible fractured hip (proximal femur). What is the minimum number of projections that should be taken for this patient?

    A. One
    B. Three

    C. Two
    D. Five

14. **Situation:** A patient enters the emergency room with a possible fractured little (fifth) toe. What is the minimum number of projections that must be taken?

    A. One
    B. Three

    C. Two
    D. Five

15. Which of the following positioning routines should be performed for a wrist study?

    A. AP, PA, and lateral projections
    B. AP and lateral projections

    C. PA, oblique, and lateral projections
    D. Oblique, axial, and lateral projections

16. Which of the following positioning routines should be performed for a chest study?

    A. PA and lateral projections
    B. PA, oblique, and lateral projections

    C. AP, PA, and lateral projections
    D. PA, RAO, and LAO projections

17. The technique for localizing bony and soft tissue of radiographic landmarks is termed:

    A. Localization
    B. Tactile localization

    C. Physical assessment
    D. Palpation

18. Which is not one of the ASRT ACE Campaign points?

    A. Announce your name.
    B. Communicate your credentials.

    C. Expediate the procedure.
    D. Explain the procedure.

19. Which of the following is not within the scope of practice of the radiologic technologist?

    A. Explain the procedure to the patient.

    B. Prepare the contrast media or other medications required during the procedure.

    C. Administer IV medication for pain prior to the procedure.

    D. Determine if the patient may be pregnant prior to the procedure.

20. True/False: Gonadal shielding may be used as long as it doesn't interfere with the clinical intent of the radiologic procedure (per department policy).

Self-Test D: Imaging Principles

1. Which of the following is defined as the exposure to the image receptor (IR)?

    A. Dose

    B. Receptor Exposure

    C. mAs

    D. Air kerma

2. Which of the following controls the quantity of x-ray photons in the x-ray beam?

    A. mA

    B. kVp

    C. SID

    D. OID

3. Which of the following is the primary controller of the energy of the x-ray beam?

    A. mAs

    B. kVp

    C. SID

    D. OID

4. Which of the following increases receptor exposure and provides the equivalent of doubling mAs?

    A. Inverse square law

    B. ALARA

    C. 15% rule

    D. Anode Heel Effect

5. **Situation:** An SID of 40 inches (100 cm) yields 1 mGy. What will increasing the SID to 80 inches (200 cm) yield?

    A. 4 mGy

    B. 2 mGy

    C. 0.5 mGy

    D. 0.25 mGy

6. Which of the following techniques or devices reduces the amount of scatter radiation striking the IR?

    A. Collimation

    B. Lower kVp

    C. Grids

    D. All of the above

7. A grid is generally recommended when a body part is thicker than:

    A. 2 inches (5 cm)

    B. 4 inches (10 cm)

    C. 8 inches (20 cm)

    D. 10 inches (25 cm)

8. True/False: A virtual grid is scatter correction software and is not a physical piece of equipment.

9. Which of the following is the most commonly used form of x-ray beam restriction?

    A. Filtration

    B. Collimation

    C. Palpation

    D. Detector Exposure Index (DEI)

10. Which of the following does the exposure indicator (EI) provide a numerical value for?

    A. Dose to the patient

    B. Dose to the technologist

    C. Exposure to the image receptor

    D. Air kerma

11. True/False: exposure indictors (EI) may be positive or inversely correlated.

12. True/False: Spatial resolution is optimal with a long OID and a short SID.

13. Which of the following factors best controls involuntary cardiac motion artifact?

    A. Careful instructions given to the patient

    B. High kVp technique

    C. Practicing with patient when to hold breath

    D. Shortening the exposure time

14. **Situation:** The technologist is asked to produce a high-quality image of the carpal (wrist) bones. The emergency room physician suspects that the patient has a very small fracture of one of the bones. Which of following sets of technical factors produces an image with the highest degree of radiographic resolution?

    A. 1.0-mm focal spot and 30-inch (80-cm) SID

    B. 2.0-mm focal spot and 36-inch (90-cm) SID

    C. 0.5-mm focal spot and 40-inch (100-cm) SID

    D. 0.3-mm focal spot and 40-inch (100-cm) SID

15. The misrepresentation of an object's size or shape projected on a radiograph is called:

    A. Magnification

    B. Blurring

    C. Unsharpness

    D. Distortion

16. Which of the following sets of factors *minimizes* radiographic distortion to the greatest degree?

    A. 40-inch (100-cm) SID and 8-inch (20-cm) OID

    B. 44-inch (110-cm) SID and 6-inch (15-cm) OID

    C. 72-inch (180-cm) SID and 3-inch (7.5-cm) OID

    D. 60-inch (150-cm) SID and 4-inch (10-cm) OID

17. The best method to reduce distortion of the joints of the hand is to keep the fingers _____ to the IR.

    A. Perpendicular

    B. Parallel

    C. At a 30-degree angle

    D. Vertical

18. Which of the following is not a primary controlling factor of distortion?

    A. SID

    B. OID

    C. CR alignment

    D. mAs

19. Which of the following projections requires the use of a grid?

    A. PA hand

    B. Axial calcaneus (heel)

    C. AP abdomen

    D. AP elbow

20. **Situation:** A patient presents to the emergency room with an injury to the hand. The hand is wrapped with gauze which increases OID. Which of the following modifications can be done to minimize distortion due to the increased OID?

    A. Increase kVp by 15%

    B. Use a large focal spot

    C. Increase SID

    D. Double the mAs

Self-Test E: Digital Imaging Characteristics

1. Each digital image is formed by two-dimensional elements termed:
   - A. Pixels
   - B. Matrix
   - C. Voxels
   - D. Bytes

2. Highly complex mathematical formulas used in creating the digital image are termed:
   - A. Digital reconstructions
   - B. Bit processing matrices
   - C. Digital displays
   - D. Algorithms

3. True/False: Changes in kVp have little impact on patient dose with digital imaging.

4. True/False: kVp and mAs do not have the same direct effect on image quality with digital imaging as they do with IR-screen imaging.

5. True/False: A wide exposure latitude associated with digital imaging systems will often reduce repeat exposures.

6. The intensity of light that represents the individual pixels in the image on the monitor is termed:
   - A. Latitude
   - B. Brightness
   - C. Contrast
   - D. Resolution

7. The primary controlling factor of contrast in the digital image is:
   - A. kVp
   - B. mAs
   - C. Processing algorithms
   - D. Use of a grid

8. The greater the bit depth of a digital system, the greater the:
   - A. Contrast resolution
   - B. Brightness
   - C. Resolution
   - D. Noise

9. Which of the following terms describes the minimum pixel size that can be displayed by a monitor?
   - A. Acquisition pixel size
   - B. Display pixel size
   - C. Monitor latent pixel size
   - D. Reconstructed pixel size

10. True/False: OID and SID have little impact on spatial resolution of the digital image.

11. True/False: The current range of spatial resolution for digital general radiographic imaging is between 2.5 and 5 line pairs per mm.

12. Which of the following describes how efficiently the digital image receptor detects and converts x-ray energy into a signal?
    - A. SID
    - B. Matrix
    - C. DQE
    - D. SNR

13. Random disturbance that obscures or reduces clarity is the definition of:
    - A. Noise
    - B. Signal
    - C. Digital fluctuation
    - D. Signal variation

14. True/False: Close collimation reduces the amount of scatter produced and increases contrast.

15. True/False: A high SNR results when an insufficient mAs is used in creating a digital image.

16. Which of the following factors results in an increase in noise?

    A. Excessive mAs

    B. Scatter radiation

    C. High kVp

    D. Decrease in pixel size

17. Which of the following can reduce scatter to the digital image receptor?

    A. Grids

    B. Collimation

    C. Selecting optimal kVp

    D. All of the above

18. What is the best way to determine overexposure on a digital image?

    A. Check the EI number

    B. Check SNR

    C. Observe the density on the image

    D. Assess the contrast

19. True/False: The electronic system, nonuniformity of the image receptor, or power fluctuations can produce electronic noise on a digital radiographic image.

20. True/False: Postprocessing can correct for a low-SNR image.

Self-Test F: Digital Imaging Equipment

1. Which of the following statements is true in regard to PSP (computed radiography) imaging?

    A. PSP provides a wide exposure latitude.

    B. AEC cannot be used with PSP.

    C. Collimation should not be used.

    D. A longer SID must be used with PSP over film-screen systems.

2. Which of the following processes is used to erase the PSP imaging plate following exposure?

    A. Ultraviolet light

    B. Low-level x-rays

    C. Bright light

    D. Laser

3. Patient information may be linked to the image on the CR imaging plate by the:

    A. Light source

    B. Laser

    C. X-ray source

    D. Bar-code reader

4. The PSP imaging plate is composed of:

    A. Calcium tungstate phosphor

    B. Zinc cadmium sulfate phosphor

    C. Silicon phosphor

    D. Photostimulable phosphor

5. The latent image recorded on the PSP image plate is read by a(n):

    A. Laser

    B. Bright light source

    C. Microwave source

    D. Ultraviolet light source

6. True/False: Close collimation must be avoided when acquiring an image on a PSP IP.

7. True/False: Grids cannot be used with a PSP system.

8. True/False: Grids are often used for extremity exams when using FPD-TFT (digital radiography).

9. True/False: FPD-TFT often requires less exposure than analog (film-screen) systems.

10. True/False: Close collimation should be avoided when using DR.

11. True/False: FPD-TFT can be either cassette-less or cassette-based systems.

12. True/False: RIS is a digital network that permits viewing and storage of both digital and analog (film-screen) produced images.

13. _____ controls the brightness of a digital image (within a certain range):

    A. Window width

    B. Window level

    C. Display pixel

    D. Bit depth

14. DICOM refers to:

    A. A set of standards to ensure communication among digital imaging systems

    B. A new direct digital "flat-plate" receptor system

    C. A digital image transmission system

    D. A new-generation CR system

15. A digital transmission system for transferring radiographic images to remote locations is termed:

    A. PACS

    B. Direct DR

    C. HIS

    D. Teleradiography

16. Any residual latent image is erased on the PSP image plate by applying:

    A. Microwaves

    B. Heat

    C. Low-level radiation

    D. Bright light

17. A series of "boxes" that give form to the image is the definition for:

    A. Pixels

    B. Voxels

    C. Display matrix

    D. Acquisition matrices

18. A 30 × 35-cm IR is equivalent to a:

    A. 14 × 17-inch IR

    B. 11 × 14-inch IR

    C. 8 × 10-inch IR

    D. 10 × 12-inch IR

19. The application of specific image processing to reduce the display of noise in an image is the definition for:

    A. Windowing

    B. Edge enhancement

    C. Window width

    D. Smoothing

20. _____ is the application of specific image processing that alters the pixel values across the image to present a more uniform image appearance.

    A. Smoothing

    B. Edge enhancement

    C. Brightness gain

    D. Equalization

Self-Test G: Radiation Protection

1. What is the SI unit of radiation measurement for an absorbed dose?
   A. Sievert
   B. Gray
   C. Coulombs per kilogram of air
   D. Roentgen

2. Which term is replacing "exposure" to describe skin dose?
   A. Sievert
   B. Gray
   C. Air kerma
   D. Rem

3. What is the annual whole-body effective dose (ED) for a technologist?
   A. 100 mSv or 10 rem
   B. 1 mSv or 0.1 rem
   C. 10 mSv or 1 rem
   D. 50 mSv or 5 rem

4. What is the cumulative lifetime ED for a 25-year-old technologist?
   A. 250 mSv
   B. 25 mSv
   C. 500 mSv
   D. 2500 mSv

5. What is the annual ED limit for an individual younger than 18 years of age?
   A. 50 mSv or 5 rem
   B. 1 mSv or 0.1 rem
   C. 1 mSv or 1 rem
   D. 100 mSv or 10 rem

6. The federal set maximum limit on exposure rates for intensified fluoroscopy units is:
   A. 3–4 R/min
   B. 0.5 R/min
   C. 1 R/min
   D. 10 R/min

7. For most modern equipment, the average fluoroscopy tabletop exposure rate is:
   A. 10 R/min
   B. 5–8 R/min
   C. 1–3 R/min
   D. 15–20 R/min

8. What is the primary purpose of x-ray tube filtration?
   A. Absorb lower (unusable) energy x-rays
   B. Reduce the x-ray intensity
   C. Increase quantity of the x-ray photons
   D. All of the above

9. Which of the following results in the highest ED for females (assuming no specific area shields or collimation are used)?
   A. Anteroposterior (AP) thoracic spine (7 × 17-inch)
   B. AP thoracic spine (14 × 17-inch)
   C. AP cervical spine (10 × 12-inch)
   D. PA chest (14 × 17-inch)

10. The use of a 1-mm lead equivalent gonadal shield reduces the gonadal dose by _____ if the gonads are within the primary x-ray field.
    A. 20%–30%
    B. 40%–50%
    C. 50%–90%
    D. 100%

11. Which of the following provides the radiation output measurement that includes combination dose and amount of tissue irradiated?

A. DQE

C. SID

B. DAP

D. PBL

12. True/False: Low kVp and high mAs techniques greatly reduce patient dose compared with high kVp and low mAs techniques.

13. True/False: The total ED for females on an AP chest projection is more than double that of a PA chest.

14. True/False: The use of a positive beam limiting (PBL) collimator is no longer required by the FDA for new x-ray equipment manufactured after 1994.

15. True/False: Collimators must be accurate to within 5% of the selected SID.

16. Which of the following is not one of the cardinal principles of radiation protection?

A. Distance

C. Time

B. Shielding

D. Collimation

17. Which of the following changes will best reduce patient dose?

A. Decrease kVp and increase mAs

C. Increase kVp and lower mAs

B. Use a grid

D. Increase mAs and lower kVp

18. Where is the safest place for the technologist to stand during a fluoroscopic procedure?

A. At the head end of the table

C. On the floor behind the fluoroscopic tower

B. At the foot end of the table

D. Behind the radiologist (flouroscopist)

19. Which of the following protection devices must be used during a fluoroscopic procedure?

A. Bucky slot shield

C. Compensating filter

B. Lead gloves

D. Restraining devices

20. The effective dose (ED) per month for a pregnant technologist is:

A. 1 mSv (0.1 rem)

C. 5 mSv (500 rem)

B. 0.5 mSv (0.05 rem)

D. 50 mSv (5 rem)

21. True/False: A fetal personnel dosimeter is worn at the level of the waist by a pregnant technologist during fluoroscopy.

22. True/False: All administrative staff in the radiology department must wear a personnel dosimeter even if not involved with actual radiographic procedure.

23. True/False: The ICRP and ACR have determined that the "10-day rule" is obsolete for procedures of the abdomen and pelvis.

24. Which of the following statements is false in regard to digital imaging?

A. The use of higher kVp and lower mAs is recommended.

C. All radiographs should be within the exposure indicator.

B. A minimal 40-inch (100-cm) SID is encouraged with all PSP and DR procedures.

D. ALARA does not apply to digital imaging.

25. True/False: Using a different algorithm to process an overexposed CR image is an acceptable and ethical practice.

1 Terminology, Positioning, and Imaging Principles

WORKBOOK SELF-TEST ANSWER KEY

Self-Test A: General, Systemic, and Skeletal Anatomy and Arthrology

1. A. Integumentary
   D. Osseous
2. C. 206
3. B. Circulatory
4. B. Urinary
5. D. Integumentary
6. B. Axial and appendicular
7. A. Spongy or cancellous
8. C. Hyaline or articular cartilage
9. D. Diploe
10. A. Diaphysis (body)
11. C. Epiphyses
12. D. Metaphysis
13. A. Fibrous
14. B. Cartilaginous
15. C. Distal tibiofibular joint
16. 1. C
    2. A
    3. B
    4. D
    5. C
    6. A
    7. D
    8. C
17. D. Fibrous
18. 1. E
    2. A
    3. F
    4. C
    5. B
    6. D
    7. G
    8. D
    9. C
    10. E

Self-Test B: Positioning Terminology

1. C. Midcoronal
2. False
3. C. Sagittal plane
4. 1. E
   2. I
   3. G
   4. J
   5. A
   6. K
   7. C
   8. H
   9. B
   10. F
   11. L
   12. D
5. 1. L
   2. G
   3. F
   4. J
   5. A
   6. H
   7. D
   8. C
   9. B
   10. K
   11. I
   12. E
6. D. Projection
7. A. LAO
8. C. Ventral decubitus
9. D. Anteroposterior
10. C. RPO
11. D. AP oblique with lateral rotation
12. A. Dorsoplantar
13. D. Fowler
14. B. PA oblique with medial rotation
15. A. Tangential
16. C. Transthoracic
17. D. Parietoacanthial
18. C. AP chest with 20-degree cephalic angle
19. A. Radiographic view
20. 1. D
    2. H
    3. I
    4. F
    5. J
    6. C
    7. A
    8. G
    9. B
    10. E

Self-Test C: Positioning Principles

1. False
2. False
3. False
4. True
5. A. Announce your name.
   B. Communicate your credentials.
   C. Explain the procedure.
6. 1. B
   2. B
   3. A
   4. A
   5. B
   6. A
   7. A
   8. B
   9. A
   10. A
7. B. Pelvis
8. C. Two
9. C. Two
10. C. Two
11. B. Three
12. C. Two
13. C. Two
14. B. Three
15. C. PA, oblique, and lateral projections
16. A. PA and lateral projections
17. D. Palpation
18. C. Expedite the procedure.
19. C. Administer IV medication for pain prior to the procedure.
20. True

Self-Test D: Imaging Principles

1. B. Receptor exposure
2. A. mA
3. B. kVp
4. C. 15% rule (Increasing kVp by 15% is similar to doubling the mAs.)
5. D. 0.25 mGy (inverse square law)
6. D. All of the above

7. B. 4 inches (10 cm), unless using virtual grid software
8. True
9. B. Collimation
10. C. Exposure to the image receptor
11. True
12. False
13. D. Shortening the exposure time
14. D. 0.3 mm focal spot and 40-inch (100-cm) SID
15. D. Distortion
16. C. 72-inch (180-cm) SID and 3-inch (7.5-cm) OID
17. B. Parallel
18. D. mAs
19. C. AP abdomen
20. C. Increase SID

Self-Test E: Digital Imaging Characteristics

1. A. Pixels
2. D. Algorithms
3. False
4. True
5. True
6. B. Brightness
7. C. Processing algorithms
8. A. Contrast resolution
9. B. Display pixel size
10. False
11. True
12. C. DQE (detective quantum efficiency)

13. A. Noise
14. True
15. False
16. B. Scatter radiation
17. D. All of the above
18. A. Check the EI number
19. True
20. False

Self-Test F: Digital Imaging Equipment

1. A. PSP provides a wide exposure latitude.
2. C. Bright light
3. D. Bar code reader
4. D. Photostimulable phosphor
5. A. Laser
6. False
7. False
8. True
9. True
10. False
11. True
12. False (radiology information system; PACS provides this capability.)
13. B. Window level
14. A. A set of standards to ensure communication among digital imaging systems
15. D. Teleradiology
16. D. Bright light
17. C. Display matrix
18. B. 11 × 14-inch IR

19. D. Smoothing
20. D. Equalization

Self-Test G: Radiation Protection

1. B. Gray
2. C. Air kerma
3. D. 50 mSv or 5 rem
4. A. 250 mSv
5. B. 1 mSv or 0.1 rem
6. D. 10 R/min
7. C. 1–3 R/min
8. A. Absorb lower (unusable) energy x-rays
9. B. AP thoracic spine (14 × 17-inch)
10. C. 50%–90%
11. B. DAP (dose area product)
12. False
13. True
14. True
15. False (2%)
16. D. Collimation
17. C. Increase kVp and lower mAs
18. D. Behind the radiologist
19. A. Bucky slot shield
20. B. 0.5 mSv (0.05 rem)
21. True
22. False
23. True
24. D. ALARA does not apply to digital imaging (false).
25. False

2 Chest

CHAPTER OBJECTIVES

After you have successfully completed the activities in this chapter, you will be able to:

_____ 1. List the parts of the bony thorax.

_____ 2. List specific topographic positioning landmarks of the chest.

_____ 3. Identify the parts and function of specific structures of the respiratory system.

_____ 4. List the four organs of the mediastinum.

_____ 5. Identify specific structures of the chest on line drawings.

_____ 6. Identify specific structures of the chest on posteroanterior (PA) and lateral radiographs.

_____ 7. Identify specific structures of the chest on a computed tomography (CT) transverse image.

_____ 8. Describe the methods to ensure a proper degree of inspiration during chest radiography.

_____ 9. Describe the importance of using close collimation, and anatomic side markers during chest radiography.

_____ 10. Identify the common kVp ranges used during chest radiography.

_____ 11. Identify alterations in positioning routine and exposure factors specific to pediatric, geriatric, and bariatric patients.

_____ 12. List three reasons for taking chest radiographs with the patient in the erect position whenever possible.

_____ 13. Describe the three important positioning criteria that must be present on chest radiographs using erect PA and lateral positions.

_____ 14. Describe the advantages of the central ray placement method compared with the traditional method of centering for the PA and lateral chest projections.

_____ 15. Identify advantages and disadvantages in using CT, diagnostic medical sonography (DMS), nuclear medicine, and magnetic resonance imaging (MR) to demonstrate specific types of pathologic conditions in the chest.

_____ 16. Match various types of clinical indications to their correct definition.

_____ 17. For specific forms of chest pathology, indicate whether manual exposure factors need to be increased, decreased, or to remain the same.

_____ 18. List the correct central ray placement, part position, and criteria for specific chest projections.

_____ 19. Given a hypothetic situation, identify the correct modifications of position, kVp level, or both to improve the radiographic image.

_____ 20. Given a hypothetic situation, identify the correct position for a radiograph of specific pathologic conditions.

POSITIONING AND RADIOGRAPHIC CRITIQUE

_____ 1. Using a peer, position the patient for PA, anteroposterior (AP), and lateral chest projections.

_____ 2. Using a chest phantom, use routine PA and lateral chest positions to produce satisfactory radiographs (if equipment is available).

_____ 3. Determine whether rotation is present on PA and lateral chest radiographs.

_____ 4. Evaluate chest radiographs based on established radiographic criteria.

_____ 5. Distinguish between acceptable and unacceptable chest radiographs based on exposure factors, motion, collimation, positioning, or other errors.

LEARNING EXERCISES

Complete the following review exercises after reading the associated pages in Chapter 2 of the textbook as indicated by each exercise. Answers to each review exercise are given at the end of the review exercises and laboratory activities.

PART I: RADIOGRAPHIC ANATOMY

REVIEW EXERCISE A: Radiographic Anatomy of the Chest (see textbook pp. 68–75)

1. The bony thorax consists of (A) the single _____ anteriorly, (B) 2

   _____, (C) 2 _____, (D) 12 pairs of

   _____, and (E) 12 _____ posteriorly.

2. The two important bony landmarks of the thorax that are used for locating the central ray on a PA and AP chest

   projection are the (A) _____ and the (B) _____, respectively.

3. The four divisions of the respiratory system are:

   A. _____   C. _____

   B. _____   D. _____

4. Identify the correct anatomic terms for the following structures.

   A. Adam's apple _____   D. Shoulder blade _____

   B. Voice box _____   E. Collarbone _____

   C. Breastbone _____

5. List the three divisions of the structure located superior to the larynx that serve as a common passageway for both food and air.

   A. _____   C. _____

   B. _____

6. What is the name of the structure that acts as a lid over the larynx to prevent foreign objects such as food particles

   from entering the respiratory system? _____

7. The trachea is located _____ (anteriorly or posteriorly) to the esophagus.

8. The _____ bone is seen in the anterior portion of the neck and is found just below the tongue or floor of the mouth.

9. If a person accidentally inhales a food particle, it is likely to enter the

   (A)_____ bronchus because it is

   (B)_____

10. A. What is the name of the prominence, or ridge, seen when looking down into the trachea where it divides into the

    right and left bronchi? _____

    B. This prominence, or ridge, is approximately at the level of the _____ vertebra.

11. What is the term for the small air sacs located at the distal ends of the bronchioles, in which oxygen and carbon

    dioxide are exchanged in the blood? _____

12. A. The delicate, double-walled sac or membrane that contains the lungs is called the

    _____.

    B. The outer layer of this membrane adhering to the inner surface of the chest wall and diaphragm is the

    _____.

    C. The inner layer adhering to the surface of the lungs is the _____ or

    _____.

    D. The potential space between these two layers (identified in B and C) is called the

    _____.

    E. Air or gas that enters the space identified in D results in a condition called _____.

13. Fill in the correct terms for the following portions of the lungs.

    A. Lower, concave portion: _____

    B. Central area in which bronchi and blood vessels enter the lungs: _____

    C. Upper, rounded portion above the level of the clavicles: _____

    D. Extreme, outermost lower corner of the lungs: _____

14. Explain why the right lung is smaller than the left lung and the right hemidiaphragm is positioned higher than the left hemidiaphragm. _____

15. List the four important structures located in the mediastinum.

    A. _____   C. _____

    B. _____   D. _____

16. Identify the following structures in Fig. 2.1.

    A. _____ gland

    B. _____

    C. _____

    D. _____

    E. _____

    F. _____ gland

    G. _____

    H. _____

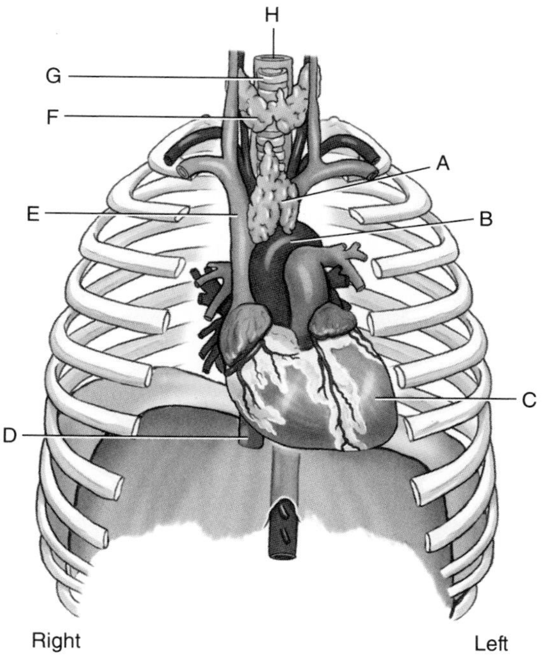

Fig. 2.1 Structures within the mediastinum.

17. The heart is enclosed in a double-walled membrane called the _____.

18. The three parts of the aorta are the _____, _____, and

_____.

19. Identify the following labeled structures as seen on PA and lateral chest radiographs in Figs. 2.2 and 2.3.

A. _____

B. _____

C. _____

D. _____

E. _____

F. _____

G. _____

H. _____

I. _____

J. _____

K. _____

L. _____

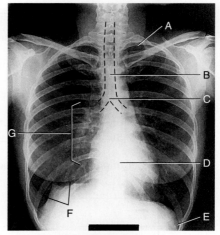

Fig. 2.2 Posteroanterior chest radiograph.

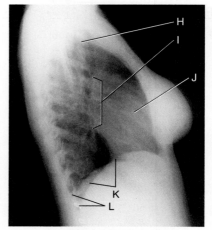

Fig. 2.3 Lateral chest radiograph.

20. Identify the labeled parts on this CT image (Fig. 2.4) of a transverse section of the thorax at the level of T5, the fifth thoracic vertebra, which is also the level of the carina. (Hint: B, G, and H are major blood vessels.)

A. _____

B. _____

C. _____

D. _____

E. _____

F. _____

G. _____

H. _____

I. _____

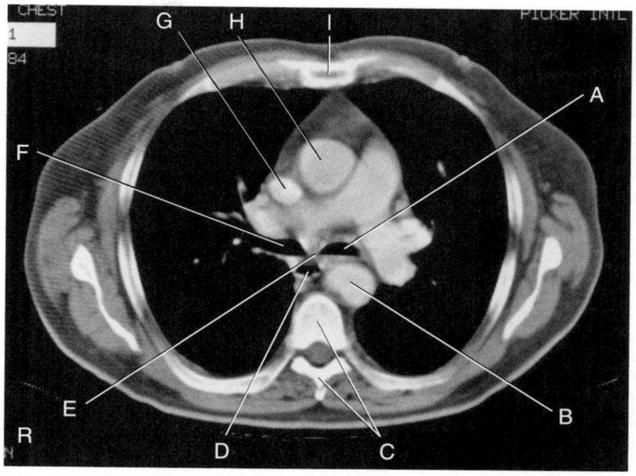

Fig. 2.4 Computed tomography transverse section of the thorax at the level of T5.

PART II: RADIOGRAPHIC POSITIONING

REVIEW EXERCISE B: Technical Considerations (see textbook pp. 76–87)

1. Which type of body habitus is associated with a broad and deep thorax? _____

2. Which of the following types of body habitus may cause the costophrenic angles to be cut off if careful vertical collimation is not used?

   A. Hypersthenic

   B. Hyposthenic

   C. Sthenic

   D. Hyposthenic and asthenic

3. What is the minimum number of ribs that should be demonstrated above the diaphragm on a PA radiograph of an average adult chest with full inspiration? _____

4. Which of the following objects should be removed (or moved) before chest radiography? (Choose all that apply.)

   A. Necklace

   B. Bra

   C. Religious medallion around neck

   D. Dentures

   E. Pants

   F. Hair fasteners

   G. Oxygen lines

5. True/False: Long hair may produce an artifact when imaging with digital radiographic systems.

6. True/False: Chest radiography is the most commonly repeated radiographic procedure because of poor positioning or exposure factor selection errors.

7. Chest radiography for the adult patient usually uses a kilovoltage range of _____ to

   _____ kVp.

8. True/False: Generally, you do not need to use radiographic grids for adult patients for PA or lateral chest radiographs.

9. Optimal technical factor selection ensures proper penetration of the:

    A. Heart
                  D. Hilar region

    B. Great vessels
          E. All of the above

    C. Lung regions

10. Describe the way optimal image exposure of the lungs and mediastinal structures can be determined on a PA chest radiograph. _____

11. True/False: Because the heart is always located in the left thorax, the use of anatomic side markers on a PA chest projection may not be necessary.

12. What is another term for the condition termed *visceral inversion?* _____

13. Which of the following devices should be used for the erect PA and lateral chest projections for an infant?

    A. Upright chest device
          C. Pigg-O-Stat

    B. Supine table Bucky
         D. Plexiglas restraint board

14. Which of the following sets of exposure factors is recommended for a chest examination of a young pediatric patient?

    A. 70–85 kVp, short exposure time
        C. 100–120 kVp, short exposure time

    B. 90–100 kVp, medium exposure time
      D. 120–150 kVp, long exposure time

15. True/False: Because they have shallower (superior–inferior dimension) lung fields, the central ray is often centered higher for geriatric patients.

16. True/False: CR centering for the PA chest projection on a bariatric patient is 1–2 inches (2.5–5 cm) lower than for a sthenic patient.

17. To ensure better lung inspiration during chest radiography, exposure should be made during the

    _____ inspiration.

18. List four possible pathologic conditions that suggest the need for inspiration and expiration PA chest projections.

    A. _____
                    C. _____

    B. _____
                    D. _____

19. List and explain briefly the three reasons chest projections should be taken with the patient in the erect position (when the patient's condition permits).

    A. _____
                    C. _____

    B. _____

20. Why do the lungs tend to expand more with the patient in an erect position than in a supine position?

_____

21. Explain the primary purpose and benefit of performing chest radiography using a 72-inch (180-cm) source image receptor distance (SID). _____

22. Which of the following anatomic structures is examined to determine rotation on a PA chest radiograph?

   A. Appearance of ribs

   B. Shape of heart

   C. Symmetric appearance and location of sternoclavicular joints

   D. Symmetric appearance and location of costophrenic angles

23. Which positioning tip will help prevent the patient's chin and neck from being superimposed over the upper airway and apices of the lungs for a PA chest radiograph?

   _____

   _____

24. For patients with the following clinical histories, which lateral projection would you perform—right or left?

   A. Patient with severe pains in left side of chest _____

   B. Patient with no chest pain but recent history of pneumonia in right lung _____

   C. Patient with no chest pain or history of heart trouble _____

25. Why is it important to raise the patient's arms above the head for lateral chest projections?

   _____

   _____

26. The traditional central ray centering technique for the chest is to place the top of the image receptor (IR) _____ inches (_____ cm) above the shoulders.

27. A recommended central ray centering technique for a PA chest projection requires the technologist to palpate the

   _____ and measure down from that bony landmark _____ inches (_____ cm) for a male

   and _____ inches (_____ cm) for a female patient.

28. A. Should the 14- × 17-inch (35- × 43-cm) image receptor be aligned in portrait or landscape orientation for a PA

   chest projection of a hypersthenic patient? _____

   B. For an asthenic patient? _____

29. Which of the following bony landmarks is palpated for centering of the AP chest projection?

   A. Vertebra prominens

   B. Jugular notch

   C. Thyroid cartilage

   D. Sternal angle

30. True/False: With most digital chest units, the question of IR placement into either the portrait or the landscape position is eliminated because of the larger IR.

31. True/False: In general for an average patient, more collimation should be visible on the lower margin of the chest image than on the top for a PA or lateral chest projection.

32. True/False: The height, or vertical dimension, of the average-to-more broad individual's chest is greater than the width or horizontal dimension.

33. True/False: Multislice CT (MSCT) can produce high-resolution images of the heart on one breath-hold.

45

34. True/False: Single-photon emission computed tomography (SPECT) is frequently used to diagnose myocardial infarction.

35. True/False: Diagnostic medical sonography (DMS) is not an effective modality to detect pleural effusion.

36. True/False: Echocardiography and electrocardiography are basically the same procedure.

37. Match each of the following descriptions of clinical indicators to its correct term.

_____	1. One of the most common inherited diseases	A. Atelectasis
_____	2. Condition most frequently associated with congestive heart failure	B. Bronchiectasis
_____	3. Dyspnea	C. Bronchitis
_____	4. Accumulation of air in pleural cavity	D. Chronic obstructive pulmonary disease
_____	5. Accumulation of pus in pleural cavity	E. Shortness of breath
_____	6. A form of occupational lung disease	F. Cystic fibrosis
_____	7. A contagious disease caused by an airborne bacterium	G. Empyema
_____	8. Irreversible dilation of bronchioles	H. Pleurisy
_____	9. Most common form is emphysema	I. Pneumothorax
_____	10. Acute or chronic irritation of bronchi	J. Pulmonary edema
_____	11. Collapse of all or portion of lung	K. Tuberculosis
_____	12. Inflammation of pleura	L. Silicosis

38. What is a common radiographic sign seen on a chest radiograph for a patient with respiratory distress syndrome (RDS)?

A. Enlargement of heart

B. Fluid in apices

C. Sail sign

D. Air bronchogram sign

39. For the following types of pathologic conditions, indicate whether manual exposure factors would be increased (+), decreased (−), or generally remain the same (0) compared with standard chest exposure factors.

_____ Left lung atelectasis

_____ Lung neoplasm

_____ Severe pulmonary edema

_____ RDS or adult respiratory distress syndrome (ARDS), known as hyaline membrane disease (HMD) in infants

_____ Reactivation (secondary) tuberculosis

_____ Advanced emphysema

_____ Large pneumothorax

_____ Pulmonary emboli

_____ Primary tuberculosis

_____ Advanced asbestosis

40. Which of the following is not a form of occupational lung disease?

    A. Anthracosis

    B. Emphysema

    C. Silicosis

    D. Asbestosis

41. Which of the following chest projections/positions is recommended to detect calcifications or cavitation within the upper lung region beneath the clavicles?

    A. Left lateral decubitus

    B. PA

    C. RPO and LPO

    D. AP lordotic

REVIEW EXERCISE C: Positioning of the Chest (see textbook pp. 88–100)

1. Why is a PA chest preferred to an AP projection? _____

2. The CR is placed at the level of the _____ vertebra for an adult PA chest projection.

3. The shoulders need to be rolled forward for the PA projection to allow the _____

   to move laterally and be clear of the lung fields.

4. Why should a left lateral be performed unless departmental protocol indicates otherwise?

   _____

5. How much separation of the posterior ribs on a lateral chest projection indicates excessive rotation from a true lateral

   position? _____ (Note: Less separation than this is caused by the divergent x-rays.)

6. To prevent the clavicles from obscuring the apices on an AP projection of the chest, the central ray should be

   angled (A) _____ (caudad or cephalad) so that it is perpendicular to the

   (B) _____.

7. What is the name of the condition characterized by fluid entering the pleural cavity?

   _____

8. Which specific position would be used if a patient were unable to stand but the physician suspected that the

   patient had fluid in the left lung? _____

9. What is the name of the condition characterized by free air entering the pleural cavity?

   _____

10. Which specific position would be used if the patient were unable to stand but the physician suspected that the patient

    had free air in the left pleural cavity? _____

11. What circumstances or clinical indications suggest that an AP lordotic projection should be ordered?

    _____

12. What position/projection would be used for a patient who is too ill or weak to stand for an AP lordotic projection?

_____

13. A. Which anterior oblique projection would best elongate the left thorax—right anterior oblique (RAO) or left anterior oblique (LAO)? _____

   B. Which posterior oblique projection would best elongate the left thorax—RPO or LPO?

_____

14. For certain studies of the heart, the _____ (right or left) anterior oblique requires a rotation

   of _____ degrees.

15. True/False: A grid is not recommended for an LPO projection of the adult chest.

16. Where is the central ray placed for a lateral projection of the upper airway? _____

17. Careful collimation during a chest radiograph will improve image quality by decreasing

   _____ radiation to the IR.

18. What are the recommended patient instructions when performing an erect PA chest on a female patient with large

   pendulous breasts? _____

19. True/False: If your facility uses a virtual grid, a physical grid is still needed.

20. An erect chest PA radiograph aids the patient to achieve full inspiration and helps to prevent

   _____ _____ and _____ of the pulmonary vessels.

REVIEW EXERCISE D: Problem Solving for Technical and Positioning Errors

The following radiographic problems involve technical and positioning errors that lead to substandard images. Other questions involve situations pertaining to various conditions and pathologic findings. As you analyze these problems and situations, use your textbook to help you find solutions to these questions.

1. A radiograph of a PA view of the chest shows that the sternoclavicular (SC) joints are not the same distance from the spine. The right SC joint is closer to the midline than is the left SC joint. What is the positioning error?

_____

2. A radiograph of a PA projection of the chest demonstrates only seven posterior ribs above the diaphragm. What caused this problem, and how could it be prevented on the repeat exposures?

_____

_____

3. A radiograph of a PA and a left lateral projection of the chest demonstrates the mediastinum of the chest is underpenetrated. The technologist used the following factors for the radiograph: a 72-inch (180-cm) SID, an upright Bucky, a full-inspiration exposure, 75-kVp and 800-mA, and a short exposure time.

   A. Which of these factors is the most likely cause of the problem? Briefly explain.

_____

B. How can the technologist improve the image when making the repeat exposure?

_____

4. A radiograph of a PA projection of the chest demonstrates the top of the apices is cut off and a wide collimation border can be seen below the diaphragm. How can this be corrected during the repeat radiograph?

_____

5. **Situation:** A patient with a clinical history of advanced emphysema comes to the radiology department for a chest x-ray. AEC will not be used. How should the technologist alter the manual exposure settings for this patient?

   A. Do not alter them. Use the standard exposure factors.

   B. Decrease the kVp moderately (−−).

   C. Increase the kVp slightly (+).

   D. Increase the kVp moderately (++).

5. **Situation:** A patient with severe pleural effusion comes to the radiology department for a chest x-ray. Automatic exposure control (AEC) will not be used. How should the technologist alter the manual exposure settings for this patient?

   A. Do not alter them. Use the standard exposure factors.

   B. Decrease the kVp moderately (−−).

   C. Increase the kVp slightly (+).

   D. Increase the kVp moderately (++).

7. **Situation:** A patient comes to the radiology department for a presurgical chest examination. The clinical history indicates a possible situs inversus of the thorax (transposition of structures within the thorax). Which positioning step or action must be taken to perform a successful chest examination?

_____

8. A radiograph of a lateral projection of the chest shows the posterior ribs and costophrenic angles are separated more than 1″ or 2.5 cm, indicating excessive rotation. Describe a possible method for determining the direction of rotation.

_____

9. **Situation:** A patient enters the emergency room with a possible hemothorax in the right lung caused by a motor vehicle accident (MVA). The patient is unable to stand or sit erect. Which specific projection would best demonstrate

   this condition, and why? _____

10. **Situation:** A young child enters the emergency room with a possible foreign body in one of the bronchi of the lung. The foreign body, a peanut, cannot be seen on the PA and lateral projections of the chest projection. Which additional projection(s) could the technologist perform to locate the foreign body?

_____

11. **Situation:** A routine chest series indicates a possible mass beneath the patient's right clavicle. The PA and lateral projections are inconclusive. What additional projection(s) could be taken to rule out this condition?

_____

12. **Situation:** A patient has a possible small pneumothorax. Routine chest projections (PA and lateral) fail to show the pneumothorax conclusively. Which additional projections could be taken to rule out this condition?

_____

49

13. **Situation:** A patient with a history of pleurisy comes to the radiology department. Which of the following radiographic series should be performed?

  A. Soft tissue lateral of the upper airway   C. Erect PA and lateral

  B. Right and left lateral decubitus   D. CT scan of the chest

14. **Situation:** A patient with a possible neoplasm in the right lung apex comes to the radiology department for a chest examination. The PA and lateral projections do not clearly demonstrate the neoplasm because of superimposition of the clavicle over the apex. The patient is unable to stand or sit erect. Which additional projection can be taken to demonstrate the neoplasm clearly and to eliminate the superimposition of the clavicle and the left lung apex?

  _____

15. **Situation:** PA and left lateral projections demonstrate a suspicious region in the left lung. The radiologist orders an oblique projection that will best demonstrate or "elongate" the left thorax. Which specific oblique projections will best elongate the left thorax? (More than one oblique projection will accomplish this goal.)

  _____

REVIEW EXERCISE E: Critique Radiographs of the Chest

The following questions relate to the radiographs found in this exercise. Evaluate these radiographs for the radiographic criteria categories (1–5). Describe the corrections needed to improve the overall image. The major, or "repeatable," errors are specific errors that indicate the need for a repeat exposure, regardless of the nature of the other errors.

A. PA chest (Fig. 2.5)

  Description of possible error:

  1. Anatomy demonstrated:

  _____

  2. Part positioning:

  _____

  3. Collimation field size and central ray:

  _____

  4. Exposure:

  _____

  5. Anatomic side markers:

  _____

  Repeatable error(s):

  _____

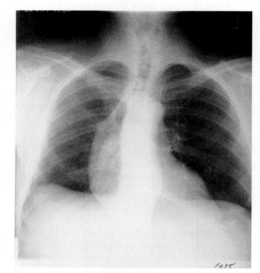

Fig. 2.5 Posteroanterior chest radiograph.

B. Lateral chest (Fig. 2.6)

Description of possible error:

1. Anatomy demonstrated:

   _____

2. Part positioning:

   _____

3. Collimation field size and central ray:

   _____

4. Exposure:

   _____

5. Anatomic side markers:

   _____

Repeatable error(s):

_____

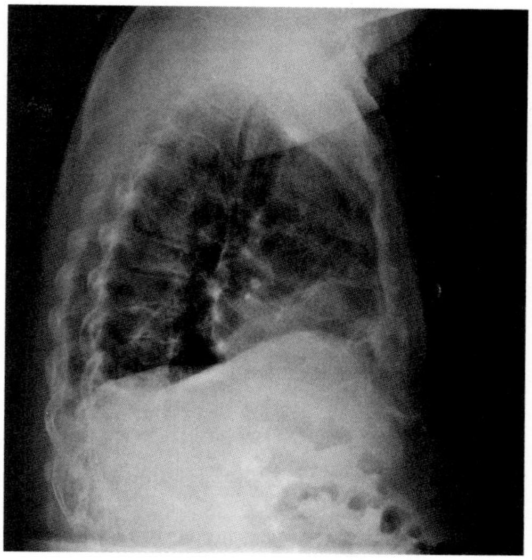

Fig. 2.6 Lateral chest radiograph.

PART III: LABORATORY ACTIVITIES

You must gain experience in chest positioning before performing the following exams on actual patients. You may gain experience with positioning and radiographic evaluation of these projections by performing exercises using radiographic phantoms and practicing on other students (although not taking actual exposures).

The following suggested activities assume your teaching institution has an energized lab and radiographic phantoms. If not, perform only Laboratory Exercise B, the physical positioning activities. (Check off each step and projection as you complete it.)

Laboratory Exercise A: Energized Laboratory

1. Using the chest radiographic phantom, produce radiographs using:

   _____ PA and AP projections   _____ Lateral projection

2. Evaluate the radiographs you produced previously, additional radiographs provided by your instructor, or both for the following criteria.

   _____ Rotation   _____ Anatomic side markers

   _____ Collimation field size   _____ Proper exposure factors

   _____ Part and central ray centering   _____ Motion

Laboratory Exercise B: Physical Positioning

1. On another person, simulate taking all of the following routine and special projections of the chest. Follow the suggested positioning steps and sequence as listed in the following and as described in Chapter 2 of your textbook:

_____ PA chest   _____ AP supine or semisupine

_____ Anterior and posterior oblique   _____ Lateral decubitus

_____ Lateral chest   _____ AP lordotic

_____ AP and lateral upper airway

Step 1. General patient positioning

_____ Select the size and number of image receptors needed.

_____ Prepare the radiographic room. Check that the x-ray tube is centered to the center of the IR holder (or the centerline of the table for Bucky exams).

_____ Correctly identify the patient and bring the patient into the room.

_____ Explain to the patient what you will be doing.

_____ Assist the patient to the proper place and position for the first radiograph.

Step 2. Measuring part thickness

_____ Measure the body part being radiographed and set correct exposure factors. (If using an AEC system, select the correct chamber cells on the control panel.)

Step 3. Part positioning

_____ Align and center the body part to the central ray or vice versa for chest positioning with the chest board. (For Bucky exams on a table, move the patient and tabletop together as needed [with floating-type tabletop].)

Step 4. Image receptor (IR) centering

_____ After the part has been centered to the central ray, the IR is also centered to the central ray. (Note: This step can be omitted on most chest units in which the x-ray tube and the IR unit are attached and move together.)

Additional steps or actions

_____ 1. Collimate accurately to include only the area of interest.

_____ 2. Place the correct side marker within the exposure field (so that you do not superimpose pertinent anatomic structures).

_____ 3. Restrain or provide support for the body part to prevent motion.

_____ 4. Use contact lead shielding when required (e.g., gonadal, breast, thyroid).

_____ 5. Give clear breathing instructions and make the exposure while watching patient through the console window.

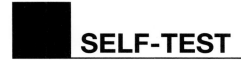

SELF-TEST

This self-test should be taken only after completing the readings, review exercises, and laboratory activities for a particular section. The purpose of this test is not only to provide a learning exercise but also to serve as a strong indicator of what your final unit evaluation exam will cover. It is strongly suggested that if you do not receive at least a 90%–95% grade on each self-test, you should review those areas in which you missed questions before going to your instructor for the final unit evaluation exam.

1. Match each of the following structures with its correct anatomic term.

    _____1. Breastbone   A. Clavicle

    _____2. Adam's apple   B. Larynx

    _____3. Shoulder blade   C. Thyroid cartilage

    _____4. Voice box   D. Scapula

    _____5. Collarbone   E. Sternum

2. Another term for the seventh cervical vertebrae is:

    A. Xiphoid process   C. Axis

    B. Jugular notch   D. Vertebra prominens

3. A notch, or depression, located on the superior portion of the sternum is called the:

    A. Sternal notch   C. Jugular notch

    B. Xiphoid notch   D. Sternal angle

4. The trachea bifurcates and forms the:

    A. Right and left bronchi   C. Costophrenic angles

    B. Right and left hilum   D. Pulmonary arteries

5. A specific prominence, or ridge, found at the point where the internal distal trachea divides into the right and left bronchi, is called the:

    A. Hilum   C. Epiglottis

    B. Carina   D. Alveoli

6. The area of each lung where the bronchi and blood vessels enter and leave is called the:

    A. Carina   C. Base

    B. Apex   D. Hilum

7. The structures within the lung in which oxygen and carbon dioxide gas exchange occurs are called:

   A. Carina
   B. Alveoli
   C. Hilum
   D. Bronchi

8. Which of the following is *not* an aspect of the pleura?

   A. Parietal pleura
   B. Hilar pleura
   C. Pleural cavity
   D. Pulmonary pleura

9. The condition in which blood fills the potential space between the layers of pleura is called:

   A. Pneumothorax
   B. Hemothorax
   C. Atelectasis
   D. Empyema

10. The extreme, outermost lower corner of each lung is called the:

    A. Costophrenic angle
    B. Apex
    C. Base
    D. Hilar region

11. Which of the following structures is *not* found in the mediastinum?

    A. Thymus gland
    B. Heart and great vessels
    C. Epiglottis
    D. Trachea

12. A narrow thorax that is shallow from the front to back but very long in the vertical dimension is characteristic of a(n) _____ body habitus.

    A. Hypersthenic
    B. Sthenic
    C. Hyposthenic
    D. Asthenic

13. Identify the best technical factors for adult chest radiography from the following choices.

    A. 70–85 kVp, 40-inch (100-cm) SID
    B. 110–120 kVp, 40-inch (100-cm) SID
    C. 110–120 kVp, 60-inch (150-cm) SID
    D. 110–125 kVp, 72-inch (180-cm) SID

14. Match the correct answers for the structures labeled on this midsagittal section of the pharynx and upper airway (Fig. 2.7).

_____ A.		1.	Laryngopharynx
_____ B.		2.	Uvula
_____ C.		3.	Epiglottis
_____ D.		4.	Esophagus
_____ E.		5.	Spinal cord
_____ F.		6.	Oral cavity
_____ G.		7.	Hyoid bone
_____ H.		8.	Nasopharynx
_____ I.		9.	Thyroid gland
_____ J.		10.	Oropharynx
_____ K.		11.	Larynx
_____ L.		12.	Hard palate
_____ M.		13.	Thyroid cartilage

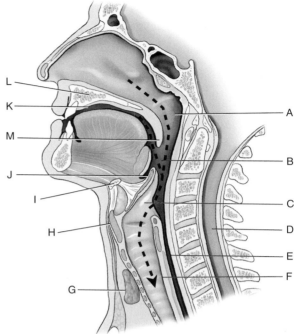

Fig. 2.7 Midsagittal section of the pharynx and upper airway.

15. Identify the structures labeled on this CT axial section of the soft-tissue neck at the level of C5 (the fifth cervical vertebra) (Fig. 2.8).

A. _____

B. _____

C. _____

D. _____

E. _____

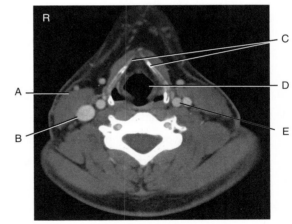

Fig. 2.8 CT axial section at the level of C5.

16. Identify the structures on this CT axial section of the thorax at the approximate level of T4–T5, 1 cm proximal to carina (Hint: B, E, and F are major blood vessels) (Fig. 2.9).

A. _____

B. _____

C. _____

D. _____

E. _____

F. _____

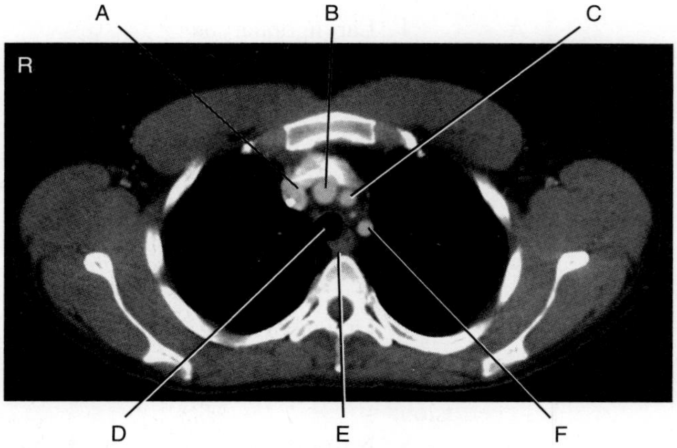

Fig. 2.9 Axial sectional level at T3.

17. What is the name of the special immobilization device used for pediatric chest studies?

A. Pigg-O-Stat

B. Restraining chair

C. Chest immobilizer

D. Franklin unit

18. Which of the following exposure factors is recommended for a chest study of a young pediatric (<4 years old) patient?

A. 110–125 kVp, short exposure time

B. 90–105 kVp, medium exposure time

C. 70–85 kVp, short exposure time

D. 60–75 kVp, long exposure time

19. Which of the following is *not* a valid reason to perform chest projections with the patient in the erect position?

A. To reduce patient dose

B. To demonstrate air and fluid levels

C. To allow the diaphragm to move down farther

D. To prevent hyperemia of pulmonary vessels

20. Why are the shoulders pressed downward and toward the IR for a PA projection of the chest?

A. To allow visualization of air-filled larynx

B. To prevent hyperemia of pulmonary vessels

C. To allow the diaphragm to move down farther

D. To reduce chest rotation

21. Why are the shoulders rolled forward for a PA projection of the chest?

A. To remove scapulae from lung fields

B. To prevent hyperemia of pulmonary vessels

C. To allow the diaphragm to move down farther

D. To reduce chest rotation

22. Where is the central ray placed for an AP supine projection of the chest?

 A. 7–8 inches (18–20 cm) below the vertebra prominens

 B. 1–2 inches (2.5–5 cm) below the jugular notch

 C. 3–4 inches (8–10 cm) below the jugular notch

 D. 3–4 inches (8–10 cm) below the thyroid cartilage

23. Which of the following terms is defined as a "shortness of breath?"

 A. Dyspnea

 B. Bronchiectasis

 C. Pleurisy

 D. Atelectasis

24. A condition in which all or a portion of the lung is collapsed is:

 A. Atelectasis

 B. Pleural effusion

 C. Pneumothorax

 D. Pneumoconiosis

25. A condition in which excess fluid builds in the lungs as a result of obstruction of the pulmonary circulation is termed:

 A. Pulmonary emboli

 B. Pneumothorax

 C. Pulmonary edema

 D. Bronchopneumonia

26. A sudden blockage of an artery in the lung is called:

 A. Pleurisy

 B. Pulmonary emboli

 C. Adult respiratory distress syndrome (ARDS)

 D. Chronic obstructive pulmonary disease (COPD)

27. Which of the following is *not* a form of occupational lung disease?

 A. Asbestosis

 B. Silicosis

 C. Anthracosis

 D. Tuberculosis

28. Which of the following is a pleural effusion where the fluid is pus?

 A. Empyema

 B. Hemothorax

 C. Pneumothorax

 D. Silicosis

29. A PA chest radiograph shows that the left sternoclavicular joint is superimposed over the spine (in comparison with the right joint). What specific positioning error is involved?

 A. Poor inspiration

 B. Rotation into a right anterior oblique (RAO) position

 C. Rotation into a left anterior oblique (LAO) position

 D. Tilting of the chest toward the left

30. A PA chest radiograph demonstrates 10 posterior ribs above the diaphragm. Is this an acceptable degree of

 inspiration? _____ Yes _____ No

31. A PA and lateral chest radiographic study has been completed. The PA projection shows the right costophrenic angle was collimated off, but both angles are included on the lateral projection. Would you repeat the PA

 projection? _____ Yes _____ No

32. A lateral chest radiograph demonstrates the soft tissue of the upper limbs is superimposed over the apices of the lungs. How can this situation be prevented?

   A. Deeper inspiration
           C. Slight rotation to the patient's left

   B. Extend chin
           D. Raise upper limbs higher

33. A lateral chest radiograph shows that the posterior ribs and costophrenic angles are separated by approximately inch (slightly less than 1″ (2.5 cm)). Should the technologist repeat this projection? _____ Yes _____ No

34. **Situation:** A radiograph of an AP lordotic projection shows that the clavicles are projected within the apices. The clinical instructor informs the student technologist that the study is unacceptable, but during the repeat exposure the patient complains of being too unsteady to lean backward for another projection. What other options are available if the student wants to complete the study?

   A. Perform the PA lordotic projection

   B. Perform an AP axial projection

   C. Perform both lateral decubitus projections

   D. Perform inspiration and expiration PA projections

35. **Situation:** An ambulatory patient with a clinical history of advanced emphysema enters the emergency room. The patient is having difficulty breathing and is receiving oxygen. The physician has ordered a PA and lateral chest study. Should the technologist alter the manual exposure factors for this patient?

   A. No. Use the standard exposure factors.

   B. Yes. Increase the exposure factors.

   C. Yes. Decrease the exposure factors.

   D. No. Increase the SID instead of changing the exposure factors.

36. **Situation:** A patient enters the ER with an injury to the chest. The ER physician suspects a pneumothorax may be present in the right lung. The patient is unable to stand or sit erect. Which specific position or projection can be performed to confirm the presence of the pneumothorax?

   A. Left lateral decubitus
           C. Right lateral decubitus

   B. Inspiration and expiration PA
           D. AP lordotic

37. **Situation:** A PA and lateral chest study shows a suspicious mass located near the heart in the right lung. The radiologist would like a radiograph of the patient in an anterior oblique position to delineate the mass from the heart. Which position or projection should the technologist use to accomplish this objective?

   A. 45° LAO
           C. 60° LAO

   B. 45° RAO
           D. AP lordotic

38. **Situation:** A patient with a history of pulmonary edema comes to the radiology department and is unable to stand. The physician suspects fluid in the left lung. Which specific projection should be used to confirm this diagnosis?

   A. Right lateral decubitus
           C. AP lordotic

   B. AP axial
           D. Left lateral decubitus

2 Chest

1. 1. E
   2. C
   3. D
   4. B
   5. A
2. D. Vertebra prominens
3. C. Jugular notch
4. A. Right and left bronchi
5. B. Carina
6. D. Hilum
7. B. Alveoli
8. B. Hilar pleura
9. B. Hemothorax
10. A. Costophrenic angle
11. C. Epiglottis
12. D. Asthenic
13. D. 110–125 kVp, 72-inch
    (180-cm) SID
14. A. 8
    B. 10
    C. 1
    D. 5
    E. 4
    F. 11
    G. 9
    H. 13
    I. 7
    J. 3
    K. 6
    L. 12
    M. 2
15. A. Sternocleidomastoid muscle
    B. Internal jugular vein
    C. Thyroid cartilage
    D. Larynx
    E. Common carotid artery
16. A. Superior vena cava
    B. Brachiocephalic artery
    C. Left common carotid artery
    D. Trachea
    E. Esophagus
    F. Left subclavian artery
17. A. Pigg-O-Stat
18. C. 70–85 kVp, short exposure
    time
19. A. To reduce patient dose
20. D. To reduce chest rotation
21. A. To remove scapulae from
    lung fields
22. C. 3–4 inches (8–10 cm) below
    the jugular notch
23. A. Dyspnea
24. A. Atelectasis
25. C. Pulmonary edema
26. B. Pulmonary emboli
27. D. Tuberculosis
28. A. Empyema
29. C. Rotation into an LAO
    position
30. Yes, 10 ribs showing is accept-
    able. (Some healthy patients can
    inhale more deeply and show 11
    ribs.)
31. Yes. The costophrenic angles
    must be visualized on both the
    PA and lateral projections.
32. D. Raise upper limbs higher.
33. No. This separation is acceptable
    and is caused by the divergent
    x-ray beam.
34. Perform an AP axial projection.
35. C. Yes. Decrease the exposure
    factors.
36. A. Left lateral decubitus
37. C. 60° LAO
38. D. Left lateral decubitus

3 Abdomen

After you have successfully completed the activities in this chapter, you will be able to:

_____ 1. List the location of the three muscles of the abdomen that are important in abdominal radiography.

_____ 2. List the major organs and structures of the digestive and urinary systems.

_____ 3. Using drawings and radiographs, identify the principal structures of the digestive system, biliary system, urinary system, and accessory organs involved in digestion.

_____ 4. Identify whether select organs of the abdomen are intraperitoneal, retroperitoneal, or infraperitoneal.

_____ 5. Identify the correct quadrant or region of the abdomen in which specific organs are located.

_____ 6. Identify specific bony topographic landmarks used for positioning of the abdomen.

_____ 7. Using drawings, radiographs, and computed tomography (CT) images, identify the major bony and soft tissue structures of the abdomen.

_____ 8. List specific types of pathology that are clinical indications for an acute abdominal series.

_____ 9. List specific methods for controlling involuntary and voluntary motion during abdominal radiography.

_____ 10. Describe the factors that affect collimation and the use of gonadal shielding "(when required by policy)" during abdominal radiography.

_____ 11. Identify the ideal kVp ranges to be used during abdominal radiography.

_____ 12. Identify alterations in positioning routine and exposure factors for pediatric, geriatric, and bariatric patients.

_____ 13. Identify the pathologic conditions and diseases of the abdomen that are best demonstrated with CT, diagnostic medical sonography (DMS), nuclear medicine, and magnetic resonance imaging (MR).

_____ 14. Match various types of abdominal pathologic findings to their correct definition.

_____ 15. Match specific types of abdominal pathologic findings to their correct radiographic appearance.

_____ 16. Describe variations in recommended field size, collimation, and central ray (CR) placement that can be used to accommodate differences in body habitus.

_____ 17. List the correct central ray placement, part position, and radiographic criteria for specific abdomen projections.

_____ 18. List the clinical indications for the acute abdominal series.

_____ 19. List the projections taken for the acute abdominal series and variations that can be used to accommodate specific patient conditions.

_____ 20. Given various hypothetic situations, identify the correct modification of position, exposure factors, or both to improve the radiographic image.

_____ 21. Given various hypothetic situations, identify the correct position for a specific pathologic feature or condition.

POSITIONING AND RADIOGRAPHIC CRITIQUE

_____ 1. Use another student as a model to practice putting a patient in supine, erect, and lateral decubitus abdominal positions.

_____ 2. Using an abdomen phantom, produce an AP projection of the abdomen that results in a satisfactory radiograph (if equipment is available).

_____ 3. Evaluate radiographic images of the abdomen for specific positioning and technical errors.

_____ 4. Evaluate abdominal radiographs based on established radiographic criteria.

_____ 5. Distinguish between acceptable and unacceptable abdominal radiographs based on exposure factors, motion, collimation, positioning, or other errors.

_____ 6. Identify specific bony and soft tissue structures seen radiographically.

_____ 7. Discriminate among radiographs taken in supine, erect, or lateral decubitus positions.

LEARNING EXERCISES

Complete the following review exercises after reading the associated pages in Chapter 3 of the textbook as indicated by each exercise. Answers to each review exercise are provided at the end of the review exercises.

PART I: RADIOGRAPHIC ANATOMY

REVIEW EXERCISE A: Abdominopelvic Anatomy (see textbook pp. 102–109)

1. The two large muscles found in the posterior abdomen adjacent to the lumbar vertebra that are usually visible on an anteroposterior (AP) radiograph are called the _____.

2. The medical prefix for stomach is _____.

3. List the three parts of the small intestine.

   A. _____   C. _____

   B. _____

4. Which portion of the small intestine is considered to be the longest? _____

5. The large intestine begins in the _____ quadrant with a saclike area called the

   _____.

6. The sigmoid colon is located between the _____ and _____ of the large intestine.

7. Which of the following organs is considered part of the lymphatic system?

    A. Liver

    B. Spleen

    C. Pancreas

    D. Gallbladder

8. List the three accessory digestive organs.

    A. _____

    B. _____

    C. _____

9. Circle the correct term. The pancreas is located anteriorly or posteriorly to the stomach.

10. Which of the following organs is *not* directly associated with the digestive system?

    A. Gallbladder

    B. Spleen

    C. Jejunum

    D. Pancreas

11. Why is the right kidney found in a more inferior position than the left kidney? _____

12. Which endocrine glands are superomedial to each kidney? _____

13. True/False: The correct term for the radiographic study of the entire urinary system is the intravenous pyelogram (IVP).

14. The double-walled membrane that lines the abdominopelvic cavity is called the _____.

15. The organs located posteriorly to, or behind, the serous membrane lining of the abdominopelvic cavity are referred

    to as _____.

16. Which of the following structures helps stabilize and support the small intestine?

    A. Omentum

    B. Peritoneum

    C. Viscera

    D. Mesentery

17. Which of the following structures is a double fold of peritoneum that connects the transverse colon to the greater curvature of the stomach?

    A. Mesocolon

    B. Lesser omentum

    C. Greater omentum

    D. Mesentery

18. Match the following structures to the correct location of the peritoneum.

_____ 1. Liver   A. Intraperitoneum

_____ 2. Urinary bladder   B. Retroperitoneum

_____ 3. Kidneys   C. Infraperitoneum

_____ 4. Spleen

_____ 5. Ovaries

_____ 6. Duodenum

_____ 7. Transverse colon

_____ 8. Testes

_____ 9. Adrenal glands

_____ 10. Stomach

_____ 11. Pancreas

_____ 12. Ascending and descending colon

19. For each of the following organs, identify the correct abdominal quadrant in which the organ is found—left upper quadrant (LUQ), left lower quadrant (LLQ), right lower quadrant (RLQ), or right upper quadrant (RUQ).

A. Liver _____

B. Spleen _____

C. Sigmoid colon _____

D. Left colic flexure _____

E. Stomach _____

F. Appendix _____

G. Two-thirds of jejunum _____

20. What is the correct name for the abdominal region found directly in the middle of the abdomen?

A. Epigastric   C. Umbilical

B. Inguinal   D. Pubic

21. Which of the following abdominal regions contains the rectum?

A. Pubic   D. Epigastric

B. Inguinal   E. Hypochondriac

C. Umbilical   F. Lumbar

22. Identify the bony landmarks in Fig. 3.1.

A. _____

B. _____

C. _____

D. _____

E. _____

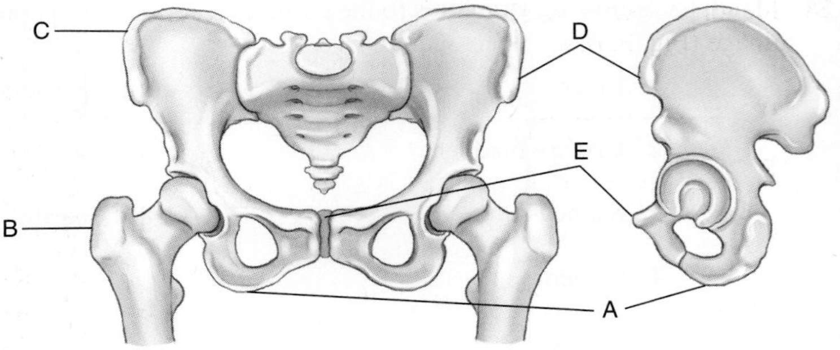

Fig. 3.1 Landmarks of the pelvis.

23. The prominence of the greater trochanter is at about the same level as the _____ symphysis pubis, and the lower margins of the ischial tuberosities are about _____ inches (_____ cm) _____ (proximal or distal) to the symphysis pubis.

24. Which topographic landmark corresponds to the inferior margin of the abdomen and is formed by the anterior junction of the two pelvic bones? _____

25. Which topographic landmark is found at the level of L2–L3? _____

26. The iliac crest is at the level of the _____ vertebra.

27. Identify the labeled parts of the digestive system (Fig. 3.2).

A. _____

B. _____

C. _____

D. _____ valve

E. _____

F. _____

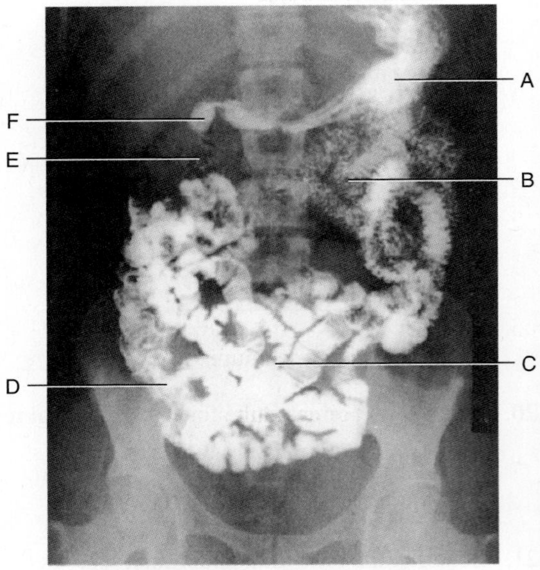

Fig. 3.2 Radiograph of the digestive tract.

28. Identify the labeled structures present on the CT image (Fig. 3.3).

A. _____

B. _____

C. _____

D. _____

E. _____

F. _____

G. _____

H. _____

I. _____

J. _____

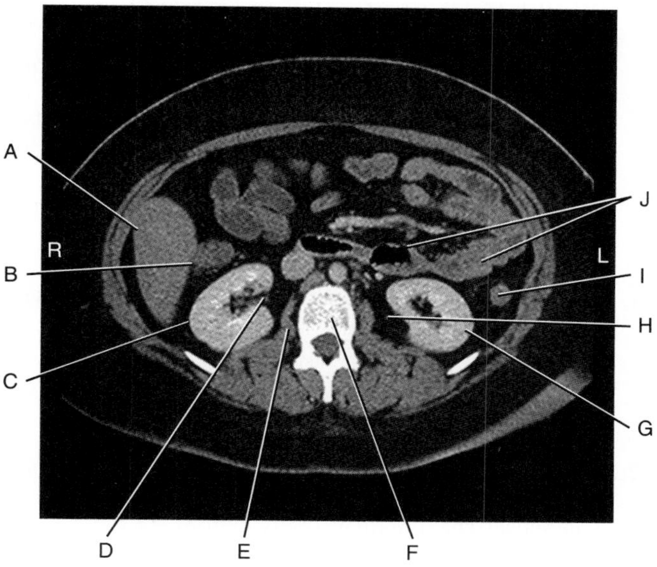

Fig. 3.3 CT image of the abdomen at the level of L1/L2.

PART II: RADIOGRAPHIC POSITIONING AND OTHER PATIENT CONSIDERATIONS

REVIEW EXERCISE B: Shielding, Exposure Factors, and Positioning (see textbook pp. 110–121)

1. What are the two causes of voluntary motion?

   A. _____   B. _____

2. Voluntary motion can best be prevented by _____ to the patient.

3. What is the primary cause for involuntary motion in the abdomen?

   _____

4. What is the best mechanism to control involuntary motion?

   _____

5. True/False: Because the liver margin is visible in the right upper quadrant of the abdomen, it is not necessary to place a right or left anatomic side marker on the cassette before exposure.

6. True/False: For an adult abdomen, a collimation margin must be visible on all four sides of the radiograph.

7. Gonadal shielding should *not* be used during abdomen radiography if:

   A. It obscures essential anatomy   C. It is against local regulations or department policy

   B. It interferes with the AEC system   D. Any of the above

8. Gonadal shielding for _____ may be impossible for studies of the lower abdominopelvic region.

   A. Males   C. Both males and females

   B. Females   D. Small children

9. Gonadal shielding for females involves placing the top of the shield at or slightly above the level of the _____, with the bottom at the _____. "(When required by policy.)"

10. Which of the following exposure considerations would be most ideal for an AP abdomen of an average-sized adult using a digital radiographic system?

    A. 110–120 kVp, grid, 40-inch (100-cm) SID

    B. 95–105 kVp, grid, 40-inch (100-cm) SID

    C. 80–85 kVp, grid, 40-inch (100-cm) SID

    D. 60–70 kVp, grid, 40-inch (100-cm) SID

11. Which of the following technical considerations is essential when performing abdomen studies on a young pediatric patient?

    A. Short exposure times

    B. High-speed image receptor

    C. Reduced kVp and mAs

    D. All of the above

12. True/False: A radiolucent pad should be placed underneath geriatric patients for added comfort.

13. True/False: The umbilicus (belly button) is a reliable, alternative landmark to use for the bariatric patient.

14. True/False: The image receptor should be placed in portrait alignment for an abdomen study on a bariatric patient.

15. With the use of iodinated contrast media, _____ is able to distinguish between a simple cyst and a tumor of the liver.

    A. DMS

    B. Nuclear medicine

    C. CT

    D. MR

16. The preferred imaging modality for examining the gallbladder quickly is:

    A. DMS

    B. Nuclear medicine

    C. Barium enema study

    D. MR

17. _____ is recommended to evaluate patients with acute appendicitis.

    A. DMS

    B. Nuclear medicine

    C. CT

    D. MR

18. Match the following definitions to the correct clinical indication:

    _____ 1. Free air or gas in the peritoneal cavity

    _____ 2. Inflammatory condition of the colon

    _____ 3. Telescoping of a section of bowel into another loop of bowel

    _____ 4. Abnormal accumulation of fluid in the peritoneal cavity

    _____ 5. Bowel obstruction caused by a lack of intestinal peristalsis

    _____ 6. A twisting of a loop of bowel creating an obstruction

    _____ 7. Chronic inflammation of the intestinal wall that may result in bowel obstruction

    A. Volvulus

    B. Adynamic (paralytic) ileus

    C. Ascites

    D. Ulcerative colitis

    E. Pneumoperitoneum

    F. Intussusception

    G. Crohn disease

19. Match each of the following radiographic appearances of the abdomen to its corresponding type of pathologic condition:

_____ 1. Distended loops of air-filled small intestine		A. Ascites
_____ 2. Air-filled "coiled spring" appearance		B. Volvulus
_____ 3. General abdominal haziness		C. Pneumoperitoneum
_____ 4. Thin crest-shaped radiolucency underneath diaphragm		D. Ulcerative colitis
_____ 5. Deep air-filled mucosal protrusions of colon wall		E. Intussusception
_____ 6. Large amount of air trapped in sigmoid colon with a tapered narrowing at the site of obstruction		F. Crohn disease

20. The central ray (CR) is centered to the level of the _____ for a supine AP projection of the abdomen.

21. Exposure for an AP projection of the abdomen should be taken on _____ (inspiration or expiration).

22. Rotation can be determined on a kidney, ureter, and bladder (KUB) radiograph by the loss of the symmetric appearance of:

A. _____   C. _____

B. _____   D. _____

23. Which type of body habitus might require two landscape-aligned image receptors to be taken so the entire abdomen is included?

24. True/False: A tall asthenic patient may require two 14- × 17-inch (35- × 43-cm) image receptor placed portrait so the entire abdomen is included.

25. True/False: For a KUB, it is accepted practice to indicate the side of the body during postprocessing after the exposure has been completed. The liver is always on the right side of the body.

_____

26. Why is it recommended to take abdominal radiographs at the end of patient expiration?

27. Which of the following abdominal structures is not visible on a properly exposed KUB?

A. Kidneys   C. Pancreas

B. Margin of liver processes   D. Lumbar transverse processes

28. Why may the PA projection of a KUB generally be less desirable than the AP projection?

_____

29. Which decubitus position of the abdomen best demonstrates intraperitoneal air in the abdomen?

_____

30. Why should a patient be placed in the decubitus position for a minimum of 5 minutes before exposure?

_____

31. Which decubitus position best demonstrates possible aneurysms, calcifications of the aorta, or umbilical hernias?

_____

32. Which projection best demonstrates a possible aortic aneurysm in the prevertebral region of the abdomen?

_____

33. List the projections commonly performed for an acute abdominal series or three-way abdomen series.

A. _____   C. _____

B. _____

34. Which projection of the (two-projection/way) acute abdominal series best demonstrates free air under the diaphragm?

_____

35. Which positioning routine should be used for an acute abdominal series if the patient is too ill to stand?

_____

36. Which of the following projections requires a kVp setting of 110–125?

A. Erect abdomen for ascites   C. PA, erect chest for free air under diaphragm

B. Supine abdomen for intra-abdominal mass   D. Dorsal decubitus abdomen for calcified aorta

37. To ensure the diaphragm is included on an erect abdomen projection, the central ray should be at the level of

_____, which places the top of the 14- × 17-inch (35- × 43-cm) image receptor at the

level of the _____.

38. What is the recommended overlap when using two landscape-placed image receptors for an AP projection of a supine

abdomen of a bariatric patient? _____

39. What scale of contrast is recommended for visualization of the abdominal structures on an abdominal x-ray?

A. Short scale   B. Long scale

40. True/False: The patient best controls peristalsis by holding his or her breath during exposure.

REVIEW EXERCISE C: Problem Solving for Technical and Positioning Errors

The following radiographic problems involve technical and positioning errors that may lead to substandard images. As you analyze these problems, review your textbook to find solutions to these questions.

Other questions involve situations pertaining to various patient conditions and pathologic findings. If you need more information about a particular pathologic condition, review your textbook or a medical dictionary to learn more about it.

1. A KUB radiograph shows that the symphysis pubis was cut off along the bottom of the image. Is this an acceptable radiograph? If it is not, how can this problem be prevented during the repeat exposure?

_____

_____

2. A radiograph of an AP projection of an average-size adult abdomen was produced using the following exposure factors: 100 kVp, 600 mA, 1/10 second, grid, and 40-inch (100-cm) SID. The exposure indicator (EI) revealed that the patient was over exposed. Which adjustment to the technical considerations should be made to ensure the EI is within the acceptable limits?

_____

_____

3. A radiographic image of an AP projection of the abdomen demonstrates motion. The following exposure factors were selected: 78 kVp, 200 mA, 2/10 second, grid, and 40-inch (100-cm) SID. The technologist is sure that the patient did not breathe or move during the exposure. What may have caused this blurriness? What can be done to correct this problem on the repeat exposure?

_____

_____

4. A radiograph of an AP abdomen shows the left iliac wing is more narrowed than the right. What specific positioning error caused this?

_____

_____

5. **Situation**: A patient with a possible dynamic ileus enters the emergency room. The patient is able to stand. The physician has ordered an acute abdominal series. What specific positioning routine should be used?

_____

_____

6. **Situation**: A patient with a possible perforated duodenal ulcer enters the emergency room (ER). The ER physician is concerned about the presence of free air in the abdomen. The patient is in severe pain and *cannot* stand. What positioning routine should be used to diagnose this condition?

_____

_____

7. **Situation**: The ER physician suspects that a patient has a kidney stone. The patient is sent to the radiology department to confirm the diagnosis. What specific positioning routine would be used to rule out the presence of a kidney stone?

_____

_____

8. **Situation**: A patient in intensive care may have developed intra-abdominal bleeding. The patient is in critical condition and cannot go to the radiology department. The physician has ordered a portable study of the abdomen. Which specific position or projection can be used to determine the extent of the bleeding?

_____

_____

9. **Situation**: A patient with a history of ascites comes to the radiology department. Which of the following positions best demonstrates this condition?

A. Erect AP abdomen

B. Erect PA chest

C. Supine KUB

D. Prone KUB

10. **Situation**: A KUB radiograph shows that the gonadal shielding is superior to the upper margin of the symphysis pubis. The female patient has a history of kidney stones. What is the next step the technologist should take?

A. Accept the radiograph because the shielding did not obscure the kidneys.

B. Repeat the exposure without using gonadal shielding.

C. Repeat the exposure only if the patient complains of pain in the lower abdomen.

D. Repeat the exposure with gonadal shielding, but position it below the symphysis pubis.

11. **Situation**: A bariatric patient comes to the radiology department for a KUB. The radiograph shows that the symphysis pubis is included on the image, but the upper abdomen, including the kidneys, is cut off. What is the next step the technologist should take?

A. Accept the radiograph.

B. Repeat the exposure, but expose it during inspiration to force the kidneys lower into the abdomen.

C. Ask the radiologist whether the upper abdomen really needs to be seen. Repeat only if requested.

D. Repeat the exposure. Use two landscape aligned 14- × 17-inch (35- × 43-cm) image receptors to include the entire abdomen.

12. **Situation**: A patient comes from the ER with a large distended abdomen caused by an ileus. The physician suspects that the distention is caused by a large amount of bowel gas that is trapped in the small intestine. The exposure factors for a KUB on an average, healthy adult is 76 kVp, 30 mAs. Should the technologist change any of these exposure factors for this patient? (Automatic exposure control [AEC] is not being used.)

A. No. Use the standard exposure settings.

B. Yes. Decrease the milliamperage seconds (mAs).

C. Yes. Increase the milliamperage seconds (mAs).

D. Yes. Increase the kilovoltage (kVp).

13. **Situation**: A child goes to radiology for an abdomen study. It is possible that he swallowed a coin. The ER physician believes it may be in the upper GI tract. Which of the following routines would best identify the location of the coin?

A. KUB and left lateral decubitus

B. Acute abdominal series

C. KUB and lateral abdomen

D. Supine and erect KUB

REVIEW EXERCISE D: Critique Radiographs of the Abdomen

The following questions relate to the radiographs found in this exercise. Evaluate these radiographs for the radiographic criteria categories (1–5). Describe the corrections needed to improve the overall image. The major, or "repeatable," errors are specific errors that indicate the need for a repeat exposure, regardless of the nature of the other errors.

A. AP KUB (Fig. 3.4)

Description of possible error:

1. Anatomy demonstrated:

_____

2. Part positioning:

_____

3. Collimation field size and central ray:

_____

4. Exposure:

_____

5. Anatomic side markers:

_____

Repeatable error(s):

_____

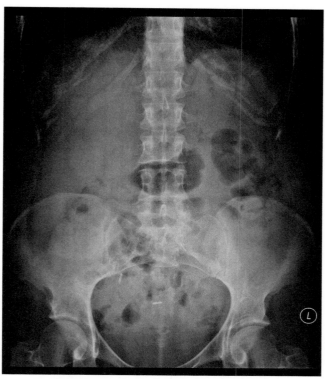

Fig. 3.4 Anteroposterior image of kidneys, ureters, and bladder. *(Case courtesy of Dr. Jeremy Jones, Radiopaedia. org, rID: 34067.)*

B. AP erect abdomen (Fig. 3.5)

Description of possible error:

1. Anatomy demonstrated:

_____

2. Part positioning:

_____

3. Collimation field size and central ray:

_____

4. Exposure:

_____

5. Anatomic side markers:

_____

Repeatable error(s):

_____

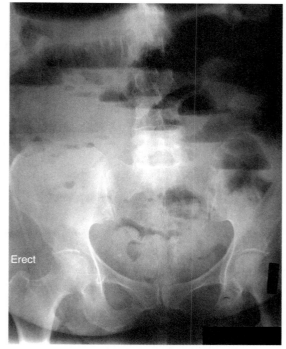

Fig. 3.5 Anteroposterior image of erect abdomen.

PART III: LABORATORY EXERCISES

You must gain experience in abdomen positioning before performing the following exams on actual patients. You may gain experience in positioning and radiographic evaluation of these projections by performing exercises using radiographic phantoms and practicing on other students (although you will not be taking actual exposures).

The following suggested activities assume your teaching institution has an energized lab and radiographic phantoms. If not, perform only Laboratory Exercise B, the physical positioning activities. (Check off each step and projection as you complete it.)

Laboratory Exercise A: Energized Laboratory

1. Using the abdominal radiographic phantom, produce a KUB radiograph.

2. Evaluate the KUB radiograph, additional radiographs provided by your instructor, or both, for the following criteria:

_____ Rotation   _____ Part and central ray centering

_____ Proper exposure factors   _____ Motion

_____ Collimation field size   _____ Anatomic side markers

Laboratory Exercise B: Physical Positioning

1. On another person, simulate taking all of the following basic and special projections of the abdomen. Follow the suggested positioning steps and sequence as listed in the following and as described in Chapter 3 of your textbook.

_____ KUB of the abdomen   _____ Dorsal decubitus

_____ Left lateral decubitus   _____ Acute abdominal series to include: AP supine, AP erect, PA chest

Step 1. General patient positioning

_____ Select the size and number of IR needed.

_____ Prepare the radiographic room. Check that the x-ray tube is centered to the center of the IR holder (or the centerline of the table for Bucky exams).

_____ Correctly identify the patient and bring the patient into the room.

_____ Explain to the patient what you will be doing.

_____ Assist the patient to the proper place and position for the first radiograph.

Step 2. Measuring part thickness

_____ Measure the body part being radiographed and set the correct exposure factors (technique). (If using an AEC system, select the correct chamber cells on the control panel.)

Step 3. Part positioning

_____ Align and center the body part to the central ray or vice versa. For Bucky exams on a table, move the patient and tabletop together as needed (with a floating type of tabletop). (Note: In cases in which the correct central ray position is of primary importance, the central ray icon is included in the textbook on the appropriate positioning page.)

Step 4. IR centering

_____ After the part has been centered to the central ray, the IR is also centered to the central ray.

Additional steps or actions

_____ 1. Collimate accurately to include only the area of interest.

_____ 2. Place the correct marker within the exposure field (so that you do not superimpose pertinent anatomic structures).

_____ 3. Restrain or provide support for the body part to prevent motion.

_____ 4. Use contact lead shielding when requested.

_____ 5. Give clear breathing instructions and make the exposure while watching the patient through the console window.

72

MY SCORE = _____%

This self-test should be taken only after completing all of the readings, review exercises, and laboratory activities for a particular section. The self-test is divided into six sections. The purpose of this test is not only to provide a good learning exercise but also to serve as a strong indicator of what your final unit evaluation exam will cover. It is strongly suggested that if you do not receive at least a 90%–95% grade on each self-test, you should review those areas in which you missed questions before going to your instructor for the final unit evaluation exam.

1. The double-walled membrane lining the abdominal cavity is called the:

   A. Greater omentum   C. Lesser omentum

   B. Mesentery   D. Peritoneum

2. Which of the following soft tissue structures are seen on a properly exposed KUB?

   A. Spleen   C. Psoas muscles

   B. Pancreas   D. Stomach

3. The first portion of the small intestine is called the:

   A. Duodenum   C. Jejunum

   B. Ileum   D. Pylorus

4. At the junction of the small and large intestine is the:

   A. Sigmoid colon   C. Ileocecal valve

   B. Rectum   D. Ascending colon

5. Match the correct answers to the structures labeled in Fig. 3.6.

   _____A. Sigmoid colon

   _____B. Liver

   _____D. Oral cavity

   _____E. Spleen

   _____F. Stomach

   _____G. Esophagus

   _____H. Oropharynx

   _____I. Pancreas

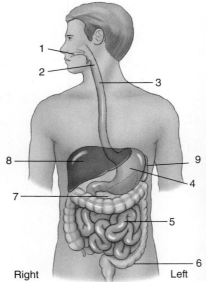

Fig. 3.6 Digestive tract and surrounding structures.

73

6. Which of the following is not an accessory organ of digestion?

   A. Liver

   B. Gallbladder

   C. Pancreas

   D. Kidney

7. The kidneys are connected to the bladder by way of the:

   A. Urethra

   B. Renal artery

   C. Ureter

   D. Renal vein

8. Which structure stores and releases bile?

   A. Liver

   B. Spleen

   C. Pancreas

   D. Gallbladder

9. Which of the following structures connects the small intestine to the posterior abdominal wall?

   A. Greater omentum

   B. Peritoneum

   C. Lesser omentum

   D. Mesentery

10. For each of the following organs, identify the correct abdominal quadrant(s) in which the organ would be found on an average sthenic patient—left upper quadrant (LUQ), left lower quadrant (LLQ), right lower quadrant (RLQ), or right upper quadrant (RUQ). (Note: Some organs may be found in more than one quadrant.)

    A. Cecum _____

    B. Liver _____

    C. Spleen _____

    D. Stomach _____

    E. Right colic flexure _____

    F. Sigmoid colon _____

    G. Appendix _____

    H. Pancreas _____

    I. Gallbladder _____

11. Which region of the abdomen contains the spleen?

    A. Epigastric

    B. Umbilical

    C. Left hypochondriac

    D. Left inguinal

12. Match the following structures to the correct compartment of the peritoneum.

_____ 1. Cecum   A. Intraperitoneum

_____ 2. Jejunum   B. Retroperitoneum

_____ 3. Ascending colon   C. Infraperitoneum

_____ 4. Liver

_____ 5. Adrenal glands

_____ 6. Gallbladder

_____ 7. Ovaries

_____ 8. Duodenum

_____ 9. Urinary bladder

_____ 10. Pancreas

13. The xiphoid process corresponds with which vertebral level?
    A. T9–T10   C. L2–L3
    B. L4–L5   D. T4–T5

14. Identify the topographic positioning landmarks as labeled in Figs. 3.7 and 3.8.

    _____ A. Iliac crest

    _____ B. Ischial tuberosity

    _____ C. Xiphoid process

    _____ D. Pubic symphysis

    _____ E. Greater trochanter

    _____ F. Lower costal margin

    _____ G. Anterior superior iliac
               spine (ASIS)

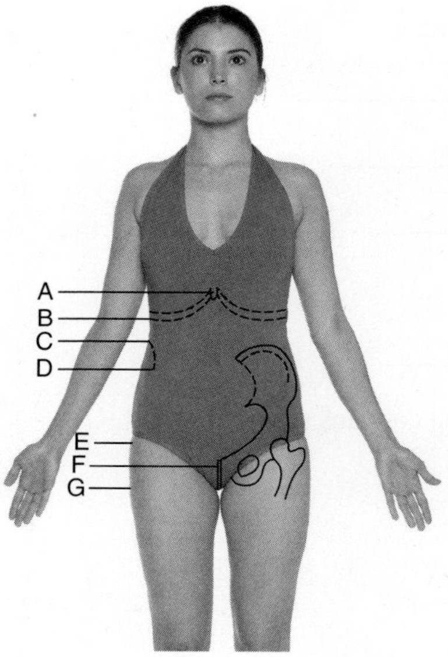

Fig. 3.7 Anterior surface landmarks.

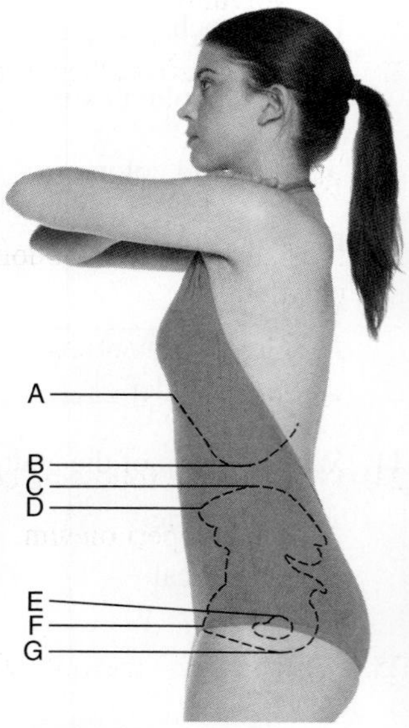

Fig. 3.8 Lateral surface landmarks.

15. To identify the inferior margin of the abdomen, the technologist can palpate the symphysis pubis or:
    A. Iliac crest   C. ASIS
    B. Greater trochanter   D. Ischial tuberosity

16. An important anatomic landmark that is commonly used to locate the center of the abdomen is the:

A. Iliac crest

C. ASIS

B. Greater trochanter

D. Ischial tuberosity

17. Which of the following factors best controls the involuntary motion of a young, pediatric patient during abdominal radiography?

A. Short exposure time

C. Clear, concise breathing instructions

B. High kVp (110–125)

D. Use of compression band across the abdomen

18. An abnormal accumulation of fluid in the abdominal cavity is called:

A. Ileus

C. Volvulus

B. Ulcerative colitis

D. Ascites

19. Another term describing a nonmechanical bowel obstruction is:

A. Pneumoperitoneum

C. Ascites

B. Paralytic ileus

D. Intussusception

20. The telescoping of a section of bowel into another loop is called:

A. Intussusception

C. Volvulus

B. Ascites

D. Ulcerative colitis

21. A chronic disease involving inflammation of the large intestine is:

A. Ascites

C. Crohn disease

B. Volvulus

D. Ulcerative colitis

22. Free air or gas in the peritoneal cavity is:

A. Pneumothorax

C. Pneumoperitoneum

B. Ileus

D. Volvulus

23. Free air in the intra-abdominal cavity rises to the level of the _____ in a patient who is in the erect position.

A. Greater omentum

C. Intraperitoneal cavity

B. Diaphragm

D. Liver

24. Which of the following conditions is demonstrated radiographically as general abdominal haziness?

A. Pneumoperitoneum

C. Ileus

B. Ascites

D. Volvulus

25. Which one of the following conditions is demonstrated radiographically as distended, air-filled loops of the small bowel?

A. Ascites

C. Pneumoperitoneum

B. Ulcerative colitis

D. Ileus

26. Identify the structures labeled on this (AP) KUB radiograph (Fig. 3.9).

A. _____

B. _____

C. _____

D. _____

E. _____

F. _____

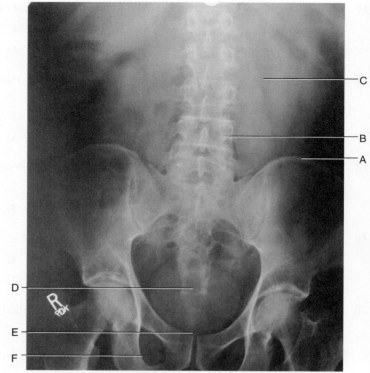

Fig. 3.9 Anteroposterior kidneys, ureters, and bladder radiograph.

27. Identify the organs or structures labeled on this CT image (Fig. 3.10) at the level of L2–L3.

A. _____

B. _____

C. _____

D. _____

E. _____

F. _____

G. _____

H. _____

I. _____

J. _____

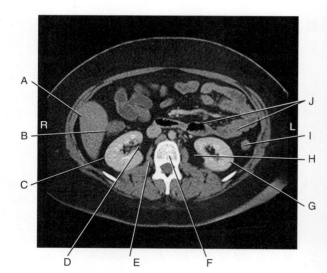

Fig. 3.10 CT image of the abdomen.

28. Which of the following sets of exposure factors would be ideal for abdominal radiography (for a sthenic adult)?

    A. 110 kVp, grid, 40-inch (100-cm) SID

    B. 78 kVp, grid, 40-inch (100-cm) SID

    C. 78 kVp, grid, 72-inch (180-cm) SID

    D. 65 kVp, grid, 40-inch (100-cm) SID

29. A radiograph of an AP projection of the abdomen shows that the right iliac wing is wider than the left. What type of positioning error was involved?

    A. Rotation toward the left

    B. Tilt to the left

    C. Rotation toward the right

    D. Tilt to the right

30. Most abdominal projections are taken:

    A. On expiration

    B. During shallow breathing

    C. On inspiration

    D. During deep breathing

31. A KUB radiograph on a large hypersthenic patient shows that the entire abdomen is not included on the 14- × 17-inch (35- × 43-cm) recommended field size. What can be done to correct this on the repeat radiograph?

    A. Use two image receptors placed in portrait orientation.

    B. Use two image receptors placed in landscape orientation.

    C. Expose during deep inspiration.

    D. Perform KUB with patient in the erect position.

32. What is the minimum amount of time a patient should be upright before taking a projection to demonstrate intra-abdominal free air?

    A. 20 minutes

    B. 30 minutes

    C. 2 minutes

    D. 5 minutes

33. If the PA chest projection is *not* performed for the acute abdomen series, centering for the erect abdomen projection *must* include the:

    A. Inferior liver margin

    B. Diaphragm

    C. Entire kidneys

    D. Bladder

34. Which specific decubitus position of the abdomen should be used in an acute abdomen series if the patient cannot stand?

    A. Left lateral decubitus

    B. Dorsal decubitus

    C. Right lateral decubitus

    D. Ventral decubitus

35. **Situation**: A patient with a possible ileus enters the emergency room. The physician orders an acute abdominal series. The patient can stand. Which specific position best demonstrates air/fluid levels in the abdomen?

    A. AP supine abdomen

    B. Right lateral decubitus

    C. Dorsal decubitus

    D. AP erect abdomen

36. **Situation**: A patient with a possible perforated bowel caused by trauma enters the ER. The patient is unable to stand. Which projection best demonstrates any possible free air within the abdomen?

    A. Dorsal decubitus

    B. Left lateral decubitus

    C. AP supine abdomen

    D. Right lateral decubitus

37. **Situation**: A patient with a clinical history of a possible umbilical hernia comes to the radiology department. The KUB is inconclusive. Which additional projection can be undertaken to help confirm the diagnosis?

    A. AP erect abdomen

    B. Left lateral decubitus

    C. Dorsal decubitus

    D. Ventral decubitus

38. **Situation**: A patient comes to the radiology department with a clinical history of pneumoperitoneum. The patient is able to stand. Which of the following projections best demonstrates this condition?

    A. AP supine abdomen

    B. AP erect abdomen

    C. Dorsal decubitus

    D. Left lateral decubitus

39. **Situation**: A patient comes to the radiology department with a clinical history of ascites. The patient is unable to stand or sit erect. Which of the following projections best demonstrates this condition?

    A. AP supine abdomen

    B. Left lateral decubitus

    C. Dorsal decubitus

    D. AP supine chest

40. **Situation**: A patient comes in the ER with possible gallstones. The patient is in severe pain. Which of the following imaging modalities or projections provides the quickest method for confirming the presence of gallstones?

    A. DMS

    B. Acute abdomen series

    C. MR

    D. KUB

41. **Situation**: A patient comes into the ER with the history of Crohn disease. An acute abdomen series is ordered on this patient. Which of the following is the reason for this order?

    A. Verify diagnosis

    B. Identify current status of intestinal inflammation

    C. Identify location of gallstones

    D. Verify current infection

42. Which of the following alternative imaging modalities is most effectively used to evaluate GI motility and reflux?

    A. CT

    B. MR

    C. DMS

    D. Nuclear medicine

43. Which of the following technical factors is essential when using digital imaging to ensure a high-quality image is produced?

    A. Low kVp

    B. 72-inch (180-cm) SID

    C. Large focal spot

    D. Close collimation

3 Abdomen

1. D. Peritoneum
2. C. Psoas muscles
3. A. Duodenum
4. C. Ileocecal (valve) sphincter
5. A. 6
   B. 8
   C. 5
   D. 1
   E. 9
   F. 4
   G. 3
   H. 2
   I. 7
6. D. Kidney
7. C. Ureter
8. D. Gallbladder
9. D. Mesentery
10. A. RLQ
    B. RUQ
    C. LUQ
    D. LUQ
    E. RUQ
    F. LLQ
    G. RLQ
    H. RUQ and LUQ
    I. RUQ
11. C. Left hypochondriac
12. 1. A
    2. A
    3. B

4. A
5. B
6. A
7. C
8. B
9. C
10. B
13. A. T9–T10
14. 1. C
    2. G
    3. A
    4. F
    5. E
    6. B
    7. D
15. B. Greater trochanter
16. A. Iliac crest
17. A. Short exposure time
18. D. Ascites
19. B. Paralytic ileus
20. A. Intussusception
21. D. Ulcerative colitis
22. C. Pneumoperitoneum
23. B. Diaphragm
24. B. Ascites
25. D. Ileus
26. A. Iliac crest
    B. L4 lumbar spine
    C. Psoas muscles
    D. Coccyx
    E. Pubic symphysis
    F. Obturator foramen

27. A. Liver
    B. Ascending colon
    C. Right kidney
    D. Right ureter
    E. Right psoas muscle
    F. L2–L3 vertebra
    G. Left kidney
    H. Left ureter
    I. Descending colon
    J. Small intestine (jejunum)
28. B. 78 kVp, grid, 40-inch (100-cm) SID
29. C. Rotation toward the right
30. A. On expiration
31. B. Use two image receptors placed in landscape orientation.
32. D. 5 minutes
33. B. Diaphragm
34. A. Left lateral decubitus
35. D. AP erect abdomen
36. B. Left lateral decubitus
37. C. Dorsal decubitus
38. B. AP erect abdomen
39. B. Left lateral decubitus
40. A. DMS
41. B. Identify current status of intestinal inflammation.
42. D. Nuclear medicine
43. D. Close collimation

A1

4 Upper Limb

CHAPTER OBJECTIVES

After you have successfully completed the activities in this chapter, you will be able to:

_____ 1. List the total number of bones in the hand and wrist.

_____ 2. Identify specific aspects of the phalanges, metacarpals, and carpal bones.

_____ 3. On drawings and radiographs, identify specific anatomic structures of the hand and wrist.

_____ 4. List and describe the location, size, and shape of each carpal bone of the wrist.

_____ 5. Match specific joints of the hand and wrist according to classification and movement type.

_____ 6. List four specific ligaments of the wrist.

_____ 7. On drawings and radiographs, identify specific fat pads and stripes of the upper limb.

_____ 8. Distinguish between ulnar and radial deviation wrist movements.

_____ 9. Identify specific parts of the forearm, elbow, and distal humerus.

_____ 10. On drawings and radiographs, identify specific anatomic structures of the forearm, elbow, and distal humerus.

_____ 11. List the technical factors commonly used for upper limb radiography.

_____ 12. Match specific clinical indications of the upper limb to their correct definition.

_____ 13. Match specific clinical indications of the upper limb to their correct radiographic appearance.

_____ 14. For select pathologic conditions of the upper limb, indicate whether manual exposure factors should be increased, decreased, or should remain the same.

_____ 15. Identify the correct central ray (CR) placement, part position, and radiographic criteria for specific positions of the fingers, thumb, hand, wrist, forearm, and elbow.

_____ 16. Identify which structures are best seen with each routine and special projection of the upper limb.

_____ 17. Based on clinical situations, describe the preferred positioning routine to assist the physician with the diagnosis of a specific condition or disease process.

_____ 18. Identify and apply the exposure conversion chart for various sizes of plaster and fiberglass casts.

_____ 19. List the three radiographic criteria for a true lateral elbow position.

_____ 20. Given various hypothetic situations, identify the correct modification of position, exposure factors, or both to improve the radiographic image.

_____ 21. Given various hypothetic situations, identify the correct position for a specific clinical indication or pathologic feature.

_____ 22. Given radiographs of specific upper limb positions, identify specific positioning and exposure factor errors.

POSITIONING AND RADIOGRAPHIC CRITIQUE

_____ 1. Using another student as a model, practice routine and special projections of the upper limb.

_____ 2. Using a hand and elbow radiographic phantom, produce satisfactory radiographs of the hand, thumb, wrist, and elbow (if equipment is available).

_____ 3. Critique and evaluate upper limb radiographs based on the five divisions of radiographic criteria: (1) anatomy demonstrated; (2) position; (3) recommended field size, collimation, and central ray; (4) exposure; and (5) anatomic side markers.

_____ 4. Distinguish between acceptable and unacceptable upper limb radiographs based on exposure factors, motion, collimation, positioning, or other errors.

LEARNING EXERCISES

Complete the following review exercises after reading the associated pages in the textbook as indicated by each exercise. Answers to each review exercise are given at the end of the review exercises.

PART I: RADIOGRAPHIC ANATOMY

REVIEW EXERCISE A: Anatomy of the Hand and Wrist (see textbook pp. 124–127)

1. Identify the number of bones for each of the following.

   A. Phalanges (fingers and thumb) _____   C. Carpals (wrist) _____

   B. Metacarpals (palm) _____   D. Total _____

2. The two portions of the thumb (first digit) are the:

   A. _____   B. _____

3. The three portions of each finger (second through fifth digits) are the:

   A. _____   B. _____

   C. _____

4. The three parts of each phalanx, starting distally, are the:

   A. _____   C. _____

   B. _____

5. List the three parts of each metacarpal, starting proximally:

   A. _____   C. _____

   B. _____

6. The name of the joint between the proximal and distal phalanges of the first digit is the _____.

7. The joints between the metacarpals and the phalanges are the _____.

8. Fill in the names and parts of the following bones and joints of the right hand as labeled in Fig. 4.1. Include abbreviations for joints if applicable.

A. _____

B. _____

C. _____

D. _____

E. _____

F. _____

G. _____

H. _____

I. _____

J. _____

K. _____

L. _____

M. _____

N. _____

O. _____

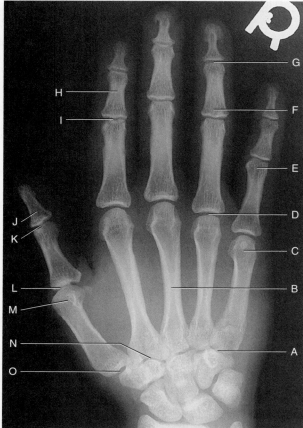

Fig. 4.1 Posteroanterior right hand.

9. Match each of the carpal bones labeled in Figs. 4.2 and 4.3 with its correct name.

_____ A.   1. Lunate

_____ B.   2. Hamate

_____ C.   3. Trapezium

_____ D.   4. Pisiform

_____ E.   5. Triquetrum

_____ F.   6. Trapezoid

_____ G.   7. Capitate

_____ H.   8. Scaphoid

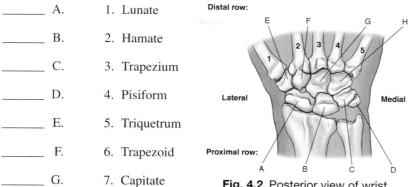

Fig. 4.2 Posterior view of wrist.

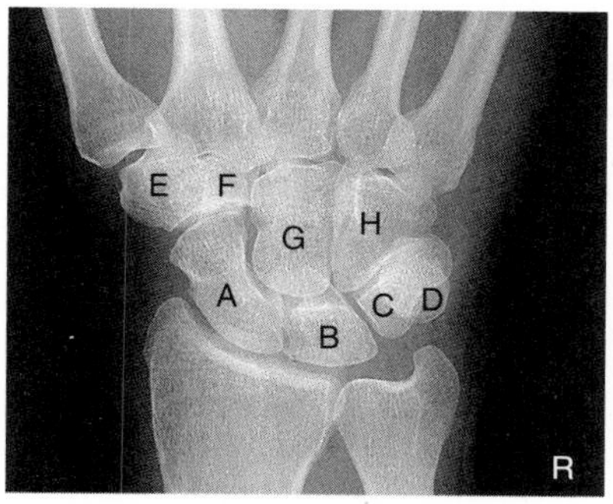

Fig. 4.3 Posteroanterior wrist.

10. Which is the largest of the carpal bones? _____

11. What is the name of the hooklike process extending anteriorly from the hamate? _____

12. Which is the most commonly fractured carpal bone? _____

13. Which is the smallest of the carpal bones?

_____

14. Match each of the structures labeled on Figs. 4.4 and 4.5 with the correct term.

_____ A.   1. Capitate

_____ B.   2. Scaphoid

_____ C.   3. Base of first metacarpal

_____ D.   4. Pisiform

_____ E.   5. Trapezoid

_____ F.   6. Hamulus (hamular process)

_____ G.   7. Triquetrum

_____ H.   8. Hamate

_____ I.   9. Trapezium

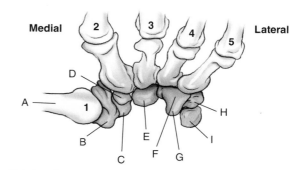

Fig. 4.4 Carpal canal, tangential inferosuperior projection.

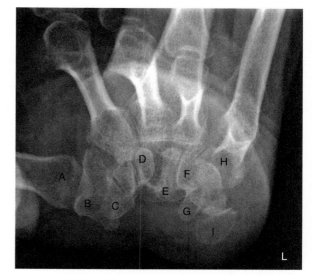

Fig. 4.5 Carpal canal, tangential inferosuperior projection.

15. Identify the carpals and other structures labeled in Fig. 4.6.

A. _____

B. _____

C. _____

D. _____

E. _____

F. _____

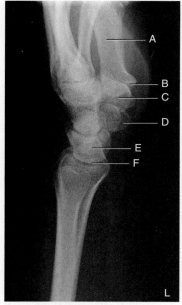

Fig. 4.6 Lateral wrist.

REVIEW EXERCISE B: Anatomy of the Forearm, Elbow, and Distal Humerus (see textbook pp. 128–133)

1. A. In the anatomic position, which of the bones of the forearm is located on the lateral (thumb) side?

   _____

   B. Which is on the medial side? _____

2. Indicate whether the following structures are part of the radius (R), ulna (U), or distal humerus (H) by listing the appropriate letter next to the structure.

   _____ A. Trochlear notch   _____ E. Coronoid tubercle

   _____ B. Radial notch   _____ F. Coronoid process

   _____ C. Olecranon fossa   _____ G. Olecranon process

   _____ D   Trochlea   _____ H. Coronoid fossa

3. Which joint permits the forearm to rotate during pronation? _____

4. A. The articular portion of the medial aspect of the distal humerus is called the _____.

   B. The similar structure found on the lateral aspect of the distal humerus is called the _____.

5. The deep depression located on the posterior aspect of the distal humerus is the _____.

6. The criteria for evaluating a true lateral position of the elbow are the appearance of three concentric arcs (Fig. 4.7). These arcs include:

   A. The first and smallest of the arcs: _____

   B. The intermediate double arc, consisting of the outer ridges of:

       (a) The smaller arc: _____

       (b) The larger arc: _____

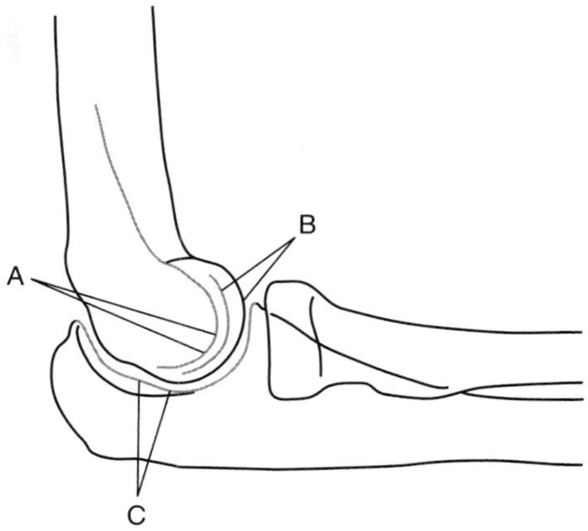

Fig. 4.7 The lateral elbow. Three concentric circles.

   C. The third arc, which is part of the ulna: _____

7. Match the following articulations with the correct joint movement types.

   _____ A. Interphalangeal   1. Ginglymus

   _____ B. Carpometacarpal of first digit   2. Ellipsoidal

   _____ C. Elbow joint (humeroulnar and humeroradial)   3. Pivot

   _____ D. Metacarpophalangeal of second to fifth digits   4. Plane

   _____ E. Radiocarpal   5. Saddle

   _____ F. Intercarpal

   _____ G. Elbow joint

   _____ H. Proximal radioulnar joint

8. Ellipsoidal joints are classified as freely movable, or _____, and allow movement in _____ directions.

9. True/False: In addition to the ulnar and radial collateral ligaments, the following five additional ligaments are also important in stabilizing the wrist joint.

   A. Dorsal radiocarpal   D. Scapholunate

   B. Palmar radiocarpal   E. Lunotriquetral

   C. Triangular fibrocartilage complex (TFCC)

10. Which ligament of the wrist extends from the styloid process of the radius to the lateral aspect of the scaphoid and trapezium bones? _____

11. What is the name of the two special turning or bending positions of the hand and wrist that demonstrate medial and lateral aspects of the carpal region?

A. _____   B. _____

12. Of the two positions listed in the previous question, which is most commonly performed to detect a fracture of the scaphoid bone? _____

13. How does the forearm appear radiographically if pronated for a posteroanterior (PA) projection?

_____

14. The two important fat stripes or bands around the wrist joint are the:

A. _____   B. _____

15. The fat pads around the elbow joint are valuable diagnostic indicators if the following three technical/positioning requirements are met with the lateral position.

A. _____

B. _____

C. _____

16. True/False: If the posterior fat pad of the elbow is not visible radiographically, it suggests that a nonobvious radial head or neck fracture is present.

17. True/False: Excessive kVp may obscure the visibility of a fat pad.

18. True/False: Trauma or infection makes the anterior fat pad more difficult to see on a lateral elbow radiograph.

19. Which routine projections best demonstrate the scaphoid fat stripe?

_____

20. Which routine projection best demonstrates the pronator fat stripe?

_____

21. Identify the parts labeled in Figs. 4.8 and 4.9.

A. _____

B. _____

C. _____

D. _____

E. _____

F. _____

G. _____

H. _____

I. _____

J. _____

K. _____

L. _____

M. _____

N. * _____

O. * _____

P. * _____

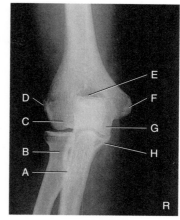

Fig. 4.8 Anteroposterior elbow.

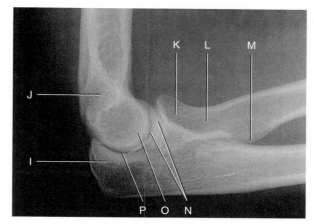

Fig. 4.9 Lateral elbow.

* Hint: These are concentric arcs as evidence of a true lateral position.

22. Identify the parts labeled in Figs. 4.10 and 4.11.

A. _____

B. _____

C. _____

D. _____

E. _____

F. _____

G. _____

H. _____

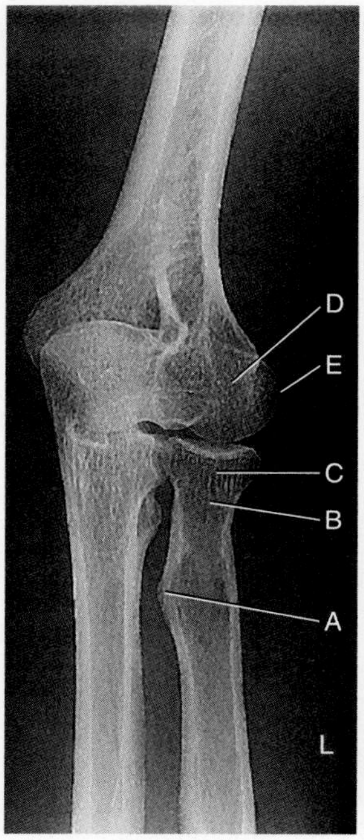

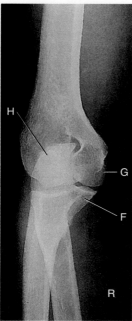

Fig. 4.10 Lateral (external) rotation of the elbow.

Fig. 4.11 Medial (internal) rotation of the elbow.

PART II: RADIOGRAPHIC POSITIONING

REVIEW EXERCISE C: Positioning of the Fingers, Thumb, Hand, and Wrist (see textbook pp. 134–160)

1. Identify the following technical factors most commonly used for upper limb radiography.

   A. kVp range: _____

   B. Long or short exposure time: _____

   C. Large or small focal spot: _____

   D. Most common minimum source–image receptor distance (SID): _____

   E. Grids (or virtual grid technology) are recommended if the body part measures greater than _____ inches (__cm).

   F. Small-to-medium dry plaster casts: Increase _____ kVp.

   G. Large plaster casts: Increase _____ kVp.

   H. Fiberglass casts: Increase _____ kVp.

   I. Correctly exposed radiographs: Visualize _____ margins and

      _____ markings of all bones.

2. The general rule for collimation for upper limb radiography states: _____.

3. Circle all pertinent factors that help reduce image distortion during upper limb radiography.

A. kVp

B. 40–44 inches (100–110 cm) SID

C. Milliamperage seconds (mAs)

D. Minimal object–image receptor distance (OID)

E. Correct central ray placement and angulation

F. Use of small focal spot

4. True/False: Trauma patients can be radiographed directly on the stretcher.

5. True/False: Guardians of young pediatric patients who are undergoing upper limb studies can be asked to hold their child during the radiographic study.

6. _____ is a radiographic procedure that uses contrast media injected into the joint capsule to visualize soft tissue pathology of the wrist, elbow, and shoulder joints.

7. What is the positioning routine for the second through fifth digits of the hand?

_____

_____

8. How much of the metacarpals should be included for PA projection of the digits?

_____

_____

9. List the two radiographic criteria used to determine whether rotation is present on the PA projection of the digits.

A. _____

B. _____

10. Identify which positioning modification(s) should be used for a study of the second digit to reduce distortion for each of the following:

A. PA oblique projection: _____

B. Lateral position: _____

11. Where is the central ray centered for a PA oblique projection of the second digit?

_____

12. Why is it important to keep the affected digit parallel to the image receptor (IR) for the PA oblique and lateral projections?

    A. To prevent distortion of the phalanx   C. To demonstrate small, nondisplaced fractures near the joint

    B. To prevent distortion of the joints   D. All of the above

13. Why is the anteroposterior (AP) projection of the thumb recommended instead of the PA?

    _____

14. Which projection of the thumb is achieved naturally by placing the palmar surface of the hand in contact with the IR?

    _____

15. What recommended field size should be used for a thumb projection? _____

16. A sesamoid bone is frequently found adjacent to the _____ joint of the thumb.

17. True/False: The entire metacarpal and trapezium must be demonstrated on all projections of the thumb.

18. Where is the central ray centered for an AP projection of the thumb?

    A. First interphalangeal (IP) joint   C. First metacarpophalangeal (MCP) joint

    B. Midaspect of proximal phalanx   D. First proximal interphalangeal (PIP) joint

19. A Bennett fracture involves:

    A. Base of first metacarpal   C. Scaphoid bone

    B. Trapezium bone   D. Fracture extending through first IP joint

20. A. Which special positioning method can be performed to better delineate a possible Bennett fracture?

    _____

    B. What degree of central ray angulation is required for this projection? _____

21. Where is the central ray centered for a PA projection of the hand?

    A. Third MCP joint   C. Second MCP joint

    B. Midaspect of third metacarpal   D. Third PIP joint

22. A minimum of _____ inch(es) (_____cm) of the forearm should be included radiographically for a PA projection of the hand.

23. True/False: Slight superimposition of the distal third, fourth, and fifth metacarpals may occur with a well-positioned PA oblique projection of the hand.

24. Which preferred lateral position of the hand best demonstrates the phalanges without excessive superimposition?

    _____

25. Which lateral projection of the hand best demonstrates a possible foreign body in the palm of the hand?

    _____

26. What type of CR angle is required for the AP axial projection (Brewerton method)?

    _____

27. The AP axial projection (Brewerton method) is commonly used to evaluate for early signs of:

A. Osteoporosis

C. Osteopetrosis

B. Osteomyelitis

D. Rheumatoid arthritis

28. Which projection best demonstrates possible scapholunate ligament tears? _____

29. How much rotation is required for an oblique projection of the wrist?

_____

30. Which alternative projection to the routine PA wrist best demonstrates the intercarpal joint spaces and wrist joint?

_____

31. Which positioning error is involved if a majority of the carpal bones are superimposed in a PA oblique wrist projection?

_____

32. Which of the following fractures is not demonstrated in a wrist routine?

A. Barton

C. Smith

B. Pott's

D. Colles

33. During the PA axial scaphoid projection with central ray angle and ulnar flexion, the central ray must be angled

_____ degrees _____ (distally or proximally).

34. How much are the hand and wrist elevated from the IR for the modified Stecher method?

A. None

C. 20 degrees

B. 10 degrees

D. 15 degrees

35. How much central ray angulation to the long axis of the hand is required for the carpal canal (tunnel) projection?

_____

36. Which special projection of the wrist best demonstrates the interspaces on the ulnar side of the wrist between the

lunate, triquetrum, pisiform, and hamate bones? _____

37. Which special projection of the wrist helps rule out abnormal calcifications in the carpal sulcus?

_____

38. How much central ray angulation from the long axis of the forearm is required for the carpal bridge (tangential)

projection?_____

39. The hand and wrist form a _____ degree angle to the forearm with the carpal bridge (tangential) projection.

REVIEW EXERCISE D: Clinical Indications of the Fingers, Thumb, Hand, and Wrist (see textbook pp. 136-137)

1. List the correct pathology term for each of the following definitions.

   A. _____ Fracture and dislocation of the posterior articular surface of the distal radius

   B. _____ Most common type of primary malignant (cancerous) tumor occurring in bone

   C. _____ Reduction in the quantity of bone or atrophy of skeletal tissue

   D. _____ Sprain or tear of the ulnar collateral ligament

   E. _____ An abnormality of the cartilage affecting long bones

   F. _____ Transverse fracture extending through the distal aspect of the metacarpal neck, most often the fifth metacarpal

   G. _____ Hereditary condition marked by abnormally dense bone

   H. _____ Transverse fracture of the distal radius with posterior displacement of the distal fragment

2. Match the clinical indication or disease to its radiographic appearance.

   _____ A. Narrowing of joint space with periosteal growths on the joint margins   1. Osteomyelitis

   _____ B. Fluid-filled joint space with possible calcification   2. Bursitis

   _____ C. Possible calcification in the carpal sulcus   3. Carpal tunnel syndrome

   _____ D. Soft tissue swelling and loss of fat-pad detail visibility   4. Osteoarthritis

   _____ E. Mixed areas of sclerotic and cortical thickening along with radiolucent lesions   5. Osteopetrosis

3. For the following pathologic conditions, indicate whether bone density will increase (+) or decrease (−).

   _____ Osteoporosis   _____ Osteopetrosis

REVIEW EXERCISE E: Positioning of the Forearm, Elbow, and Humerus (see textbook pp. 161–171)

1. Which routine projections are required for a study of the forearm? _____

2. True/False: For a forearm study, the technologist needs to include only the joint closest to the site of the injury.

3. To position the patient properly for an AP projection of the elbow, the epicondyles must be _____ to the IR.

4. If the patient cannot fully extend the elbow for the AP projection, what alternative projection(s) should be performed?

   _____

5. Which routine projection of the elbow best demonstrates the radial head, neck, and tuberosity with slight (if any) superimposition of the ulna? _____

6. To position the patient properly for an AP forearm, the hand should be _____.

7. Which projection of the elbow best demonstrates the coronoid process in profile?

    _____

8. The best position to evaluate the posterior fat pads of the elbow joint is:

    _____.

9. Which special projection(s) of the elbow should be performed instead of the routine AP if the patient's elbow is tightly flexed and cannot extend at all?

    _____

10. How much is the upper limb rotated for a lateral (rotation) oblique projection of the elbow?

    _____

11. How much and in which direction should the central ray be angled for the trauma axial lateral projection (Coyle method) involving the radial head?

    _____

12. How much and in which direction should the central ray be angled for the trauma axial lateral projection (Coyle method) involving the coronoid process?

    _____

13. What is the amount of elbow flexion required for the trauma lateral projection (Coyle method) to demonstrate the coronoid process?

    _____

14. What is the only difference among the four radial head lateral projections of the elbow?

    _____

REVIEW EXERCISE F: Problem Solving for Technical and Positioning Errors

The following radiographic problems involve technical and positioning errors that may lead to substandard images. As you analyze these problems, review your textbook to find solutions to these questions.

Other questions involve situations pertaining to various patient conditions and clinical indications. If you need more information about a particular pathologic condition, review your textbook or a medical dictionary to learn more about it.

1. A three-projection study of the hand was taken using the following exposure factors: 64 kVp, 1000 mA, 1/100 second, large focal spot, and 36-inch (90-cm) SID. Which of these factors should be changed on future hand studies to produce more optimal images?

    _____

2. A radiograph of a PA projection of the second digit shows that the phalanges are not symmetric on both sides of the bony shafts. Which specific positioning error is involved?

    _____

3. A radiograph of a PA oblique projection of the hand shows that the fourth and fifth metacarpals are superimposed. Which specific positioning error is involved?

_____

4. In a radiographic study of the forearm, the proximal radius crossed over the ulna in the frontal projection. Which specific positioning error led to this radiographic outcome?

_____

5. A PA axial scaphoid projection of the wrist using a 15-degree distal central ray angle and ulnar flexion was performed. The resultant radiograph shows that the scaphoid bone is foreshortened. How must this projection be modified to produce a more diagnostic image of the scaphoid?

_____

6. A radiograph of an AP elbow projection shows considerable superimposition between the proximal radius and ulna. Which specific positioning error is involved?

_____

7. A routine radiograph of an AP oblique elbow with lateral rotation shows that the radial tuberosity is superimposed on the ulna. In what way must this position be modified during the repeat exposure?

_____

8. A radiograph of a lateral projection of the elbow shows that the humeral epicondyles are not superimposed and the trochlear notch is not clearly demonstrated. Which specific type of positioning error is involved?

_____

9. **Situation:** A patient with a possible fracture of the radial head enters the emergency room. When the technologist attempts to place the arm in the AP oblique with lateral rotation, but the patient is unable to extend or rotate the elbow laterally. Which other positions can be used to demonstrate the radial head and neck without superimposition on the proximal ulna?

_____

10. **Situation:** A patient with a metallic foreign body in the palm of the hand enters the emergency room. Which specific positions should be used to locate the foreign body?

_____

11. **Situation:** A patient with a trauma injury enters the ER with an evident Colles fracture. Which positioning routine should be used to determine the extent of the injury?

_____

12. **Situation:** A patient with a dislocated elbow enters the ER. The patient has the elbow tightly flexed and is careful not to move it. Which specific positioning routine can be used to determine the extent of the injury?

_____

13. **Situation:** A patient with a possible fracture of the trapezium enters the ER. The routine projections do not clearly demonstrate a possible fracture. Which other special projection can be taken?

_____

14. **Situation:** A patient with a history of carpal tunnel syndrome comes to the radiology department. The orthopedic physician suspects that bony changes in the carpal sulcus may be causing compression of the median nerve. Which special projection best demonstrates this region of the wrist?

_____

15. **Situation:** A patient comes to the radiology department for a hand series to evaluate early evidence of rheumatoid arthritis. Which special position can be used in addition to the routine hand projections to evaluate this patient?

_____

16. **Situation:** A patient is referred to radiology with a possible injury to the ulnar collateral ligament. The patient complains of pain near the first MCP joint. Initial radiographs of the hand do not indicate any fracture or dislocation. Which special projection can be performed to rule out an injury to the ulnar collateral ligament?

_____

17. **Situation:** A patient enters the ER with a possible foreign body in the dorsal aspect of the wrist. Initial wrist radiographs are inconclusive in demonstrating the location of the foreign body. What additional projection can be performed to demonstrate this region of the wrist?

_____

18. **Situation:** A patient has a routine elbow series performed. The AP projection indicates a possible deformity or fracture of the coronoid process. However, the patient is unable to pronate the upper limb for the AP oblique-medial rotation projection because of an arthritic condition. What other projection could be performed to demonstrate the coronoid process?

_____

REVIEW EXERCISE G: Critique Radiographs of the Upper Limb

The following questions relate to the radiographs found in this exercise. Evaluate these radiographs for the radiographic criteria categories (1 through 5) that follow. Describe the corrections needed to improve the overall image. The major, or "repeatable," errors are specific errors that indicate the need for a repeat exposure, regardless of the nature of the other errors.

A. PA hand (Fig. 4.12)

Description of possible error:

1. Anatomy demonstrated:

_____

2. Part positioning:

_____

3. Collimation field size and central ray:

_____

4. Exposure:

_____

5. Anatomic side markers:

_____

Repeatable error(s): _____

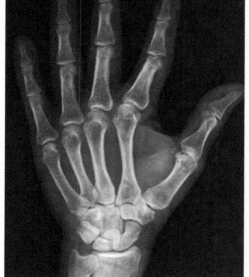

Fig. 4.12 Posteroanterior hand.

B. Lateral wrist (Fig. 4.13)

Description of possible error:

   1. Anatomy demonstrated:

   _____

   2. Part positioning:

   _____

   3. Collimation field size and central ray:

   _____

   4. Exposure:

   _____

   5. Anatomic side markers:

   _____

Repeatable error(s): _____

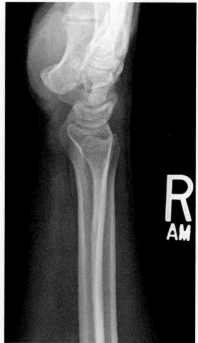

Fig. 4.13 Lateral wrist.

C. AP elbow (Fig. 4.14)

Description of possible error:

   1. Anatomy demonstrated:

   _____

   2. Part positioning:

   _____

   3. Collimation field size and central ray:

   _____

   4. Exposure:

   _____

   5. Anatomic side markers:

   _____

Repeatable error(s): _____

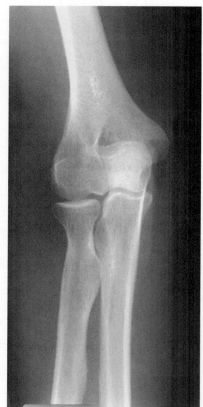

Fig. 4.14 Anteroposterior elbow.

D. PA wrist with ulnar deviation (Fig. 4.15)

Which special wrist projection is demonstrated in this radiograph?

Description of possible error:

    1. Anatomy demonstrated:

    _____

    2. Part positioning:

    _____

    3. Collimation field size and central ray:

    _____

    4. Exposure:

    _____

    5. Anatomic side markers:

    _____

Repeatable error(s): _____

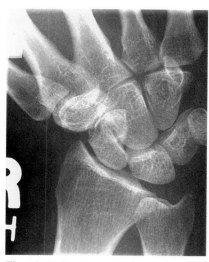

Fig. 4.15 Posteroanterior wrist with ulnar deviation.

E. Pediatric PA forearm (Fig. 4.16)

Description of possible error:

    1. Anatomy demonstrated:

    _____

    2. Part positioning:

    _____

    3. Collimation field size and central ray:

    _____

    4. Exposure:

    _____

    5. Anatomic side markers:

    _____

Repeatable error(s): _____

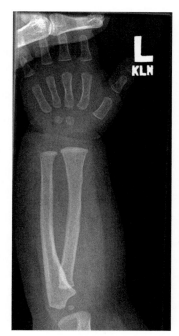

Fig. **4.16** Pediatric posteroanterior forearm.

F. Lateral elbow (Fig. 4.17)

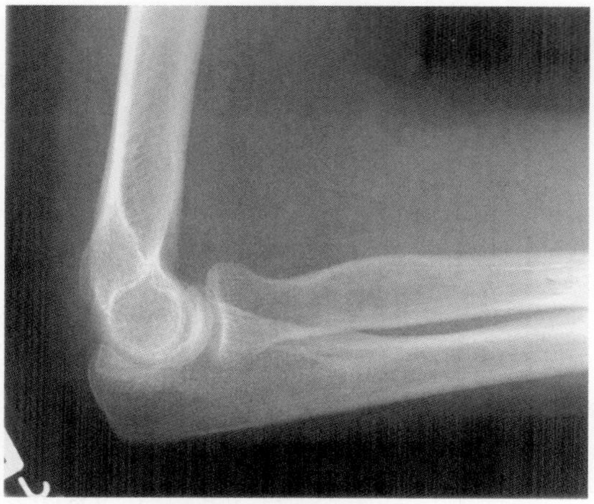

Description of possible error:

1. Anatomy demonstrated:

   _____

2. Part positioning:

   _____

3. Collimation field size and central ray:

   _____

4. Exposure:

   _____

5. Anatomic side markers:

   _____

Fig. 4.17 Lateral elbow.

Repeatable error(s): _____

PART III: LABORATORY EXERCISES

You must gain experience in upper limb positioning before performing the following exams on actual patients. You can obtain experience in positioning and radiographic evaluation of these projections by performing exercises using radiographic phantoms and by practicing on other students (although you will not be taking actual exposures).

The following suggested activities assume that your teaching institution has an energized lab and radiographic phantoms. If not, perform Laboratory Exercises B and C, the radiographic evaluation and the physical positioning exercises. (Check off each step and projection as you complete them.)

Laboratory Exercise A: Energized Laboratory

1. Using the hand radiographic phantom, produce radiographs of the following positioning routines:

   _____Hand (PA, oblique, lateral)   _____Thumb (AP, oblique, lateral)

   _____Wrist (PA, oblique, lateral)

2. Using the elbow radiographic phantom, produce radiographs of the following positioning routines:

   _____AP   _____AP oblique, medial rotation

   _____Lateral elbow   _____AP oblique, lateral rotation

Laboratory Exercise B: Radiographic Evaluation

1. Evaluate and critique the radiographs produced previously, additional radiographs provided by your instructor, or both. Evaluate each radiograph for the following points:

_____ Evaluate the completeness of the study. (Are all of the pertinent anatomic structures included on the radiograph?)

_____ Evaluate for positioning or centering errors (e.g., rotation, off centering).

_____ Evaluate for correct exposure factors and possible motion. (Are the image receptor exposure and contrast of the images acceptable?)

_____ Determine whether anatomic side markers and an acceptable degree of collimation are seen on the images.

Laboratory Exercise C: Physical Positioning

1. On another person, simulate performing all of the following routines and special projections of the upper limb. Include the six steps listed here and described in the textbook. (Check off each step when completed satisfactorily.)

Step 1. Appropriate collimation field size with correct side markers

Step 2. Correct central ray placement and centering of part to central ray and/or IR

Step 3. Accurate collimation

Step 4. Area shielding of patient where required

Step 5. Use of proper immobilizing devices when needed

Step 6. Approximate correct exposure factors, breathing instructions where applicable, and initiating exposure

Projections	Step 1	Step 2	Step 3	Step 4	Step 5	Step 6
• Second to fifth digit routines (PA, oblique, lateral)	_____	_____	_____	_____	_____	_____
• Thumb routine (AP, oblique, lateral)	_____	_____	_____	_____	_____	_____
• Hand (PA, oblique, lateral)	_____	_____	_____	_____	_____	_____
• Wrist routine (PA, oblique, lateral)	_____	_____	_____	_____	_____	_____
• Scaphoid, carpal canal, carpal bridge, and bilateral PA stress projections	_____	_____	_____	_____	_____	_____
• Elbow routine (AP, oblique, lateral)	_____	_____	_____	_____	_____	_____
• AP–partial flexion	_____	_____	_____	_____	_____	_____
• AP–acute flexion	_____	_____	_____	_____	_____	_____
• Trauma axial lateral (Coyle)	_____	_____	_____	_____	_____	_____
• Radial head projections	_____	_____	_____	_____	_____	_____
• Forearm routine (AP, lateral)	_____	_____	_____	_____	_____	_____

This self-test should be taken only after completing all of the readings, review exercises, and laboratory activities for a particular section. The purpose of this test is not only to provide a good learning exercise but also to serve as a strong indicator of what your final unit evaluation exam will cover. It is strongly suggested that if you do not achieve at least a 90%–95% grade on each self-test, you should review those areas in which you missed questions before going to your instructor for the final unit evaluation exam.

1. A. How many bones make up the phalanges of the hand?

    A. 14

    B. 8

    C. 5

    D. 16

  B. How many bones make up the carpal region?

    A. 14

    B. 8

    C. 5

    D. 7

  C. What is the total number of bones that make up the hand and wrist?

    A. 21

    B. 27

    C. 26

    D. 32

2. Match the following joint locations with the correct term.

  _____ A. Between the two phalanges of the first digit (thumb)   1. Radiocarpal

  _____ B. Between the first metacarpal and the proximal phalanx of the thumb   2. Fourth DIP

  _____ C. Between the middle and distal phalanges of the fourth digit   3. Fourth PIP

  _____ D. Between the carpals and the first metacarpal   4. First MCP

  _____ E. Between the forearm and the carpals   5. First CMC

  _____ F. Between the distal radius and ulna   6. Distal radioulnar

        7. IP

3. Match each of the structures labeled in Fig. 4.18 with its correct term.

_____ A.   1. Distal phalanx of fourth digit

_____ B.   2. Head of fifth metacarpal

_____ C.   3. Base of fourth metacarpal

_____ D.   4. Scaphoid

_____ E.   5. Base of first metacarpal

_____ F.   6. Pisiform

_____ G.   7. Trapezoid

_____ H.   8. Body of proximal phalanx of fifth digit

_____ I.   9. Fifth carpometacarpal joint

_____ J.   10. Triquetrum

_____ K.   11. Radius

_____ L.   12. Proximal phalanx of first digit

_____ M.   13. Radiocarpal joint

_____ N.   14. Hamate

_____ O.   15. Capitate

_____ P.   16. Distal interphalangeal joint of fifth digit

_____ Q.   17. Trapezium

_____ R.   18. First metacarpophalangeal joint

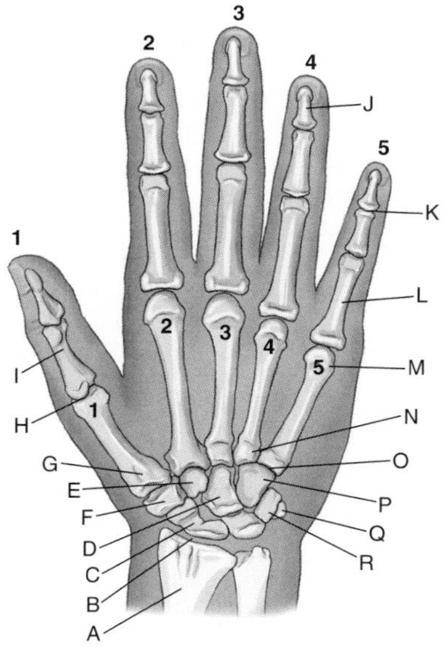

Fig. 4.18 Osteology of the hand and wrist.

4. Which carpal contains a "hooklike" process?

   A. Scaphoid   C. Hamate
   B. Trapezium   D. Pisiform

5. Which carpal articulates with the base of thumb?

   A. Scaphoid   C. Trapezoid
   B. Lunate   D. Trapezium

6. Which carpal is most commonly fractured?

   A. Scaphoid   C. Trapezium
   B. Capitate   D. Triquetrum

7. Which two carpal bones are located most anteriorly as seen on a lateral wrist radiograph? (Hint: They are on the radial side of the wrist.)

   A. Hamate and pisiform   C. Capitate and lunate
   B. Trapezium and trapezoid   D. Scaphoid and trapezium

8. Match each of the structures of the wrist labeled in Figs. 4.19, 4.20, and 4.21 to its correct term.

_____ A.   1. Pisiform

_____ B.   2. Trapezoid

_____ C.   3. Scaphoid

_____ D.   4. Triquetrum

_____ E.   5. Base of first metacarpal

_____ F.   6. Radius

_____ G.   7. Lunate

_____ H.   8. Trapezium

_____ I.   9. Hamate

_____ J.   10. Ulna

_____ K.   11. Capitate

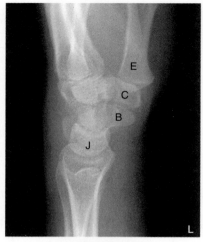

Fig. 4.19 Lateral wrist.

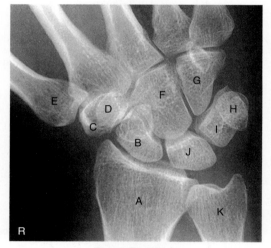

Fig. 4.20 Wrist.

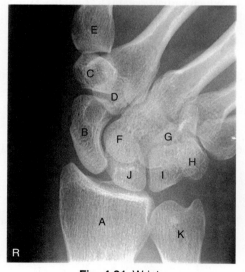

Fig. 4.21 Wrist.

9. Which wrist projection does Fig. 4.20 represent?

   A. PA wrist

   B. PA–ulnar deviation

   C. PA–radial deviation

   D. Carpal canal

10. Which of the following carpals is *not* seen clearly in the projection in Fig. 4.20?

    A. Pisiform

    B. Lunate

    C. Scaphoid

    D. Triquetrum

11. Which projection does Fig. 4.21 represent?

    A. PA–ulnar deviation

    B. Carpal canal

    C. PA–radial deviation

    D. Modified Stecher method

12. Which of the following carpal bones is best demonstrated in the projection in Fig. 4.21?

    A. Trapezium

    B. Scaphoid

    C. Trapezoid

    D. Hamate

13. Which bone of the upper limb contains the coronoid process?

    A. Humerus

    B. First metacarpal

    C. Radius

    D. Ulna

14. Where are the coronoid and radial fossae located?

    A. Anterior aspect of distal humerus

    B. Posterior aspect of distal humerus

    C. Proximal radius and ulna

    D. Distal end of radius

15. Which two bony landmarks are palpated to assist with positioning of the upper limb?

    A. Coronoid and olecranon processes

    B. Pisiform and hamate

    C. Lateral and medial epicondyles

    D. Radial and ulnar styloid processes

16. Where is the coronoid tubercle located?

    A. Medial aspect of coronoid process

    B. Anterior aspect of distal humerus

    C. Lateral aspect of proximal radius

    D. Posterior aspect of distal humerus

17. In an erect anatomic position, which of the following structures is considered most inferior or distal?

    A. Head of ulna

    B. Olecranon process

    C. Radial tuberosity

    D. Head of radius

18. Match the following articulations to the correct joint movement type. (Each joint movement type may be used more than once.)

    _____ A. Intercarpal joints

    _____ B. Radiocarpal joint

    _____ C. Elbow joint

    _____ D. First carpometacarpal joint

    _____ E. Third carpometacarpal joint

    1. Saddle

    2. Ginglymus

    3. Ellipsoidal

    4. Plane

19. The following four radiographs represent the most common routine projections for the elbow. Match each of these projections to the correct figure number.

　　_____ A. Fig. 4.22　　1. AP projection

　　_____ B. Fig. 4.23　　2. Lateral position

　　_____ C. Fig. 4.24　　3. AP oblique–lateral rotation

　　_____ D. Fig. 4.25　　4. AP oblique–medial rotation

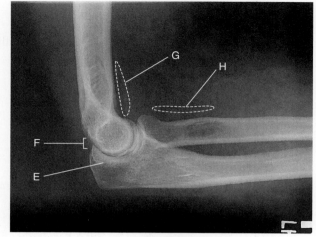

Fig. 4.22

Identify the soft tissue and bony structures labeled on Figs. 4.22, 4.23, 4.24, and 4.25. (Terms may be used more than once.)

_____E.　　　1. Trochlea

_____F.　　　2. Olecranon process

_____G.　　　3. Coronoid process

_____H.　　　4. Medial epicondyle

_____I.　　　5. Supinator fat pad

_____J.　　　6. Capitulum

_____K.　　　7. Region of anterior fat pad

_____L.　　　8. Radial head and neck

_____M.　　　9. Region of posterior fat pad

_____N.　　　10. Coronoid tubercle

_____O.

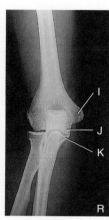

Fig. 4.23

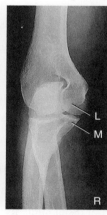

Fig. 4.24

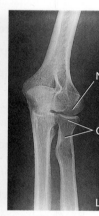

Fig. 4.25

20. Identify each of the structures labeled on Figs. 4.26 and 4.27 with its correct term.

_____ A.   1. Coronoid fossa

_____ B.   2. Medial epicondyle

_____ C.   3. Head of radius

_____ D.   4. Trochlea

_____ E.*   5. Radial tuberosity

_____ F.*   6. Coronoid process

_____ G.   7. Lateral epicondyle

_____ H.   8. Capitulum

_____ I.   9. Trochlear sulcus

_____ J.   10. Coronoid tubercle

_____ K.   11. Radial fossa

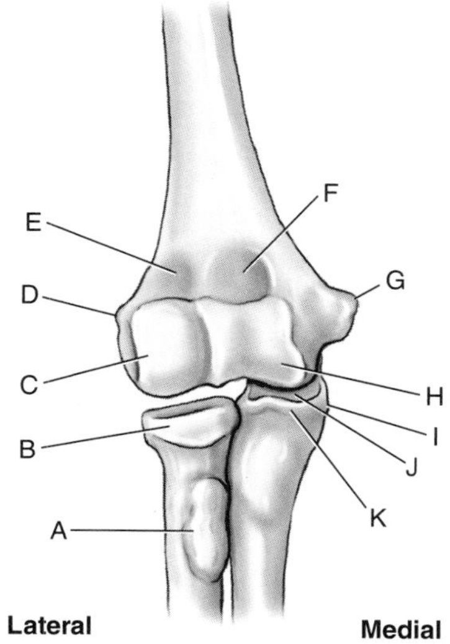

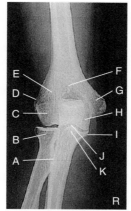

Fig. 4.26 Anteroposterior projection of the elbow.

Fig. 4.27 Elbow. Anteroposterior extended.

21. True/False: To visualize fat pads surrounding the elbow, exposure factors must be adjusted to see both bony and soft tissue structures.

22. True/False: Anterior and posterior fat pads of the elbow are best seen on correctly positioned and correctly exposed AP elbow projections.

23. Why should a forearm never be taken as a PA projection?

    A. Too painful for the patient

    B. Causes the proximal radius to cross over the ulna

    C. Causes the distal radius to cross over the ulna

    D. Increases the OID of the distal radius

*_____Not visible on radiograph.

105

24. In what position should the hand be for an AP elbow projection?

    A. Supinated (palm up)
    B. Pronated (palm down)
    C. Rotated 20 degrees from supinated position
    D. True lateral position

25. In what position should the hand be for an AP medial rotation oblique elbow position?

    A. Supinated
    B. Pronated
    C. Rotated 20 degrees from supinated position
    D. True lateral position

26. Match the projection of the elbow that best demonstrates each of the following structures:

    _____ A. Coronoid process in profile
    _____ B. Radial head and tuberosity without superimposition
    _____ C. Olecranon process in profile
    _____ D. Coronoid tubercle
    _____ E. Trochlear notch in profile
    _____ F. Capitulum and lateral epicondyle in profile
    _____ G. Olecranon process seated in olecranon fossa

    1. Lateral elbow
    2. AP elbow
    3. AP, oblique w/ medial rotation
    4. AP oblique w/ lateral rotation

27. True/False: Placing multiple images on the same digital IP is recommended as long as close collimation is applied for each projection.

28. The long axis of the anatomic part being imaged should be placed:

    A. Perpendicular to the long axis of the IR
    B. Parallel to the long axis of the IR
    C. 30-degree angle to the long axis of the IR
    D. Any way that will accommodate multiple images being placed on a single IR

29. *Arthrography* is a radiographic study of:

    A. Fat pads and stripes
    B. Epiphyses of long bones
    C. Medullary aspect of long bones
    D. Soft-tissue structures within certain synovial joints

30. Match each of the following pathologic terms to its correct definition.

_____ 1. Accumulated fluid within the joint cavity   A. Skier's thumb

_____ 2. A reduction in the quantity of bone or atrophy of skeletal tissue   B. Bursitis

_____ 3. Local or generalized infection of bone or bone marrow   C. Carpal tunnel syndrome

_____ 4. Reverse of a Colles fracture   D. Bennett fracture

_____ 5. Inflammation of the fluid-filled sacs enclosing the joints   E. Smith fracture

_____ 6. Fracture of the base of the first metacarpal   F. Joint effusion

_____ 7. Sprain or tear of the ulnar collateral ligament   G. Osteomyelitis

_____ 8. Painful disorder of hand and wrist from compression of the median resulting nerve   H. Osteoporosis

31. Where is the CR centered for a Bilateral PA Stress Projection (Clenched PA) of the wrist?

A. Midpoint between both 2nd MP joints

B. Midpoint between both 1st IP joints

C. Midpoint between both carpal regions

D. 1" distal to the radial styloid process of the left wrist

32. Where is the central ray centered for a PA projection of the second digit?

A. Affected PIP joint

B. Affected middle phalanx

C. Affected MCP joint

D. Affected CMC joint

33. Why is it important to keep the long axis of the digit parallel to the IR?

A. To reduce distortion of the phalanges

B. To visualize joints properly

C. To demonstrate small fractures

D. All of the above

34. Where is the central ray placed for a PA projection of the hand?

A. Second MCP joint

B. Third MCP joint

C. Middle phalanx of third digit

D. Third PIP joint

35. What is the major disadvantage of performing a PA projection of the thumb rather than an AP?

A. Increased OID

B. Increase in patient dose

C. Painful for patient

D. Awkward position for patient

36. What type of fracture is best demonstrated with a modified Robert method?

A. Barton fracture

B. Colles fracture

C. Bennett fracture

D. Smith fracture

37. True/False: The Brewerton method requires a CR angle of 15-degree proximal

38. True/False: The hand(s) is(are) placed in a true PA position when using the Brewerton method.

39. Choose the *best* set of exposure factors for upper limb radiography.

    A. 75 kVp, 200 mA, 1/20 second, small focal spot, and 40-inch (100-cm) SID

    B. 75 kVp, 600 mA, 1/60 second, large focal spot, and 40-inch (100-cm) SID

    C. 64 kVp, 100 mA, 1/10 second, small focal spot, and 40-inch (100-cm) SID

    D. 64 kVp, 200 mA, 1/20 second, small focal spot, and 40-inch (100-cm) SID

40. A radiograph of a PA oblique of the hand shows that the third, fourth, and fifth metacarpals are superimposed. What must be done to correct this positioning problem on the repeat exposure?

    A. Increase obliquity of the hand   C. Decrease obliquity of the hand

    B. Spread fingers out further   D. Form a tight fist with the fingers

41. A radiograph of an AP elbow projection demonstrates total separation between the proximal radius and ulna. What must be done to correct this positioning error on the repeat exposure?

    A. Rotate upper limb medially   C. Angle central ray 5–10-degree caudad

    B. Rotate upper limb laterally   D. Fully extend elbow

42. A radiograph of the carpal canal (inferosuperior) projection shows that the pisiform and hamulus are superimposed. What can be done to correct this problem on the repeat exposure?

    A. Flex wrist slightly   C. Rotate wrist laterally 5–10 degrees

    B. Extend wrist slightly   D. Rotate wrist medially 5–10 degrees

43. A radiograph of an AP oblique-medial rotation shows that the coronoid process is not in profile and the radial head is not superimposed over the ulna. What specific positioning error was involved?

    A. Insufficient medial rotation   C. Excessive extension of elbow

    B. Excessive medial rotation   D. Excessive flexion of elbow

44. A radiograph of a lateral projection of the elbow shows that the epicondyles are not superimposed and the trochlear notch is not clearly seen. What must be done to correct this positioning error during the repeat exposure?

    A. Angle central ray 45 degrees toward shoulder   C. Angle central ray 45 degrees away from shoulder

    B. Place humerus/forearm in same horizontal plane   D. Extend elbow to form an 80-degree horizontal plane angle

45. **Situation:** A patient with a possible Barton fracture enters the emergency room. Which positioning routine should be performed to confirm the diagnosis?

    A. Elbow   C. Hand

    B. Wrist   D. Thumb

46. **Situation:** A patient with a possible Smith fracture enters the emergency room. Which positioning routine should be performed to confirm this diagnosis?

    A. Hand   C. Wrist/forearm

    B. Thumb   D. Elbow

47. **Situation:** A patient has a Colles fracture reduced, and a large plaster cast is placed on the upper limb. The orthopedic surgeon orders a post reduction study. The original technique, used before the cast placement, involved 60 kVp and 5 mAs. How should the exposure factors be altered with a large plaster cast?

   A. Same exposure factors

   B. 75–78 kVp

   C. 65 kVp

   D. 68–70 kVp

48. **Situation:** A pediatric patient with a possible radial head fracture is brought into the emergency room. It is too painful for the patient to extend the elbow beyond 90 degrees or to rotate the hand. What type of special (i.e., optional) projection could be performed on this patient to confirm the diagnosis without causing further discomfort?

   A. Coyle method

   B. Modified Robert method

   C. Brewerton method

   D. Modified Stecher method

4 Upper Limb

1. A. A. 14
   B. B. 8
   C. B. 27
2. A. 7
   B. 4
   C. 2
   D. 5
   E. 1
   F. 6
3. A. 11
   B. 13
   C. 4
   D. 15
   E. 7
   F. 17
   G. 5
   H. 18
   I. 12
   J. 1
   K. 16
   L. 8
   M. 2
   N. 3
   O. 9
   P. 14
   Q. 6
   R. 10
4. C. Hamate
5. D. Trapezium
6. A. Scaphoid
7. D. Scaphoid and trapezium
8. A. 6
   B. 3
   C. 8
   D. 2
   E. 5
   F. 11
   G. 9
   H. 1
   I. 4
   J. 7
   K. 10
9. C. PA—radial deviation
10. C. Scaphoid
11. A. PA—ulnar deviation
12. B. Scaphoid
13. D. Ulna
14. A. Anterior aspect of distal humerus
15. C. Lateral and medial epicondyles
16. A. Medial aspect of coronoid process
17. A. Head of ulna
18. A. 4
    B. 3
    C. 2
    D. 1
    E. 4
19. A. 2
    B. 1
    C. 4
    D. 3
    E. 2
    F. 9
    G. 7
    H. 5
    I. 4
    J. 1
    K. 10
    L. 1
    M. 3
    N. 6
    O. 8
20. A. 5
    B. 3
    C. 8
    D. 7
    E. 11
    F. 1
    G. 2
    H. 4
    I. 10
    J. 9
    K. 6
21. True
22. False (lateral)
23. B. Causes the proximal radius to cross over the ulna.
24. A. Supinated (palm up)
25. B. Pronated (palm down)
26. A. 3
    B. 4
    C. 1
    D. 2
    E. 1
    F. 4
    G. 2
27. False. It is recommended that only one projection be placed on a digital IP. The anatomy should be centered on the IP.
28. B. Parallel to long axis of the IR
29. D. Soft-tissue structures within certain synovial joints
30. 1. F
    2. H
    3. G
    4. E
    5. B
    6. D
    7. A
    8. C
31. C. Midpoint between both carpal regions
32. A. Affected PIP joint
33. D. All of the above
34. B. Third MCP joint
35. A. Increased OID (to include base of first metacarpal, thumb must be raised)
36. C. Bennett fracture
37. True
38. False
39. D. 64 kVp, 200 mA, 1/20 second, small focal spot, and 40-inch (100-cm) SID
40. C. Decrease obliquity of hand.
41. A. Rotate upper limb medially.
42. C. Rotate wrist laterally 5–10 degrees.
43. A. Insufficient medial rotation
44. B. Place humerus/forearm in same horizontal plane.
45. B. Wrist
46. C. Wrist/forearm
47. D. 68–70 kVp
48. A. Coyle method

5 | Humerus and Shoulder Girdle

CHAPTER OBJECTIVES

After you have successfully completed the activities in this chapter, you will be able to:

_____ 1. Identify the bones and specific features of the humerus and shoulder girdle.

_____ 2. On drawings and radiographs, identify specific anatomic structures of the humerus and shoulder girdle.

_____ 3. Match specific joints of the shoulder girdle to their structural classification and movement type.

_____ 4. Describe anatomic relationships of prominent structures of the humerus and shoulder girdle.

_____ 5. On radiographic images, identify rotational positions of the humerus.

_____ 6. List the technical and shielding considerations (when required) commonly used for humerus and shoulder girdle radiography.

_____ 7. Match specific clinical indications of the shoulder girdle to the correct definition.

_____ 8. Match specific clinical indications of the shoulder girdle to the correct radiographic appearance.

_____ 9. For select forms of pathologic conditions of the shoulder girdle, indicate whether manual exposure factors should be increased, decreased, or should remain the same.

_____ 10. Identify alterations in positioning routine and exposure factors for pediatric, geriatric, and bariatric patients.

_____ 11. List routine and special projections of the humerus and shoulder, including the type and recommended field size, the central ray location with correct angles, and the structures best demonstrated.

_____ 12. Given various hypothetic situations, identify the correct modification of a position and/or exposure factors to improve the radiographic image.

_____ 13. Given various hypothetic situations, identify the correct position for a specific pathologic feature or condition.

_____ 14. Given radiographs of specific humerus and shoulder girdle projections, identify specific positioning and exposure factor errors.

POSITIONING AND RADIOGRAPHIC CRITIQUE

_____ 1. Using a peer, position the patient for routine and special projections of the humerus and shoulder girdle.

_____ 2. Using a shoulder radiographic phantom, produce satisfactory radiographs of the shoulder girdle (if equipment is available).

_____ 3. Critique and evaluate shoulder girdle radiographs based on the five divisions of radiographic criteria: (1) anatomy demonstrated, (2) position, (3) collimation and central ray, (4) exposure, and (5) anatomic side markers.

_____ 4. Distinguish between acceptable and unacceptable shoulder girdle radiographs based on exposure factors, motion, collimation, positioning, or other errors.

LEARNING EXERCISES

Complete the following review exercises after reading the associated pages in the textbook as indicated by each exercise. Answers to each review exercise are given at the end of the review exercises.

PART I: RADIOGRAPHIC ANATOMY

REVIEW EXERCISE A: Radiographic Anatomy of the Humerus and Shoulder Girdle (see textbook pp. 176–180)

1. The shoulder girdle consists of (A) _____, (B) _____, and (C) _____.

2. Identify the labeled parts in Figs. 5.1 and 5.2. Include secondary terms in parentheses where indicated.

    A. _____ (_____)

    B. _____ (_____)

    C. _____

    D. _____

    E. _____ (_____)

    F. _____

    G. Which projection (internal, external, or neutral rotation) of the proximal humerus is represented by this drawing and radiograph?

    _____

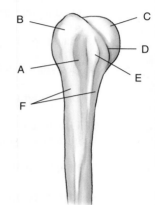

Fig. 5.1 Frontal view, proximal humerus.

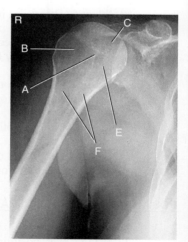

Fig. 5.2 Radiograph, proximal humerus.

3. The three aspects of the clavicle are the (A) _____, (B) _____, and (C) _____.

4. The _____ (male or female) clavicle tends to be thicker and more curved in shape.

5. The three angles of the scapula include the (A) _____, (B) _____, and (C) _____.

6. The anterior surface of the scapula is referred to as the _____ surface.

7. What is the anatomic name for the armpit? _____

8. What are the names of the two fossae located on the posterior scapula?

   A. _____   B. _____

9. All of the joints of the shoulder girdle are classified as being _____.

10. List the movement types for the following joints:

    A. Scapulohumeral: _____

    B. Sternoclavicular: _____

    C. Acromioclavicular: _____

11. Match each of the following anatomic structures with its correct location.

    _____ 1. Greater tubercle   A. Scapula

    _____ 2. Coracoid process   B. Clavicle

    _____ 3. Crest of spine   C. Proximal humerus

    _____ 4. Sternal extremity

    _____ 5. Acromial extremity

    _____ 6. Intertubercular groove

    _____ 7. Glenoid cavity (fossa)

    _____ 8. Surgical neck

12. Identify the following structures labeled in Figs. 5.3 and 5.4. Include secondary terms in parentheses where indicated.

A. _____

B. _____

  (_____)

C. _____

D. _____

E. _____

F. _____

G. _____

  (_____) border

H. _____

  (_____) border

I. _____

  (_____) surface

J. _____

  (_____) surface

K. _____

L. _____

M. _____

N. _____

  (_____)

O. _____

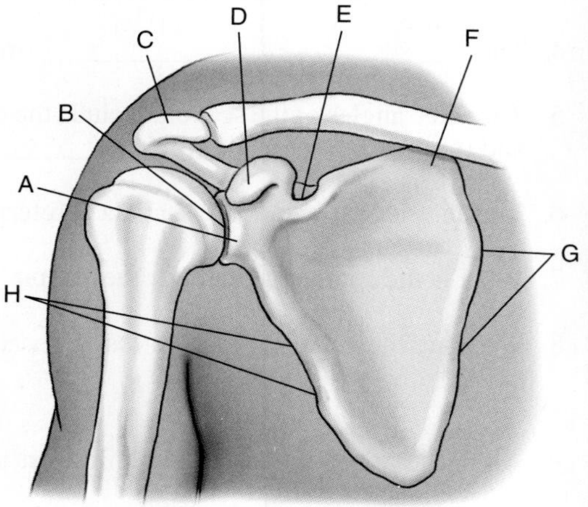

Fig. 5.3 Frontal view, scapula.

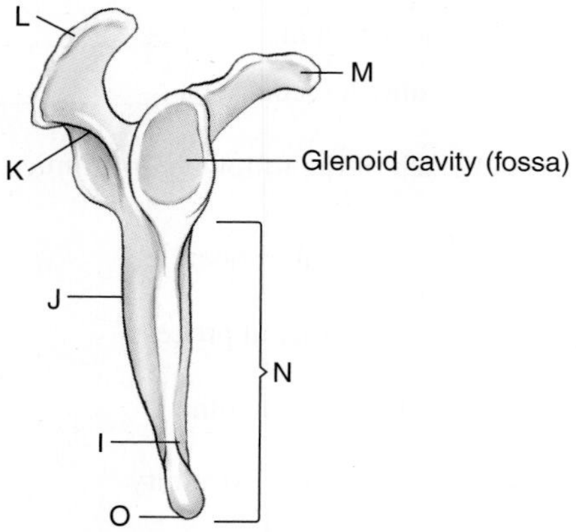

Fig. 5.4 Lateral view, scapula.

13. Identify the structures labeled in Fig. 5.5.

A. _____

B. _____ joint

C. _____

D. _____

E. _____

F. _____

G. Is this an internal or external rotation anteroposterior (AP) projection of the proximal humerus and shoulder?

_____

H. Does Fig. 5.5 represent an AP or a lateral perspective of the proximal humerus?

_____

I. Are the epicondyles of the distal humerus parallel or perpendicular to the IR on this projection?

_____

Identify the structures labeled in Fig. 5.6.

J. _____

K. _____

L. _____

M. _____

N. What is the correct term to describe the projection shown

in Fig. 5.6? _____

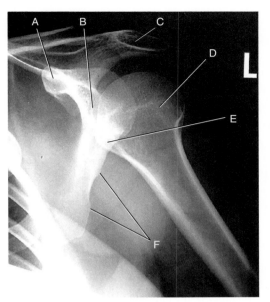

Fig. 5.5 Radiograph.

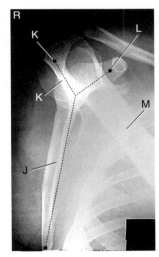

Fig. 5.6 Radiograph.

14. Identify the structures labeled in Fig. 5.7.

   A. _____

   B. _____

   C. _____

   D. _____

   E. What is the name of the projection shown in Fig. 5.7?

   _____

   F. How much (at what angle) should the affected arm be abducted from the body for this projection?

   _____

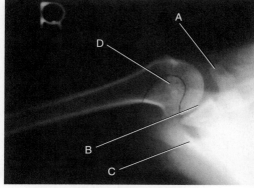

Fig. 5.7 Radiograph.

PART II: RADIOGRAPHIC POSITIONING

REVIEW EXERCISE B: Positioning of the Humerus and Shoulder Girdle (see textbook pp. 181–208)

1. Identify the correct proximal humerus rotation for the each of the following.

   _____ 1. Greater tubercle profiled laterally

   _____ 2. Humeral epicondyles angled 45 degrees to image receptor (IR)

   _____ 3. Epicondyles perpendicular to IR

   _____ 4. Supination of hand

   _____ 5. Palm of hand against thigh

   _____ 6. Epicondyles parallel to IR

   _____ 7. Lesser tubercle profiled medially

   _____ 8. Proximal humerus in a lateral position

   _____ 9. Proximal humerus in position for an AP projection

   A. External rotation

   B. Internal rotation

   C. Neutral rotation

2. Identify the proximal humerus rotation represented on the radiographs in Figs. 5.8–5.10.

   A. Fig. 5.8 represents _____ rotation.

   B. Fig. 5.9 represents _____ rotation.

   C. Fig. 5.10 represents _____ rotation.

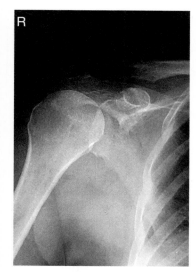
Fig. 5.8 Proximal humerus.

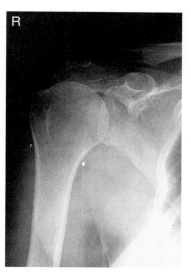
Fig. 5.9 Proximal humerus.

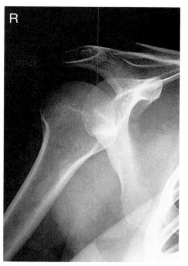
Fig. 5.10 Proximal humerus.

3. Indicate whether each of the following positioning and technical considerations is true or false for the shoulder girdle.

   A. True/False: The use of a grid is not required for shoulder studies that measure less than 4 inches (10 cm).

   B. True/False: The kVp range for adult shoulder projections is between 100 and 110 kVp.

   C. True/False: Low mA with long exposure times should be used for adult shoulder studies.

   D. True/False: Large focal spot setting should be selected for most adult shoulder studies.

   E. True/False: Shoulder projections are best performed erect when possible.

   F. True/False: A 72-inch (180-cm) source image distance (SID) is recommended for most shoulder girdle studies.

   G. True/False: Selection of the center cell if using the AEC.

4. Which of the following kVp ranges should be used for a shoulder series on an average adult using a grid?

   A. 100–120 kVp

   B. 55–60 kVp

   C. 80–90 kVp

   D. 65–70 kVp

5. Which of the following devices permits good visualization of soft-tissue and bony anatomy for adult shoulder radiography?

   A. Wedge compensating filter

   B. Aluminum added filtration

   C. Trough compensating filter

   D. Boomerang compensating filter

6. If physical immobilization is required, which individual should be asked to restrain a child for a shoulder series?

   A. Parent or guardian

   B. Radiologic technologist

   C. Radiography student

   D. Nurse aide

7. True/False: It is recommended to perform shoulder positions on bariatric patients in the erect position when possible.

8. True/False: CT arthrography of the shoulder joint often requires the use of iodinated contrast media injected into the joint space.

9. True/False: Magnetic resonance imaging (MR) can be used to evaluation soft tissue injuries.

10. True/False: Nuclear medicine bone scans can demonstrate signs of osteomyelitis and cellulitis.

11. True/False: Radiography is more sensitive than nuclear medicine for demonstrating physiologic aspects of the shoulder girdle.

12. True/False: Diagnostic medical sonography (DMS) can provide a functional (dynamic) evaluation of joint movement that MR cannot.

13. Match each of the following clinical indications to its correct definition.

    _____ 1. Compression between the greater tuberosity and soft tissues on the coracoacromial ligamentous and osseous arch

    _____ 2. Injury of the anteroinferior glenoid labrum

    _____ 3. Inflammatory condition of the tendon

    _____ 4. Superior displacement of the distal clavicle

    _____ 5. Compression fracture of the articular surface of the humeral head

    _____ 6. Traumatic injury to one or more of the supportive muscles of the shoulder girdle

    _____ 7. Atrophy of skeletal tissue

A. Acromioclavicular joint dislocation

B. Bankart lesion

C. Hill-Sachs defect

D. Impingement syndrome

E. Osteoporosis

F. Rotator cuff tear

G. Tendonitis

14. Match the following radiographic appearances to the correct pathology.

    _____ 1. Subacromial spurs

    _____ 2. Fluid-filled joint space

    _____ 3. Thin bony cortex

    _____ 4. Abnormal widening of acromioclavicular joint space

    _____ 5. Calcified tendons

    _____ 6. Avulsion fracture of the glenoid rim

    _____ 7. Narrowing of joint space

    _____ 8. Closed joint space

    _____ 9. Compression fracture of humeral head

A. Rheumatoid arthritis

B. Bankart lesion

C. Hill-Sachs defect

D. Osteoarthritis

E. Bursitis

F. Osteoporosis

G. Impingement syndrome

H. Acromioclavicular joint separation

I. Tendonitis

15. Which of the following clinical indications requires a decrease in manual exposure factors?

A. Impingement syndrome

B. Bursitis

C. Bankart lesion

D. Osteoporosis

16. True/False: The shoulder is the most common joint to develop bursitis due to repetitive motion.

17. True/False: Rheumatoid arthritis is more prevalent in men over women.

18. The most common injury to the rotator cuff is to the _____ tendon.

    A. Supraspinatus

    C. Teres minor

    B. Infraspinatus

    D. Subscapularis

19. Which two shoulder projections are taken routinely for a shoulder (with no traumatic injury) and proximal humerus?

    A. _____

    B. _____

20. Specifically, where is the central ray placed for an AP projection of the shoulder?

    _____

21. Which lateral projection can be performed to demonstrate the *entire* humerus for a patient with a midhumeral fracture?

    _____

22. To best demonstrate a possible Hill-Sachs defect, which additional positioning technique can be added to the inferosuperior axial (Lawrence method) projection?

    A. Angle central ray 10–15 degrees caudad

    C. Angle central ray 3–5 degrees caudad

    B. Rotate affected arm externally approximately 45 degrees

    D. Place humeral epicondyles parallel to IR

23. What type of central ray angulation is required for the inferosuperior axial projection (Lawrence method) for the shoulder?

    A. 25–30 degrees medially

    C. 25-degree anterior and 25 degrees medially

    B. 35–45-degrees medially

    D. Central ray perpendicular to IR

24. The _____ projection of the shoulder produces an image of the glenoid process in profile.

    This projection is also referred to as the _____ method.

25. Which of the following projections produces a tangential projection of the intertubercular sulcus (groove)?

    A. Fisk modification

    C. Hobbs modification

    B. Grashey method

    D. Lawrence method

26. The CR for the superoinferior transaxillary projection is directed _____.

27. Which of the following projections is best for demonstrating a possible dislocation of the proximal humerus?

    A. Anterior oblique (Grashey method)

    C. Inferosuperior axial (Clements modification) projection

    B. Fisk modification

    D. Posterior oblique (scapular Y) projection

28. The _____ projection is the special projection of the shoulder that best demonstrates the acromio-humeral space for possible subacromial spurs, which create shoulder impingement symptoms (more than one answer possible).

29. What type of CR angle is required for the apical AP axial shoulder projection?

    A. 10–15 degrees caudad

    B. 30 degrees caudad

    C. 45 degrees caudad

    D. 5–10 degrees cephalad

30. Which of the following nontrauma projections can be performed erect to provide a lateral perspective of the proximal humerus in relationship to the scapulohumeral joint?

    A. Tangential projection (Fisk modification)

    B. AP projection–neutral rotation

    C. Posteroanterior (PA) axial transaxillary projection (Bernageau method)

    D. Anterior oblique position (Grashey method)

31. How much is the CR angled for the inferosuperior axial projection (Clements modification) if the patient cannot fully abduct the arm 90 degrees?

    A. 5–15 degrees

    B. 45 degrees

    C. 25–30 degrees

    D. 20 degrees

32. What CR angle is required for the AP axial projection (Zanca method) for acromioclavicular (AC) joints?

    A. 25 degrees cephalad

    B. 45 degrees caudad

    C. 5–10 degrees caudad

    D. 10–15 degrees cephalad

33. True/False: The PA axial transaxillary projection (Bernageau method) requires no CR angle.

34. True/False: The transthoracic lateral projection can be performed for possible fractures or dislocations of the proximal humerus.

35. True/False: The use of a breathing technique can be performed for the transthoracic lateral humerus projection.

36. True/False: The affected arm must be placed into external rotation for the transthoracic lateral projection.

37. True/False: A central ray angle of 10–15 degrees caudad may be used for the transthoracic lateral shoulder projection if the patient is unable to elevate the uninjured arm and shoulder sufficiently.

38. True/False: The scapular Y lateral (posterior oblique) position requires the body to be rotated 25–30 degrees anteriorly toward the affected side.

39. Which two landmarks are placed perpendicular to the IR for the scapular Y lateral projection?

    _____

40. Which special projection of the shoulder requires that the affected side be rotated 45 degrees toward the cassette and uses a 45 degrees caudad central ray angle?

    _____

41. A posterior dislocation of the humerus projects the humeral head _____ (superior or inferior) to the glenoid cavity with the special projection described in the previous question.

42. An asthenic patient requires _____ (more or less) CR angle for an AP axial clavicle projection than a hypersthenic patient.

43. What must be ruled out before performing the weight-bearing study for AC joints?

    _____

44. Match each of the following projections with its corresponding method name. Method names may be used more than once.

   _____ 1. Inferosuperior axial   A. Neer method

   _____ 2. Anterior oblique for glenoid cavity   B. Grashey method

   _____ 3. Tangential for intertubercular (bicipital) sulcus   C. Bernageau method

   _____ 4. Supraspinatus outlet tangential   D. Fisk modification

   _____ 5. PA axial transaxillary   E. Garth method

   _____ 6. AP apical oblique axial

45. What is the most common clinical indication to perform the Alexander method for the AC joints?

A. Possible fracture of distal clavicle   C. Suspected AC joint separation

B. Possible fracture of coracoid process   D. Suspected subacromial spurs

46. What type of CR angle is required for the Pearson method for AC joints?

A. 20 degrees cephalad   C. 25–30 degrees cephalad

B. 10 degrees caudad   D. No CR angle

47. Where is the CR centered for the AP scapula projection?

_____

48. What type of CR angle is required for the lateral scapula position?

A. 10–15 degrees cephalad   C. 10–15 degrees caudad

B. 5–15 degrees caudad   D. None

49. True/False: Orthostatic (breathing) technique is recommended for the transthoracic lateral projection.

50. True/False: The lateral scapula and posterior oblique (scapular Y) projections are the same projection.

Review Exercise C: Problem Solving for Technical and Positioning Errors

1. A radiography of a lateral humerus was taken using 70 kVp, 20 mAs, 40-inch (100 cm) SID, and a physical grid. The exposure indicator revealed the patient was overexposed. The radiograph revealed that the lesser tubercle was not in profile. What must be done to correct the overexposure and positioning errors on the repeat exposure?

_____

2. A radiograph of an AP axial clavicle projection reveals that the clavicle is projected below the superior border of the scapula. What can the technologist do to correct this problem during the repeat exposure?

_____

3. A radiograph of an AP recumbent scapula reveals that the scapula is within the lung field and difficult to see. Which two things can the technologist do to improve the visibility of the scapula during the repeat exposure?

_____

4. A radiograph of an AP projection (with external rotation) of a shoulder (with no traumatic injury) reveals that neither the greater nor lesser tubercles are profiled. What must be done to correct this during the repeat exposure?

_____

5. A radiograph of a lateral scapula position reveals that it is not a true lateral projection. (Considerable separation exists between the axillary and vertebral borders.) The projection was taken using the following factors: erect position, 40-inch (100-cm) SID, 45-degree rotation toward IR from PA, central ray centered to midscapula, and no central ray angulation. Based on these factors, how can this position be improved during the repeat exposure?

_____

6. A radiograph of the AP oblique (Grashey method) taken with a 30-degree rotation of the affected shoulder toward the IR reveals that the borders of the glenoid cavity are not superimposed. The patient has broad, rounded shoulders. What must be done to get better superimposition of the cavity during the repeat exposure?

_____

7. **Situation:** A patient with a possible right shoulder dislocation enters the emergency room. The technologist attempts to perform an erect transthoracic lateral projection, but the patient is unable to raise the left arm and shoulder high enough. The resultant radiograph reveals that the shoulders are superimposed, and the right shoulder and humeral head are not well visualized. What can be done to improve this image during the repeat exposure?

_____

8. **Situation:** A patient with a possible fracture of the right proximal humerus from an automobile accident enters the emergency room. The patient has other injuries and is unable to stand or sit erect. Which positioning routine should be used to determine the extent of the injury?

_____

9. **Situation:** A patient with a clinical history of chronic shoulder dislocation comes to the radiology department. The orthopedic physician suspects that a Hill-Sachs defect may be present. Which specific position(s) may be used to best demonstrate this pathologic feature?

_____

10. **Situation:** A patient with a possible Bankart lesion comes to the radiology department. List three projections that can be performed that may demonstrate signs of this injury.

   A. _____

   B. _____

   C. _____

11. **Situation:** A patient with a possible rotator cuff tear comes to the radiology department. Which of the following imaging modalities would best demonstrate this injury?

   A. Arthrography

   B. MR

   C. Nuclear medicine

   D. Radiography

12. **Situation:** A patient with a clinical history of tendon injury in the shoulder region comes to the radiology department. The orthopedic physician needs a functional study of the shoulder joint performed to determine the extent of the tendon injury. Which of the following modalities would best demonstrate this injury?

   A. Arthrography

   B. MR

   C. Diagnostic medical sonography (DMS)

   D. Nuclear medicine

13. A radiograph of an AP projection with internal rotation of the shoulder does not demonstrate either the greater or lesser tubercle in profile. What is the most likely cause for this radiographic outcome?

_____

14. A radiograph of a transthoracic lateral projection demonstrates considerable superimposition of lung markings and ribs over the region of the proximal shoulder. What can the technologist do to minimize this problem during the repeat exposure?

_____

15. **Situation:** A patient enters the ER with a definite fracture to the midhumerus. Because of other trauma the patient is unable to stand. Which lateral projection would demonstrate the entire humerus?

_____

16. **Situation:** The AP apical oblique axial projection (Garth method) is performed on a patient with a shoulder injury. The resultant radiograph demonstrates the proximal humeral head projected below the glenoid cavity. What type of trauma or pathology is indicated with this radiographic appearance?

_____

Review Exercise D: Critique Radiographs of the Shoulder Girdle

The following questions relate to the radiographs found in this exercise. Evaluate these radiographs for the radiographic criteria categories (1 through 5) that follow. Describe the corrections needed to improve the overall image. The major or "repeatable" errors are specific errors that indicate the need for a repeat exposure, regardless of the nature of the other errors.

A. AP clavicle (Fig. 5.11)

Description of possible error:

1. Anatomy demonstrated:

    _____

2. Part positioning:

    _____

3. Collimation field size and central ray:

    _____

4. Exposure:

    _____

5. Anatomic side markers:

    _____

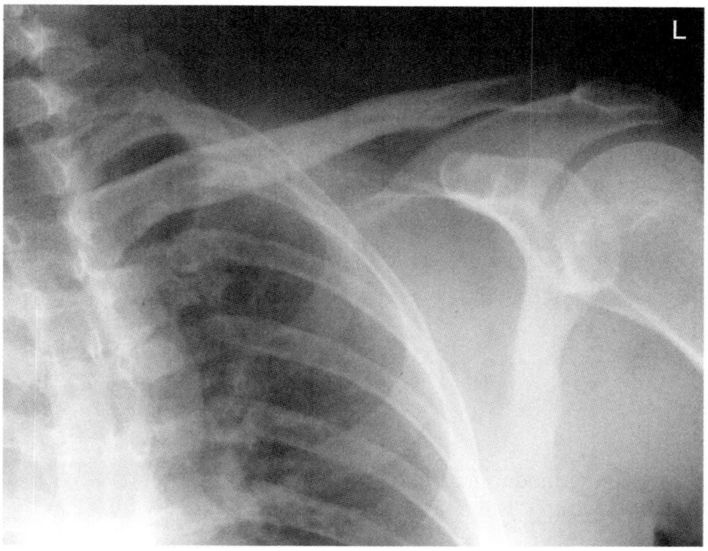

Fig. 5.11 Anteroposterior clavicle.

Repeatable error(s):_____

B. AP shoulder—external rotation (Fig. 5.12)

Description of possible error:

    1. Anatomy demonstrated:

    _____

    2. Part positioning:

    _____

    3. Collimation field size and central ray:

    _____

    4. Exposure:

    _____

    5. Anatomic side markers:

    _____

Repeatable error(s):

_____

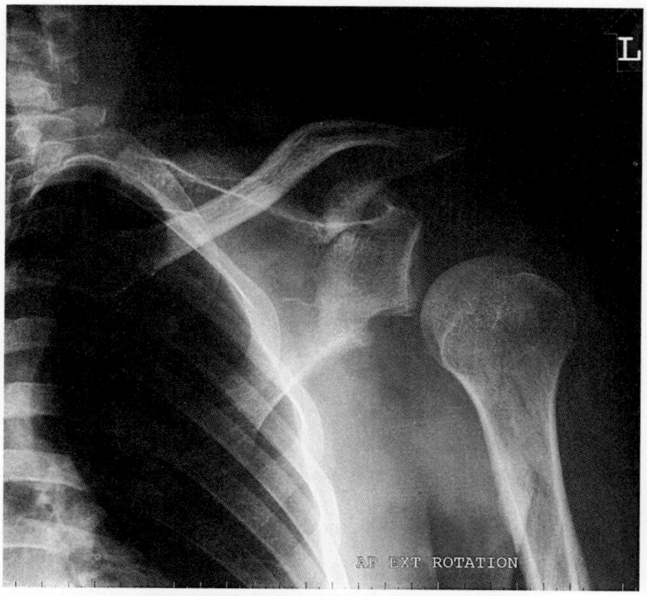

Fig. 5.12 Anteroposterior shoulder—external rotation.

C. AP scapula (Fig. 5.13)

Description of possible error:

    1. Anatomy demonstrated:

    _____

    2. Part positioning:

    _____

    3. Collimation field size and central ray:

    _____

    4. Exposure:

    _____

    5. Anatomic side markers:

    _____

Repeatable error(s): _____

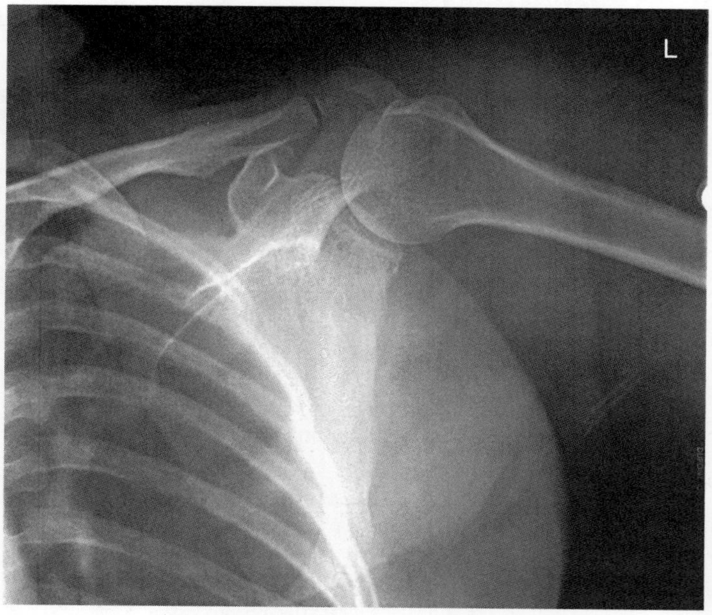

Fig. 5.13 Anteroposterior scapula.

D. AP humerus (Fig. 5.14)

Description of possible error:

1. Anatomy demonstrated:

   _____

2. Part positioning:

   _____

3. Collimation field size and central ray:

   _____

4. Exposure:

   _____

5. Anatomic side markers:

   _____

Repeatable error(s):

   _____

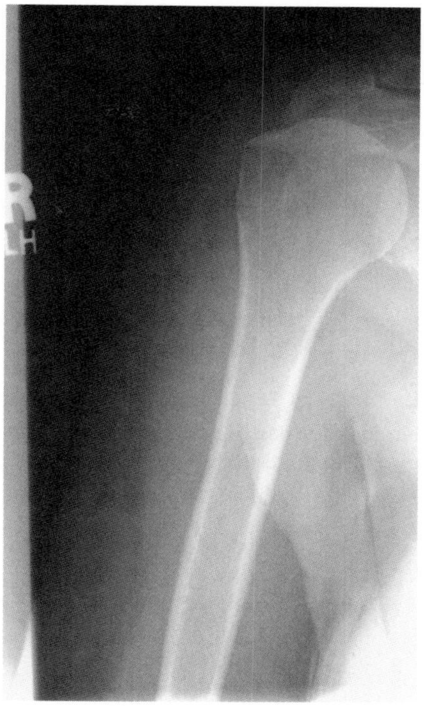

Fig. 5.14 Anteroposterior humerus.

Which projection (AP, lateral, or oblique) and which rotation (internal, external, or neutral) of the proximal humerus

are evident?_____

PART III: LABORATORY EXERCISES

You must gain experience in positioning each part of the humerus and shoulder girdle before performing the following exams on actual patients. You can get experience in positioning and radiographic evaluation of these projections by performing exercises using radiographic phantoms and practicing on other students (although you will not be taking actual exposures).

   The following suggested activities assume that your teaching institution has an energized lab and radiographic phantoms. If not, perform Laboratory Exercises B and C, the radiographic evaluation, and the physical positioning exercises. (Check off each step and projection as you complete it.)

Laboratory Exercise A: Energized Laboratory

1. Using the thorax radiographic phantom, produce radiographs of the following basic routines:

   _____AP shoulder   _____AP and lateral scapula

   _____Anterior oblique (Grashey method)   _____Apical AP axial projection

   _____AP and AP axial clavicle

Laboratory Exercise B: Radiographic Evaluation

1. Evaluate and critique the radiographs produced in the preceding, additional radiographs provided by your instructor, or both. Evaluate each radiograph for the following points:

_____Evaluate the completeness of the study. (Are all of the pertinent anatomic structures included on the radiograph?)

_____Evaluate for positioning or centering errors (e.g., rotation, off centering).

_____Evaluate for correct image receptor exposure factors and possible motion.

_____Determine whether markers and an acceptable degree of collimation and/or area shielding (when required) are seen on the images.

Laboratory Exercise C: Physical Positioning

On another person, simulate performing all of the following basic and special projections of the humerus and shoulder girdle. Include the six steps listed in the following and described in the textbook. (Check off each step when completed satisfactorily.)

Step 1. Appropriate recommended field size with correct markers

Step 2. Correct central ray placement and centering of part to central ray and/or IR

Step 3. Accurate collimation

Step 4. Area shielding of patient when required

Step 5. Use of proper immobilizing devices when needed

Step 6. Approximate correct exposure factors, breathing instructions where applicable, and initiating the exposure

Projections	Step 1	Step 2	Step 3	Step 4	Step 5	Step 6
• Humerus (AP and lateral)	_____	_____	_____	_____	_____	_____
• Transthoracic lateral for humerus	_____	_____	_____	_____	_____	_____
• Shoulder series (nontrauma) (AP internal and external rotation)	_____	_____	_____	_____	_____	_____
• Inferosuperior axial (Lawrence)	_____	_____	_____	_____	_____	_____
• Anterior oblique (Grashey)	_____	_____	_____	_____	_____	_____
• Apical AP axial and oblique projection	_____	_____	_____	_____	_____	_____
• Tangential (Fisk) for intertubercular sulcus	_____	_____	_____	_____	_____	_____
• Posterior oblique–scapular Y	_____	_____	_____	_____	_____	_____
• Transthoracic lateral (Lawrence)	_____	_____	_____	_____	_____	_____
• Superoinferior transaxillary	_____	_____	_____	_____	_____	_____
• AP and AP axial clavicle	_____	_____	_____	_____	_____	_____
• AP and lateral scapula	_____	_____	_____	_____	_____	_____
• AC joints (with and without weights)	_____	_____	_____	_____	_____	_____

This self-test should be taken only after completing all of the readings, review exercises, and laboratory activities for a particular section. The purpose of this test is not only to provide a good learning exercise but also to serve as a strong indicator of what your final unit evaluation exam will cover. It is strongly suggested that if you do not get at least a 90% to 95% grade on each self-test, you should review those areas in which you missed questions before going to your instructor for the final unit evaluation exam.

1. Select the term(s) that correctly describe(s) the shoulder joint.

   A. Humeroscapular
   B. Scapulohumeral
   C. Glenohumeral
   D. B and C

2. Which specific joint is found on the lateral end of the clavicle?

   A. Scapulohumeral
   B. Sternoclavicular
   C. Acromioclavicular
   D. Glenohumeral

3. Which of the following is not an angle found on the scapula?

   A. Inferior angle
   B. Medial angle
   C. Lateral angle
   D. Superior angle

4. Which of the following structures of the scapula extends most anteriorly?

   A. Glenoid cavity
   B. Acromion
   C. Scapular spine
   D. Coracoid process

5. True/False: The male clavicle is shorter and less curved than the female clavicle.

6. Which bony structure separates the supraspinous and infraspinous fossae?

   A. Scapular spine
   B. Glenoid cavity
   C. Acromion
   D. Superior border of scapula

7. Which of the following structures is considered the most posterior?

   A. Scapular notch
   B. Coracoid process
   C. Acromion
   D. Glenoid process

8. What is the type of joint movement for the scapulohumeral joint?

   A. Plane
   B. Ball and socket
   C. Ellipsoidal
   D. Pivot (trochoidal)

9. Identify the labeled structures in Fig. 5.15. (Terms may be used more than once.)

_______A. 1. Spine of scapula

_______B. 2. Lesser tubercle

_______C. 3. Coracoid process

_______D. 4. Lateral (axillary) border of scapula

_______E. 5. Scapulohumeral joint

_______F. 6. Clavicle

_______G. 7. Intertubercular sulcus

_______H. 8. Acromion of scapula

_______I. 9. Neck of scapula

_______J. 10. Greater tubercle

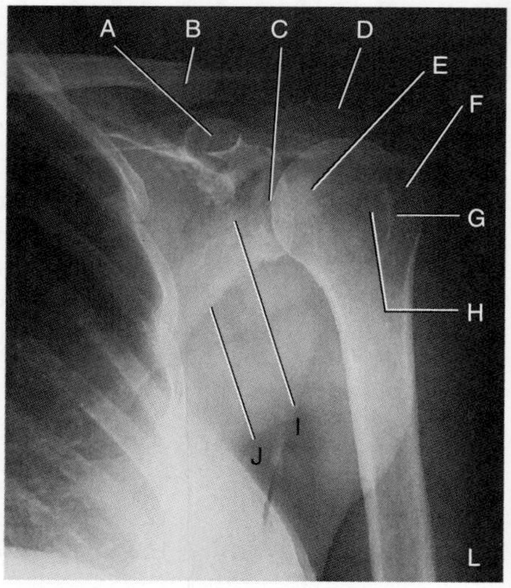
A
B
C
D
E
F
G
H
I
J
L
Fig. 5.15 Shoulder projection.

K. Does Fig. 5.15 represent an AP projection with: (A) an internal, (B) an external, or (C) a neutral rotation of the humerus? __________________Identify the labeled structures in Fig. 5.16. (Terms may be used more than once.)

_______L. 11. Lateral extremity of clavicle

_______M. 12. Head of humerus

_______N. 13. Glenoid cavity

_______O.

_______P.

_______Q.

_______R.

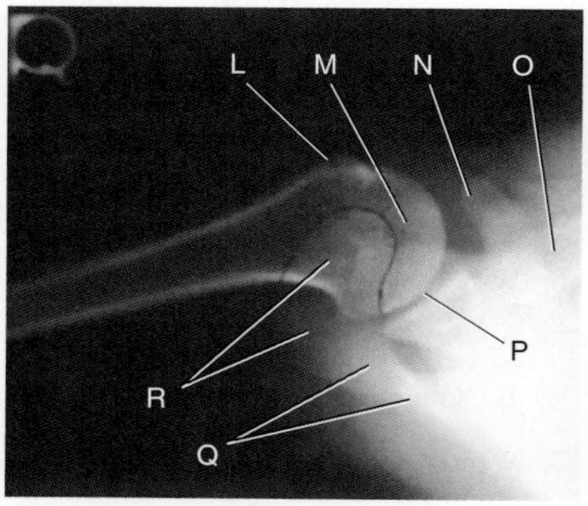
L
M
N
O
P
R
Q
Fig. 5.16 Shoulder projection.

S. What is the correct term and method for the projection seen in Fig. 5.16?

A. Inferosuperior axial projection

B. Transthoracic lateral— (Lawrence method)

C. Anterior oblique— (Grashey method)

D. PA axial transaxillary projection— (Bernageau method)

10. Which of the following technical considerations does not apply for adult shoulder radiography?

A. Nongrid

B. Center cell AEC

C. 40- to 44-inch (100- to 110-cm) SID

D. 70–80 kVp

11. True/False: If a virtual grid is used, a physical grid is not needed.

12. True/False: The greatest technical concern during a pediatric shoulder study is voluntary motion.

13. Which of the following imaging modalities or procedures assesses physiologic aspects instead of anatomic?

   A. Diagnostic medical sonography (DMS)   C. CT arthrography

   B. MR   D. Nuclear medicine

14. Which of the following imaging modalities or procedures provides a functional, or dynamic, study of the shoulder joint?

   A. DMS   C. Nuclear medicine

   B. Radiography   D. MR

15. Match each of the following clinical indications to its correct definition.

   _____ 1. Disability of the shoulder joint caused by chronic   A. Rotator cuff tear
              inflammation in and around the joint
                                                                           B. Osteoporosis
   _____ 2. Injury to the anteroinferior glenoid labrum
                                                                           C. Rheumatoid arthritis
   _____ 3. Chronic systemic disease with arthritic inflammatory
              changes throughout the body   D. Idiopathic chronic adhesive capsulitis

   _____ 4. Superior displacement of distal clavicle   E. Bankart lesion

   _____ 5. Compression fracture of humeral head   F. AC joint dislocation

   _____ 6. Traumatic injury to one or more muscles of the shoulder   G. Hill-Sachs defect
              joint

   _____ 7. Reduction in the quantity of bone

16. Which of the following projections and/or positions best demonstrates signs of impingement syndrome in the acromiohumeral space?

   A. AP and lateral shoulder external rotation   C. Inferosuperior axial with exaggerated rotation

   B. Inferosuperior axial   D. Apical AP axial projection

17. Which of the following pathologic conditions often produces narrowing of the joint space?

   A. Osteoarthritis   C. Osteoporosis

   B. Bursitis   D. Idiopathic chronic adhesive capsulitis

18. Which of the following pathologic conditions results in systemic inflammatory changes to connective tissues?

   A. Bursitis   C. Rotator cuff tear

   B. Rheumatoid arthritis   D. Bankart lesion

19. What is an alternative CR centering technique for an AP shoulder projection on a bariatric patient if unable to palpate the coracoid process?

   A. Center at level of jugular notch   C. Center 2 inches (5 cm) below AC joint

   B. Center 2 inches (5 cm) below level of vertebra   D. Center at level of xiphoid process
      prominens

128

20. What type of compensating filter is recommended for use on an AP shoulder projection for a hypersthenic patient?

   A. Boomerang

   B. Trough

   C. Wedge

   D. Gradient

21. Which routine projection of the shoulder requires that the humeral epicondyles be parallel to the IR?

   A. External rotation

   B. Neutral rotation

   C. Internal rotation

   D. Anterior oblique (Grashey method)

22. Where is the central ray centered for an AP projection—external rotation of the shoulder?

   A. Acromion

   B. 1 inch (2.5 cm) superior to coracoid process

   C. 1 inch (2.5 cm) inferior to coracoid process

   D. 2 inches (5 cm) inferior to acromioclavicular joint

23. Which position of the shoulder and proximal humerus projects the lesser tubercle in profile medially?

   A. External rotation

   B. Neutral rotation

   C. Internal rotation

   D. Exaggerated rotation

24. What type of central ray angle should be used for the inferosuperior axial projection for the scapulohumeral joint space?

   A. 15 degrees medially

   B. 25–30 degrees medially

   C. 25 degrees anteriorly and medially

   D. 35–45 degrees medially

25. To best demonstrate the Hill-Sachs defect on the inferosuperior axial projection, which additional positioning maneuver must be used?

   A. Angle central ray 35 degrees medially

   B. Use exaggerated external rotation

   C. Use exaggerated internal rotation

   D. Abduct arm 120-degree rotation from midsagittal plane

26. How are the humeral epicondyles aligned for a rotational lateromedial projection of the humerus?

   A. 45 degrees to IR

   B. Perpendicular to IR

   C. Parallel to IR

   D. 20-degree angle to IR

27. Which special projection of the shoulder places the glenoid cavity in profile for an "open" scapulohumeral joint?

   A. Garth method

   B. Transthoracic lateral (Lawrence method)

   C. Fisk modification

   D. Grashey method

28. What type of CR angle is required for the apical AP axial shoulder (Garth method) projection?

   A. 15 degrees cephalad

   B. 10–15 degrees caudad

   C. 30 degrees caudad

   D. 45 degrees caudad

29. For the erect version of the tangential projection for the intertubercular sulcus, the patient leans forward _____ from vertical.

   A. 5–7 degrees

   B. 20–25 degrees

   C. 10–15 degrees

   D. 35–45 degrees

30. What is the major advantage of the supine, tangential version of the intertubercular sulcus projection over the erect version?

   A. Less radiation exposure

   B. Reduced object-image receptor distance

   C. Less risk for motion

   D. Ability to use automatic exposure control

31. Which of the following projections best demonstrates the supraspinatus outlet region?

   A. Tangential projection (Neer method)

   B. Fisk method

   C. Inferosuperior axial projection

   D. PA axial transaxillary projection (Bernageau method)

32. With which of the following projections can an orthostatic (breathing) technique be used?

   A. Grashey method

   B. Transthoracic lateral for humerus

   C. Scapular Y lateral

   D. Garth method

33. What central ray angulation is required for the tangential projection-supraspinatus outlet (Neer method)?

   A. 10–15 degrees caudad

   B. 45-degree caudad

   C. 25 degrees anteriorly and medially

   D. None; central ray is perpendicular

34. Which clinical indication is best demonstrated with the Garth method?

   A. Bursitis

   B. Rheumatoid arthritis

   C. Scapulohumeral dislocations

   D. Signs of shoulder impingement

35. Which anatomy of the shoulder is best demonstrated with superoinferior transaxillary projection?

   A. Coracoid process of the scapula on end

   B. Scapular spine

   C. Greater tubercle

   D. Intertubercular (bicipital) sulcus

36. If the patient cannot fully abduct the affected arm 90 degrees for the inferosuperior axial transaxillary projection (Clements modification), the technologist can angle the CR _____ degrees toward the axilla.

   A. 5–15 degrees

   B. 20–25 degrees

   C. 25–30 degrees

   D. 45 degrees

37. Which of the following projections requires the CR to be centered 2 inches (5 cm) inferior and medial from the superolateral border of the shoulder?

   A. Tangential projection (Fisk modification)

   B. Inferosuperior axial (Clements projection)

   C. Anterior oblique (Grashey method)

   D. Posterior oblique (scapula Y lateral projection)

38. Which anatomy is best demonstrated by the Alexander method?

   A. Scapulohumeral joint

   B. Coracoid process

   C. Proximal humerus

   D. AC joints

39. Which type of injury must be ruled out before the weight-bearing phase of an AC joint study?

   A. Shoulder separation

   B. Fractured clavicle

   C. Bursitis of the scapulohumeral joint

   D. Bankart lesion

40. What is the **minimal** amount of weight a large adult should have strapped to each wrist for the weight-bearing phase of an AC joint study?

   A. 5–7 lb (2–3 kg)

   B. 8–10 lb (3–4 kg)

   C. 12–15 lb (5–6 kg)

   D. 20–30 lb (9–13 kg)

130

41. True/False: A PA axial projection of the clavicle requires a 35- to 45-degree caudal central ray angle.

42. True/False: A 72-inch (180-cm) SID is recommended for adult AC joint studies.

43. Which two positioning landmarks are aligned perpendicularly to the IR for the lateral scapula projection?

    A. Scapular spine and greater tubercle   C. AC joint and greater tubercle

    B. Superior angle and AC joint   D. Acromion and coracoid process

44. A radiograph of an anterior oblique (Grashey method) shows that the anterior and posterior glenoid rims are not superimposed. The following positioning factors were used: erect position, body rotated 25–30 degrees toward the affected side, central ray perpendicular to scapulohumeral joint space, and affected arm slightly abducted in neutral rotation. Which of the following modifications will superimpose the glenoid rims during the repeat exposure?

    A. Angle central ray 10–15 degrees caudad   C. Place affected arm in external rotation position

    B. Rotate body less toward affected side   D. Rotate body more toward affected side

45. **Situation:** A patient with a possible shoulder dislocation enters the emergency room. A neutral AP projection of the shoulder has been taken, confirming a dislocation. Which additional projection should be taken?

    A. Inferosuperior axial (Clements modification)   C. AP apical oblique axial (Garth method)

    B. Alexander method   D. AP, external rotation

46. A radiograph of an AP axial clavicle taken on an asthenic patient shows that the clavicle is projected in the lung field below the top of the shoulder. The following positioning factors were used: erect position, central ray angled 15-degree cephalad, 40-inch (100-cm) SID, and respiration suspended at end of expiration. Which of the following modifications should be made during the repeat exposure?

    A. Increase central ray angulation   C. Reverse central ray angulation

    B. Suspend respiration at end of inspiration   D. Use 72-inch (180-cm) SID

47. **Situation:** A patient with a possible right-shoulder separation enters the emergency room. Which of the following routines should be performed?

    A. AC joint series: non–weight-bearing and weight-bearing projections

    B. AP neutral projection and AP apical oblique axial (Garth method)

    C. AP neutral and transthoracic lateral projections

    D. AP internal and external projections

48. **Situation:** A patient comes to the radiology department with a history of tendonitis of the bicep tendon. Which of the following projections will best demonstrate calcification of the tendon within the intertubercular sulcus?

    A. AP apical oblique axial (Garth method)

    B. AP oblique (Grashey method)

    C. PA axial transaxillary projection (Bernageau method)

    D. Tangential projection (Fisk modification)

49. An AP apical oblique axial (Garth method) radiographic image demonstrates poor visibility of the shoulder joint. The technologist used the following factors: patient erect, facing the x-ray tube, 45 degrees of rotation of affected shoulder toward the IR, 45-degree cephalad angle, and the CR centered to the scapulohumeral joint. Which of the following factors would have contributed to this substandard Garth position?

    A. Wrong direction of CR angle

    B. Incorrect CR centering

    C. Position must be performed recumbent

    D. Shoulder rotated in wrong direction

50. **Situation:** A patient is referred to radiology for an AC joint series. The routine calls for an AP axial projection (Zanca method) to be included. How is this projection performed?

    A. Ask another technologist to hold the patient erect for the projection.

    B. Perform the position AP erect with 10- to 15-degree cephalic angle

    C. Perform an AP recumbent with 35–45 degrees angled toward the image receptor

    D. AP erect projections with and without weights

51. **Situation:** A patient enters the ER with a proximal and midhumeral fracture. The patient is in extreme pain. Which of the following positioning routines would demonstrate the entire humerus without excessive movement of the limb?

    A. AP and mediolateral humerus

    B. AP and transthoracic lateral

    C. AP and transthoracic lateral of humerus

    D. AP and scapular Y lateral

5 | Humerus and Shoulder Girdle

WORKBOOK SELF-TEST ANSWER KEY

1. D. (Although both terms are correct [B and C], *scapulo-humeral joint* is the preferred term)
2. C. Acromioclavicular
3. B. Medial angle
4. D. Coracoid process
5. False
6. A. Scapular spine
7. C. Acromion
8. B. Ball and socket
9. A. 3
   B. 6
   C. 5
   D. 8
   E. 12
   F. 10
   G. 7
   H. 2
   I. 9
   J. 4
   K. B. External rotation
   L. 2
   M. 12
   N. 3
   O. 6 or 11
   P. 13 or 5
   Q. 1
   R. 8
   S. A. Inferosuperior axial projection
10. A. Nongrid. (Most, if not all, adult shoulders measure

greater than 4 inches [10 cm] and require a grid unless using virtual grid software.)

11. True
12. True
13. D. Nuclear medicine
14. A. DMS
15. 1. D
    2. E
    3. C
    4. F
    5. G
    6. A
    7. B
16. D. Apical AP axial projection
17. A. Osteoarthritis
18. B. Rheumatoid arthritis
19. C. Center 2 inches (5 cm) below AC joint
20. A. Boomerang
21. A. External rotation
22. C. 1 in (2.5 cm) inferior to cora-coid process
23. C. Internal rotation
24. B. 25–30 degrees medially
25. B. Use exaggerated external rotation (MSP).
26. B. Perpendicular to IR
27. D. Grashey method
28. D. 45 degrees caudad
29. C. 10–15 degrees
30. B. Reduced OID
31. A. Tangential projection (Neer method)
32. B. Transthoracic lateral for humerus

33. A. 10–15 degrees caudad
34. C. Scapulohumeral dislocations
35. A. Coracoid process of the scapula on end
36. A. 5–15 degrees toward axilla
37. C. Anterior oblique (Grashey method)
38. D. AC joints (see alternative AP axial projection in text)
39. B. Fractured clavicle
40. B. 8–10 lb (3–4 kg)
41. False
42. True
43. B. Superior angle of scapula and AC joint
44. D. Rotate body more toward affected side.
45. C. AP apical oblique axial (Garth method)
46. A. Increase central ray angulation.
47. A. Acromioclavicular joint series: non–weight-bear-ing and weight-bearing projections
48. D. Tangential projection (Fisk method)
49. A. Wrong direction of CR angle
50. B. Perform the AP position erect with 10- to 15-degree cephalic angle.
51. C. AP and transthoracic lateral of humerus

A1

6 Lower Limb

CHAPTER OBJECTIVES

After you have successfully completed the activities in this chapter, you will be able to:

_____ 1. Identify the bones and specific features of the toes, foot, ankle, lower leg, knee, patella, and distal femur.

_____ 2. On drawings and radiographs, identify specific anatomic features of the foot, ankle, leg, knee, patella, and distal femur.

_____ 3. Identify specific joints of the foot, ankle, leg, and knee according to the correct classification and movement type.

_____ 4. Match specific clinical indications of the lower limb to the correct definition.

_____ 5. Match specific clinical indications of the lower limb to the correct radiographic appearance.

_____ 6. Describe the basic and special projections of the toes, foot, ankle, calcaneus, knee, patella, intercondylar fossa, and femur, including central-ray (CR) placement and angulation, correct recommended field size, part positioning, technical factors, and evaluation criteria.

_____ 7. List the various patient dose ranges for each projection of the lower limb.

_____ 8. Given various hypothetic situations, identify the correct modification of a position and/or exposure factors to improve the radiographic image.

_____ 9. Given various hypothetic situations, identify the correct position for a specific pathologic form or condition.

_____ 10. Given radiographs of specific lower limb projections, identify specific positioning and exposure-factor errors.

POSITIONING AND RADIOGRAPHIC CRITIQUE

_____ 1. Using a peer, perform basic and special projections of the lower limb.

_____ 2. Using foot and knee phantoms, produce satisfactory radiographs of the lower limb (if equipment is available).

_____ 3. Critique and evaluate lower limb radiographs based on the five divisions of radiographic criteria: (1) anatomy demonstrated, (2) position, (3) collimation and central ray, (4) exposure, and (5) anatomic side markers.

_____ 4. Distinguish between acceptable and unacceptable lower limb radiographs based on exposure factors, motion, collimation, positioning, or other errors.

LEARNING EXERCISES

Complete the following review exercises after reading the associated pages in the textbook as indicated by each exercise. Answers to each review exercise are given at the end of the review exercises.

133

Copyright © 2025 by Elsevier Inc.
All rights are reserved, including those for text and data mining, AI training, and similar technologies.

Chapter **6** **Lower Limb**

REVIEW EXERCISE A: Radiographic Anatomy of the Foot and Ankle (see textbook pp. 212–217)

1. Fill in the number of bones for the following:

   A. Phalanges _____

   B. Metatarsals _____

   C. Tarsals _____

   D. Total _____

2. What are two differences in the phalanges of the foot as compared to the phalanges of the hand?

   A. _____

   B. _____

3. Which tuberosity of the foot is palpable and is a common site of fracture?

4. Where are the sesamoid bones of the foot most commonly located? _____

5. What is the largest and strongest tarsal bone? _____

6. What is the name of the joint found between the talus and the calcaneus? _____

7. List the three specific articular facets found in the joint described in the previous question.

   A. _____

   B. _____

   C. _____

8. The small opening, or space, found in the middle of the joint identified in question 6 is called the _____
   _____.

9. Match each of the following characteristics to the correct tarsal bone. (Answers may be used more than once.)

   _____ 1. Forms an aspect of the ankle joint

   _____ 2. The smallest of the cuneiforms

   _____ 3. Found on the medial side of the foot between the talus and the three cuneiforms

   _____ 4. The largest of the cuneiforms

   _____ 5. Articulates with the second, third, and fourth metatarsal

   _____ 6. The most superior tarsal bone

   _____ 7. Articulates with the first metatarsal

   _____ 8. Common site for bone spurs

   _____ 9. A tarsal found anterior to the calcaneus and lateral to the lateral (third) cuneiform

   _____ 10. The second largest tarsal bone

   A. Calcaneus

   B. Talus

   C. Cuboid

   D. Navicular

   E. Lateral (third) cuneiform

   F. Intermediate (second) cuneiform

   G. Medial (first) cuneiform

10. Identify the labeled structures found in Figs. 6.1 and 6.2.

A. _____

B. _____

C. _____

D. _____

E. _____

F. _____

G. _____

H. _____

I. _____

J. _____

K. _____

L. _____

M. Fig. 6.1 represents a radiograph of which projection of the foot?

_____

N. _____

O. _____

P. _____

Q. _____

R. _____

S. _____

T. Fig. 6.2 represents a radiograph of which projection?

_____

11. True/False: The cuboid articulates with the four bones of the foot.

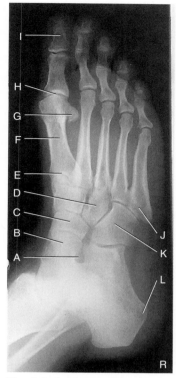

Fig. 6.1 Anatomy of the foot.

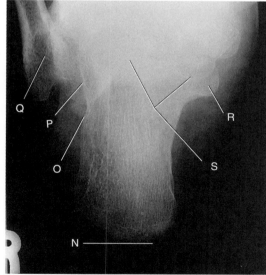

Fig. 6.2 Anatomy of the foot.

12. The calcaneus articulates with the talus and the:

    A. Navicular

    C. Medial (first) cuneiform

    B. Cuboid

    D. Lateral (third) cuneiform

13. List the two arches of the foot.

    A. _____

    B. _____

14. Which large tendon attaches to the tuberosity of the calcaneus?

    _____.

15. Which three bones make up the ankle joint?

    A. _____

    B. _____

    C. _____

16. The three bones of the ankle form a deep socket into which the talus fits. This socket is called the

    _____.

17. The distal tibial joint surface forming the roof of the distal ankle joint is called the:

    A. Tibial plafond

    C. Tibial plateau

    B. Articular facet

    D. Ankle mortise

18. True/False: The medial malleolus is approximately one-half inch (1 cm) posterior to the lateral malleolus.

19. The ankle joint is classified as a synovial joint with _____-type movement.

20. Identify the structures labeled in Figs. 6.3 and 6.4.

    Fig. 6.3

    A. _____

    B. _____

    C. _____

    D. _____

    E. _____

    Fig. 6.4

    F. _____

    G. _____

    H. _____

    I. _____

    J. _____

    K. _____

    L. _____

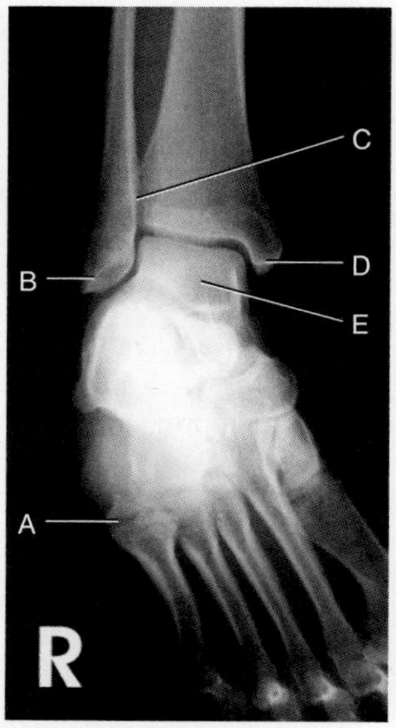

Fig. 6.3 Anatomy of the ankle.

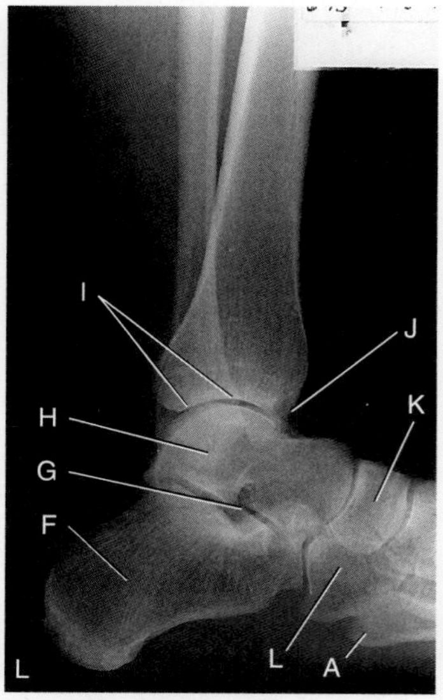

Fig. 6.4 Anatomy of the ankle.

    M. Fig. 6.3 represents a radiograph of which projection of the ankle?

REVIEW EXERCISE B: Radiographic Anatomy of the Lower Leg, Knee, and Distal Femur (see textbook pp. 218–223)

1. The _____ is the weight-bearing bone of the lower leg.

2. What is the name of the large prominence located on the mid-anterior surface of the proximal tibia that serves as a distal attachment for the patellar tendon? _____

3. What is the name of the small prominence located on the posterolateral aspect of the medial condyle of the femur that is an identifying landmark to determine possible rotation of a lateral knee? _____

4. A small, triangular depression located on the tibia that helps form the distal tibiofibular joint is called the

   _____.

5. The articular facets of the proximal tibia are also referred to as the _____.

6. The articular facets slope _____ degrees posteriorly in relation to the long axis of the tibia.
   A. 25   C. 35
   B. 45   D. 10–20

7. The most proximal aspect of the fibula is the _____.

8. The extreme distal end of the fibula forms the _____.

9. What is the name of the largest sesamoid bone in the body?

10. What are two other names for the patellar surface of the femur?
    A. _____   B. _____

11. What is the name of the depression located on the posterior aspect of the distal femur? _____

12. Why must the central ray be angled 5–7 degrees cephalad for a lateral knee position? _____

13. The slightly raised area located on the posterolateral aspect of the medial femoral condyle is called the:
    A. Trochlear tubercle   C. Adductor tubercle
    B. Anterior crest   D. Tibial tuberosity

14. What are the two palpable bony landmarks found on the distal femur?
    A. _____   B. _____

15. The general region of the posterior knee is called the _____.

16. True/False: A 20-degree flexion of the knee forces the patella firmly against the patellar surface of the femur.

17. True/False: The patella acts as a pivot to increase the leverage of a large muscle found in the anterior thigh.

18. True/False: The posterior surface of the patella is normally rough.

19. For which large muscle does the patella serve as a pivot to increase the leverage?

_____.

20. List the correct terms for the following joints:

A. Between the patella and distal femur _____

B. Between the two condyles of the femur and tibia _____

21. List the four major ligaments of the knee.

A. _____   C. _____

B. _____   D. _____

22. The crescent-shaped fibrocartilage disks that act as shock absorbers in the knee joint are called _____.

23. List the two bursae found in the knee joint.

A. _____   B. _____

24. Match each of the following structures to the correct bone. (Answers may be used more than once.)

_____ 1. Tibial plafond   A. Tibia

_____ 2. Medial malleolus   B. Fibula

_____ 3. Lateral epicondyle   C. Distal femur

_____ 4. Patellar surface   D. Patella

_____ 5. Articular facets

_____ 6. Fibular notch

_____ 7. Styloid process

_____ 8. Base

_____ 9. Intercondyloid eminence

_____ 10. Neck

138

Chapter **6 Lower Limb**

Copyright © 2025 by Elsevier Inc.
All rights are reserved, including those for text and data mining, AI training, and similar technologies.

25. Match each of the following articulations to the correct joint classification or movement type. (Answers may be used more than once.)

_____ 1. Ankle joint

_____ 2. Patellofemoral

_____ 3. Proximal tibiofibular

_____ 4. Tarsometatarsal

_____ 5. Knee joint (femorotibial)

_____ 6. Distal tibiofibular

A. Synarthrodial (gomphoses type)

B. Ginglymus (hinge)

C. Saddle (sellar)

D. Plane (gliding)

E. Amphiarthrodial (syndesmosis type)

F. Bicondylar

26. Identify the labeled structures in Figs. 6.5–6.7.

Fig. 6.5

A. _____

B. _____

C. _____

D. _____

E. _____

F. _____

G. _____

H. _____

I. _____

Fig. 6.6

J. _____

K. _____

L. _____

M. _____

N. _____

O. _____ (-degree angle)

P. _____

Q. _____

R. _____

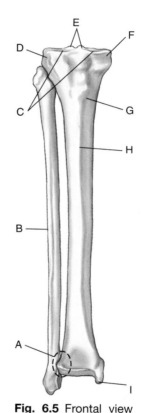

Fig. 6.5 Frontal view of tibia and fibula.

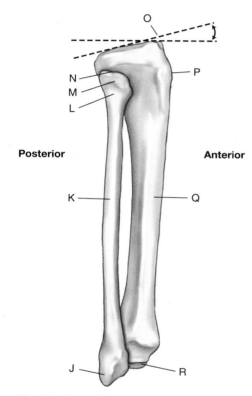

Posterior

Anterior

Fig. 6.6 Lateral view of tibia and fibula.

Fig. 6.7

S. _____

T. _____

U. _____

V. _____

W. _____

X. Which projection does the radiograph in

  Fig. 6.7 represent? _____

27. Identify the bony structures labeled in Figs. 6.8 and 6.9.

Fig. 6.8

A. _____

B. _____

C. _____

D. _____

E. _____

F. _____

G. _____

H. _____

Fig. 6.9

I. _____

J. _____

K. _____

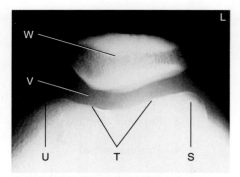

Fig. 6.7 Anatomy of the knee and patella.

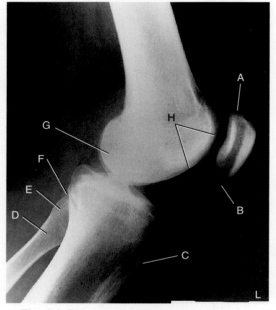

Fig. 6.8 True lateral radiograph of the knee.

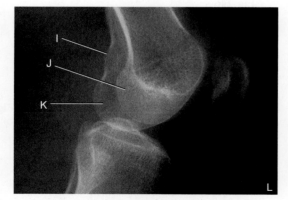

Fig. 6.9 Lateral radiograph of the knee.

28. Match the following foot and ankle movements to the correct definition.

_____A. Inward turning or bending of ankle

_____B. Decreasing the angle between the dorsum pedis and the anterior lower leg

_____C. Extending the ankle or pointing the foot and toe downward

_____D. Outward turning or bending of ankle

1. Inversion (varus)

2. Plantar flexion

3. Eversion (valgus)

4. Dorsiflexion

PART II: RADIOGRAPHIC POSITIONING

REVIEW EXERCISE C: Positioning of the Foot and Ankle (see textbook pp. 224–244)

1. True/False: The recommended source image receptor distance (SID) for lower limb radiography is 40 inches (100 cm).

2. True/False: The use of a grid for foot and ankle studies is required.

3. True/False: With digital imaging, multiple exposures on the same imaging are not suggested.

4. True/False: With digital radiography, it is recommended that the anatomy should be centered to the IR.

5. True/False: A kVp range between 50 to 55 should be used for knee radiography.

6. True/False: Technologists should hold pediatric patients rather than use immobilization devices to reduce repeat projections.

7. True/False: It is recommended that bariatric patients be allowed to wear pants for lower limb radiography.

8. Match the following clinical indications to the correct definition.

_____A. An inflammatory condition involving the anterior, proximal tibia

_____B. Also known as osteitis deformans

_____C. Malignant tumor of the cartilage

_____D. Inherited type of arthritis that commonly affects males

_____E. Benign, neoplastic bone lesion caused by overproduction of bone at a joint

_____F. Benign bone lesion usually developing in teens or young adults

_____G. Most prevalent primary bone malignancy in pediatric patients

_____H. Benign, neoplastic bone lesion filled with clear fluid

_____I. Injury to a large ligament located between the bases of the first and second metatarsal

_____J. Condition affecting the sacroiliac joints and lower limbs of young men, especially the posterosuperior margin of the calcaneus

1. Exostosis

2. Lisfranc joint injury

3. Bone cyst

4. Reiter syndrome

5. Osteoid osteoma

6. Ewing sarcoma

7. Gout

8. Paget disease

9. Osgood-Schlatter disease

10. Chondrosarcoma

9. The formal name for "runner's knee" is _____.

10. What is another term for osteomalacia? _____

11. Match the following radiographic appearances to the correct clinical indication.

_____   A. Asymmetric erosion of joint spaces with calcaneal erosion   1. Osteoid osteoma

_____   B. Uric acid deposits in joint spaces   2. Ewing sarcoma

_____   C. Well-circumscribed lucency   3. Gout

_____   D. Small, round/oval density with lucent center   4. Osgood-Schlatter disease

_____   E. Narrowed, irregular joint surfaces with sclerotic articular surfaces   5. Osteoarthritis

_____   F. Fragmentation or detachment of the tibial tuberosity   6. Osteomalacia

_____   G. Ill-defined area of bone destruction with surrounding "onion peel"   7. Reiter syndrome

_____   H. Decreased bone density and bowing deformities of weight-bearing   8. Bone cyst
limbs

12. A Lisfranc injury involves the:

A. Foot   C. Calcaneus

B. Ankle   D. Distal femur

13. Why is the central ray angled 10–15 degrees toward the calcaneus for an anteroposterior (AP) projection of the toes?

_____

14. Where is the central ray centered for an AP oblique projection of the foot? _____

15. Which projection is best for demonstrating the sesamoid bones of the foot? _____

16. The foot should be dorsiflexed so that the plantar surface of the foot is _____ degrees from vertical for the sesamoid projection.

17. Why should the central ray be perpendicular to the metatarsals for an AP projection of the foot?

_____.

18. True/False: A foot with a high, anterior arch may require an increase of CR to 15 degrees posteriorly.

19. Rotation can be determined on a radiograph of an AP foot projection by the near-equal distance between the

_____ metatarsals.

20. Which oblique projection of the foot best demonstrates the majority of the tarsal bones?

_____.

21. Which oblique projection of the foot best demonstrates the navicular and the first and second cuneiforms with minimal superimposition?

_____.

22. Which projection places the foot into a more natural, true lateral position: mediolateral or lateromedial?

    _____.

23. Which type of study should be performed to best evaluate the status of the longitudinal arches of the foot?

    _____.

24. How should the central ray be angled from the long axis of the foot for the plantodorsal (axial) projection of the

    calcaneus? _____

25. Where is the central ray directed for a dorsoplantar (axial) weight-bearing projection of the calcaneus?

    _____   _____

26. Where is the central ray placed for a mediolateral projection of the calcaneus?

    _____.

27. Which joint surface of the ankle is not typically visualized with a correctly positioned AP projection of the ankle?

    A. Medial aspect of joint   C. Lateral aspect of joint

    B. Superior aspect of joint   D. All of the listed aspects of the joint are visualized.

28. Why should AP, 45-degree oblique, and lateral ankle radiographs include the proximal metatarsals?

    _____.

29. How much (if any) should the foot and ankle be rotated for an AP mortise projection of the ankle?

    _____.

30. Which positioning line or plane is parallel to IR for an AP mortise projection of the ankle?

    _____.

31. Which projection of the ankle best demonstrates a possible fracture of the lateral malleolus and the base of the fifth metatarsal?

32. With a true lateral projection of the ankle, the lateral malleolus is:

    A. Projected over the anterior aspect of the distal tibia

    B. Projected over the posterior aspect of the distal tibia

    C. Directly superimposed over the distal tibia

    D. Directly superimposed over the medial malleolus

33. Which projections of the ankle require forced inversion and eversion movements?

34. True/False: The AP stress projections are performed to demonstrate stress fractures of the distal fibula.

35. True/False: The AP stress projections of the ankle must have a physician or health care professional stress the ankle during exposures.

REVIEW EXERCISE D: Positioning of the Tibia, Fibula, Knee, and Distal Femur (see textbook pp. 245–262)

1. What is the basic positioning routine for a study of the tibia and fibula?

   _____.

2. Why is it important to include the knee joint for an initial study of tibia trauma, even if the patient's symptoms involve the middle and distal aspect?

   _____

3. To include both joints for a lateral projection of the tibia and fibula for an adult, the technologist may place the IR _____ in relation to the part.

   A. Parallel   C. Diagonal

   B. Perpendicular   D. Transverse

4. What is the recommended central-ray angulation for an AP projection of the knee when the ASIS to table distance is greater than 24 cm (9.5 inches)?

   A. 3–5 degrees caudad   C. Central ray perpendicular to IR

   B. 3–5 degrees cephalad   D. Central ray perpendicular to patellar plane

5. Where is the central ray centered for an AP projection of the knee?

   A. 0.5 inch (1.25 cm) distal to apex of patella   C. Midpatella

   B. 1 inch (2.5 cm) proximal to apex of patella   D. Level of tibial tuberosity

6. Which basic projection of a knee best demonstrates the proximal fibula free of superimposition?

   A. True AP   C. AP oblique, 45-degree medial rotation

   B. True lateral   D. AP oblique, 45-degree lateral rotation

7. For the AP oblique projection of the knee, the _____ rotation (medial [internal] or lateral [external]) best visualizes the lateral condyle of the tibia and the head and neck of the fibula.

8. What is the recommended central-ray placement for a lateral knee position on a tall, slender male patient with a narrow pelvis (without support of the lower leg)?

   A. 5–10 degrees caudad   C. Central ray perpendicular to IR

   B. 5 degrees cephalad   D. Central ray perpendicular to patellar plane

9. How much flexion is recommended for a lateral projection of the knee to best demonstrate the patellofemoral joint space?

   A. No flexion   C. 30–35 degrees

   B. 20–30 degrees   D. 45 degrees

10. Which positioning error(s) is (are) present if the distal borders of the femoral condyles are not superimposed on a radiograph of a lateral knee on an average-sized knee? (More than one answer possible.) _____

11. Which positioning error is present if the posterior portions of the femoral condyles are not superimposed on a mediolateral knee radiograph? _____

12. Which anatomic structure on the posterior femur can be used to determine if a rotation error (overrotation or underrotation) is present on a lateral knee radiograph?

    _____.

13. Which special projection of the knee is best to evaluate the knee joint for cartilage degeneration or deformities?

    _____.

14. What is the best modality to examine ligament injuries to the knee?

    A. CT

    B. Nuclear medicine

    C. MR

    D. Diagnostic medical sonography (DMS)

15. Which of the following special projections of the knee best demonstrates the intercondylar fossa?

    A. Holmblad method

    B. Merchant method

    C. AP weight-bearing, bilateral projections

    D. Settegast method

16. How much flexion of the lower leg is required for the PA axial projection (Camp Coventry method) when the central ray is angled at 40 degrees caudad? _____

17. Why are posteroanterior (PA) axial projections for the intercondylar fossa recommended instead of AP axial projections (Béclere method)?

18. What type of CR angulation is required for the PA axial weight-bearing projection (Rosenberg method)?

    A. None. CR is perpendicular

    B. 10 degrees caudad

    C. 10 degrees cephalad

    D. 5–7 degrees cephalad

19. How much flexion of the knees is required for the PA axial weight-bearing projection (Rosenberg method)?

    A. 20–30 degrees

    B. 35–40 degrees

    C. 5–10 degrees

    D. 45 degrees

20. How much knee flexion is required for the PA axial projection (Holmblad method)?

    A. 45 degrees

    B. 35 degrees

    C. 60–70 degrees

    D. None. Lower limb is fully extended

21. What type of CR angle is required for the PA projection (Holmblad method)?

    A. 10 degrees caudad

    B. 10 degrees cephalad

    C. 15–20 degrees cephalad

    D. None. CR is perpendicular to IR

22. True/False: To place the interepicondylar line parallel to the IR for a PA projection of the patella, the lower limb must be rotated approximately 5 degrees internally.

    _____.

23. How much flexion of the knee is recommended for a lateral projection of the patella?

    _____.

24. How much central ray angle from the long axis of the femora is required for the tangential (Merchant method) bilateral projection? _____

25. How much part flexion is required for the following methods?

    A. Hughston method _____

    B. Settegast method _____

26. What type of CR angle is required for the superoinferior sitting tangential method for the patella?

    A. 40 degrees cephalad   C. Depends on degree of flexion

    B. 5–10 degrees caudad   D. None. CR is perpendicular to IR

27. Match each of the following descriptions of positioning for projections of the knee and/or patella to its correct name or term. (Use each answer only once.)

    _____1. Can be performed using a wheelchair or lowered radio-graphic table

    _____2. Patient prone; requires 90-degree knee flexion

    _____3. Patient prone with 40- to 50-degree knee flexion and equal 40- to 50-degree caudad CR angle

    _____4. IR is placed on a footstool to minimize the OID

    _____5. Patient prone with 55-degree knee flexion and 45-degree cephalic CR angle

    _____6. Patient supine with cassette resting on midthighs

    _____7. Patient supine with 40-degree knee flexion and 30-degree caudad CR angle from horizontal

    A. Inferosuperior for patellofemoral joint

    B. Merchant method

    C. Hughston method

    D. Camp Coventry method

    E. Settegast method

    F. Holmblad method (variation)

    G. Hobbs modification

28. Which of the following special projections of the knee must be performed erect?

    A. Rosenberg method   C. Settegast method

    B. Camp Coventry method   D. Hughston method

29. True/False: The recommended SID is 48 inches (120 cm) to 72 inches (180 cm) for the tangential (bilateral Merchant) projection.

30. How much knee flexion is required for the horizontal beam lateral patella projection?

    A. 5 or 10 degrees   C. 25 or 30 degrees

    B. 15–20 degrees   D. None

REVIEW EXERCISE E: Problem Solving for Technical and Positioning Errors

1. **Situation:** A radiograph of an AP projection of the foot shows that the metatarsophalangeal joints are not open and the metatarsals are somewhat foreshortened. But there is equal spacing between the mid metatarsals. What positioning error was involved, and what modification should be made to improve this image on the repeat exposure?

    _____

2. **Situation:** A radiograph of an AP oblique–medial rotation projection of the foot shows that the proximal third to fifth metatarsals are superimposed. What type of positioning error led to this radiographic outcome?

    _____

3. **Situation:** A radiograph of a plantodorsal (axial) projection of the calcaneus shows considerable foreshortening of the calcaneus. What type of positioning modification is needed on the repeat exposure?

    _____

4. **Situation:** A radiograph of an AP projection of the ankle shows that the lateral surface of the ankle joint is totally open. (It should not be open on a true AP projection.) The technologist is positive that the ankle was in the correct, true AP position with the long axis of the foot perpendicular to the IR. What else could have led to this joint space being open?

_____

5. **Situation:** A radiograph of an intended AP mortise projection shows that the lateral malleolus is superimposed over the talus, and the distal tibiofibular joint is not well demonstrated. What is the most likely reason for this radiographic outcome?

_____

6. **Situation:** A radiograph of an AP knee projection demonstrates that the femorotibial joint space is not open at all. The patient is young and has no history of degenerative disease. What type of positioning modification may improve the outcome of this projection?

_____

7. **Situation:** A radiograph of an AP oblique with medial rotation of the knee to demonstrate the proximal fibula shows that there is total superimposition of the proximal tibia and the fibula. What must be modified to correct this projection?

_____

8. **Situation:** A radiograph of a lateral recumbent knee shows that the posterior border of the medial femoral condyle (identified by the adductor tubercle) is not superimposed but is slightly posterior to the lateral condyle. The fibular head is also completely superimposed by the tibia. What type of positioning error led to this radiographic outcome?

_____

9. **Situation:** A patient with trauma to the medial aspect of the foot comes to the emergency room. A heavy object was dropped on the foot near the base of the first metatarsal. Basic foot projections do not clearly demonstrate this region. What other projection of the foot could be used to delineate this area better?

_____

10. **Situation:** A radiograph of an AP and lateral tibia and fibula shows that the ankle joint is not included on the AP projection, but both the knee and the ankle are included on the lateral projection. What should the technologist do in this situation?

_____

11. **Situation:** A radiograph obtained by using the PA axial (Camp Coventry method) shows that the distal femoral condyles, articular facets, and intercondylar fossa are asymmetric. What possible positioning errors might have produced this distortion of the anatomy?

_____

12. **Situation:** A radiograph of a lateral patella shows that the patella is drawn tightly against the intercondylar sulcus. Which positioning modification should be performed to improve the quality of the image during the repeat exposure?

_____

13. **Situation:** A patient with a history of degenerative disease of the left knee joint comes to the radiology department. The orthopedic surgeon orders a radiographic study to determine the extent of damage to the joint space. Which projection(s) should be performed?

_____

14. **Situation:** A patient with a possible Lisfranc joint injury comes to the radiology department. Which radiographic position(s) best demonstrate(s) this type of injury?

_____

15. **Situation:** A patient with a history of pain in the feet comes to the radiology department. The referring physician orders a study to evaluate the longitudinal arches of the feet. Which positioning routine should be used?

_____

16. **Situation:** A patient with bony, loose bodies (or "joint mice") within the knee joint comes to radiology for a knee series. The AP and lateral knee projections fail to demonstrate any loose bodies. What additional knee projection can be taken to better demonstrate them?

_____

17. **Situation:** A young male patient comes to the radiology department with a clinical history of Osgood-Schlatter disease. Which single projection of the basic knee series will best demonstrate this condition?

_____

18. **Situation:** A radiograph of a mediolateral knee projection demonstrates that the medial femoral condyle is projected inferior to the lateral condyle. What can the technologist do to correct this problem during the repeat exposure?

_____

19. **Situation:** A physician orders a bilateral, tangential projection of the patella and patellofemoral joint space. But the patient is restricted to a wheelchair and cannot lie on the radiographic table because of chronic pain. Which projection could be performed with the patient remaining in the wheelchair?

_____

20. **Situation:** A tangential (inferosuperior) projection of the patellofemoral joint space shows that the patella is seated into the intercondylar sulcus and the joint space is not demonstrated. What possible positioning errors might have produced this radiographic outcome?

_____

REVIEW EXERCISE F: Critique Radiographs of the Lower Limbs

The following questions relate to the radiographs found in this exercise. Evaluate these radiographs for the radiographic criteria categories (1 through 5) that follow. Describe the corrections needed to improve the overall image. The major, or "repeatable," errors are specific errors that indicate the need for a repeat exposure, regardless of the nature of the other errors.

Comparing these radiographs with the correctly positioned and exposed radiographs in this chapter of the textbook will help you evaluate each of them for errors.

A. Bilateral tangential patella (Fig. 6.10)

Description of possible error:

    1. Anatomy demonstrated:

    _____

    2. Part positioning:

    _____

    3. Collimation field size and central ray:

    _____

    4. Exposure:

    _____

    5. Anatomic side markers:

    _____

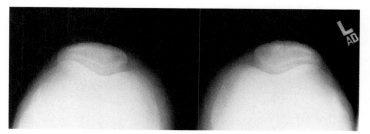

Fig. 6.10 Bilateral tangential patella.

Repeatable error(s): _____

B. Plantodorsal (axial) calcaneus (Fig. 6.11)

Description of possible error:

    1. Anatomy demonstrated:

    _____

    2. Part positioning:

    _____

    3. Collimation field size and CR:

    _____

    4. Exposure:

    _____

    5. Anatomic side markers:

    _____

Repeatable error(s): _____

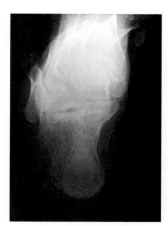

Fig. 6.11 Plantodorsal (axial) calcaneus.

C. AP mortise ankle (Fig. 6.12)

Description of possible error:

1. Anatomy demonstrated:

   _____

2. Part positioning:

   _____

3. Collimation field size and CR:

   _____

4. Exposure:

   _____

5. Anatomic side markers:

   _____

Repeatable error(s): _____

D. AP lower leg (Fig. 6.13)

Description of possible error:

1. Anatomy demonstrated:

   _____

2. Part positioning:

   _____

3. Collimation field size and central ray:

   _____

4. Exposure:

   _____

5. Anatomic side markers:

   _____

Repeatable error(s): _____

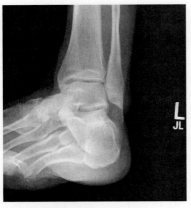

Fig. 6.12 Anteroposterior mortise ankle.

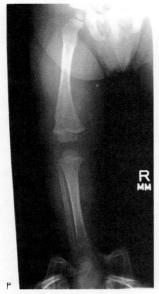

Fig. 6.13 Anteroposterior lower leg (pediatric).

E. Mediolateral knee (Fig. 6.14)

Description of possible error:

    1. Anatomy demonstrated:

    _____

    2. Part positioning:

    _____

    3. Collimation field size and central ray:

    _____

    4. Exposure:

    _____

    5. Anatomic side markers:

    _____

Repeatable error(s): _____

F. AP medial oblique knee (Fig. 6.15)

Description of possible error:

    1. Anatomy demonstrated:

    _____

    2. Part positioning:

    _____

    3. Collimation field size and central ray:

    _____

    4. Exposure:

    _____

    5. Anatomic side markers:

    _____

Repeatable error(s): _____

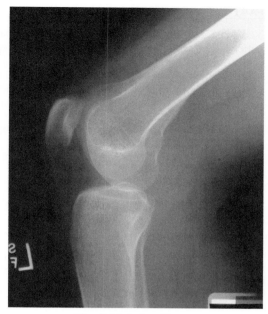

Fig. 6.14 Lateral knee.

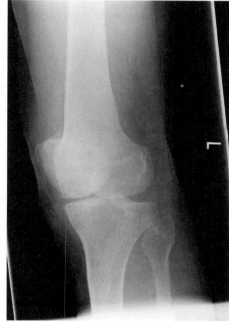

Fig. 6.15 Anteroposterior medial oblique knee.

151

PART III: LABORATORY ACTIVITIES

You must gain experience in positioning each part of the lower limb before performing the following exams on actual patients. You can obtain experience in positioning and radiographic evaluation of these projections by performing exercises using radiographic phantoms and practicing on other students (although you will not be taking actual exposures).

The following suggested activities assume that your teaching institution has an energized lab and radiographic phantoms. If not, perform Laboratory Exercises B and C, the radiographic evaluation and the physical positioning exercises. (Check off each step and projection as you complete it.)

Laboratory Exercise A: Energized Laboratory

1. Using the foot/ankle radiographic phantom, produce radiographs of the basic routines for the following:

   _____ Foot

   _____ Ankle

   _____ Calcaneus

2. Using the knee radiographic phantom, produce radiographs of the following basic routines:

   _____ AP

   _____ AP oblique, medial rotation

   _____ Lateral (horizontal beam lateral if flexed knee is not available)

Laboratory Exercise B: Radiographic Evaluation

1. Evaluate and critique the radiographs produced in the preceding, additional radiographs provided by your instructor, or both. Evaluate each radiograph for the following points:

   _____ Evaluate the completeness of the study. (Are all of the pertinent anatomic structures included on the radiograph?)

   _____ Evaluate for positioning or centering errors (e.g., rotation, off centering).

   _____ Evaluate for correct exposure factors and possible motion. (Are the density and contrast of the images acceptable?)

   _____ Determine whether anatomic side markers and an acceptable degree of collimation are seen on the images.

Laboratory Exercise C: Physical Positioning

On another person, simulate performing all basic and special projections of the lower limb as follows. Include the six steps listed here and described in the textbook. (Check off each step when completed satisfactorily.)

Step 1. Appropriate recommended field size with correct markers

Step 2. Correct central-ray placement and centering of part to central ray and/or IR

Step 3. Accurate collimation

Step 4. Area shielding of patient when required

Step 5. Use of proper immobilizing devices when needed

Step 6. Approximate correct exposure factors, breathing instructions where applicable, and "making" exposure

Projections	*Step 1*	*Step 2*	*Step 3*	*Step 4*	*Step 5*	*Step 6*
• Positioning routine for a specific toe	_____	_____	_____	_____	_____	_____
• Basic foot routine	_____	_____	_____	_____	_____	_____
• Special projection for sesamoid bones	_____	_____	_____	_____	_____	_____
• Basic projections of the calcaneus including weight-bearing	_____	_____	_____	_____	_____	_____
• Weight-bearing foot projections	_____	_____	_____	_____	_____	_____
• Basic ankle routine, including mortise and 45-degree oblique projections	_____	_____	_____	_____	_____	_____
• AP and lateral tibia and fibula	_____	_____	_____	_____	_____	_____
• Basic knee routine	_____	_____	_____	_____	_____	_____
• Special projections for intercondylar fossa	_____	_____	_____	_____	_____	_____
• Weight-bearing AP knee projections	_____	_____	_____	_____	_____	_____
• Special projections for patellofemoral joint space	_____	_____	_____	_____	_____	_____

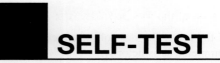

SELF-TEST

This self-test should be taken only after completing all of the readings, review exercises, and laboratory activities for a particular section. The purpose of this test is not only to provide a good learning exercise but also to serve as a strong indicator of what your final evaluation exam will be. It is strongly suggested that if you do not get at least a 90%–95% grade on this self-test, you should review those areas in which you missed questions before going to your instructor for the final evaluation exam for this chapter.

1. Which of the following is not an aspect of the metatarsal?

   A. Head

   B. Tail

   C. Body

   D. Base

2. True/False: The distal portion of the fifth metatarsal is a common fracture site.

3. Where are the sesamoid bones of the foot most commonly located?

   A. Plantar surface near head of first metatarsal

   B. Plantar surface at first tarsometatarsal joint

   C. Dorsum aspect near base of first metatarsal

   D. Plantar surface near cuboid bone

4. What is the name of the tarsal bone found on the medial side of the foot between the talus and three cuneiforms?

   A. Calcaneus

   B. Lateral malleolus

   C. Cuboid

   D. Navicular

5. Which is considered the smallest tarsal bone?

   A. Medial cuneiform

   B. Navicular

   C. Intermediate cuneiform

   D. Lateral cuneiform

6. What is another term for the talocalcaneal joint?

   A. Tarsometatarsal joint

   B. Subtalar joint

   C. Mortise joint

   D. Tibiocalcaneal joint

7. The distal tibial joint surface is called the:

   A. Medial malleolus

   B. Tibial plafond

   C. Lateral malleolus

   D. Anterior tubercle

8. True/False: The mortise of the ankle should be totally open and visible on a correctly positioned AP projection of the ankle.

9. Match each of the following structures or characteristics to the correct bone of the foot or ankle. (Use each choice only once.)

_____1. Trochlear process

_____2. Lateral malleolus

_____3. The second largest tarsal bone

_____4. Found between the navicular and base of first metatarsal

_____5. Base

_____6. Found between the calcaneus and talus

_____7. Anterior tubercle

A. Metatarsal

B. Talus

C. Tibia

D. Calcaneus

E. Sinus tarsi

F. Medial cuneiform

G. Fibula

10. Match the structures labeled in Fig. 6.16. (Use each choice only once.)

_____A.   1. Talus

_____B.   2. First metatarsal

_____C.   3. Lateral malleolus

_____D.   4. Distal tibiofibular joint

_____E.   5. Medial malleolus

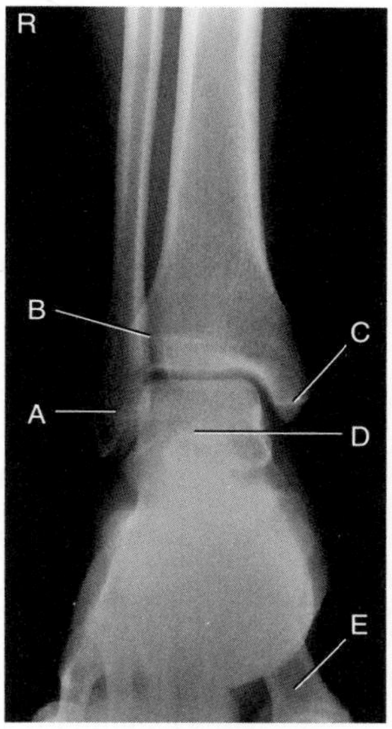

Fig. 6.16 Anatomy of the ankle.

11. What projection does Fig. 6.16 represent?

A. AP mortise ankle

B. AP stress ankle–inversion

C. AP ankle

D. AP stress ankle–eversion

12. Match the structures labeled on the radiographs in Figs. 6.17–6.19. (Answers may be used more than once.)

_____A.

_____B.

_____C.

_____D.

_____E.

_____F.

_____G.

_____H.

_____I.

_____J.

_____K.

1. Distal phalanx, second digit

2. Proximal phalanx, first digit

3. Interphalangeal joint

4. Head of second metatarsal

5. Metatarsophalangeal joint of first digit

6. Base of first metatarsal

7. Proximal phalanx, second digit

8. Head of first metatarsal

9. Distal phalanx, first digit

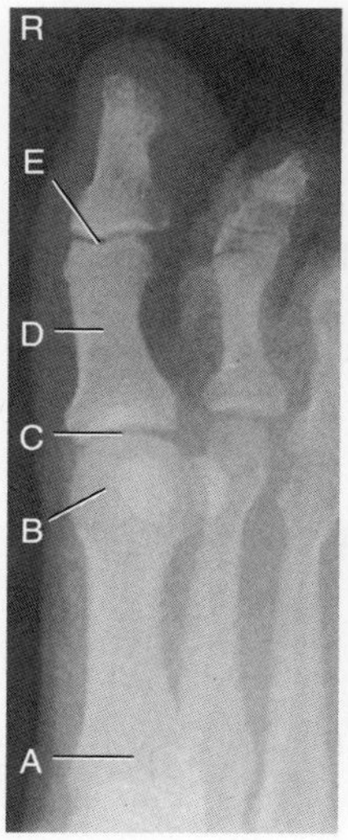

Fig. 6.17 Anatomy of the metatarsal bones and digits.

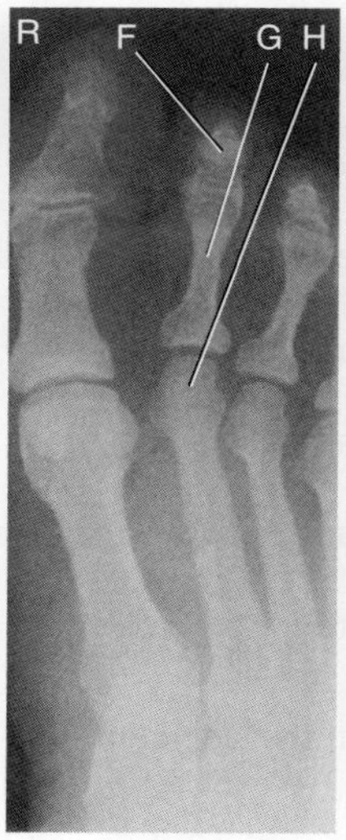

Fig. 6.18 Anatomy of the metatarsal bones and digits.

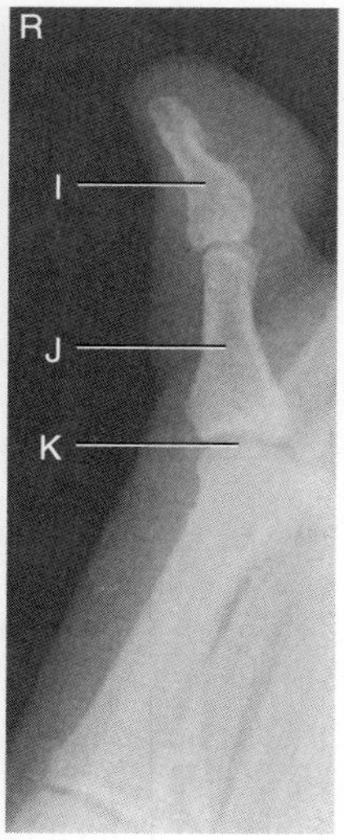

Fig. 6.19 Anatomy of the metatarsal bones and digits.

13. Which of the radiographs in the previous question represents an AP oblique projection of the toes?

A. Fig. 6.17

B. Fig. 6.19

C. Fig. 6.18

D. None of the above

14. What is the correct central-ray centering placement for an AP projection of the toes?

A. Affected metatarsophalangeal joint

B. Affected distal interphalangeal joint

C. Affected proximal interphalangeal joint

D. Head of affected metatarsal

15. Which type of central-ray angle is required for an AP projection of the toes?

A. None (central ray is perpendicular)

B. 10- to 15-degree posterior

C. 5-degree posterior

D. 20- to 25-degree posterior

16. Which of the following projections is used for the sesamoid bones of the foot?

A. AP and lateral weight-bearing

B. Camp Coventry

C. Tangential

D. AP mortise

17. How much foot rotation is required for the AP oblique, medial rotation projection of the foot?

A. 3–5 degrees

B. 45 degrees

C. 15–20 degrees

D. 30–40 degrees

18. What is another term for the AP projection of the foot?

    A. Mortise projection

    B. Plantodorsal (axial) projection

    C. Weight-bearing study

    D. Dorsoplantar projection

19. What CR angle is generally required for the AP projection of the foot?

    A. 10-degree posterior

    B. 10-degree anterior

    C. 15-degree posterior

    D. None (central ray is perpendicular)

20. Which projection of the foot best demonstrates the cuboid?

    A. AP

    B. AP oblique–lateral rotation

    C. AP oblique–medial rotation

    D. Lateromedial

21. What is another term for the intercondyloid eminence?

    A. Tibial plateaus

    B. Intercondylar fossa

    C. Tibial tuberosity

    D. Intercondylar tubercles

22. What is the name of the deep depression found on the posterior aspect of the distal femur?

    A. Intercondylar fossa

    B. Intercondylar sulcus

    C. Patellar surface

    D. Articular facets

23. A line drawn across the most distal aspect of the medial and lateral femoral condyles would be _____ from being at a right angle (90 degrees) to the long axis of the femur.

    A. 5–7 degrees

    B. 3–5 degrees

    C. 0 degree

    D. 10–20 degrees

24. True/False: The angle referred to in question #23 would be less on a tall, slender person.

25. The upper, or superior, portion of the patella is called the:

    A. Apex

    B. Base

    C. Styloid process

    D. Patellar head

26. Which two ligaments of the knee joint help stabilize the knee from the anterior and posterior perspective?

    A. Collaterals

    B. Patellar

    C. Cruciates

    D. Quadriceps femoris

27. Which structures serve as shock absorbers within the knee joint?

    A. Articular facets

    B. Infrapatellar and suprapatellar bursae

    C. Menisci

    D. Infrapatellar fat pads

28. Match the structures labeled in Figs. 6.20 and 6.21. (Use each choice only once.)

_____A.   1. Medial condyle of tibia

_____B.   2. Neck of fibula

_____C.   3. Head of fibula

_____D.   4. Articular facets

_____E.   5. Patella

_____F.   6. Lateral condyle of femur

_____G.   7. Proximal tibiofibular joint

_____H.   8. Intercondyloid eminence

_____I.   9. Femorotibial joint space

_____J.   10. Lateral condyle of tibia

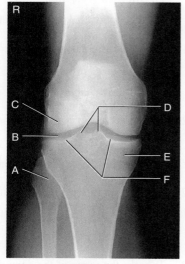

Fig. 6.20 Anteroposterior radiograph of the knee.

29. Which knee projection does Fig. 6.21 represent?

A. AP

B. AP oblique–medial rotation

C. AP oblique–lateral rotation

D. AP weight-bearing

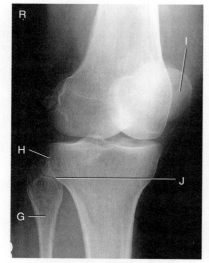

Fig. 6.21 Radiograph of the knee.

30. Match the parts labeled in Figs. 6.22 and 6.23. (Answers may be used more than once.)

_____A.

_____B.

_____C.

_____D.

_____E.

_____F.

_____G.

_____H.

_____I.

_____J.

1. Adductor tubercle

2. Head of fibula

3. Medial femoral condyle

4. Anterior aspect of medial condyle

5. Lateral femoral condyle

6. Anterior aspect of lateral femoral condyle

7. Tibial tuberosity

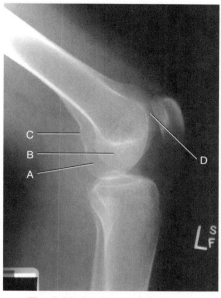

Fig. 6.22 Anatomy of the knee.

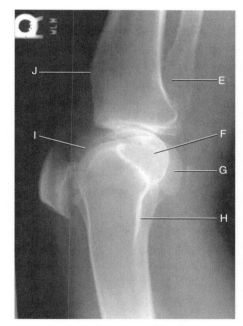

Fig. 6.23 Anatomy of the knee.

31. What is the primary positioning error present in Fig. 6.22 (mediolateral projection)?

    A. Overangulation of central ray
          C. Overrotation of knee toward IR

    B. Underrotation of knee toward IR
        D. Underangulation of central ray

32. True/False: The mediolateral knee position in Fig. 6.22 is excessively flexed.

33. What is the primary positioning error in Fig. 6.23 (mediolateral projection)?

    A. Overangulation of central ray
          C. Overrotation of knee toward IR

    B. Underrotation of knee toward IR
        D. Underangulation of central ray

34. Which of the following conditions may cause the tibial tuberosity to be pulled away from the tibial shaft?

    A. Gout
          C. Osteomalacia

    B. Reiter syndrome
        D. Osgood-Schlatter disease

35. Which of the following pathologic conditions involves a large band ligament found in the forefoot?

    A. Reiter syndrome
          C. Exostosis

    B. Paget disease
        D. Lisfranc injury

36. Which of the following conditions may produce the radiographic appearance of a destructive lesion with an irregular periosteal reaction?

    A. Osteogenic sarcoma
          C. Bone cyst

    B. Gout
        D. Osteoid osteoma

37. What is the common term for chondromalacia patellae?

    A. Brittle bone disease
          C. Degenerative joint disease

    B. Runner's knee
        D. Giant cell tumor

38. Where is the central ray placed for a plantodorsal axial projection of the calcaneus?

    A. Calcaneal tuberosity
          C. Base of third metatarsal

    B. Sustentaculum tali
        D. 1 inch (2.5 cm) inferior to medial malleolus

39. Which ankle projection is best for demonstrating the mortise of the ankle?

    A. AP
          C. AP oblique (15- to 20-degree lateral rotation)

    B. AP oblique (15- to 20-degree medial rotation)
        D. Mediolateral

40. Which imaginary plane should be placed parallel to the IR for an AP projection of the knee?

    A. Intermalleolar
          C. Midsagittal

    B. Midcoronal
        D. Interepicondylar

41. Which joint space should be open or almost open for a well-positioned AP oblique knee projection with medial rotation?

    A. Both sides of knee joint
          C. Distal tibiofibular

    B. Proximal tibiofibular
        D. Patellofemoral

42. True/False: A 5- to 7-degree cephalad angle of the central ray for a mediolateral projection of the knee helps super-impose the distal borders of the medial and lateral condyles of the femur when the lower leg has not been supported.

43. Why is a PA projection of the patella preferred to an AP projection?

    A. Less object–image receptor distance (OID)   C. Less magnification of patella

    B. Less distortion of patella   D. All of these

44. **Situation:** A projection is performed for the patellofemoral joint with the patient supine and the knee flexed at 40 degrees. The central ray is angled 30 degrees caudad from horizontal. The cassette is resting on the lower legs supported by a special cassette-holding device. Which of the following methods has been described?

    A. Camp Coventry method   C. Hughston method

    B. Settegast   D. Bilateral Merchant method

45. What is the major disadvantage of the Settegast method?

    A. Requires use of specialized equipment   C. Requires hyperflexion of knee

    B. Requires AP positioning   D. Requires the use of a long OID

46. **Situation:** A radiograph of an AP knee shows that the joint spaces are not equally open and the proximal fibula is completely superimposed over the tibia. Which specific positioning error leads to this radiographic outcome?

    A. Underangulation of central ray   C. Overangulation of central ray

    B. Lateral rotation of lower limb   D. Medial rotation of lower limb

47. **Situation:** A radiograph of the Camp Coventry method was produced, but the intercondylar fossa is not open and is foreshortened. The following positioning factors were used: prone position, lower leg flexed 45 degrees, and central ray angled 30 degrees caudad and centered to the popliteal crease. Which of the following should be done during the repeat exposure to produce a more diagnostic image?

    A. Decrease lower leg flexion to 30 degrees

    B. Rotate lower limb 5 degrees internally

    C. Increase CR angle to 45 degrees caudad

    D. Increase flexion of lower limb to between 50 and 60 degrees

48. **Situation:** A radiograph of a plantodorsal (axial) projection of the calcaneus shows that the calcaneus is foreshortened. The following positioning factors were used: supine position, foot dorsiflexed perpendicular to IR, and central ray angled 30 degrees cephalad and centered to the base of the third metatarsal. Which of the following should be done during the repeat exposure to produce a more diagnostic image?

    A. Increase central-ray angulation to 40 degrees cephalad   C. Reduce dorsiflexion of foot

        D. Center central ray to sustentaculum tali

    B. Reverse direction of central-ray angulation

49. **Situation:** A bilateral patellofemoral joint space study is ordered. The patient is paraplegic and cannot stand. Which of the following projections is best suited for this patient?

    A. Hobbs modification   C. Bilateral Merchant method

    B. Bilateral inferosuperior axial   D. Bilateral Settegast method

50. **Situation:** A radiograph of an AP mortise projection of the ankle shows that the lateral joint space is not open with the lateral malleolus superimposed over the talus. The talus is distorted. What positioning error leads to this outcome?

   A. Insufficient medial rotation

   B. Excessive medial rotation

   C. Excessive dorsiflexion of the foot

   D. Excessive plantar flexion of the foot

51. **Situation:** A patient is referred to radiology for a possible Lisfranc injury. Which of the following positioning routines best demonstrates this condition?

   A. Weight-bearing knee study

   B. AP and lateral lower leg

   C. Knee routine to include intercondylar fossa projection

   D. Weight-bearing foot study

6 Lower Limb

1. B. Tail
2. False (proximal aspect or tuberosity is commonly fractured)
3. A. Plantar surface near head of first metatarsal
4. D. Navicular
5. C. Intermediate cuneiform
6. B. Subtalar joint
7. B. Tibial plafond
8. False (the lateral aspect of the ankle joint would not be open)
9. 1. D
   2. G
   3. B
   4. F
   5. A
   6. E
   7. C
10. A. 3
    B. 4
    C. 5
    D. 1
    E. 2
11. C. AP ankle
12. A. 6
    B. 8
    C. 5
    D. 2
    E. 3
    F. 1
    G. 7
    H. 4
    I. 9
    J. 2
    K. 5
13. A. Fig. 6.17
14. A. Affected metatarsophalangeal joint
15. B. 10- to 15-degree posterior (toward calcaneus)
16. C. Tangential
17. D. 30–40 degrees
18. D. Dorsoplantar projection
19. A. 10-degree posterior (more or less angle may be applied based on the height of the arch)
20. C. AP oblique—medial rotation
21. D. Intercondylar tubercles
22. A. Intercondylar fossa
23. A. 5–7 degrees
24. True
25. B. Base
26. C. Cruciates
27. C. Menisci
28. A. 3
    B. 9
    C. 6
    D. 8
    E. 1
    F. 4
    G. 2
    H. 10
    I. 5
    J. 7
29. B. AP oblique—medial rotation
30. A. 3
    B. 5
    C. 1
    D. 6
    E. 2
    F. 3
    G. 5
    H. 1
    I. 4
    J. 7
31. B. Under-rotation toward IR
32. True (patella is drawn into the patellar surface-sulcus)
33. C. Overrotation of knee toward IR
34. D. Osgood-Schlatter disease
35. D. Lisfranc injury
36. A. Osteogenic sarcoma
37. B. Runner's knee
38. C. Base of third metatarsal
39. B. AP oblique (15- to 20-degree medial rotation)
40. D. Interepicondylar
41. B. Proximal tibiofibular
42. True
43. D. All of these
44. D. Bilateral Merchant
45. C. Requires hyperflexion of knee.
46. B. Lateral rotation of lower limb
47. C. Increase CR angle to 45 degrees caudad.
48. A. Increase central-ray angulation to 40 degrees cephalad.
49. A. Hobbs modification
50. B. Excessive medial rotation
51. D. Weight-bearing foot study

A1

7 Femur and Pelvic Girdle

CHAPTER OBJECTIVES

After you have successfully completed the activities in this chapter, you will be able to:

_____ 1. Identify the bones and specific features of the femur and pelvic girdle on drawings and radiographs.

_____ 2. Identify the location of the major landmarks of the pelvis and hip and describe two methods of locating the femoral head and neck on an anteroposterior (AP) hip and pelvis radiograph.

_____ 3. List the structural and functional differences of the greater and lesser pelvis and the structural difference between the male and female pelvis.

_____ 4. List the correct classification and movement type for the pelvic joints.

_____ 5. Identify the specific pediatric, geriatric, and bariatric patient applications for pelvis and hip radiographic examinations as described in the textbook.

_____ 6. Match specific clinical indications of the pelvic girdle to the correct definition.

_____ 7. Match specific clinical indications of the pelvic girdle to the correct radiographic appearance.

_____ 8. Determine whether a pelvis or hip is in a true AP position based on the established radiographic criteria.

_____ 9. Given various hypothetic clinical situations, identify the correct modification of a position and/or exposure factors to improve the radiographic image.

_____ 10. Given radiographs of specific femur, hip, and pelvis projections, identify positioning and exposure factor errors.

POSITIONING AND RADIOGRAPHIC CRITIQUE

_____ 1. Using a peer, position for the basic and special projections of the femur and pelvic girdle.

_____ 2. Using a pelvic radiographic phantom, produce satisfactory radiographs of specific positions (if equipment is available).

_____ 3. Critique and evaluate pelvic girdle radiographs based on the five divisions of radiographic criteria: (1) anatomy demonstrated, (2) position, (3) collimation field size and central ray (CR), (4) exposure, and (5) anatomic side markers.

_____ 4. Distinguish between acceptable and unacceptable pelvic girdle radiographs based on exposure factors, motion, collimation field size, positioning, or other errors.

LEARNING EXERCISES

Complete the following review exercises after reading the associated pages in the textbook as indicated by each exercise. Answers to each review exercise are given at the end of the review exercises.

PART I: RADIOGRAPHIC ANATOMY

REVIEW EXERCISE A: Radiographic Anatomy of the Femur, Hips, and Pelvis (see textbook pp. 268–274)

1. The largest and strongest bone of the body is the _____.

2. A small depression located in the center of the femoral head is the _____.

3. The lesser trochanter is located on the _____ (medial or lateral) aspect of the proximal femur.

   It projects _____ (anteriorly or posteriorly) from the junction between the neck and shaft.

4. Because of the alignment between the femoral head and pelvis, the lower limb must be rotated

   _____ degrees internally to place the femoral neck parallel to the plane of the image receptor to achieve a true AP projection.

5. True/False: The terms *pelvis* and *pelvic girdle* are not synonymous.

   A. List the four bones that make up the pelvis. _____

   B. List the two bones that make up the pelvic girdle. _____

   C. List two additional terms used for the bones identified in B.

   (a) _____

   (b) _____

6. List the three divisions of the hip bone.

   A. _____   C. _____

   B. _____

7. All three divisions of the hip bone eventually fuse at the _____ at the age of _____.

8. What are the two important radiographic landmarks found on the ilium?

   A. _____   B. _____

9. Which bony landmark is found on the most inferior aspect of the posterior pelvis?

   _____

10. What is the name of the joint found between the superior rami of the pubic bones?

   _____

11. The _____ of the pelvis is the largest foramen in the skeletal system.

12. The upper margin of the greater trochanter is approximately (A) _____ inches above the level of the superior border of the symphysis pubis, and the ischial tuberosity is about (B)

   _____ inches below.

13. An imaginary plane that divides the pelvic region into the greater and lesser pelvis is called the

   _____.

14. List the alternate terms for the greater and lesser pelvis.

   A. Greater pelvis _____   B. Lesser pelvis _____

15. List the major function of the greater pelvis and the lesser pelvis.

   A. Greater pelvis _____   B. Lesser pelvis _____

16. List the three aspects of the lesser pelvis, which also describe the birth route during the delivery process.

   A. _____   C. _____

   B. _____

17. Match the following structures or characteristics to the correct hip bone. (Answers may be used more than once.)

   _____ 1. Possesses a large tuberosity found at the most inferior aspect of the pelvis   A. Ilium

   _____ 2. Lesser sciatic notch   B. Ischium

   _____ 3. Ala   C. Pubis

   _____ 4. Posterior superior iliac spine (PSIS)

   _____ 5. Possesses a slightly movable joint

   _____ 6. Anterior superior iliac spine (ASIS)

   _____ 7. Forms the anterior, inferior aspect of the lower pelvic girdle

   _____ 8. Articulates with the sacrum to form the sacroiliac (SI) joints

18. In the past, which radiographic examination was performed to measure the fetal head in comparison with the maternal pelvis to predict possible birthing problems? _____

19. What imaging modality has replaced the procedure identified in question 18? _____

20. Indicate whether the following radiographic characteristics apply to a male (M) or female (F) in relation to an AP projection of the pelvis.

_____ 1. Wide, more flared ilia

_____ 2. Pubic arch angle of 110 degrees

_____ 3. A heart-shaped pelvic inlet

_____ 4. Narrow ilia that are less flared

_____ 5. Pubic arch angle of 75 degrees

_____ 6. Ischial spines protruding less into pelvic inlet

21. List the joint classification, mobility type, and movement type for the joints of the pelvis. Write *N/A* (not applicable) if the mobility or movement type does not apply.

	Classification	*Mobility Type*	*Movement Type*
A. Hip joint	_____	_____	_____
B. Sacroiliac	_____	_____	_____
C. Symphysis pubis	_____	_____	_____
D. Acetabulum (union)	_____	_____	_____

22. Identify the structures labeled in Figs. 7.1 and 7.2. Where indicated, use the following abbreviations to identify with which bone of the pelvis each labeled part is associated: *IL*, ilium; *IS*, ischium; *P*, pubis.

Structure	*Bone*
A. _____	_____
B. _____	_____
C. _____	_____
D. _____	_____
E. _____	_____
F. _____	_____
G. _____	_____
H. _____	_____
I. _____	_____
J. _____	_____
K. _____	_____
L. _____	_____
M. _____	_____
N. _____	_____
O. _____	_____
P. _____	_____
Q. _____	_____
R. _____	_____
S. _____	_____
T. _____	_____
U. _____	_____
V. _____	_____
W. _____	_____
X. _____	_____
Y. _____	_____
Z. _____	_____

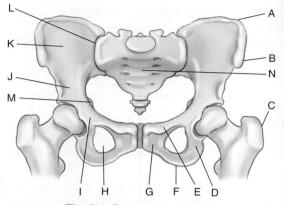

Fig. 7.1 Frontal view, pelvis.

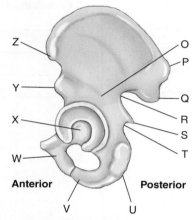

Anterior   **Posterior**

Fig. 7.2 Lateral view, pelvis.

REVIEW EXERCISE B: Positioning of the Femur, Hips, and Pelvis (see textbook pp. 275–295)

1. Which two bony landmarks need to be palpated for hip localization?

   A. _____   B. _____

2. From the midpoint of the imaginary line created by the two landmarks identified in the previous question, where

   would the femoral neck be located? _____

3. A second method for locating the femoral head is to palpate the _____ and go

   _____ inches (_____ cm) medial at the level of the

   _____, which is _____ inches

   (_____ cm) distal to the original palpation point.

4. To achieve a true AP position of the proximal femur, the lower limb must be

   rotated _____ internally.

5. Which structures on an AP pelvis or hip radiograph indicate whether the proximal head and neck are in position

   for a true AP projection? _____

6. Which physical sign may indicate that a patient has a hip fracture? _____

7. Which projection should be taken first and reviewed by a radiologist before attempting to rotate the hip into a lateral

   position (if trauma is suspected)? _____

8. If gonadal shield is used for a hip study on a young female, how should it be placed? _____

9. If gonadal shield is used for a hip study on a young female, how should it be placed?

   _____

10. What are the three types of Femoroacetabular Impingement (FAI)?

    _____, _____, _____

11. What is the advantage of using 90 kVp rather than a lower kVp range for hip and pelvis studies on younger

    patients? _____

12. What is the disadvantage of using 90 kVp for hip and pelvis studies for geriatric patients with some bone mass

    loss? _____

13. Which of the following conditions is a common clinical indication for performing pelvic and hip examinations on a
    pediatric (newborn) patient?

    A. Osteoporosis   C. Ankylosing spondylitis

    B. Developmental dysplasia of hip (DDH)   D. Osteoarthritis

14. True/False: Geriatric patients are often more prone to hip fractures because of their increased incidence of osteoporosis.

15. True/False: The soft tissue of a bariatric patient is indicative of the actual size of the bony pelvis.

16. Which of the following imaging modalities can be used on a newborn to assess hip joint stability during movement of the lower limbs?

    A. Diagnostic medical sonography (DMS)   C. Magnetic resonance (MR)

    B. Computed tomography (CT)   D. Nuclear medicine (NM)

17. Which of the following imaging modalities is most sensitive in diagnosing early signs of metastatic carcinoma of the pelvis?

    A. Diagnostic medical sonography (DMS)   C. MR

    B. CT   D. Nuclear medicine (NM)

18. Match each of the following clinical indications to the correct definition. (Use each choice only once.)

    _____ A. A degenerative joint disease

    _____ B. Most common fracture in older patients because of high incidence of osteoporosis or avascular necrosis

    _____ C. A malignant tumor of the cartilage of hip

    _____ D. A disease producing extensive calcification of the longitudinal ligament of the spinal column

    _____ E. A fracture resulting from a severe blow to one side of the pelvis

    _____ F. Malignancy spread to bone via the circulatory and lymphatic systems or direct invasion

    _____ G. Now referred to as developmental dysplasia of the hip

    1. Metastatic carcinoma

    2. Ankylosing spondylitis

    3. Congenital dislocation

    4. Chondrosarcoma

    5. Proximal hip fracture

    6. Pelvic ring fracture

    7. Osteoarthritis

19. Which of the following devices will improve overall visibility of the proximal hip demonstrated on an axiolateral (inferosuperior) projection?

    A. Small focal spot   C. Compensating filter

    B. Increased added filtration   D. Shadow shield

20. Which of the following modalities will best demonstrate a possible pelvic ring fracture?

    A. CT   C. MR

    B. Nuclear medicine (NM)   D. Diagnostic medical sonography (DMS)

21. True/False: Both joints must be included on an AP and lateral projection of the femur even if a fracture of the proximal femur is evident.

22. Where is the central ray placed for an AP pelvis projection? _____

23. The central ray for the AP pelvis projection is approximately _____ inch(es) (_____cm) inferior to the level of the ASIS.

24. Which specific positioning error is present when the left iliac wing is elongated on an AP pelvis radiograph?

    _____

169

25. Which specific positioning error is present when the left obturator foramen is more open than the right side on an

    AP pelvis radiograph? _____

26. Indicate whether each of the following projections is used for patients with traumatic (T) injuries or nontraumatic (NT) injuries.

    _____ A. Axiolateral, inferosuperior (Danelius-Miller method) projection

    _____ B. Unilateral modified Cleaves method

    _____ C. AP bilateral modified Cleaves method

    _____ D. Modified axiolateral (Clements-Nakayama method)

    _____ E. AP axial for pelvic outlet (Taylor method)

27. Which of the following projections is recommended to demonstrate the superoposterior wall of the acetabulum?

    A. AP axial inlet

    B. Posteroanterior (PA) axial oblique

    C. Axiolateral inferosuperior

    D. Modified axiolateral

28. How many degrees are the dependent lower limb and foot rotated away from the IR in a modified false profile projection?

29. How many degrees are the femurs abducted (from the vertical plane) for the bilateral modified Cleaves projection?

    _____

30. Where is the central ray placed for a bilateral modified Cleaves method projection?

    _____

31. What recommended field size should be used for an adult bilateral modified Cleaves projection?

    _____

32. Where is the central ray placed for an AP unilateral modified Cleaves method projection? _____

33. Which central ray angle is required for the AP axial for pelvic outlet (Taylor method) projection for a female patient?

    A. 15–25 degrees caudad

    B. 30–45 degrees cephalad

    C. 20–35 degrees cephalad

    D. None (central ray is perpendicular)

34. Which type of pathology is best demonstrated with the posterior oblique (Judet method)?

    A. Acetabular fractures

    B. Anterior pelvic bone fractures

    C. Proximal femur fractures

    D. Femoral neck fractures

35. How much obliquity of the body is required for the posterior oblique projection (Judet method)?

    A. None (central ray is perpendicular)

    B. 20 degrees

    C. 30 degrees

    D. 45 degrees

36. What type of CR angle is used for a PA axial oblique (Teufel) projection?

    A. 15 degrees cephalad

    B. 15–20 degrees cephalad

    C. 5 degrees caudad

    D. 12 degrees cephalad

170

37. How is the pelvis (body) positioned for a PA axial oblique (Teufel) projection?

    A. PA with 45 degrees rotated away from affected side   C. PA 35–40 degrees rotated toward affected side

    B. Prone or erect PA—no rotation   D. AP with 40 degrees rotated away from affected side

38. True/False: Any orthopedic device or appliance of the hip should be seen in its entirety on an AP hip radiograph.

39. The axiolateral (inferosuperior) projection is designed for _____ (traumatic or nontraumatic) situations.

40. How is the unaffected leg positioned for the axiolateral hip projection?_____

41. Which of the following factors does *not* apply to an axiolateral (inferosuperior) projection of the hip on a male patient?

    A. IR parallel to femoral neck   C. Use of gonadal shielding

    B. 80 to 90 kVp   D. Use of a stationary grid

42. True/False: An AP pelvis projection using 90 kVp and 8 mAs results in less patient dose than a projection using 80 kVp and 12 mAs (for both males and females).

43. True/False: The unaffected foot during an axiolateral (inferosuperior) projection can be burned if allowed to rest on the collimator.

44. The modified axiolateral (Clements-Nakayama method) projection requires the CR to be angled

    _____ degrees posteriorly from horizontal.

45. Which special projection of the hip demonstrates the anterior and posterior rims of the acetabulum and the ilioischial and iliopubic columns? (Include the projection name and the method name.)

    A. _____

    B. Which central ray angle (if any) is used for this projection?_____

46. What is the name of a special projection of the pelvis used to assess trauma to pubic and ischial structures?

    (Include the projection name and the method name.) _____

47. Match each of the following projections with its corresponding proper name. (Use each choice only once.)

    _____ 1. Axiolateral (inferosuperior)   A. Judet

    _____ 2. Modified axiolateral   B. Taylor

    _____ 3. AP bilateral or unilateral hip and proximal femur   C. Clements-Nakayama

    _____ 4. Posterior axial oblique for acetabulum   D. Danelius-Miller

    _____ 5. AP axial for pelvic outlet bones   E. Teufel

    _____ 6. Posterior oblique for acetabulum   F. Modified Cleaves

48. What is the optimal amount of hip abduction applied for the unilateral modified Cleaves method projection to demonstrate the femoral neck without distortion?

A. 45 degrees from vertical

C. 10 degrees from vertical

B. 90 degrees from vertical

D. 20–30 degrees from vertical

49. True/False: The Lauenstein/Hickey method for the unilateral hip and proximal femur projection will produce distortion of the femoral neck.

50. How much is the IR tilted for the modified axiolateral projection of the hip? _____

REVIEW EXERCISE C: Problem Solving for Technical and Positioning Errors

1. **Situation:** A radiograph of an AP pelvis projection shows that the lesser trochanters are readily demonstrated on the medial side of the proximal femurs. The patient is ambulatory but has a history of early osteoarthritis in both hips. Which positioning modification needs to be made to prevent this positioning error?

_____

_____

2. **Situation:** A radiograph of an AP pelvis shows that the right iliac wing is foreshortened as compared with the left side. Which specific positioning error was made?

_____

_____

3. **Situation:** A radiograph of a unilateral modified Cleaves projection produces distortion of the femoral neck. Based on the AP hip projection, the radiologist suspects a nondisplaced fracture of the femoral neck. What can the technologist do to define this region better?

_____

_____

4. **Situation:** A radiograph of an axiolateral (Danelius-Miller method) projection shows that the posterior aspect of the acetabulum and femoral head were cut off of the bottom of the image. The emergency room physician requests that the projection be repeated. What can be done to avoid this problem on the repeat exposure?

_____

_____

5. **Situation:** A radiograph of an AP axial projection for anterior pelvic bones shows that the pubic and ischial bones are not elongated sufficiently. The following exposure factors were used for this study: 86 kVp, 7 mAs, Bucky, 20- to 30-degree central ray cephalad angle, and 40-inch (100-cm) source image receptor distance (SID). The female patient was placed in a supine position on the table. What must be changed to improve the quality of the image during the repeat exposure?

_____

_____

172

6. **Situation:** A patient enters the ER with a pelvis injury resulting from a motor vehicle accident. The initial AP pelvis projection demonstrates a possible defect or fracture of the left acetabulum. No other fractures are detected and the patient is able to move comfortably. What additional projections can be taken to demonstrate a possible acetabular fracture?

_____

_____

7. **Situation:** A radiograph of an AP pelvis shows overall the image is underexposed (underpenetrated). The following exposure factors were used: 80 kVp, 40-inch (100-cm) SID, Bucky, and automatic exposure control with the center chamber activated. Which of these factors should be changed to produce increased image density?

_____

_____

8. **Situation:** A radiograph from a modified axiolateral projection of the hip shows excessive grid lines on the image, which also appears underexposed. What can be done to avoid this problem during the repeat exposure?

_____

_____

9. **Situation:** A portable AP and lateral hip study is ordered for a patient who is in recovery following hip replacement surgery. The radiograph of the AP hip shows that the upper portion of the acetabular prosthesis is slightly cut off but is included on the lateral projection. Should the technologist repeat the AP projection? Why or why not?

_____

_____

10. **Situation:** A patient with hip pain from a fall enters the emergency room. The physician orders a left hip study. When moved to the radiographic table, the patient complains loudly about the pain in the left hip. Which positioning routine should be used for this patient?

_____

_____

11. **Situation:** A patient has just been moved to his hospital room after a bilateral hip replacement surgery. The surgeon has ordered a postoperative hip routine for both hips. Which specific positioning routine should be used? (The patient can be brought to the radiology department.)

_____

_____

12. **Situation:** A patient with a possible pelvic ring fracture from a trauma enters the emergency room. The AP pelvis projection, which was taken to determine whether the right acetabulum was fractured, is inconclusive. Which other radiographic projection can be taken to better visualize the acetabulum? What other imaging modality can be used to determine the presence of a pelvic ring fracture?

_____

_____

13. **Situation:** A physician orders a study for inlet and outlet projections of the pelvis. Which projections could be performed to meet this request?

_____

_____

14. **Situation:** A technologist notices that his AP pelvis projections often demonstrate a moderate degree of rotation. What positioning technique can the technologist perform to eliminate (or at least minimize) rotation on his AP pelvis projections?

_____

_____

15. **Situation:** A very young child comes to the radiology department with a clinical history of DDH. What is the most common positioning routine for this condition?

_____

_____

REVIEW EXERCISE D: Critique Radiographs of the Femur and Pelvis

The following questions relate to the radiographs found in this exercise. Evaluate these radiographs for the radiographic criteria categories (1 through 5) that follow. Describe the corrections needed to improve the overall image. The major, or "repeatable," errors are specific errors that indicate the need for a repeat exposure, regardless of the nature of the other errors.

A. AP Pelvis (Fig. 7.3)

Description of possible error:

    1. Anatomy demonstrated:

    _____

    2. Part positioning:

    _____

    3. Collimation field size and central ray:

    _____

    4. Exposure:

    _____

    5. Anatomic Side Markers:

    _____

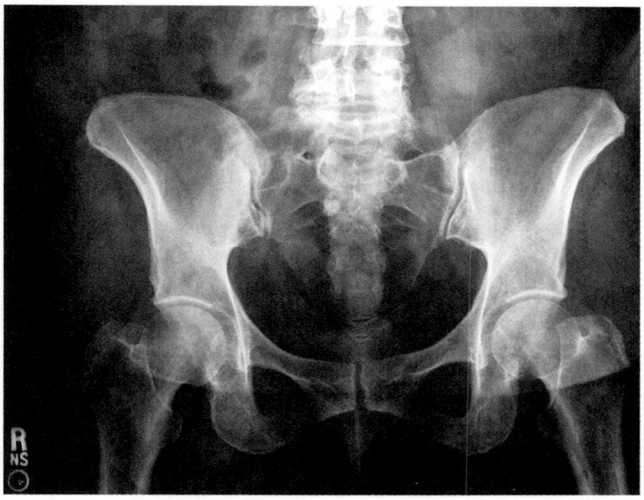

Fig. 7.3 Anteroposterior Pelvis.

Repeatable error(s):

_____

B. AP Pelvis (Fig. 7.4)

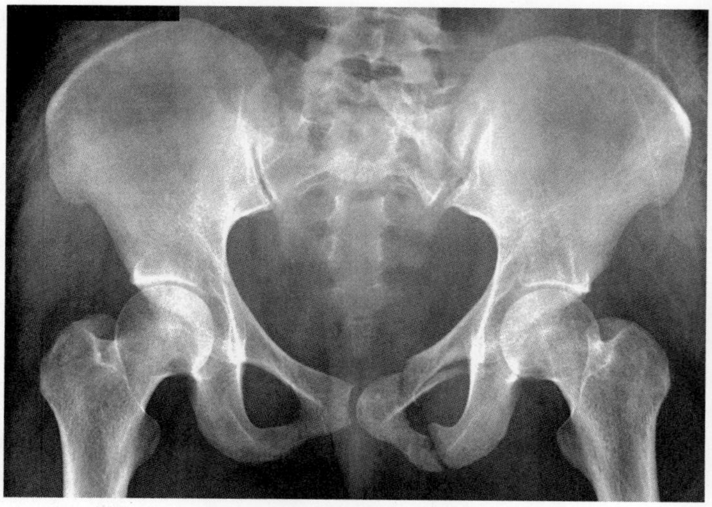

Description of possible error:

    1. Anatomy demonstrated:

    _____

    2. Part positioning:

    _____

    3. Collimation field size and central ray:

    _____

    4. Exposure:

    _____

    5. Anatomic Side Markers:

    _____

Repeatable error(s):

    _____

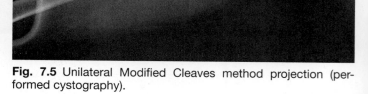

Fig. 7.4 Anteroposterior Pelvis.

C. Unilateral modified Cleaves method projection (performed cystography) (Fig. 7.5)

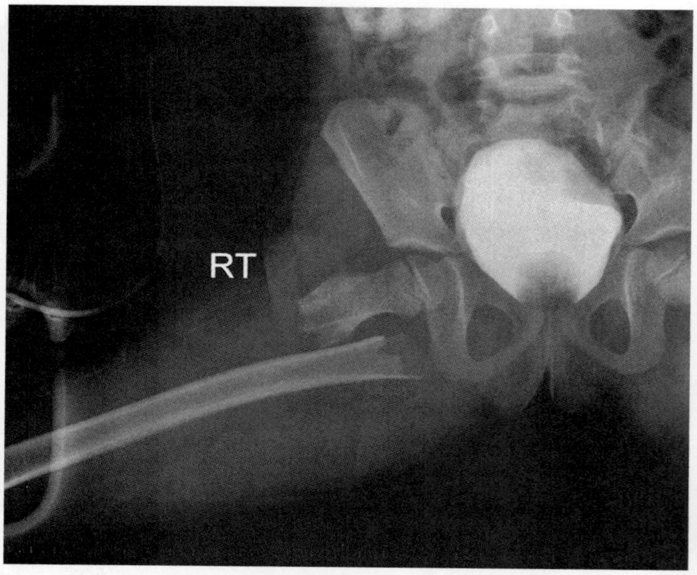

Description of possible error:

    1. Anatomy demonstrated:

    _____

    2. Part positioning:

    _____

    3. Collimation field size and central ray:

    _____

    4. Exposure:

    _____

    5. Anatomic Side Markers:

    _____

Repeatable error(s):

    _____

Fig. 7.5 Unilateral Modified Cleaves method projection (performed cystography).

D. Bilateral modified Cleaves method (2-year-old) (Fig. 7.6)

Description of possible error:

1. Anatomy demonstrated:

_____

2. Part positioning:

_____

3. Collimation field size and central ray:

_____

4. Exposure:

_____

5. Anatomic Side Markers:

_____

Repeatable error(s):

_____

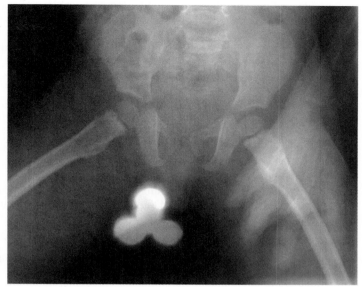

Fig. 7.6 Bilateral Modified Cleaves method (2-year-old).

PART III: LABORATORY EXERCISES

You must gain experience in positioning each part of the proximal femur and pelvis before performing the following exams on actual patients. You can obtain experience in positioning and radiographic evaluation of these projections by performing exercises using radiographic phantoms and by practicing positioning on other students (although you will not be taking actual exposures).

The following suggested activities assume that your teaching institution has an energized lab and radiographic phantoms. If not, perform Laboratory Exercises B and C, the radiographic evaluation and the physical positioning exercises. (Check off each step and projection as you complete it.)

Laboratory Exercise A: Energized Laboratory

1. Using the pelvic radiographic phantom, produce radiographs of the following basic routines:

_____AP pelvis projection

_____Posterior oblique positions for acetabulum (Judet method)

_____AP axial projection (Taylor method)

Laboratory Exercise B: Radiographic Evaluation

1. Evaluate and critique the radiographs produced previously, additional radiographs provided by your instructor, or both. Evaluate each radiograph for the following points:

_____ Evaluate the completeness of the study. (Are all of the pertinent anatomic structures included on the radiograph?)

_____ Evaluate for positioning or centering errors (e.g., rotation, off centering).

_____ Evaluate for correct exposure factors and possible motion. (Are the optimal image exposure and contrast of the images acceptable?)

_____ Determine whether markers and an acceptable degree of collimation are visible on the images.

Laboratory Exercise C: Physical Positioning

On another person, simulate performing all basic and special projections of the proximal femur and pelvic girdle as follows. Include the six steps listed in the following and described in the textbook. (Check off each step when completed satisfactorily.)

Step 1. Appropriate collimation field size with correct markers

Step 2. Correct central ray placement and centering of part to central ray and/or IR

Step 3. Accurate collimation field size

Step 4. Area shielding of patient when required

Step 5. Use of proper immobilizing devices when needed

Step 6. Approximate correct exposure factors, breathing instructions when applicable, and initiating exposure

Projections	*Step 1*	*Step 2*	*Step 3*	*Step 4*	*Step 5*	*Step 6*
AP and lateral femur	_____	_____	_____	_____	_____	_____
AP pelvis	_____	_____	_____	_____	_____	_____
AP hip, unilateral	_____	_____	_____	_____	_____	_____
Unilateral modified Cleaves method	_____	_____	_____	_____	_____	_____
Bilateral modified Cleaves method	_____	_____	_____	_____	_____	_____
Axiolateral (Danelius-Miler method) projection	_____	_____	_____	_____	_____	_____
Modified axiolateral	_____	_____	_____	_____	_____	_____
Oblique acetabulum (Judet, Teufel, False Profile)	_____	_____	_____	_____	_____	_____
AP axial for outlet	_____	_____	_____	_____	_____	_____

SELF-TEST

MY SCORE = _____ %

This self-test should be taken only after completing all of the readings, review exercises, and laboratory activities for a particular section. The purpose of this test is not only to provide a good learning exercise but also to serve as a strong indicator of what your final evaluation exam for this chapter will cover. It is strongly suggested that if you do not get at least a 90% to 95% grade on each self-test, you should review those areas in which you missed questions before going to your instructor for the final evaluation exam.

1. List the four bones of the pelvis.

   A. _____   C. _____

   B. _____   D. _____

2. List the three divisions of the hip bone.

   A. _____   C. _____

   B. _____

3. *Innominate bone* is another name for:

   A. One half of pelvic girdle   C. Ossa coxae

   B. Hip bone   D. All of the above

4. What is the largest foramen in the body?

5. Which of the following landmarks is not a palpable bony landmark?

   A. Greater trochanter   C. Ischial tuberosity

   B. Lesser trochanter   D. ASIS

6. What are the two aspects of the ischium?

   A. _____   B. _____

7. What is the name of the imaginary plane that separates the false from the true pelvis? _____

8. Match the following structures or characteristics to the correct division of the pelvis.

   _____ 1. Lesser pelvis   A. False pelvis

   _____ 2. Supports the lower abdominal organs   B. True pelvis

   _____ 3. Formed primarily by the ala of the ilium

   _____ 4. Cavity

   _____ 5. Greater pelvis

   _____ 6. Forms the actual birth canal

   _____ 7. Found below the pelvic brim

9. The pubic arch angle on an average male pelvis is an _____ (acute or obtuse) angle that

   is _____ (greater than or less than) 90 degrees.

10. Identify the labeled structures found on the following radiographs.

   A. _____

   B. _____

   C. _____

   D. _____

   E. _____

   F. _____

   G. _____

   H. _____

   I. _____

   J. Is Fig. 7.7 a male or female pelvis?

   _____

   K. _____

   L. _____

   M. _____

   N. _____

   O. Which projection of the hip is represented

   in Fig. 7.8? _____

   P. _____

   Q. _____

   R. _____

   S. _____

   T. _____

   U. _____

   V. _____

   W. Which projection of the hips is represented in

   Fig. 7.9? _____

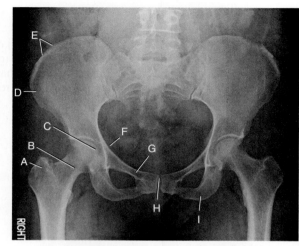

Fig. 7.7 Anteroposterior pelvis radiograph.

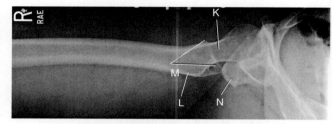

Fig. 7.8 Lateral hip radiograph.

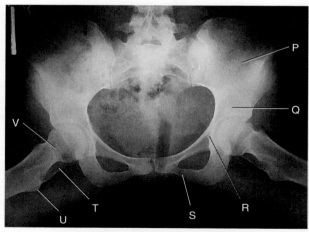

Fig. 7.9 Bilateral hip radiograph.

11. Indicate whether the following radiographic characteristics are those of a male (M) or a female (F) pelvis.

_____ 1.   Heart-shaped (oval) inlet

_____ 2.   Acute pubic arch (less than 90 degrees)

_____ 3.   Iliac wings that are more flared

_____ 4.   Obtuse pubic arch (greater than 90 degrees)

_____ 5.   Larger and more rounded inlet

_____ 6.   Iliac wings that are less flared

12. Which of the following structures is considered as the most posterior?

A. Ischial spines

B. ASIS

C. Symphysis pubis

D. Acetabulum

13. The small depression near the center of the femoral head where a ligament is attached is called the

_____.

14. Which of the following joints are synovial joints but with amphiarthrodial mobility?

A. Union of acetabula

B. Hip joints

C. SI joints

D. Symphysis pubis

15. Which of the following devices should be used for an axiolateral (inferosuperior) projection of the hip to equalize brightness of the hip region?

A. Grid

B. Small focal spot

C. Boomerang compensating filter

D. Wedge compensating filter

16. Which of the following modalities is used to assess joint stability during movement of the lower limbs on infants?

A. DMS

B. MR

C. CT

D. Weight-bearing pelvis radiographic projections

17. A geriatric patient with an externally rotated lower limb may have:

A. A normal hip joint

B. Osteoarthritis

C. A fractured proximal femur

D. Slipped capital femoral epiphysis (SCFE)

18. Which of the following pathologic indications may result in the early fusion of the SI joints?

A. Chondrosarcoma

B. Metastatic carcinoma

C. Developmental dysplasia of the hip

D. Ankylosing spondylitis

19. Match each of the following radiographic appearances with the correct clinical indications. (Use each choice only once.)

_____ 1. Usually consists of numerous small lytic lesions

_____ 2. Increased hip joint space and misalignment

_____ 3. Bilateral radiolucent lines across bones and misalignment of SI joints

_____ 4. Early fusion of SI joints and "bamboo spine"

_____ 5. Epiphyses appear shorter and epiphyseal plate wider

_____ 6. Hallmark sign of spurring and narrowing of joint space

_____ 7. Reduced smooth articulation of the hip joint

A. Pelvic ring fracture

B. DDH

C. Osteoarthritis

D. SCFE

E. Ankylosing spondylitis

F. Metastatic carcinoma

G. Femoroacetabular Impingement (FAI)

20. Which of the following radiographic signs indicates that the proximal femurs are in position for a true AP projection?

A. Appearance of the greater trochanter in profile
B. Limited visibility of fovea capitis
C. Limited visibility of the lesser trochanter in profile
D. Symmetric appearance of iliac wings

21. What is another term for the outlet of the true pelvis?

A. Ischial spines
B. Inferior aperture
C. Pelvic brim
D. Cervix

22. The typical physical sign for a possible hip fracture is the _____ of the involved foot.

A. External rotation
B. Abduction
C. Internal rotation
D. Adduction

23. Which of the following projections or methods is often performed to evaluate a pediatric patient for a congenital hip dislocation?

A. Bilateral modified Cleaves methos
B. Clements-Nakayama method
C. Taylor method
D. Judet method

24. What type of central ray angle is required when using the AP axial for outlet (Taylor method) for a male patient?

A. None (central ray is perpendicular)
B. 10–15 degrees caudad
C. 20–35 degrees cephalad
D. 30–45 degrees cephalad

25. How much is the pelvis and/or thorax rotated for a PA axial oblique (Teufel method) for acetabulum?

A. 15 degrees toward affected side
B. 30–35 degrees away from affected side
C. 20 degrees away from affected side
D. 35–40 degrees toward affected side

26. How posterior oblique rotation of the pelvis and thorax is needed for a false profile method?

A. 30 degrees
B. 45 degrees
C. 55 degrees
D. 65 degrees

27. True/False: The unilateral modified Cleaves method is intended for nontraumatic hip situations.

28. True/False: Centering for the AP pelvis projection is 1 inch, or 2.5 cm, superior to the symphysis pubis.

29. True/False: The modified axiolateral (Clements-Nakayama method) is classified as a nontraumatic lateral hip projection.

30. What type of CR angle is required for the Judet method?

   A. 12 degrees cephalad

   B. 5–10 degrees caudad

   C. 15 degrees cephalad

   D. None. CR is perpendicular

31. Which of the following projections or methods is used to evaluate the pelvic inlet for possible fracture?

   A. Danelius-Miller method

   B. AP axial projection

   C. Taylor method

   D. Clements-Nakayama method

32. **Situation:** An initial AP pelvis radiograph shows possible fractures involving the lower anterior pelvis. The emergency room physician asks for another projection to better demonstrate this area of the pelvis. The patient is traumatized and must remain in a supine position. Which projection should be taken?

_____

_____

33. **Situation:** A radiograph of an axiolateral (inferosuperior) projection of a hip demonstrates a soft tissue density that is visible across the affected hip and acetabulum. This artifact is obscuring the image of the proximal femur. What is the most likely cause of the artifact, and how can it be prevented from showing up on the repeat exposure?

_____

_____

34. **Situation:** A unilateral modified Cleaves demonstrates foreshortening of the femoral necks. The physician is unsure if there is a defect within the anatomic neck. What can be done to minimize distortion of the neck during a repeat exposure?

_____

_____

35. **Situation:** A radiograph of an AP hip shows that the lesser trochanter is not visible. Should the technologist repeat the projection? _____ If yes, what should be modified to improve the image during the repeat exposure?

_____

_____

36. **Situation:** A young patient with a clinical history of SCFE comes to the radiology department. Which projection(s) are most often taken for this condition?

_____

_____

182

37. **Situation:** A radiograph produced using the AP axial (Taylor method) demonstrates that the anterior pelvic bones of a female patient are foreshortened. The following positioning factors were used: supine position, 40-inch (100-cm) SID, and central ray angled 30 degrees caudad and centered 1 to 2 inches (3 to 5 cm) distal to symphysis pubis. Which of the following modifications should be made during the repeat exposure?

    A. Increase central ray angle

    B. Reverse central ray angle

    C. Center central ray at level of ASIS

    D. Place patient prone on table

38. **Situation:** A radiograph of an AP projection of the pelvis demonstrates the left obturator foramen is narrowed and the right one is open. What is the specific positioning error present on this radiograph?

_____

_____

39. **Situation:** A patient enters the emergency room with a possible pelvic ring fracture. The AP pelvis projection is inclusive on the extent and location of the fracture(s). What additional pelvis projection(s) can be taken on this patient to demonstrate possible pelvic fractures? (More than one correct answer is possible.)

_____

_____

40. **Situation:** A radiograph of the PA axial oblique (Teufel method) demonstrates distortion of the acetabulum. During positioning, the patient was rotated 35–40 degrees toward the affected side and CR was angled 20 degrees cephalad. What modifications are needed during the repeat exposure?

_____

_____

183

7 Femur and Pelvic Girdle

1. A. Left hip bone
   B. Right hip bone
   C. Sacrum
   D. Coccyx
2. A. Ilium
   B. Ischium
   C. Pubis
3. D. All of the above
4. Obturator foramen
5. B. Lesser trochanter
6. A. Body
   B. Ramus
7. Brim of the pelvis (pelvic brim)
8. 1. B
   2. A
   3. A
   4. B
   5. A
   6. B
   7. B
9. Acute; less than 90 degrees
10. A. Greater trochanter
    B. Neck of femur
    C. Acetabulum
    D. Anterior superior iliac spine (ASIS)
    E. Crest of ilium
    F. Ischial spine
    G. Superior ramus of pubis
    H. Symphysis pubis
    I. Ischial tuberosity
    J. Female
    K. Neck of femur
    L. Lesser trochanter
    M. Greater trochanter
    N. Ischial tuberosity
    O. Axiolateral (inferosuperior) projection or Danelius-Miller method
    P. Ala (wing) of left ilium
    Q. Body of left ilium
    R. Body of left pubis
    S. Inferior ramus of left ischium
    T. Greater trochanter
    U. Lesser trochanter
    V. Neck of right femur
    W. AP bilateral modified Cleaves method projection (modified Cleaves method)
11. 1. M
    2. M
    3. F
    4. F
    5. F
    6. M
12. A. Ischial spines
13. Fovea capitis
14. C. Sacroiliac joints
15. D. Wedge compensating filter
16. A. DMS
17. C. Fractured proximal femur
18. D. Ankylosing spondylitis
19. 1. F
    2. B
    3. A
    4. E
    5. D
    6. C
    7. G
20. C. Limited visibility of the lesser trochanter in profile
21. B. Inferior aperture
22. A. External rotation
23. A. Bilateral modified Cleaves
24. C. 20–35 degrees cephalad
25. D. 35–40 degrees toward affected side
26. D. 65 degrees
27. True
28. False. (Midway between ASIS and symphysis pubis)
29. False. (Trauma projection)
30. D. None. CR is perpendicular.
31. B. AP axial projection
32. The AP axial "outlet" projection (Taylor method) will elongate the pubis and ischium and will define this region more completely.
33. It is soft tissue from the unaffected thigh. This leg must be flexed and elevated high enough to keep it from superimposing the affected hip.
34. Only abduct the femurs 20–30 degrees from the vertical rather than 45 degrees to minimize the distortion of the femoral neck.
35. No. It is an acceptable image because the lesser trochanters should not be visible at all or should be only minimally visible on a well-positioned AP hip projection.
36. AP pelvis and bilateral modified Cleaves method
37. B. Reverse central ray angle.
38. Rotation of pelvis toward the patient's left. The elevated or upside (right) obturator foramen will become more open as compared to the opposite or downside.
39. Multiple answers are correct: Posterior oblique projections (Judet method) will demonstrate possible pelvic ring and acetabular fractures, and AP axial "outlet" and AP axial "inlet" projections will demonstrate possible fractures involving the ischium and pubis.
40. Reduce CR angle to 12 degrees cephalad.

8 Cervical and Thoracic Spine

CHAPTER OBJECTIVES

After you have successfully completed the activities in this chapter, you will be able to:

_____ 1. Using drawings and radiographs, identify specific anatomic structures of the cervical and thoracic spine.

_____ 2. Identify specific features of the cervical and thoracic vertebrae that distinguish them from other aspects of the vertebral column.

_____ 3. Identify the location, angulation, classification, and type of movement for specific joints of the cervical and thoracic spine.

_____ 4. List additional terms for the first, second, and seventh cervical vertebrae.

_____ 5. Identify topographic landmarks that can be palpated to locate specific thoracic and cervical vertebrae.

_____ 6. Match specific clinical indications of the cervical and thoracic spine to the correct definitions.

_____ 7. Identify the radiographic projection and/or procedure that best demonstrates specific pathologic indications.

_____ 8. Identify structures that are best demonstrated with each position of the cervical and thoracic spine.

_____ 9. Identify basic and special projections of the cervical and thoracic spine and list the collimation field size and the central ray (CR) location, direction, and angulation for each position.

_____ 10. Given various hypothetic situations, identify the correct modification of a position and/or exposure factors to improve the radiographic image.

_____ 11. Given radiographs of specific cervical and thoracic spine projections, identify positioning and exposure-factor errors.

POSITIONING AND RADIOGRAPHIC CRITIQUE

_____ 1. Using a peer, position for basic and special projections of the cervical and thoracic spine.

_____ 2. Using appropriate radiographic phantoms, produce satisfactory radiographs of specific positions (if equipment is available).

_____ 3. Critique and evaluate cervical and thoracic spine radiographs based on the five divisions of radiographic criteria: (1) anatomy demonstrated, (2) position, (3) collimation field size and central ray, (4) exposure, and (5) anatomic side markers.

_____ 4. Distinguish between acceptable and unacceptable spine radiographs based on exposure factors, motion, collimation, positioning, or other errors.

LEARNING EXERCISES

Complete the following review exercises after reading the associated pages in the textbook as indicated by each exercise. Answers to each review exercise are provided at the end of the review exercises.

PART I: RADIOGRAPHIC ANATOMY

REVIEW EXERCISE A: Radiographic Anatomy of the Cervical and Thoracic Spine (see textbook pp. 300–311)

1. List the number of bones found in each division in the adult vertebral column.

   A. Cervical _____

   B. Thoracic _____

   C. Lumbar _____

   D. Sacrum _____

   E. Coccyx _____

   F. Total _____

   Refer to Fig. 8.1 to answer Questions 2–4.

2. List the two primary or posterior convex curves seen in the vertebral column.

   A. _____

   B. _____

3. Indicate which two portions of the vertebral column are classified as secondary or compensatory curves.

   A. _____

   B. _____

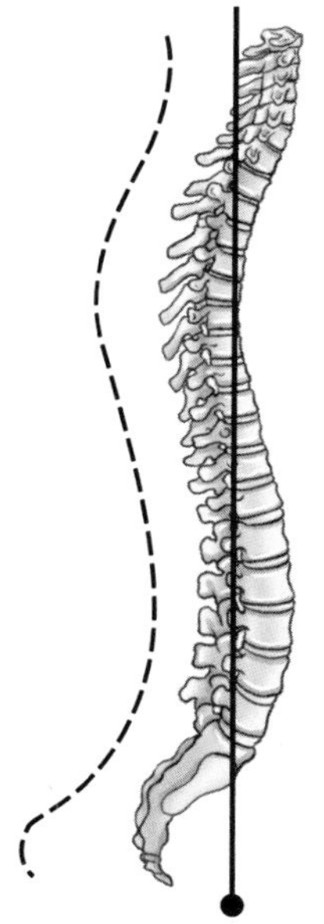

Posterior　　Centerline of gravity　　**Anterior**

Fig. 8.1 Lateral view, spinal column.

4. Match the correct aspect(s) of the vertebral column with the following characteristics. (There may be more than one correct answer.)

   _____ 1. Convex curve (with respect to posterior)　　A. Cervical spine

   _____ 2. Concave curve (with respect to posterior)　　B. Thoracic spine

   _____ 3. Secondary curve　　C. Lumbar spine

   _____ 4. Primary curve　　D. Sacrum

   _____ 5. Develops as child learns to hold head erect

5. An abnormal, or exaggerated, "sway back" lumbar curvature is called _____.

6. An abnormal lateral curvature seen in the thoracolumbar spine is called _____.

7. The two main parts of a typical vertebra are the _____ and the

_____.

8. The _____ are two bony aspects of the vertebral arch that extend posteriorly from each pedicle to join at the midline.

9. Two small notches on the superior and inferior aspects of the pedicles create the _____ foramina.

10. The opening, or passageway, for the spinal cord is the _____.

11. The spinal cord begins with the (A) _____ of the brain and extends down to the (B)

_____ vertebra, where it tapers and ends. This tapered ending is called the (C)

_____.

12. Which structures pass through the intervertebral foramina? _____

186

Chapter **8** **Cervical and Thoracic Spine**

Copyright © 2025 by Elsevier Inc.
All rights reserved, including those for text and data mining, AI training, and similar technologies.

13. Identify the following structures labeled on these drawings of typical thoracic vertebrae (Fig. 8.2).

Superior view

A. _____

B. _____

C. _____

D. _____

E. _____

F. _____

Lateral view

G. _____

H. _____

I. _____

J. _____

K. _____

Lateral oblique view

L. _____

M. _____ joint

N. _____

O. _____

P. _____

Q. The joints between the ribs and vertebrae at N are called

_____.

R. The joints between the ribs and vertebrae at P are called

_____.

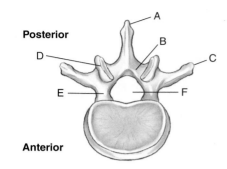

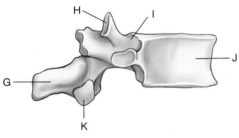

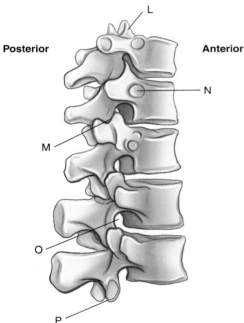

Fig. 8.2 Typical thoracic vertebrae.

14. Which of the following is found between the superior and inferior articular processes?

    A. Intervertebral joints

    B. Articular joints

    C. Zygapophyseal joints

    D. Intervertebral facets

15. True/False: Only T11 and T12 have *full* facets for articulation with ribs.

16. True/False: The zygapophyseal joints of *all* cervical vertebrae are visualized only in a true lateral position.

17. List the outer and inner aspects of the intervertebral disk.

    A. Outer aspect _____

    B. Inner aspect _____

18. The condition involving a "slipped disk" is correctly referred to as _____.

19. List the alternative names for the following cervical vertebrae.

    A. C1: _____

    B. C2: _____

    C. C7: _____

20. List three features that make the cervical vertebrae unique.

    A. _____

    B. _____

    C. _____

21. A short column of bone found between the superior and articular processes in a typical cervical vertebra is called

_____.

22. What is the term for the same structure, identified in Question 21, for the C1 vertebra?

23. The zygapophyseal joints for the second through seventh cervical vertebrae are at a

_____-degree angle to the midsagittal plane; the thoracic vertebrae are at a

_____-degree angle to the midsagittal plane.

24. What is the name of the joint found between the superior articular processes of C1 and the occipital condyles of the skull?

_____

25. The modified body of C2 is called the _____ or _____.

26. A lack of symmetry of the zygapophyseal joints between C1 and C2 may be caused by injury or may be

associated with _____ (hint: positioning error).

27. What is the unique feature of all thoracic vertebrae that distinguishes them from other vertebrae?

_____

28. Which specific thoracic vertebrae are classified as typical thoracic vertebrae (i.e., they least resemble cervical or lumbar vertebrae)?

_____

29. Identify the labeled structures on the radiographs of the cervical spine in Figs. 8.3 and 8.4. (Indicate the specific structure and the vertebra of which it is a part.)

Structure	*Vertebra*
A. _____	_____
B. _____	_____
C. _____	_____
D. _____	_____
E. _____	_____
F. _____	_____
G. _____	_____
H. _____	_____

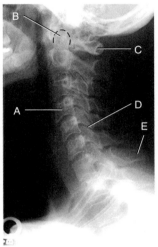

Fig. 8.3 Lateral view, cervical spine.

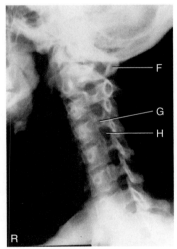

Fig. 8.4 A 45-degree oblique view, cervical spine.

30. For the central ray to pass through and "open" the intervertebral spaces on a 45-degree posterior oblique projection of the cervical vertebrae, what central ray angle (if any) is required?

_____

REVIEW EXERCISE B: Positioning of the Cervical and Thoracic Spine (see textbook pp. 312–330)

1. Name the following parts of the sternum or associated topographic landmarks.

   A. Upper portion of sternum: _____

   B. Superior margin of this upper section (landmark): _____

   C. Center portion of sternum: _____

   D. Joint between top and center portions (landmark): _____

   E. Most inferior aspect of sternum (landmark): _____

2. Match the following topographic landmarks to the correct vertebral level. (Use each choice only once.)

   _____1. Gonion   A. C7–T1

   _____2. Xiphoid process (tip)   B. T2–T3

   _____3. Thyroid cartilage   C. C1

   _____4. Jugular notch   D. T4–T5

   _____5. Sternal angle   E. T9–T10

   _____6. Mastoid tip   F. C4–C6

   _____7. Vertebra prominens   G. T7

   _____8. 3–4 inches (8–10 cm) below jugular notch   H. C3

3. In addition to the gonads, which other radiosensitive organs are of greatest concern during cervical and thoracic spine radiography?

   _____

4. List the two advantages of using higher kVp exposure factors for spine radiography on an anteroposterior (AP) thoracic spine radiograph.

   A. _____   B. _____

5. True/False: When using digital imaging for spine radiography, it is important to use close collimation, grids (physical or virtual), and lead masking.

6. True/False: If close collimation is used for the spine, the use of lead masking (blockers) is generally not required.

7. True/False: To a certain degree, magnetic resonance imaging (MR) and computed tomography (CT) are replacing myelography as the imaging modalities of choice for the diagnosis of a ruptured intervertebral disk.

8. True/False: Nuclear medicine is often performed to diagnose bone tumors of the spine.

9. To ensure that the intervertebral joint spaces are open for lateral thoracic spine projections, it is important to:

   A. Keep the vertebral column parallel to the IR

   B. Use a small focal spot

   C. Use a breathing technique

   D. Angle the central ray caudad

10. For lateral and oblique projections of the cervical spine, it is important to minimize magnification and maximize detail. This can be done by (more than one answer may be used):

    A. Keeping the vertebral column parallel to the image receptor

    B. Using a small focal spot

    C. Increasing the source image receptor distance (SID)

    D. Using an orthostatic (breathing) technique

11. Match each the following clinical indications of the spine to the correct definition. (Use each choice only once.)

    _____ A. Fracture through the pedicles and anterior arch of C2 with forward displacement on C3

    _____ B. Inflammation of the vertebrae

    _____ C. Abnormal or exaggerated convex curvature of the thoracic spine

    _____ D. Comminuted fracture of the vertebral body with posterior fragments displaced into the spinal canal

    _____ E. Avulsion fracture of the spinous process of C7

    _____ F. Abnormal lateral curvature of the spine

    _____ G. A form of rheumatoid arthritis

    _____ H. Impact fracture from axial loading of the anterior and posterior arch of C1

    _____ I. Mild form of scoliosis and kyphosis developing during adolescence

    _____ J. Produces the "bow tie" sign

    1. Ankylosing spondylitis
    2. Clay shoveler's fracture
    3. Unilateral subluxation
    4. Kyphosis
    5. Scheuermann disease
    6. Scoliosis
    7. Jefferson fracture
    8. Teardrop burst fracture
    9. Hangman's fracture
    10. Spondylitis

12. List the conventional radiographic examination and/or projections performed for the following clinical indications.

    A. Scoliosis: _____

    B. Teardrop burst fracture: _____

    C. Jefferson fracture: _____

    D. Scheuermann disease: _____

    E. Unilateral subluxation of cervical spine: _____

    F. Herniated nucleus pulposus (HNP): _____

13. What are the major differences between spondylosis and spondylitis?

_____

14. True/False: Many geriatric patients have a fear of falling off the radiographic table.

15. True/False: Performing the cervicothoracic projection is often required to demonstrate the C7/T1 region for the bariatric patient.

16. What is the name of the radiographic procedure that requires the injection of contrast media into the subarachnoid space? _____

17. Which imaging modality is ideal for detecting early signs of osteomyelitis?

_____

18. Which two landmarks must be aligned for an AP open mouth projection?_____

19. True/False: The tip of the odontoid process does not have to be demonstrated on the AP open mouth projection, because it is best seen on the lateral projection.

20. What is the purpose of the 15- to 20-degree cephalad angle for the AP axial projection of the cervical spine?

_____

21. For an AP axial of the cervical spine, a plane through the tip of the mandible and the

_____ should be parallel to the angled central ray.

    A. Mastoid process   C. Base of skull

    B. Gonion   D. External auditory meatus

22. True/False: Less CR angle is required for the AP axial projection of the cervical spine if the examination is performed supine rather than erect.

23. What are two important benefits of using an SID of 60–72 inches (150–180 cm) for the lateral cervical spine projection?

    A. _____   B. _____

24. What central ray angulation (amount and direction) must be used with a posterior oblique projection of the

    cervical spine? _____

25. Which foramina are demonstrated with a left posterior oblique (LPO) position of the cervical spine?

_____

26. Which foramina are demonstrated with a left anterior oblique (LAO) position of the cervical spine?

_____

27. In addition to extending the chin, which additional positioning technique can be performed to ensure that the mandible is not superimposed over the upper cervical vertebrae for oblique projections?

_____

28. What is the recommended SID for the cervicothoracic position of the cervical spine?

_____

29. The lateral projection of the cervical spine should be taken during _____ (inspiration, expiration, or suspended respiration). Why?

_____

30. Which specific projection must be taken first if trauma to the cervical spine is suspected and the patient is in a supine position on a backboard?

_____

31. The common name of the method for the cervicothoracic lateral position is the _____

_____

32. Where should the central ray be placed for a cervicothoracic lateral position?

_____

33. Which region of the spine must be demonstrated with a cervicothoracic lateral position?

_____

34. Which of the following projections is considered "functional studies" of the cervical spine?

    A. AP "wagging jaw" projection
                  C. Fuchs or Judd method

    B. AP open mouth position
                   D. Hyperextension and hyperflexion lateral positions

35. When should the Judd or Fuchs method be performed?

_____

36. Which AP projection of the cervical spine demonstrates the entire upper cervical spine with one single projection?

_____

37. Which two things can be done to produce equal density along the entire thoracic spine for an AP projection (especially for a patient with a thick chest)?

_____

38. What is the purpose of using an orthostatic (breathing) technique for a lateral projection of the thoracic spine?

_____

39. Which zygapophyseal joints are demonstrated in a right anterior oblique (RAO) projection of the thoracic spine?

_____

40. Which of the following projections delivers the greatest skin dose to the patient?

    A. AP thoracic spine projection

    B. Lateral cervical spine projection

    C. Cervicothoracic lateral position

    D. Fuchs or Judd method

41. True/False: The thyroid dose delivered during a posterior oblique cervical spine (LPO or RPO) projection is greater than the thyroid dose for an anterior oblique (RAO or LAO) projection of the cervical spine.

42. Which of the following structures is best demonstrated with an AP axial vertebral arch projection?

    A. Spinous processes of the lumbar spine

    B. Articular pillars (lateral masses) of the cervical spine

    C. Zygapophyseal joints of the thoracic spine

    D. Cervicothoracic spine region

43. What central ray angle must be used with the AP axial–vertebral arch (pillars) projection?

    A. 15–20 degrees cephalad

    B. 5–10 degrees cephalad

    C. 20–30 degrees caudad

    D. None. Central ray is perpendicular to IR.

44. What ancillary device should be placed behind the patient on the tabletop for a recumbent lateral projection of the thoracic spine?_____

45. Which skull positioning line is aligned perpendicular to the IR for a posteroanterior redundant (Judd) projection for the odontoid process?

_____

46. Which zygapophyseal joints are best demonstrated with an LPO position of the thoracic spine?

_____

47. How much rotation of the body is required for an oblique position of the thoracic spine from a true lateral position?

_____

REVIEW EXERCISE C: Problem Solving for Technical and Positioning Errors

1. A radiograph of an AP open mouth projection of the cervical spine shows the base of the skull is superimposed over the upper odontoid process. Which *specific* positioning error is present on this radiograph?

_____

2. A radiograph of an AP axial projection of the cervical spine shows the intervertebral disk spaces are not open. The following positioning factors were used: extension of the skull, central ray angled 10-degree cephalad, central ray centered to the thyroid cartilage, and no rotation or tilt of the spine. Which of these factors must be modified to produce a more diagnostic image?

_____

3. A radiograph of an RPO cervical spine projection shows the lower intervertebral foramina are *not* open. The upper intervertebral foramina are well visualized. What positioning error most likely led to this radiographic outcome?

_____

4. A radiograph on a lateral projection of the cervical spine shows that C7 is not clearly demonstrated. The following factors were used: erect position, 44-inch (110-cm) SID, arms down by the patient's side, and exposure made during inspiration. Which two of these factors should be changed to produce a more diagnostic image during the repeat exposure?

_____

5. A radiograph of an AP wagging jaw (Ottonello method) projection taken at 75 kVp, 10 mAs, and 0.5 second demonstrates that part of the image of the mandible is still visible and is obscuring the upper cervical spine. Which modification needs to be made to produce a more diagnostic image during the repeat exposure?

_____

6. A radiograph of a lateral thoracic spine shows that lung markings and ribs make it difficult to visualize the vertebral bodies. The following factors were used: recumbent position, 40-inch (100-cm) SID, short exposure time, and exposure made during full expiration. Which of these factors must be modified to produce a more diagnostic image during the repeat exposure?

_____

7. A radiograph of an AP projection of the thoracic spine shows the upper thoracic spine is greatly overexposed but the lower vertebrae are well visualized. The head of the patient was placed at the anode end of the table. What can be used during the repeat exposure to produce a more diagnostic image?

_____

8. A radiograph of a cervicothoracic lateral position demonstrates superimposition of the humeral heads over the upper thoracic spine. Because of an arthritic condition, the patient is unable to rotate the shoulders any farther apart. What can the technologist do to separate the shoulders further during the repeat exposure?

_____

9. **Situation:** A patient with a possible cervical spine injury enters the emergency room. The patient is on a backboard. Which projection of the cervical spine should be taken first?

_____

10. **Situation:** A patient who has been in a motor vehicle accident (MVA) enters the emergency room. The basic projections of the cervical spine show no subluxation (partial dislocation) or fracture. The physician wants the spine evaluated for whiplash injury. Which additional projections would best demonstrate this type of injury?

_____

11. **Situation:** A patient comes to the radiology department for a cervical spine series. An AP open mouth radiograph indicates that the base of the skull and the lower edge of the front incisors are superimposed, but the top of the dens is not clearly demonstrated. What should the technologist do to demonstrate the upper portion of the dens? (A horizontal beam lateral projection has ruled out a C-spine fracture or subluxation.)

_____

12. **Situation:** A broad shouldered patient comes to the radiology department for a routine cervical spine series. The lateral projection demonstrates only the C1–C5 region. The radiologist wants to see C6–T1. What additional projection can be taken to demonstrate this region of the spine?

_____

13. **Situation:** A patient enters the ER with a possible cervical spine fracture, but the initial projections do not demonstrate any gross fracture or subluxation. After reviewing the initial radiographs, the ER physician suspects either a congenital defect or a fracture of the articular pillars of C4. He wants an additional projection taken to better see this aspect of the vertebrae. What additional projection can be taken to demonstrate the articular pillars of C4?

_____

14. **Situation:** A patient comes to the ER with a possible Jefferson fracture. Other than a lateral projection or a CT scan, what specific radiographic projection will best demonstrate this type of fracture?

_____

15. **Situation:** A patient comes to the radiology department with a clinical history of Scheuermann disease. Which radiographic procedure is often performed for this condition?

_____

REVIEW EXERCISE D: Critique Radiographs of the Cervical and Thoracic Spine

The following questions relate to the radiographs found at the end of Chapter 8 of the textbook. Evaluate these radiographs for the radiographic criteria categories (1–5) that follow. Describe the corrections needed to improve the overall image. The major, or "repeatable," errors are specific errors that indicate the need for a repeat exposure, regardless of the nature of the other errors.

A. AP open mouth (Fig. 8.5)

Description of possible error:

   1. Anatomy demonstrated:

     _____

   2. Part positioning:

     _____

   3. Collimation field size and central ray:

     _____

   4. Exposure:

     _____

   5. Anatomic side markers:

     _____

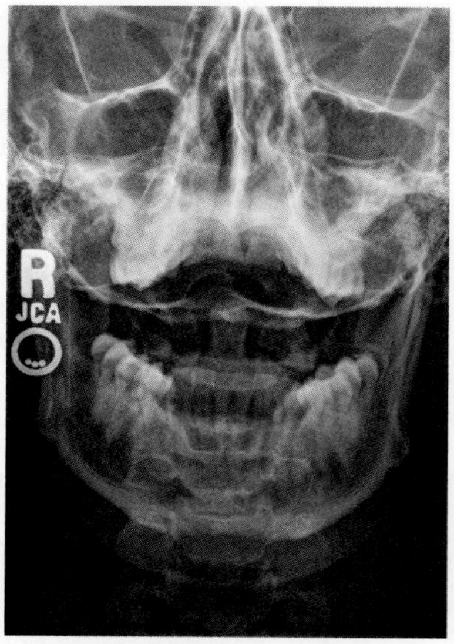

Fig. 8.5 Anteroposterior open mouth.

Repeatable error(s): _____

B. AP open mouth (Fig. 8.6)

Description of possible error:

    1. Anatomy demonstrated:

    _____

    2. Part positioning:

    _____

    3. Collimation field size and central ray:

    _____

    4. Exposure:

    _____

    5. Anatomic side markers:

    _____

Repeatable error(s): _____

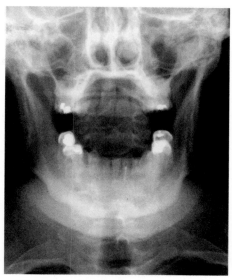

Fig. 8.6 Anteroposterior open mouth.

C. AP axial projection (Fig. 8.7)

Description of possible error:

    1. Anatomy demonstrated:

    _____

    2. Part positioning:

    _____

    3. Collimation field size and central ray

    _____

    4. Exposure:

    _____

    5. Anatomic side markers:

    _____

Repeatable error(s): _____

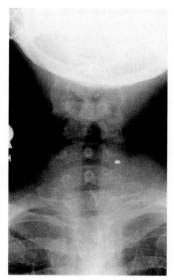

Fig. 8.7 Anteroposterior axial projection.

Chapter **8 Cervical and Thoracic Spine**

D. Right posterior oblique (Fig. 8.8)

Description of possible error:

1. Anatomy demonstrated:

   _____

2. Part positioning:

   _____

3. Collimation field size and central ray:

   _____

4. Exposure:

   _____

5. Anatomic side markers:

   _____

Repeatable error(s): _____

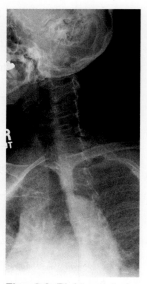

Fig. 8.8 Right posterior oblique.

E. Horizontal beam lateral (trauma) (Fig. 8.9)

Description of possible error:

1. Anatomy demonstrated:

   _____

2. Part positioning:

   _____

3. Collimation field size and central ray:

   _____

4. Exposure:

   _____

5. Anatomic side markers:

   _____

Repeatable error(s): _____

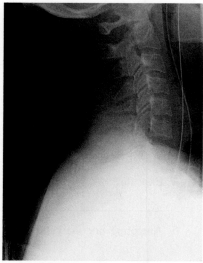

Fig. 8.9 Horizontal beam lateral (trauma).

F.   AP for odontoid process (Fuchs method) (Fig. 8.10)

Description of possible error:

1. Anatomy demonstrated:

   _____

2. Part positioning:

   _____

3. Collimation field size and central ray:

   _____

4. Exposure:

   _____

5. Anatomic side markers:

   _____

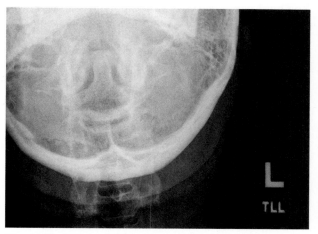

Fig. 8.10 Anteroposterior for odontoid process (Fuchs method).

Repeatable error(s): _____

G.   AP thoracic spine (Fig. 8.11)

Description of possible error:

1. Anatomy demonstrated:

   _____

2. Part positioning:

   _____

3. Collimation field size and central ray:

   _____

4. Exposure:

   _____

5. Anatomic side markers:

   _____

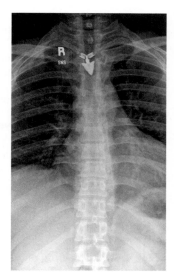

Fig. 8.11 Anteroposterior thoracic spine.

Repeatable error(s): _____

You must gain experience in positioning each part of the cervical and thoracic spine before performing the following exams on actual patients. You can get experience in positioning and radiographic evaluation of these projections by performing exercises using radiographic phantoms and by practicing positioning on other students (although you will not be taking actual exposures).

The following suggested activities assume that your teaching institution has an energized lab and radiographic phantoms. If not, perform Laboratory Exercises B and C, the radiographic evaluation and the physical positioning exercises, respectively. (Check off each step and projection as you complete it.)

Laboratory Exercise A: Energized Laboratory

1. Using the radiographic phantom, produce radiographs of the following basic routines.

    A. AP, lateral, and oblique cervical spine

    B. AP, lateral, and oblique thoracic spine

Laboratory Exercise B: Radiographic Evaluation

1. Evaluate and critique the radiographs produced previously, additional radiographs provided by your instructor, or both. Evaluate each radiograph for the following points.

    _____ Evaluate the completeness of the study. (Are all of the pertinent anatomic structures included on the radiograph?)

    _____ Evaluate for positioning or centering errors (e.g., rotation, off-centering).

    _____ Evaluate for correct exposure factors and possible motion. (Is the optimal image exposure and contrast of the images acceptable?)

    _____ Determine whether anatomic side markers and an acceptable degree of collimation are present.

Laboratory Exercise C: Physical Positioning

On another person, simulate performing all basic and special projections of the cervical and thoracic spine as follows. Include the six steps listed in the following and described in the textbook. (Check off each step when completed satisfactorily.)

Step 1. Appropriate size and type of image receptor with correct markers

Step 2. Correct central ray placement and centering of part to central ray and/or IR

Step 3. Accurate collimation

Step 4. Area shielding of patient (when required)

Step 5. Use of proper immobilizing devices when needed

Step 6. Approximate correct exposure factors, breathing instructions where applicable, and initiating exposure

Projections	Step 1	Step 2	Step 3	Step 4	Step 5	Step 6
• Cervical spine series (AP axial, AP open-mouth and lateral projections)	_____	_____	_____	_____	_____	_____
• Thoracic spine series (AP and lateral)	_____	_____	_____	_____	_____	_____
• Cervicothoracic lateral	_____	_____	_____	_____	_____	_____
• Hyperextension and flexion laterals	_____	_____	_____	_____	_____	_____
• AP wagging jaw projection	_____	_____	_____	_____	_____	_____
• AP (Fuchs) projection for dens	_____	_____	_____	_____	_____	_____
• PA (Judd) projection for dens	_____	_____	_____	_____	_____	_____
• Thoracic spine oblique projections	_____	_____	_____	_____	_____	_____

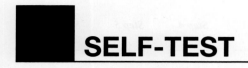 **SELF-TEST** MY SCORE = _____ %

This self-test should be taken only after completing all of the readings, review exercises, and laboratory activities for a particular section. The purpose of this test is not only to provide a good learning exercise but also to serve as a strong indicator of what your final evaluation exam for this chapter will cover. It is strongly suggested that if you do not get at least a 90%–95% grade on each self-test, you should review those areas in which you missed questions before going to your instructor for the final evaluation exam.

1. At which vertebral level does the solid spinal cord terminate? _____

2. How many segments make up the sacrum in the neonate? _____

3. Which of the following divisions of the spine is described as possessing a primary curve? (There may be more than one correct answer.)

    A. Thoracic   C. Lumbar

    B. Cervical   D. Sacral

4. True/False: The lumbar possesses a concave posterior spinal curvature.

5. An abnormal or exaggerated thoracic spinal curvature with increased convexity is called _____.

6. An abnormal or exaggerated lateral spinal curvature is called _____.

7. What is the correct term for the condition involving a "slipped disk"? _____

8. The superior and inferior vertebral notches create which foramina? _____

9. Which joints are found between the superior and inferior articular processes? _____

10. Which of the following structures makes up the inner aspect of the intervertebral disk?

    A. Annulus fibrosus   C. Annulus pulposus

    B. Nucleus pulposus   D. Nucleus fibrosus

11. The _____ artery and vein pass through the cervical transverse foramina.

12. True/False: The thoracic spine possesses facets for rib articulations and bifid spinous processes.

13. The intervertebral foramina for the cervical spine lie at a _____-degree angle to the mid-sagittal plane.

14. Which ligament holds the dens against the anterior arch of C1? _____

15. The large joint space between C1 and C2 is called the _____.

16. Two partial facets found on the thoracic vertebrae are called _____.

202

17. Which of the following thoracic vertebrae do not possess a facet for the costotransverse joint? (There may be more than one correct answer.)

    A. T1   C. T11

    B. T7   D. T12

18. What are three distinctive features of all cervical vertebrae that make them different from any other vertebrae?

    A. _____   C. _____

    B. _____

19. What is the one feature of all thoracic vertebrae that makes them different from all other vertebrae?

_____

20. Which position of the thoracic spine best demonstrates the intervertebral foramina?

_____

21. Identify the following structures labeled on Figs. 8.12–8.14 (include the specific vertebra of which each structure is a part).

Anterior

Fig. 8.12 Superior view.

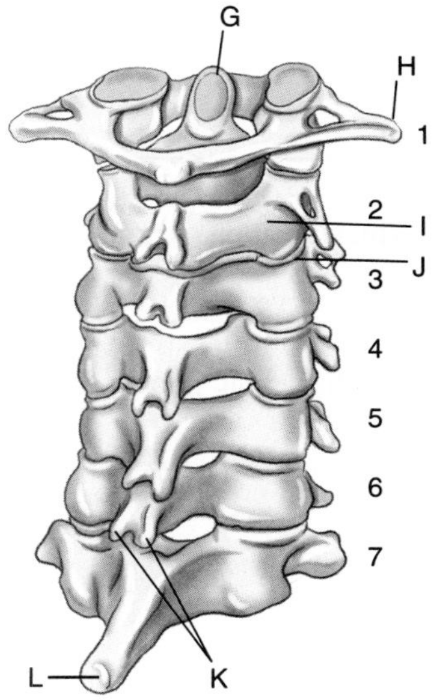

Posterior

Structure	*Vertebra*
Fig. 8.12	
A. _____	_____
B. _____	_____
C. _____	_____
D. _____	_____
E. _____	_____
F. _____	_____
Fig. 8.13	
G. _____	_____
H. _____	_____
I. _____	_____
J. _____	_____
K. _____	_____
L. _____	_____

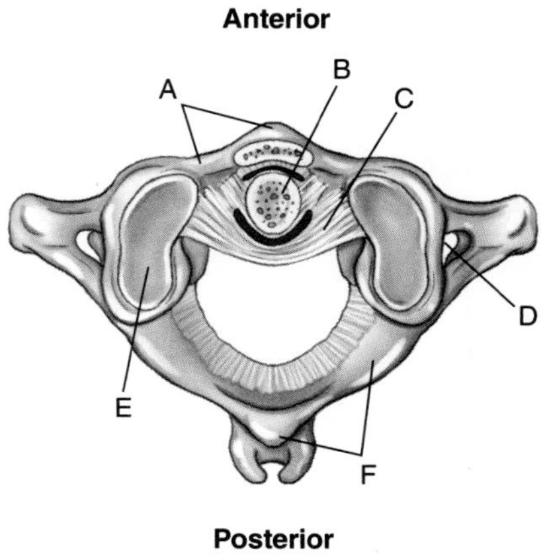

Fig. 8.13 Posterolateral view, cervical spine.

Structure   **Vertebra**

Fig. 8.14

M. _____   _____

N. _____   _____

O. _____   _____

P. _____   _____

Q. _____   _____

R. _____   _____

S. This drawing represents which vertebrae?

_____.

T. How can these specific vertebrae be identified?

_____.

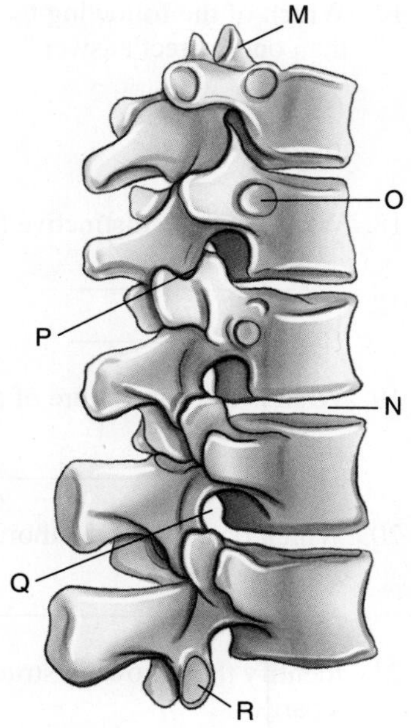

Fig. 8.14 Lateral oblique view.

22. Identify the following structures and vertebrae labeled on this AP open mouth cervical spine radiograph (Fig. 8.15).

Structure   **Vertebra**

A. _____   _____

B. _____   _____

C. _____   _____

D. _____   _____

E. _____   _____

F. _____   _____

G. _____   _____

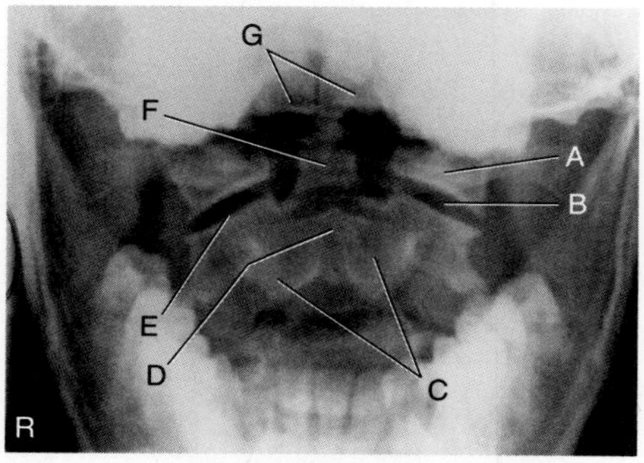

Fig. 8.15 AP open mouth cervical spine radiograph.

23. Which position or projection of the cervical spine best demonstrates the zygapophyseal joints (between C3 and C7)?

_____

24. Which specific joint spaces are visualized with an LAO projection of the thoracic spine?

_____

25. Match each of the following topographic landmarks to the correct vertebral level (using each choice only once).

_____ 1. Vertebra prominens   A. T2–T3

_____ 2. Jugular notch   B. C7–T1

_____ 3. 3–4 inches (8–10 cm) below jugular notch   C. T7

_____ 4. Gonion   D. C3

_____ 5. Sternal angle   E. C4–C6

_____ 6. Thyroid cartilage   F. T4–T5

26. Which of the following imaging modalities is **not** normally performed to rule out an HNP?

A. CT

B. Myelography

C. MR

D. Nuclear medicine (NM)

27. An avulsion fracture of the spinous processes of C6–T1 is called a:

A. Hangman's fracture

B. Clay shoveler's fracture

C. Jefferson fracture

D. Teardrop burst fracture

28. Scheuermann disease is a form of:

A. Scoliosis and/or kyphosis

B. Subluxation

C. Arthritis

D. Fracture

29. True/False: HNP most frequently develops at the L2–L3 vertebral level.

30. Which two things can be done to minimize the effects of scatter radiation on lateral projections of the thoracic and lumbar spine?

A. _____

B. _____

31. Which position or projection best demonstrates the zygapophyseal joints between C1 and C2?

_____

32. How much and in which direction (caudad or cephalad) should the central ray be angled for each of the following projections?

A. An AP axial projection of the cervical spine: _____

B. An anterior oblique projection of the cervical spine: _____

C. A posterior oblique projection of the cervical spine: _____

33. Which of the following projections of the cervical spine demonstrates the left intervertebral foramen?

A. LPO

B. LAO

C. Lateral projection

D. RAO

34. In addition to using a long SID, list the two positioning techniques you can use to lower the shoulders to visualize C7–T1 for a lateral projection of the cervical spine.

A. _____

B. _____

35. Which position or projection demonstrates the lower cervical and upper thoracic spine (C4–T3) in a lateral perspective? (Fracture/subluxation has been ruled out.)

36. List the two positions or projections that will project the dens in the center of the foramen magnum.

    A. _____   B. _____

37. **Situation:** A lateral cervical spine radiograph demonstrates the zygapophyseal joint spaces are not superimposed. Which type of positioning error(s) may lead to this radiographic outcome?

    _____

38. **Situation:** A radiograph of a lateral thoracic spine projection shows the intervertebral foramina and intervertebral joint spaces are not clearly demonstrated. Which type of problems can lead to this radiographic outcome?

    _____

39. **Situation:** A patient who was involved in an MVA 3 days earlier is experiencing severe neck pain and comes to the radiology department for a cervical spine series. The patient is not wearing a cervical collar. Should the technologist take a horizontal beam lateral projection and have it cleared before proceeding with the study? Explain.

    _____

40. **Situation:** A patient with a possible Jefferson fracture enters the ER. Which specific radiographic position best demonstrates this type of fracture?

    _____

41. **Situation:** A radiograph of an AP open mouth projection of the cervical spine demonstrates the upper incisors superimposed over the top of the dens. What specific positioning error is present on this radiograph?

    _____

42. **Situation:** A patient comes to the radiology department for a follow-up study for a clay shoveler's fracture. Which spine projections will best demonstrate this type of fracture?

    _____

43. **Situation:** A patient comes to the radiology department for a follow-up study 6 months after having spinal fusion surgery of the lower cervical spine (C5–C6). The surgeon wants to check for anteroposterior mobility of the fused spine. Beyond the basic cervical spine projections, what additional projections can be taken to assess the mobility of the spine?

44. Which of the following technical factors is most important in producing a high-quality CR image?

    A. Decrease SID whenever possible   C. Decrease kVp as much as possible

    B. Minimize the use of grids   D. Collimate as closely as possible

45. Which of the following imaging modalities is recommended for a teardrop burst fracture?

    A. CT   C. Nuclear medicine (NM)

    B. MR   D. Diagnostic medical sonography (DMS)

8 Cervical and Thoracic Spine

1. Lower border of first lumbar (L1) vertebra
2. Five
3. A. Thoracic; D. Sacral
4. True
5. Kyphosis
6. Scoliosis
7. Herniated nucleus pulposus (HNP)
8. Intervertebral foramina
9. Zygapophyseal joints
10. B. Nucleus pulposus
11. Vertebral
12. False (C-spine possesses bifid spinous processes)
13. 45
14. Transverse atlantal ligament
15. Atlantoaxial (zygapophyseal) joint
16. Demifacets
17. C. T11; D. T12
18. A. Each has three foramina (one in each transverse process in addition to the vertebral foramina).
    B. Bifid spinous processes
    C. Overlapping vertebral bodies
19. Presence of facets for articulation with ribs
20. Lateral position
21. A. Anterior arch (with anterior tubercle), C1 (atlas)
    B. Dens (odontoid process), C2
    C. Transverse atlantal ligament, C2
    D. Transverse foramen, C1
    E. Superior facet (atlanto-occipital articulation), C1
    F. Posterior arch, C1
    G. Dens (odontoid process), C2
    H. Transverse process, C1
    I. Articular pillar (lateral mass), C2
    J. Right zygapophyseal joint, C2–C3

K. Bifid, spinous process, C4
L. Vertebra prominens (spinous process), C7
M. Superior articular process, T10
N. Intervertebral disk space, T10–T11
O. Facet for costovertebral joint, T11
P. Right zygapophyseal joint, T11–T12
Q. Right intervertebral foramen, T12–L1
R. Facet of inferior articular process, L2
S. Lower thoracic (T10, T11, and T12) and upper lumbar (L1 and L2)
T. Evident by facets for articulation with ribs on upper three but not on lower two. (Note also that the last two thoracic vertebrae do not have facets on transverse processes for costotransverse joints, characteristic of T11 and T12.)

22. A. Lateral mass (articular pillar), C1
    B. Atlantoaxial (zygopophyseal) joint (between) C1 and C2
    C. Body, C2
    D. Spinous process (superimposed by body), C2
    E. Inferior articular process, C2
    F. Dens (odontoid process), C2
    G. Upper incisors (teeth)
23. Lateral position
24. Left zygapophyseal joints (downside joints)
25. 1. B
    2. A
    3. C
    4. D
    5. F
    6. E
26. D. Nuclear medicine

27. B. Clay shoveler's fracture
28. A. Scoliosis and/or kyphosis
29. False. Most common at the L4–L5 level
30. A. Close side collimation
    B. Place a lead mat or masking on tabletop behind patient.
31. AP open-mouth projection
32. A. 15–20 degrees cephalad
    B. 15 degrees caudad
    C. 15 degrees cephalad
33. B. Left anterior oblique (LAO)
34. A. Suspend respiration on full expiration
    B. Have 5- to 10-lb (3- to 4-kg) weights suspended from each wrist
35. Cervicothoracic lateral or "swimmer's" position
36. A. AP projection—Fuchs method
    B. PA projection—Judd method
37. Tilt and/or rotation of the spine
38. Not keeping spine parallel to the IR and/or not aligning the CR perpendicular to spine
39. Yes. (The technologist needs to assume there may be a fracture present. A horizontal beam lateral projection should be taken for all suspected trauma to the cervical spine. A physician must examine the radiograph and clear the patient for the remaining projections.)
40. AP open-mouth projection. Note that a horizontal beam lateral projection must be taken and cleared first.
41. Excessive flexion of skull
42. AP and lateral cervical spine projections
43. Hyperflexion and hyperextension lateral positions
44. D. Collimate as closely as possible
45. A. CT

A1

9 Lumbar Spine, Sacrum, and Coccyx

CHAPTER OBJECTIVES

After you have successfully completed the activities in this chapter, you will be able to:

_____ 1. Using drawings and radiographs, identify specific anatomic structures of the lumbar spine, sacrum, and coccyx.

_____ 2. Identify the anatomic structures that make up the "Scottie dog" sign.

_____ 3. Identify the classification and type of movement of the joints found in the lumbar spine.

_____ 4. List topographic landmarks that can be palpated to locate specific aspects of the lumbar spine, sacrum, and coccyx.

_____ 5. Define specific types of pathologic features of the spine as described in the textbook.

_____ 6. Identify radiographic appearances related to these specific types of pathologic spine features.

_____ 7. Identify basic and special projections of the lumbar spine, sacrum, coccyx, and sacroiliac joints, including the correct collimation field size and central ray (CR) location, direction, and angulation of the central ray for each projection.

_____ 8. Identify the structures that are best seen with specific projections of the lumbar spine.

_____ 9. Identify the approximate difference in patient doses between anteroposterior (AP) compared with posteroanterior (PA) projections and the approximate difference between anterior compared with posterior oblique positions of the lumbar spine.

_____ 10. Given various hypothetic situations, identify the correct modification of a position and/or exposure factors to improve the radiographic image.

_____ 11. Given radiographs of specific lumbosacral spine projections or positions, identify positioning and exposure factor errors.

POSITIONING AND RADIOGRAPHIC CRITIQUE

_____ 1. Using a peer, position for basic and special projections of the lumbosacral spine.

_____ 2. Using a lumbar spine radiographic phantom, produce satisfactory radiographs of specific positions (if equipment is available).

_____ 3. Critique and evaluate lumbar spine and SI joint radiographs based on the five divisions of radiographic criteria: (1) anatomy demonstrated, (2) position, (3) collimation field size and central ray, (4) exposure, and (5) anatomic side markers.

_____ 4. Distinguish between acceptable and unacceptable lumbosacral spine radiographs based on exposure factors, motion, collimation, positioning, or other errors.

LEARNING EXERCISES

Complete the following review exercises after reading the associated pages in the textbook as indicated by each exercise. Answers to each review exercise are provided at the end of the review exercises.

PART I: RADIOGRAPHIC ANATOMY

REVIEW EXERCISE A: Radiographic Anatomy of the Lumbar Spine, Sacrum, and Coccyx (see textbook pp. 334–339)

1. A portion of the lamina located between the superior and inferior articular processes is called the

    ____________________________.

2. The superior and inferior vertebral notches join together to form the:

    A. Vertebral foramen
    B. Intervertebral foramina
    C. Pedicle
    D. Lamina

3. Which radiographic position best demonstrates the structure identified in the previous question?

    ____

4. Identify the parts of a typical lumbar vertebra as labeled in Fig. 9.1.

    A. ______________
    B. ______________
    C. ______________
    D. ______________
    E. ______________
    F. The central ray projection, labeled F in this drawing, best demonstrates the

    ____

    ____

    G. The central ray projection, labeled G, best demonstrates the

    ____

    ____

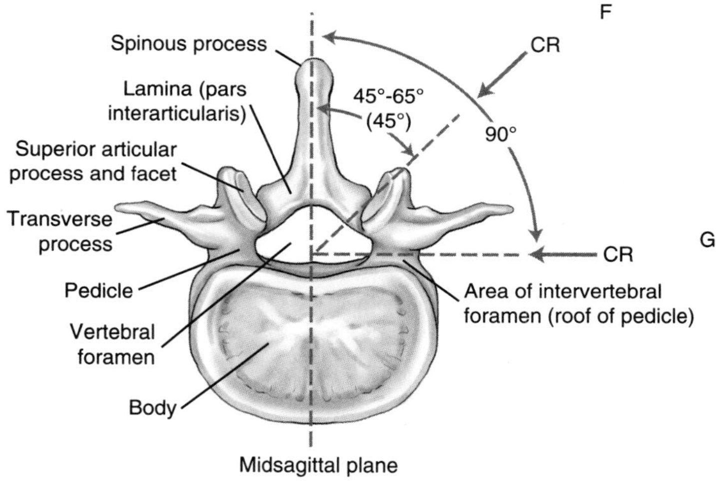

Fig. 9.1 Typical L3 vertebra. CR, central ray.

5. Would the degree of angle to demonstrate the structures identified in F in the previous question be greater or less for the lower lumbar vertebrae as compared with the upper? ____________________________

6. The small foramina found in the sacrum are called ____________________________

7. The anterior and superior aspect of the sacrum that forms the posterior wall of the pelvic inlet is called the

_____.

8. What is another term for the sacral horns? _____

9. The sacroiliac joints lie at an oblique angle of _____ degrees to the coronal plane.

10. What is the formal term for the tailbone? _____

11. What is the name of the superior broad aspect of the coccyx? _____

12. List the structure classification and movement classification and type for the following joints of the vertebrae.

	Classification	Mobility Type	Movement Type
A.	Zygapophyseal	_____	_____
B.	Intervertebral	_____	_____

13. Identify the following structures labeled on the radiographs of the lumbar spine (Figs. 9.2 and 9.3).

A. _____

B. _____

C. _____

D. _____

E. _____

F. _____ joint

G. _____

H. _____

I. _____

J. _____

K. _____

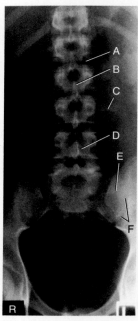
Fig. 9.2 Anteroposterior.

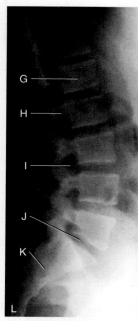
Fig. 9.3 Lateral.

Identify parts of the Scottie dog image, which should be visible on an oblique lumbar spine image (Figs. 9.4 and 9.5).

L. _____

M. _____ joint

N. _____

O. _____

P. _____

Q. _____

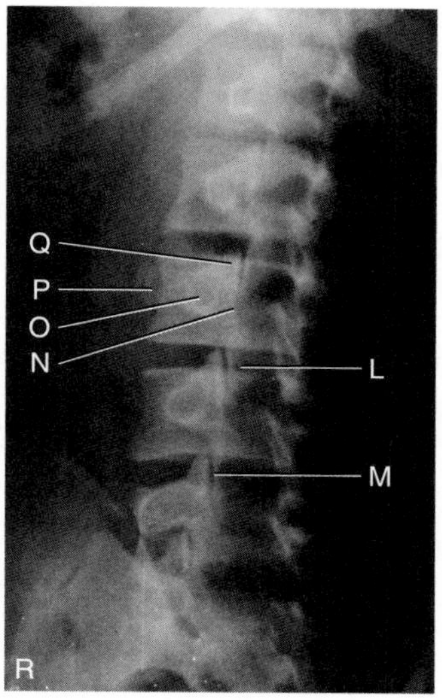

Fig. 9.4 Oblique.

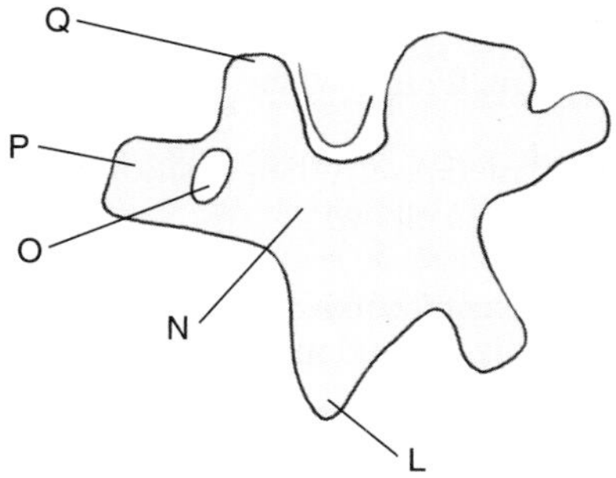

Fig. 9.5 Scottie dog image.

14. List the specific joints or foramina that are demonstrated with the following lumbar spine positions.

    A. Left posterior oblique (LPO): _____

    B. Right anterior oblique (RAO): _____

    C. Lateral: _____

    D. Right posterior oblique (RPO): _____

    E. Left anterior oblique (LAO): _____

15. The degree of obliquity required for an oblique projection at the T12–L1 level is approximately

    _____, whereas the L5–S1 spine level requires a(n) _____ oblique.

PART II: RADIOGRAPHIC POSITIONING

REVIEW EXERCISE B: Positioning of the Lumbar Spine, Sacrum, Coccyx, and Sacroiliac Joints (see textbook pp. 340–362)

1. Match each of the following topographic landmarks to the correct vertebral level. (Use each choice only once.)

    _____ 1. Anterior superior iliac spines (ASIS)   A. L2–L3

    _____ 2. Xiphoid process   B. L4–L5

    _____ 3. Lower costal margin   C. S1–S2

    _____ 4. Iliac crest   D. Prominence of greater trochanter

    _____ 5. Symphysis pubis   E. T9–T10

2. True/False: The use of higher kVp and lower mAs for lumbar spine radiography improves radiographic contrast but increases patient dose.

3. True/False: Placing a lead blocker mat behind the patient for lateral lumbar spine positions improves image quality.

4. True/False: For lumbar spine imaging, close collimation is an important factor for dose reduction to the gonads.

5. True/False: The AP projection of the lumbar spine opens the intervertebral joint spaces better than the PA projection.

6. True/False: The knees and hips should be extended for a recumbent AP projection of the lumbar spine.

7. True/False: An increased source image receptor distance (SID) of 44–48 inches (110–120 cm) reduces magnification of the spine anatomy.

8. True/False: When imaging a pediatric patient, motion is not a primary concern.

9. True/False: When positioning a bariatric patient, the iliac crest is typically at the level of the inferior margin of the flexed elbow.

10. Select the imaging modality that best demonstrates each of the following pathologic features or conditions. (Answers may be used more than once.)

    _____ A. Osteoporosis   1. Magnetic resonance imaging (MR)

    _____ B. Soft tissues of lumbar spine   2. Computed tomography (CT)

    _____ C. Structures within subarachnoid space   3. Myelography

    _____ D. Inflammatory conditions such as Paget disease   4. Bone densitometry

    _____ E. Compression fractures of the lumbar spine   5. Nuclear medicine (NM)

11. Match each of the following clinical indications to the correct definition or statement. (Use each choice only once.)

    _____ A. Lateral curvature of the vertebral column   1. Spina bifida

    _____ B. Fracture of the vertebral body caused by hyperflexion force   2. Herniated nucleus pulposus (HNP)

    _____ C. Congenital defect in which the posterior elements of the   3. Chance fracture
              vertebrae fail to unite
                                                                                4. Spondylolisthesis
    _____ D. Most common at the L4–L5 level and may result in sciatica
                                                                                5. Compression fracture
    _____ E. Forward displacement of one vertebra onto another vertebra
                                                                                6. Spondylolysis
    _____ F. Inflammatory condition that is most common in males in their
              30s   7. Ankylosing spondylitis

    _____ G. Dissolution and separation of the pars interarticularis   8. Scoliosis

    _____ H. A type of fracture that rarely causes neurologic deficits

12. With a 14- × 17-inch (35- × 43-cm) field size, the central ray is centered at the level of the

    _____ for AP and lateral lumbar spine projections.

13. Which two structures can be evaluated to determine whether rotation is present on a radiograph of an AP projection of the lumbar spine?

A. _____ B. _____

14. How much rotation is required to visualize the zygapophyseal joints properly at the L5–S1 level?

_____

15. Which specific set of zygapophyseal joints is demonstrated with an LAO position?

_____

16. The _____, which is the eye of the Scottie dog, should be near the center of the vertebral body on a correctly oblique lumbar spine position.

17. Which positioning error has been committed if the structures described in the previous question are projected too far posterior with a 45-degree oblique position of the lumbar spine? _____

18. Which position or projection of the lumbar spine series best demonstrates a possible compression fracture?

_____

19. A patient with a wide pelvis and narrow thorax may require a central ray angle of _____ degrees _____ (caudad or cephalad) for a lateral position of the lumbar spine.

20. How should the spine of a patient with scoliosis be positioned for a lateral position of the lumbar spine?

_____

21. Why should the knees and hips be flexed for a recumbent AP lumbar spine projection?

_____

22. True/False: The female ovarian dose used for a PA lumbar spine projection is approximately 25%–30% less than the dose for an AP projection.

23. Where is the central ray centered for a lateral L5–S1 projection of the lumbar spine?

_____

24. What amount and direction of central ray angulation is required for an AP axial L5–S1 projection on a male patient? _____

25. True/False: A PA or an AP projection for a scoliosis series frequently includes one erect and one recumbent position for comparison.

26. True/False: The lower margin of the image receptor must include the symphysis pubis for a scoliosis series.

27. True/False: A PA projection for a scoliosis series produces only about one-tenth of the dose to the breast tissue as compared with the AP projection, even if proper collimation is used.

28. Which of the following techniques or devices produces a more uniform density along the vertebral column for an AP/PA scoliosis projection?
   A. Use of a 14- × 36-inch (35- × 90-cm) field size
   B. Lower kVp
   C. Higher mAs
   D. Compensating filter

29. Which side of the spine should be elevated for the second exposure for the AP/PA projection (Ferguson method) scoliosis series (by having the patient stand on a block with one foot)? _____

30. For the Ferguson method, the elevated foot must be raised a minimum of _____ (inches/cm)

31. During the AP (PA) right and left bending projections of the lumbar spine, the _____ serves as a fulcrum during positioning.

32. Which projections should be taken to evaluate flexibility following spinal fusion surgery?

   _____

33. What is the recommended kVp range for lateral hyperflexion and hyperextension positions of the spine for a digital imaging system?
   A. 60–65   C. 70–75
   B. 80–95   D. 100–110

34. How much central ray angulation is required for an AP projection of the sacrum for a typical male patient?

   _____

35. Where is the CR centered for an AP axial projection of the sacrum?

   _____.

36. If a patient cannot lie on his back for the AP sacrum because it is too painful, what alternate projection can be taken to achieve a similar view of the sacrum?

   _____.

37. Where is the central ray centered for an AP projection of the coccyx?

   _____

38. How much is the CR angled for the AP axial coccyx projection? _____.

39. True/False: The AP projections of the sacrum and coccyx can be taken as one single projection to decrease gonadal dose.

40. Patients should be asked to empty the urinary bladder before performing which projection(s) of the vertebral column? _____

41. In addition to good collimation, what should be done to minimize scatter radiation on a lateral lumbar spine or lateral sacrum and coccyx radiograph?

   _____

42. Which sacroiliac (SI) joint is visualized with an RPO position?

_____

43. How much rotation of the body is required for oblique positions of the SI joints?

_____

44. What type of CR angle is recommended for the AP axial projection of the SI joints on a female patient?

A. 20 degrees cephalad   C. 30 degrees caudad

B. 30 degrees cephalad   D. 35 degrees cephalad

45. Where is the CR centered for an oblique projection of the SI joints?

_____

REVIEW EXERCISE C: Problem Solving for Technical and Positioning Errors

1. A radiograph of an AP projection of the lumbar spine shows the spinous processes are not midline to the vertebral column and distortion of the vertebral bodies is present. Which specific positioning error is present on this radiograph?

_____

2. A radiograph of an LPO projection of the lumbar spine shows the downside pedicles and zygapophyseal joints are projected over the anterior portion of the vertebral bodies. Which specific positioning error is present on this radiograph?

_____

3. A radiograph of a lateral projection of a female lumbar spine shows the mid- to lower intervertebral joint spaces are not open. The technologist supported the midsection of the spine with sponges to straighten the spine. What else can be done to open the joint spaces during the repeat exposure?

_____

4. A radiograph of a lateral L5–S1 projection shows the joint space is not open. The technologist did support the middle aspect of the spine with a sponge. What else can the technologist do to open up the joint space during the repeat exposure?

_____

5. A radiograph of an AP axial projection of the coccyx shows the distal tip is superimposed over the symphysis pubis. What must the technologist do to eliminate this problem during the repeat exposure?

_____

6. A radiograph of an oblique position of the lumbar spine shows the downside pedicle and zygapophyseal joint are posterior in relation to the vertebral body. What modification of the position must be made during the repeat exposure to produce a more diagnostic image?

_____

7. **Situation:** A patient comes to the radiology department for a follow-up study for a compression fracture of L3. The radiologist requests that collimated projections be taken of L3. Which specific projections and centering would provide a quality study of L3 and the intervertebral joint spaces?

_____

214

8. **Situation:** A young female patient comes to the radiology department for a scoliosis series. She has had repeated radiation exposure throughout a period of time and is understandably concerned about the radiation. What three things can the technologist do to minimize the dose delivered to the breast tissue?

   A. _____

   B. _____

   C. _____

9. **Situation:** A patient with an injury to the coccyx enters the emergency room. When attempting the AP projection, the patient complains that it is too uncomfortable to lie on his back. He is unable to stand. What other options are available to complete the study?

   _____

10. **Situation:** A patient with a clinical history of spondylolisthesis at the L5–S1 level comes to the radiology department. Which specific lumbar spine position is most diagnostic in demonstrating the extent of this condition?

   _____

11. **Situation:** A positioning series for SI joints is performed on a patient. The resultant radiographs do not demonstrate the inferior portion of the joints. What can be done during the repeat exposure to demonstrate this aspect of the SI joints?

   _____

12. **Situation:** A patient comes to the radiology department for a lumbar spine series. He has a clinical history of advanced spondylolysis. Which specific projection(s) of the lumbar spine series will best demonstrate this condition?

   _____

13. **Situation:** A patient comes to the radiology department with a clinical history of HNP. Which of the following imaging modalities provide the most diagnostic study for this condition?

   A. Diagnostic medical sonography (DMS)   C. Nuclear medicine

   B. MR   D. Radiography

14. **Situation:** A patient comes to the radiology department for a lumbar spine study following spinal fusion surgery. Her surgeon wants a study to assess mobility of the spine at the fusion site. Which radiographic positions provide this information?

   _____

15. **Situation:** A patient comes to the radiology department for a lumbar spine series. She has a clinical history of severe kyphosis. How should the lumbar spine series be modified for this patient?

   _____

REVIEW EXERCISE D: Critique Radiographs of the Lumbar Spine, Sacrum, and Coccyx

The following questions relate to the radiographs found in this exercise. Evaluate these radiographs for the radiographic criteria categories (1–5) that follow. Describe the corrections needed to improve the overall image. The major, or "repeatable," errors are specific errors that indicate the need for a repeat exposure, regardless of the nature of the other errors.

A. Lateral lumbar spine (Fig. 9.6)

1. Anatomy demonstrated:

   _____

2. Part positioning:

   _____

3. Collimation field size and central ray:

   _____

4. Exposure:

   _____

5. Anatomic side markers:

   _____

Repeatable error(s): _____

B. Lateral lumbar spine (Fig. 9.7)

1. Anatomy demonstrated:

   _____

2. Part positioning:

   _____

3. Collimation field size and central ray:

   _____

4. Exposure:

   _____

5. Anatomic side markers:

   _____

Repeatable error(s): _____

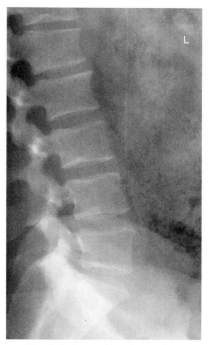

Fig. 9.6 Lateral lumbar spine.

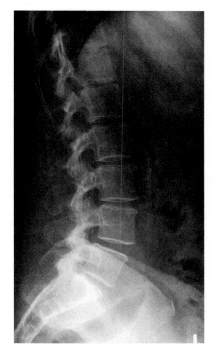

Fig. 9.7 Lateral lumbar spine.

C. Lateral L5–S1 (Fig. 9.8)

1. Anatomy demonstrated:

   _____

2. Part positioning:

   _____

3. Collimation field size and central ray:

   _____

4. Exposure:

   _____

5. Anatomic side markers:

   _____

Repeatable error(s): _____

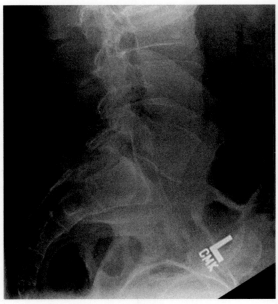

Fig. 9.8 Lateral L5–S1.

D. RPO lumbar spine (Fig. 9.9)

1. Anatomy demonstrated:

   _____

2. Part positioning:

   _____

3. Collimation field size and central ray:

   _____

4. Exposure:

   _____

5. Anatomic side markers:

   _____

Repeatable error(s): _____

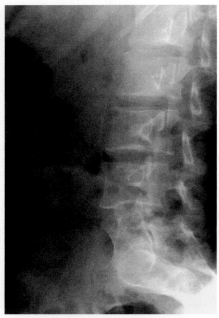

Fig. 9.9 RPO lumbar spine.

Chapter **9 Lumbar Spine, Sacrum, and Coccyx**

E. RPO lumbar spine (Fig. 9.10)

1. Anatomy demonstrated:

_____

2. Part positioning:

_____

3. Collimation field size and central ray:

_____

4. Exposure:

_____

5. Anatomic side markers:

_____

Repeatable error(s): _____

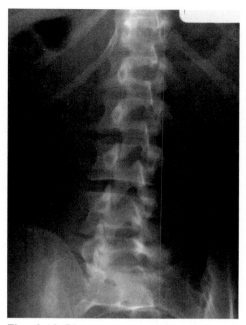

Fig. 9.10 Right posterior oblique lumbar spine.

F. LPO lumbar spine (Fig. 9.11)

1. Anatomy demonstrated:

_____

2. Part positioning:

_____

3. Collimation field size and central ray:

_____

4. Exposure:

_____

5. Anatomic side markers:

_____

Repeatable error(s): _____

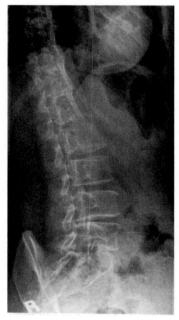

Fig. 9.11 Left posterior oblique lumbar spine.

G. AP lumbar spine (Fig. 9.12)

1. Anatomy demonstrated:

_____

2. Part positioning:

_____

3. Collimation field size and central ray:

_____

4. Exposure:

_____

5. Anatomic side markers:

_____

Repeatable error(s): _____

H. PA erect lumbar spine—scoliosis study (Fig. 9.13)

1. Anatomy demonstrated:

_____

2. Part positioning:

_____

3. Collimation field size and central ray:

_____

4. Exposure:

_____

5. Anatomic side markers:

_____

Repeatable error(s): _____

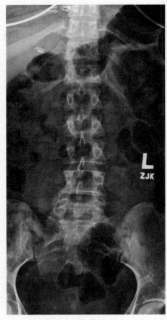

Fig. 9.12 Anteroposterior lumbar spine.

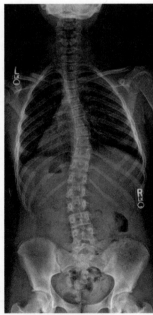

Fig. 9.13 Posteroanterior erect lumbar spine—scoliosis study.

I. Lateral erect lumbar spine—scoliosis study (Fig. 9.14)

1. Anatomy demonstrated:

   _____

2. Part positioning:

   _____

3. Collimation field size and central ray:

   _____

4. Exposure:

   _____

5. Anatomic side markers:

   _____

Repeatable error(s): _____

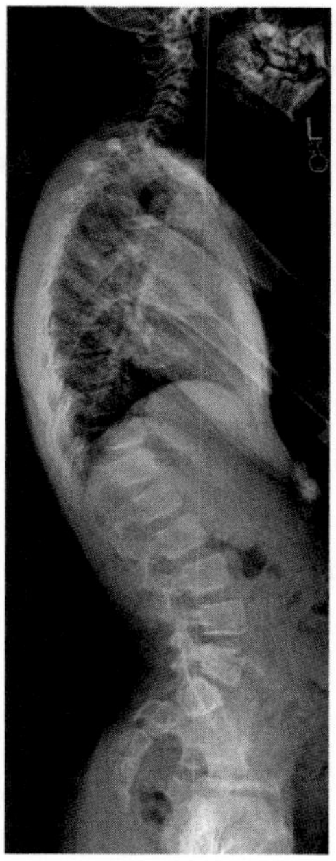

Fig. 9.14 Lateral erect lumbar spine—scoliosis study.

PART III: LABORATORY EXERCISES

You must gain experience in positioning each part of the lumbar spine, sacrum, and coccyx before performing the following exams on actual patients. You can get experience in positioning and radiographic evaluation of these projections by performing exercises using radiographic phantoms and by practicing positioning on other students (although you will not be taking actual exposures).

The following suggested activities assume that your teaching institution has an energized lab and radiographic phantoms. If not, perform Laboratory Exercises B and C, the radiographic evaluation and the physical positioning exercises, respectively. (Check off each step and projection as you complete it.)

Laboratory Exercise A: Energized Laboratory

1. Using the abdomen/lumbosacral radiographic phantom, produce radiographs of the following basic routines:

   _____ AP lumbar spine   _____ AP sacrum   _____ Posterior oblique lumbar spine

   _____ Lateral lumbar spine   _____ AP coccyx   _____ Anterior oblique lumbar spine

   _____ Lateral L5–S1   _____ Lateral sacrum and coccyx   _____ AP axial L5–S1

   _____ Oblique SI joints   _____ AP axial SI joints

Laboratory Exercise B: Radiographic Evaluation

1. Evaluate and critique the radiographs produced during the previous experiments, additional radiographs provided by your instructor, or both. Evaluate each radiograph for the following points.

   _____ Evaluate the completeness of the study. (Are all pertinent anatomic structures included on the radiograph?)

   _____ Evaluate for positioning or centering errors (e.g., rotation, off-centering).

   _____ Evaluate for correct exposure factors and possible motion. (Are the density and contrast of the images acceptable?)

   _____ Determine whether anatomic side markers and an acceptable degree of collimation are visible on the images.

Laboratory Exercise C: Physical Positioning

On another person, simulate performing all basic and special projections of the lumbar spine, sacrum, and coccyx as follows. (Check off each when completed satisfactorily.) Include the following six steps as described in the textbook.

Step 1. Appropriate size and type of image receptor with correct markers

Step 2. Correct central ray placement and centering of part to central ray and/or IR

Step 3. Accurate collimation

Step 4. Area shielding of patient (when required)

Step 5. Use of proper immobilizing devices when needed

Step 6. Approximate correct exposure factors, breathing instructions where applicable, and initiating exposure

Projections	Step 1	Step 2	Step 3	Step 4	Step 5	Step 6
• AP lumbar spine	_____	_____	_____	_____	_____	_____
• Lateral lumbar spine	_____	_____	_____	_____	_____	_____
• Lateral L5–S1	_____	_____	_____	_____	_____	_____
• AP sacrum	_____	_____	_____	_____	_____	_____
• AP coccyx	_____	_____	_____	_____	_____	_____
• Lateral sacrum and coccyx	_____	_____	_____	_____	_____	_____
• Posterior oblique lumbar spine	_____	_____	_____	_____	_____	_____
• Anterior oblique lumbar spine	_____	_____	_____	_____	_____	_____
• AP axial L5–S1	_____	_____	_____	_____	_____	_____
Spinal fusion series						
• AP (PA) R and L bending	_____	_____	_____	_____	_____	_____
• Lateral hyperextension and hyperflexion	_____	_____	_____	_____	_____	_____
Scoliosis series						
• PA (AP) and lateral erect	_____	_____	_____	_____	_____	_____
SI joint series						
• AP axial SI joints	_____	_____	_____	_____	_____	_____
• RPO and LPO SI joints	_____	_____	_____	_____	_____	_____

This self-test should be taken only after completing all of the readings, review exercises, and laboratory activities for a particular section. The purpose of this test is not only to provide a good learning exercise but also to serve as a strong indicator of what your final evaluation exam for this chapter will cover. It is strongly suggested that if you do not get at least a 90%–95% grade on each self-test, you should review those areas in which you missed questions before going to your instructor for the final evaluation exam.

1. Compared with the spinous processes of the cervical and thoracic spine, the lumbar spinous processes are:

   A. Smaller

   B. Pointed downward more

   C. Larger and more blunt

   D. Absent

2. The anterior/superior ridge of the upper sacrum is called the:

   A. Median sacral crest

   B. Cornua

   C. Promontory

   D. Sacral horns

3. Each SI joint opens obliquely _____ degrees posteriorly

   A. 20

   B. 25–30

   C. 45

   D. 50

4. The angle of the midlumbar spine zygapophyseal joints in relation to the midsagittal plane is

   _____.

5. Where is the pars interarticularis found?

   A. Superior and inferior aspect of the pedicle

   B. Between the intervertebral disk and vertebra

   C. Between the superior and inferior articular processes

   D. Between the lamina and body spinous processes

6. Identify the labeled parts of the sacrum and coccyx in the following drawings (Figs. 9.15 and 9.16).

A. _____

B. _____

C. _____

D. _____

E. _____

F. _____

G. _____

H. _____

I. _____

J. _____

K. _____

L. _____

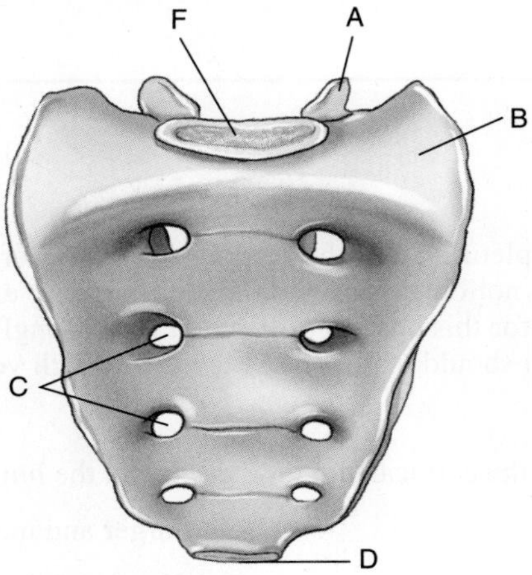

Fig. 9.15 Sacrum.

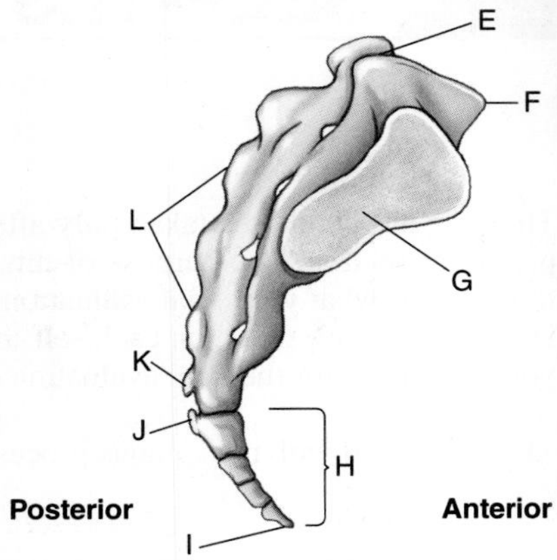

Fig. 9.16 Sacrum and coccyx.

7. Identify the labeled parts on these radiographs of individual vertebrae (Figs. 9.17 and 9.18).

A. _____

B. _____

C. _____

D. _____

E. _____

F. _____

G. _____

H. _____

I. _____

J. _____

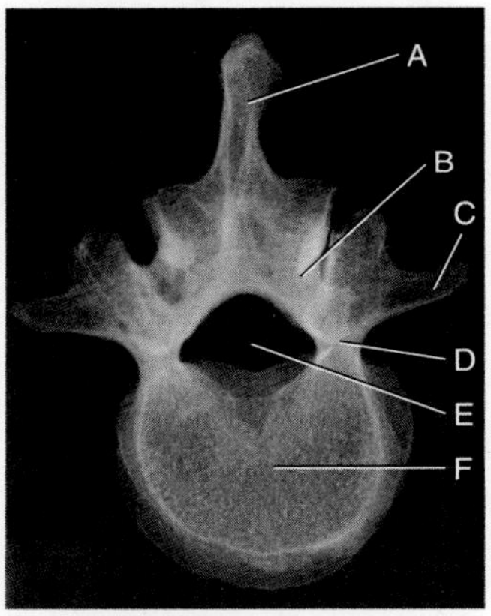

Fig. 9.17 Individual vertebra, A–F.

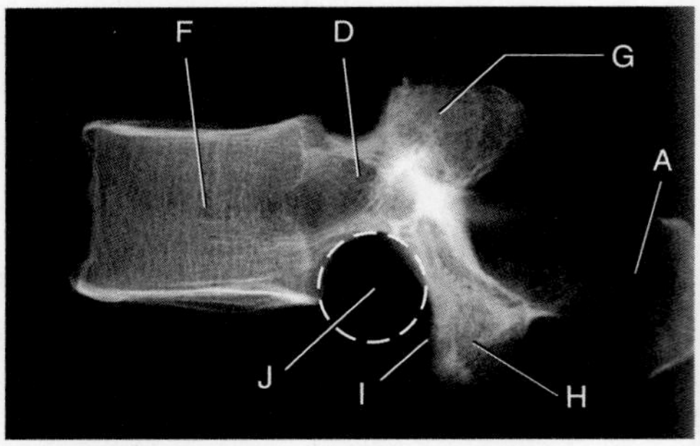

Fig. 9.18 Individual vertebra, G–J.

8. What are the characteristics of the vertebra in Fig. 9.18 that identify it as a lumbar rather than as a thoracic vertebra?

_____

9. The zygapophyseal joints of the lumbar spine are classified as _____, as joints with _____

type of joint movement.

10. List the correct terms of the lumbar vertebra that correspond to the following labeled parts of the Scottie dog as seen on an oblique radiograph of the lumbar spine (Fig. 9.19).

A. _____

B. _____

C. _____

D. _____

E. _____

F. _____ joint

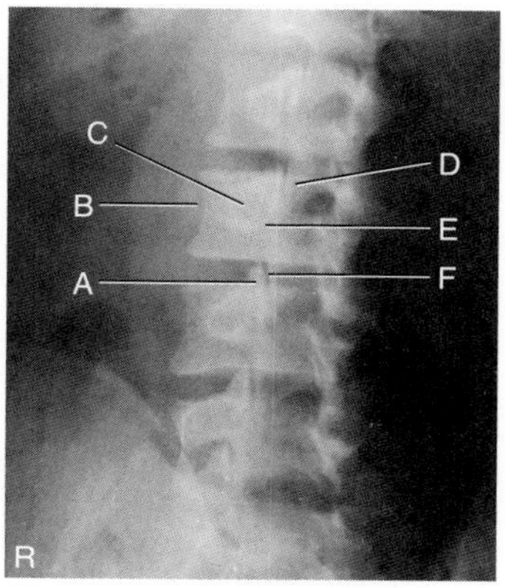

Fig. 9.19 Oblique lumbar spine.

11. The ear and front leg of the Scottie dog make up the _____ joint, best seen in the oblique position.

12. Which of the following topographic landmarks corresponds to the L2–L3 level?

   A. Xiphoid process
   B. Lower costal margin
   C. Iliac crest
   D. ASIS

13. True/False: It is possible to shield females for an AP projection of the sacrum or coccyx if the gonadal shields are correctly placed.

14. True/False: The female gonadal dose is approximately equal for either AP or PA projections of the lumbar spine.

15. Why should the knees and hips be flexed for a recumbent AP projection of the lumbar spine?

_____

16. True/False: A lead mat or masking for lateral positions of the lumbar spine should not be used with digital imaging.

17. True/False: The efficiency of CT and MR of the spine is reducing the number of myelograms being performed.

18. Anterior wedging and loss of vertebral body height are characteristic of:

   A. Chance fracture
   B. Spina bifida
   C. Compression fracture
   D. Spondylolysis

19. Which of the following conditions is often diagnosed by prenatal diagnostic medical sonography?

   A. Scoliosis
   B. Spina bifida
   C. Spondylolisthesis
   D. Ankylosing spondylitis

20. True/False: Ankylosing spondylitis usually requires an increase in manual exposure factors.

21. Where is the central ray centered for an AP projection of the lumbar spine with a 11- × 14-inch (30- × 35-cm) field size?

_____

22. Which set of zygapophyseal joints of the lumbar spine is best demonstrated with an LAO position?

_____

23. How much rotation of the spine is required to demonstrate the lumbar zygapophyseal joint space and?

_____

24. Describe the body build that might require central ray angulation to open the intervertebral joint spaces with a lateral projection of the lumbar spine, even if the patient has some support under the waist.

_____

25. What type of central ray angulation should be used for the lateral L5–S1 projection if the waist is not supported?

A. Central ray perpendicular to IR

B. 5–8 degrees caudad

C. 10–15 degrees cephalad

D. 3–5 degrees cephalad

26. For the lateral L5–S1 projection, the CR is parallel to the _____ plane.

A. Oblique

B. Midcoronal

C. Midsagittal

D. Interiliac

27. Where is the central ray centered for an AP axial projection for L5–S1?

_____

28. True/False: A kVp range of 90–100 can be used for a lateral L5–S1 projection when using a digital imaging system.

29. Which projection or method is designed to demonstrate the degree of scoliosis deformity between the primary and compensatory curves as part of a scoliosis study?

_____

30. Which projections are designed to measure mobility of the vertebral column at the site of a spinal fusion?

_____

31. Where is the central ray centered for an AP axial projection of the sacrum?

_____

32. What two things can be done to reduce the high amounts of scatter reaching the IR during a lateral projection of the sacrum and coccyx?

A. _____   B. _____

33. Why should a single lateral projection of the sacrum and coccyx be performed rather than separate lateral projections of the sacrum and coccyx?

_____

34. True/False: The pelvis must remain as stationary as possible when positioning for the hyperextension and hyperflexion projections.

35. A radiograph of an AP projection of the lumbar spine shows the SI joints are not equidistant from the spine. The right ala of the sacrum appears wider, and the left SI joint is more open than the left. Which specific positioning error is evident on this radiograph?

_____

36. A radiograph of an LPO projection of the lumbar spine shows the downside pedicles are projected toward the posterior aspect of the vertebral bodies. What must be done to correct this error during the repeat exposure?

_____

37. An AP projection of the sacrum shows that the sacrum is foreshortened and the foramina are not open. What positioning error may have led to this radiographic outcome?

_____

38. **Situation:** A patient with a possible compression fracture of L3 enters the emergency room. Which projection(s) of the lumbar spine best demonstrate(s) the extent of this injury?

_____

39. **Situation:** A patient with a clinical history of spondylolisthesis of the L5–S1 region comes to the radiology department. What basic (i.e., routine) and special (i.e., optional) projections should be included in this study? (Hint: If the oblique positions are included, how much spine rotation should be used?)

_____

40. **Situation:** A study of the SI joints demonstrates that the joints are not open and the upper iliac wings are nearly superimposing the joints. The technologist performed 35-degree RPO and LPO positions with a perpendicular CR. What can be done during the repeat exposure to open the joints?

_____

WORKBOOK SELF-TEST ANSWER KEY

1. C. Larger and more blunt
2. C. Promontory
3. B. 30
4. 45 degrees
5. C. Between the superior and inferior articular processes
6. A. Left superior articular process
   B. Left ala or wing of sacrum
   C. Pelvic (anterior) sacral foramina
   D. Apex of sacrum
   E. Sacral canal (between superior articular processes)
   F. Sacral promontory (also seen on frontal view)
   G. Auricular surface (for sacroiliac joint)
   H. Coccyx
   I. Apex of coccyx
   J. Horn (cornu) of coccyx
   K. Horn (cornu) of sacrum
   L. Median sacral crest
7. A. Spinous process
   B. Lamina
   C. Transverse process
   D. Pedicle (also shown on lateral view)
   E. Vertebral foramen
   F. Body (also shown on lateral view)
   G. Superior articular process
   H. Inferior articular process
   I. Region of articular facets (R and L sides superimposed as seen on a lateral view)
   J. Intervertebral notch or foramen
8. Large vertebral body and large, blunt spinous process
9. Synovial, plane (gliding)
10. A. Superior articular process (ear)
    B. Transverse process (nose)
    C. Pedicle (eye)
    D. Inferior articular process (leg)
    E. Pars interarticularis (neck)
    F. Zygapophyseal (between L4 and L5)
11. Zygapophyseal
12. B. Lower costal margin
13. False (would obscure essential anatomy because the ovaries are located near the lower lumbar spine)
14. False (ovaries are slightly anterior, thus AP results in about 30% greater gonadal dose than PA)
15. Opens the intervertebral disk space by reducing the normal lumbar curvature of the spine.
16. False. The lead mat should be used with digital imaging to prevent secondary scatter from reaching the sensitive image receptor. Scatter radiation produces greater "noise" in the processed image.
17. True
18. C. Compression fracture
19. B. Spina bifida
20. False
21. Level of L3 (approximately level of lower costal margin)
22. Right, or the upside joints
23. 45 degrees
24. A patient with a wide pelvis and narrow thorax
25. B. 5-degree to 8-degree caudad (CR parallel to interiliac plane)
26. D. Interiliac (plane)
27. 1.5 inches (4 cm) inferior to iliac crest, 2 inches (5 cm) posterior to ASIS
28. True (higher kilovolt ranges are encouraged when using digital systems)
29. PA (AP) projection, AP/PA projection–Ferguson method (with and without block under convex side of curve)
30. Hyperextension and hyperflexion lateral projections
31. 2 inches (5 cm) superior to symphysis pubis
32. A. Close collimation
    B. Place a lead mat or masking on tabletop behind patient
33. To reduce gonadal dose
34. True. The pelvis acts as a fulcrum (pivot point) during changes in position.
35. Rotation to the patient's right
36. Decrease rotation or obliquity of the spine
37. Insufficient cephalad CR angulation or the CR was angled in the wrong direction
38. A lateral projection (may include a coned-down spot AP/PA [preferred] and lateral of the L3 region)
39. AP, lateral, L5–S1 spot lateral, and right and left 30-degree oblique positions
40. Decrease rotation of body for oblique positions to no more than 25–30 degrees with the CR centered to the upside SI joint

A1

10 Bony Thorax—Sternum and Ribs

CHAPTER OBJECTIVES

After you have successfully completed the activities in this chapter, you will be able to:

_____ 1. Using drawings and radiographs, identify specific anatomic structures of the sternum and ribs.

_____ 2. Classify ribs as either true, false, or floating ribs.

_____ 3. Classify specific joints in the bony thorax according to their structural classification, mobility classification, and movement type.

_____ 4. Define specific types of clinical indications of the bony thorax as described in the textbook.

_____ 5. Identify basic and special projections of the ribs and sternum, including the correct collimation field size, and the location, direction, and angulation of the central ray (CR) for each position.

_____ 6. Identify the structures that are best seen with specific projections of the ribs and sternum.

_____ 7. Identify the technical considerations important in radiography of the ribs and sternum, including breathing instructions, general body position, kVp range, and other imaging options.

_____ 8. Given various hypothetic situations, identify the correct modification of a position and/or exposure factors to improve the radiographic image.

_____ 9. Given radiographs of specific bony thorax projections or positions, identify specific positioning and exposure factor errors.

POSITIONING AND RADIOGRAPHIC CRITIQUE

_____ 1. Using a peer, position for basic and special projections of the bony thorax.

_____ 2. Using a chest radiographic phantom, produce satisfactory radiographs of specific positions (if equipment is available).

_____ 3. Critique and evaluate bony thorax radiographs based on the five divisions of radiographic criteria: (1) anatomy demonstrated, (2) position, (3) collimation field size and central ray, (4) exposure, and (5) anatomic markers.

_____ 4. Distinguish between acceptable and unacceptable bony thorax radiographs based on exposure factors, motion, collimation, positioning, or other errors.

LEARNING EXERCISES

Complete the following review exercises after reading the associated pages in the textbook as indicated by each exercise. Answers to each review exercise are given at the end of the review exercises.

PART I: RADIOGRAPHIC ANATOMY

REVIEW EXERCISE A: Radiographic Anatomy of the Bony Thorax, Sternum, and Ribs (see textbook pp. 366–368)

1. List the three structures that make up the bony thorax.

   A. ______________

   B. ______________

   C. ______________

2. Identify the parts of the sternum and ribs labeled in Fig. 10.1.

   A. ______________

   B. ______________

   C. ______________

   D. ______________

   E. ______________

   F. ______________

   G. ______________

   H. ______________

   I. ______________

   J. ______________

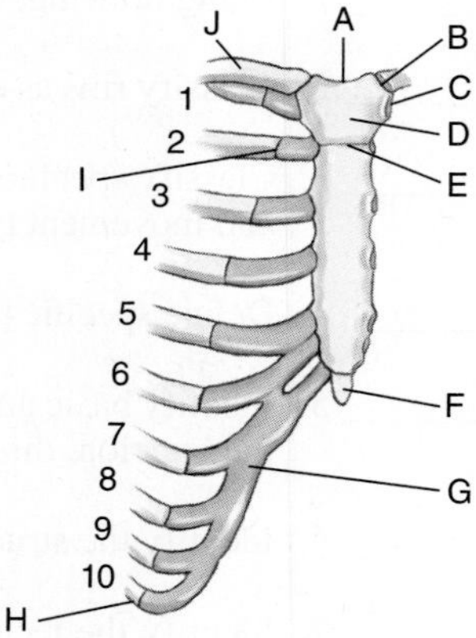

Fig. 10.1 Sternum and ribs.

3. What is the term for the long, middle aspect of the sternum? ________________________

4. The most distal aspect of the sternum does not ossify until a person is approximately

   ________________________ years of age.

5. The total sternum length on an average adult is about ________________________ inches

   (______________ cm).

6. A. The xiphoid process of the sternum is at the approximate level of the ________________________ vertebra.

   B. The sternal angle is at the level of ________________________.

   C. What is another term for the sternal angle? ________________________

7. What is the name of the joint that connects the upper limb to the bony thorax (the only bony connection between the bony thorax and upper limbs)? ________________________

8. What is the name of the section of cartilage that connects the anterior end of the rib to the sternum?

   ____

9. What distinguishes a true rib from a false rib? ________________________

10. True/False: The 11th and 12th ribs are classified as false and floating ribs.

11. True/False: The anterior aspect of the ribs is called the vertebral end.

12. Which aspect of the ribs articulates with the transverse process of the thoracic vertebrae?

    A. Head   C. Neck

    B. Costal angle   D. Tubercle

13. List the three structures found within the costal groove of each rib.

    A. _____   B. _____   C. _____

14. Answer the following questions as you study Fig. 10.2.

    A. Which end of the ribs is most superior—the posterior vertebral ends or the anterior sternal ends?

    _____

    B. Approximately how much difference in height is there between these two ends of the ribs?

    _____

    C. Which ribs articulate with the upper lateral aspect of the manubrium of the sternum?

    _____

    D. The bony thorax is widest at the lateral margins of which

    ribs? _____

    E. How many posterior ribs are shown above the diaphragm? (Hint: Recall from Chapter 2 that a minimum of 9–10 posterior ribs must be seen on an average inspiration posteroanterior [PA] chest projection.)

    _____

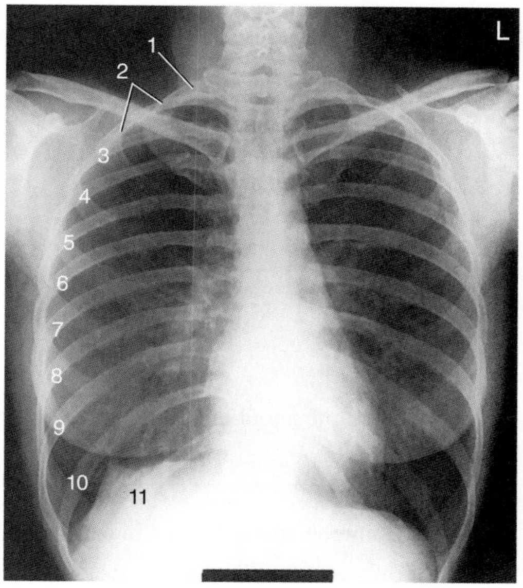

Fig. 10.2 Rib radiograph.

15. Match each of the following joints with the correct movement type.

    A. Movable—diarthrodial (plane or gliding)

    B. Immovable—synarthrodial

    C. Fibrous—syndesmosis

    _____ 1. First sternocostal

    _____ 2. First through 12th costovertebral joints

    _____ 3. First through 10th costochondral unions (between costal cartilage and ribs)

    _____ 4. First through 10th costotransverse joints (between ribs and transverse processes of T vertebrae)

    _____ 5. Second through seventh sternocostal joints (between second and seventh ribs and sternum)

_____ 6. Sixth through ninth interchondral joints (between anterior sixth and ninth costal cartilage)

_____ 7. Ninth and 10th interchondral joints between the cartilages

16. The joints from the previous question that have diarthrodial movement are classified as

_____.

17. Classify the following groups of ribs (labeled on the diagram as A, B, and C) and identify the number of the ribs in each category (Fig. 10.3).

A. _____

B. _____

C. _____

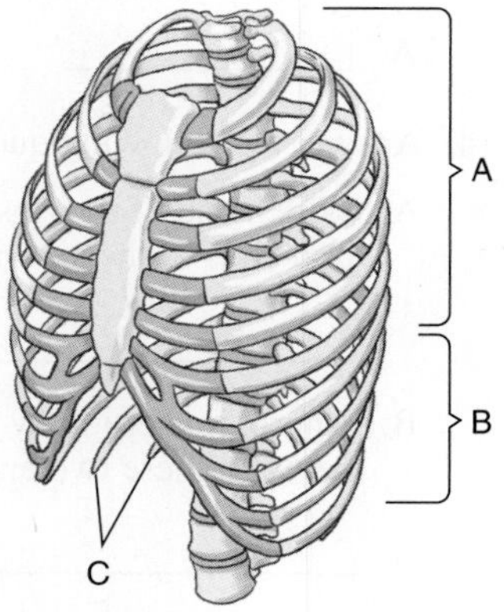

Fig. 10.3 Rib groups.

18. What is unique about the ribs in category A in the previous question?

_____

19. What is unique about the ribs in category C in the previous question?

_____

20. Identify the labeled parts of this posterior view of a typical rib (Fig. 10.4).

A. _____

B. _____

C. _____

D. _____

E. _____

F. _____

G. _____

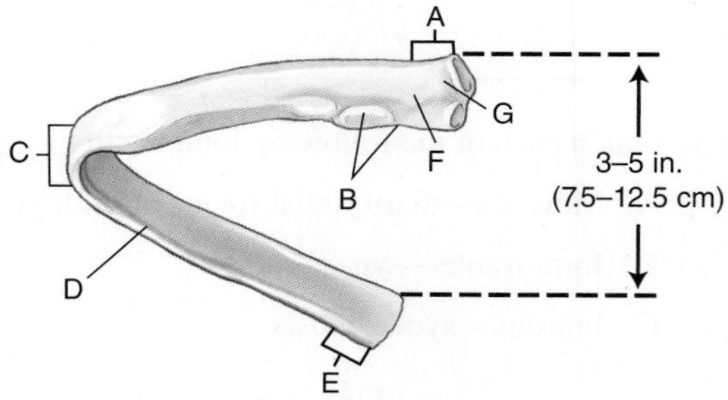

Fig. 10.4 Posterior view of a typical rib.

PART II: RADIOGRAPHIC POSITIONING

REVIEW EXERCISE B: Positioning of the Ribs and Sternum (see textbook pp. 369–382)

1. True/False: It is virtually impossible to visualize the sternum with a true PA or anteroposterior (AP) projection.

2. True/False: A broad framed (hypersthenic) patient requires more obliquity (rotation) for a frontal view of the sternum as compared with a slender (asthenic) patient.

3. How much rotation should be used for the oblique position of the sternum for a

   broad framed patient? _____

4. List the recommended ranges for the following exposure factors as they apply to an oblique position of the sternum (orthostatic-breathing technique).

   A. kVp range: _____

   B. mA (low or high): _____

   C. Exposure time (short or long): _____

5. What is the advantage of performing an orthostatic (breathing) technique for radiography of the sternum?

   _____

6. What is the primary reason that a source image receptor distance (SID) of less than 40 inches (100 cm) should not be

   used for sternum radiography? _____

7. What other imaging option is available to study the sternum if routine right anterior oblique (RAO) and lateral radi-

   ographs do not provide sufficient information? _____

8. Identify the preferred positioning factors to demonstrate an injury to the ribs found below the diaphragm:

   A. General body position (erect or recumbent): _____

   B. Breathing instructions (inspiration or expiration): _____

   C. Recommended kVp range: _____

9. An injury to the region of the eighth or ninth rib requires the _____ (above or below) diaphragm technique.

10. To elongate and visualize the axillary aspect of the ribs properly, the patient's spine should be rotated

    _____ (toward or away from) the area of interest.

11. Which projections (AP or PA and anterior or posterior oblique) should be performed for an injury to the anterior

    aspect of the ribs? _____

12. Which two rib projections should be performed for an injury to the right posterior ribs?

    _____

13. How can the site of injury be marked for a rib series?

    _____

14. If the physician suspects a pneumothorax or hemothorax has occurred as a result of a rib fracture, which additional radiographic projection(s) should be performed in addition to the routine rib projections?

    _____

15. A flail chest is defined as a(n):

  A. Asthenic body habitus

  B. Pulmonary injury caused by blunt trauma to two or more ribs

  C. Chronic obstructive pulmonary disease (e.g., emphysema)

  D. Cardiac injury caused by blunt trauma

16. If a flail chest injury is suspected, the technologist should perform rib study in which position?

  A. Supine only   C. Prone only

  B. Erect   D. Trendelenburg

17. Osteolytic metastases of the ribs produce which of the following radiographic appearances?

  A. Irregular bony margins   C. Sharp lucent lines through the ribs

  B. Increased bony density of the ribs   D. Smooth lucent "holes" in the ribs

18. Which of the following definitions applies to pectus excavatum?

  A. Multiple fractures of the sternum with fragments in the pericardium

  B. Abnormally prominent lower aspect of sternum

  C. Depressed sternum caused by congenital defect

  D. Separation between ribs and sternum resulting from trauma

19. A proliferative bony lesion of increased density is generally termed:

  A. Osteoblastic   C. Osteolytic

  B. Osteoporotic   D. Osteostenotic

20. True/False: MR provides a more diagnostic image of rib metastases as compared with a nuclear medicine scan.

21. True/False: Patients can develop osteomyelitis as a postoperative complication following open-heart surgery.

22. Which bony landmark is most easily palpated on the bariatric patient for sternum and rib projections?

  A. Jugular notch   C. Xiphoid process

  B. Sternal angle   D. Vertebra prominens

23. Which oblique position is preferred for a study of the sternum: RAO or left anterior oblique (LAO)

  _____ Why?

  _____

24. True/False: The most common error for the oblique position of the sternum is over-rotation of the thorax.

25. Where is the central ray centered for the oblique and lateral projections of the sternum?

   _____

26. What other position can be performed if the patient cannot assume a prone position for the oblique position of the sternum?

   _____

27. What is the recommended SID for a lateral projection of the sternum?

   _____ Why? _____

28. Which of the following criteria apply to a radiograph for an evaluation of the oblique sternum?

   A. The entire sternum should be adjacent to the spine and adjacent to the heart shadow.

   B. The entire sternum should lie over the heart shadow and should be adjacent to the spine.

   C. The left sternoclavicular joint should be adjacent to the spinal column.

   D. The second rib should lie directly over the manubrium of the sternum.

29. Where is the central ray centered for a PA projection of the sternoclavicular joints?

   A. Level of T7   C. At the vertebra prominens

   B. Level of T2–T3   D. Level of xiphoid process

30. What type of breathing instructions should be provided to the patient for a PA projection of the sternoclavicular joints?

   A. Suspend respiration on inspiration.

   B. Use an orthostatic-breathing technique.

   C. Suspended breathing is not necessary.

   D. Suspend respiration on expiration.

31. How much rotation of the thorax is recommended for an anterior oblique of the sternoclavicular joints?

   _____

32. Which specific oblique position best demonstrates the left sternoclavicular joint adjacent to the spine?

   _____

33. What are the three points that must be included in the patient's clinical history before a rib series?

   A. _____

   B. _____

   C. _____

34. Where is the central ray centered for an AP projection of the ribs for an injury located above the diaphragm?

_____

35. Which two specific oblique positions can be used to elongate the left axillary portion of the ribs?

_____

36. Which two basic projections or positions should be performed for an injury to the right anterior ribs?

_____

37. How many degrees of rotation are required for an oblique projection of the axillary ribs?

_____

38. What is the recommended SID for a bilateral lower rib study on an adult?

_____

39. True/False: The recommended kVp range for a study of the unilateral, upper anterior ribs is 70–85 kVp.

40. Which region of the ribs is best demonstrated with an RAO projection?

_____

41. True/False: A left lateral decubitus chest position (patient cannot stand) should be performed for a possible pneumothorax in the left thorax.

42. True/False: A right lateral decubitus chest position (patient cannot stand) should be performed for a possible hemothorax in the right thorax.

43. True/False: An RAO of the sternoclavicular joints projects the left joint closest to the spine.

44. To minimize the patient dose for an RAO projection of the sternum, the patient's skin should be at least

_____ below the collimator.

A. 40 inches (100 cm)   C. 15 inches (40 cm)

B. 72 inches (180 cm)   D. 2 inches (5 cm)

45. Which of the following conditions may require that a chest routine be included along with a study of the ribs?

A. Pectus carinatum   C. Pectus excavatum

B. Hemothorax   D. Osteomyelitis

REVIEW EXERCISE C: PROBLEM SOLVING FOR TECHNICAL AND POSITIONING ERRORS

1. A radiograph of an RAO sternum shows part of the sternum is superimposed over the thoracic spine. Which specific positioning error is visible on this radiograph?

_____

2. A radiograph of an RAO sternum shows the sternum is difficult to visualize because of excessive density. The following exposure factors were used for this image: 100 kVp, 25 mA, 3-second exposure, 40-inch (100-cm) SID, and Bucky. Which of these factors should be modified during the repeat exposure to produce a more diagnostic image?

_____

3. A radiograph of an RAO sternum shows the sternum is poorly visualized because of excessive lung markings superimposed over the sternum. The following exposure factors were used for this image: 75 kVp, 200 mA, 1-second exposure, 40-inch (100-cm) SID, and Bucky. Which of these factors can be altered to increase the visibility of the sternum?

_____

4. A radiograph of a lateral projection of the sternum shows the breast tissue is obscuring the sternum. What can be done to minimize the breast artifact over the sternum?

_____

5. Repeat PA projections of the sternoclavicular joints do not clearly demonstrate them. What other imaging modality may produce a more diagnostic image of these joints?

_____

6. **Situation:** A patient with trauma to the sternum and the left sternoclavicular joint region enters the emergency room. In addition to the sternum routine, the ER physician asks for a specific projection to better demonstrate the left sternoclavicular joint. Describe the positioning routine that you would use, including the breathing instructions. (Hint: Three projections are required.)

_____

_____

7. A radiograph of the upper ribs demonstrates that the diaphragm is superimposed over the seventh to eighth ribs, which is in the area of interest. The following exposure factors were used for the initial exposure: 75 kVp, 400 mA, 1/40 second, suspended respiration on expiration, erect position, 40-inch (100-cm) SID. Which of these factors can be modified to increase the visibility of the area of interest?

_____

8. **Situation:** A patient enters the emergency room on a trauma board after being involved in a motor vehicle accident. Because of the condition of the patient, the physician orders a portable study of the sternum in the ER. Which two projections of the sternum would be most diagnostic yet would minimize movement of the patient? (See Chapter 15 in the textbook for alternative projections.)

_____

9. **Situation:** A patient with trauma to the right upper anterior ribs enters the ER. He is able to sit in an erect position. Which positioning routine of the ribs should be performed? (Include general body position, breathing instructions, and specific projections or positions performed.)

_____

10. **Situation:** A patient with trauma to the left lower anterior ribs enters the ER. Which positioning routine of the ribs should be performed? (Include general body position, breathing instructions, and specific positions performed.)

_____

11. **Situation:** An elderly patient comes to the radiology department for a complete rib series with an emphasis on the posterior ribs. She has advanced osteoporosis and has difficulty moving and lying down. Her physician wants both upper and lower ribs examined. What type of positions should be performed? How would you adjust the technical factors for this patient?

_____

12. **Situation:** A patient enters the ER with blunt trauma to the chest. He is restricted on a trauma board. The ER physician suspects a flail chest. Beyond the initial chest projections, what positioning routine would confirm the flail chest diagnosis?

_____

REVIEW EXERCISE D: Critique Radiographs of the Bony Thorax

The following questions relate to the radiographs found in this exercise. Evaluate these radiographs for the radiographic criteria categories (1–5) that follow. Describe the corrections needed to improve the overall image. The major, or "repeatable," errors are specific errors that indicate the need for a repeat exposure, regardless of the nature of the other errors.

A. Bilateral ribs above diaphragm (Fig. 10.5)

1. Anatomy demonstrated:

_____

2. Part positioning:

_____

3. Collimation field size and central ray:

_____

4. Exposure:

_____

5. Anatomic side markers:

_____

Repeatable error(s):

_____

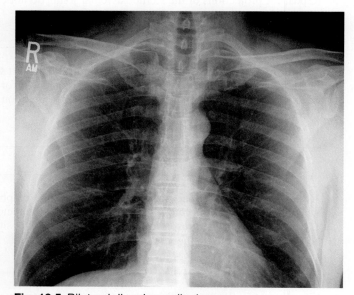

Fig. 10.5 Bilateral ribs above diaphragm.

B. Oblique sternum (Fig. 10.6)

   1. Anatomy demonstrated:

   _____

   2. Part positioning:

   _____

   3. Collimation field size and central ray:

   _____

   4. Exposure:

   _____

   5. Anatomic side markers:

   _____

Repeatable error(s):

_____

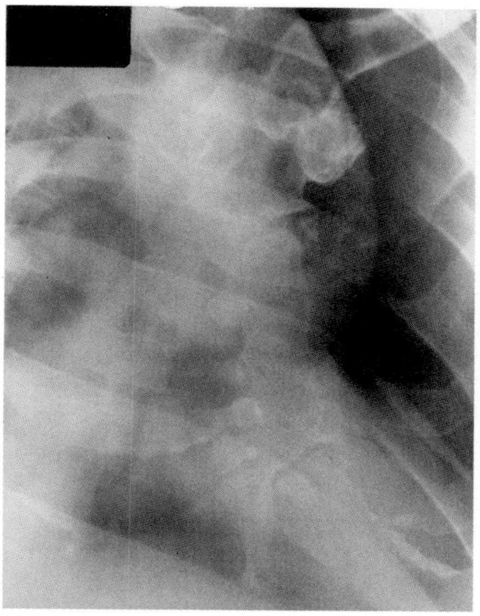

Fig. 10.6 Oblique sternum.

C. AP ribs below diaphragm (Fig. 10.7)

   1. Anatomy demonstrated:

   _____

   2. Part positioning:

   _____

   3. Collimation field size and central ray:

   _____

   4. Exposure:

   _____

   5. Anatomic side markers:

   _____

Repeatable error(s):

_____

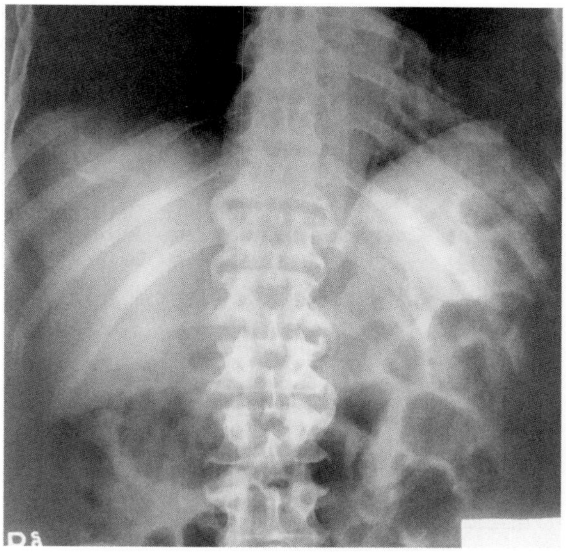

Fig. 10.7 Anteroposterior ribs below diaphragm.

D. Lateral sternum (Fig. 10.8)

   1. Anatomy demonstrated:

   _____

   2. Part positioning:

   _____

   3. Collimation field size and central ray:

   _____

   4. Exposure:

   _____

   5. Anatomic side markers:

   _____

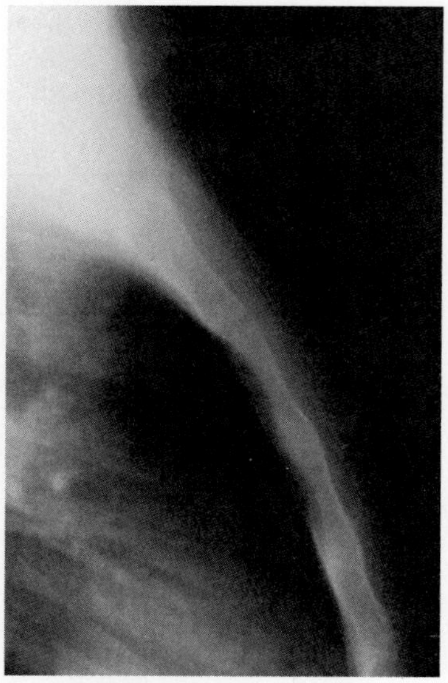

Fig. 10.8 Lateral sternum.

Repeatable error(s): _____

PART III: LABORATORY EXERCISES

You must gain experience in positioning each part of the sternum and ribs before performing the following exams on actual patients. You can get experience in positioning and radiographic evaluation of these projections by performing exercises using radiographic phantoms and by practicing positioning on other students (although you will not be taking actual exposures).

The following suggested activities assume your teaching institution has an energized lab and radiographic phantoms. If not, perform Laboratory Exercises B and C, the radiographic evaluation, and the physical positioning exercises, respectively. (Check off each step and projection as you complete it.)

Laboratory Exercise A: Energized Laboratory

1. Using the chest radiographic phantom, produce radiographs of the following basic routines:

   _____RAO sternum

   _____PA sternoclavicular joints

   _____AP (PA) ribs

   _____AP (PA) ribs, above and below diaphragm

   _____Lateral sternum

   _____RAO (LAO) sternoclavicular joints

   _____Posterior and anterior oblique ribs, above the diaphragm

   _____Horizontal beam lateral sternum

[image 1 appears here]

238

Laboratory Exercise B: Radiographic Evaluation

1. Evaluate and critique the radiographs produced in the preceding, additional radiographs provided by your instructor, or both. Evaluate each radiograph for the following points.

_____ Evaluate the completeness of the study. (Are all of the pertinent anatomic structures included on the radiograph?)

_____ Evaluate for positioning or centering errors (e.g., rotation, off-centering).

_____ Evaluate for correct exposure factors and possible motion. (Is image receptor exposure and contrast of the images acceptable?)

_____ Determine whether markers and an acceptable degree of collimation are visible on the images.

Laboratory Exercise C: Physical Positioning

On another person, simulate performing all basic and special projections of the sternum and ribs as follows. Include the six steps listed in the following and described in the textbook. (Check off each step when completed satisfactorily.)

Step 1. Appropriate size and type of image receptor with correct markers

Step 2. Correct central ray placement and centering of part to central ray and/or image receptor

Step 3. Accurate collimation

Step 4. Area shielding of patient (when required)

Step 5. Use of proper immobilizing devices when needed

Step 6. Approximate correct exposure factors, breathing instructions where applicable, and initiating exposure

Projections	Step 1	Step 2	Step 3	Step 4	Step 5	Step 6
• RAO sternum	_____	_____	_____	_____	_____	_____
• Erect lateral sternum	_____	_____	_____	_____	_____	_____
• Recumbent left posterior oblique (LPO) sternum	_____	_____	_____	_____	_____	_____
• Horizontal beam lateral sternum	_____	_____	_____	_____	_____	_____
• PA sternoclavicular joints	_____	_____	_____	_____	_____	_____
• Oblique sternoclavicular joints	_____	_____	_____	_____	_____	_____
• Rib routine for injury to right upper anterior ribs	_____	_____	_____	_____	_____	_____
• Rib routine for injury to left lower posterior ribs	_____	_____	_____	_____	_____	_____

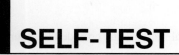

SELF-TEST

This self-test should be taken only after completing all of the readings, review exercises, and laboratory activities for a particular section. The purpose of this test is not only to provide a good learning exercise but also to serve as a strong indicator of what your final evaluation exam for this chapter will cover. It is strongly suggested that if you do not get at least a 90%–95% grade on each self-test, you should review those areas in which you missed questions before going to your instructor for the final evaluation exam.

1. List the three parts of the sternum.

   A. _____

   B. _____

   C. _____

2. What is the most distal aspect of the sternum? _____

3. What is the name of the palpable junction between the upper and midportion of the sternum? _____

   _____

4. Which aspect of the sternum possesses the jugular (suprasternal or manubrial) notch?

   A. Body

   B. Sternal angle

   C. Xiphoid process

   D. Manubrium

5. What distinguishes a true rib from a false rib?

   A. A true rib attaches directly to the sternum with its own costal cartilage.

   B. A true rib possesses a costovertebral and a costotransverse joint.

   C. A false rib does not possess a head.

   D. A false rib is composed primarily of cartilage.

6. What distinguishes a floating rib from a false rib?

   A. A floating rib is found only at the T1, T10, and T11 levels.

   B. A floating rib does not possess a head.

   C. A floating rib has no costal groove.

   D. A floating rib does not possess costal cartilage.

7. The fifth rib is an example of a _____ (true rib or false rib).

8. Which part of the sternum do the second ribs articulate?

   A. Midbody

   B. Upper manubrium

   C. Middle manubrium

   D. Sternal angle

Chapter **10** Bony Thorax—Sternum and Ribs: Self-Test

Copyright © 2025 by Elsevier Inc.
All rights reserved, including those for text and data mining, AI training, and similar technologies.

9. Which of the following structures is (are) found in the costal groove of each rib?

   A. Nerve

   B. Artery

   C. Vein

   D. All of the above

10. Match each of the following joints with the correct type of movement.

   _____ 1. Sternoclavicular

   _____ 2. Costovertebral joint

   _____ 3. First sternocostal joint

   _____ 4. Eighth interchondral joint

   _____ 5. Third costochondral union

   A. Plane (gliding)—diarthrodial

   B. Immovable—synarthrodial

11. Identify the structures labeled on the following radiographs of the sternum (Figs. 10.9 and 10.10).

   Fig. 10.9

   A. _____

   B. _____ (joint)

   C. _____

   D. _____

   E. _____

   F. _____

   G. _____

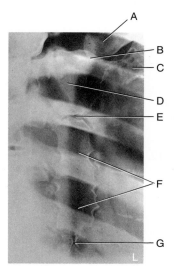

Fig. 10.9 The sternum, A–G.

Fig. 10.10

H. _____

I. _____

J. _____

K. _____

L. _____

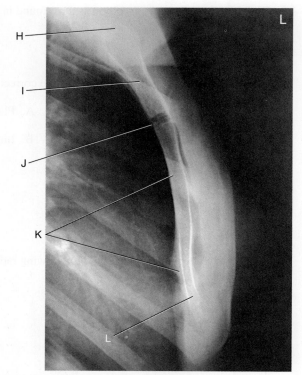

Fig. 10.10 The sternum, H–L.

12. List the correct positioning considerations for a study of the ribs above the diaphragm.

    A. Breathing instructions: _____

    B. kVp range: _____

    C. General body position: _____

13. What is the minimum SID for radiography of the sternum? (Note: This is a radiation safety concern.)

_____

14. Which of the following breathing instructions should be used for an RAO position of the sternum to maximize its visibility?

    A. Suspended inspiration   C. Suspended expiration

    B. Orthostatic-breathing technique   D. Valsalva maneuver

15. List the two factors to consider when determining which specific projections to include in the rib routine.

    A. _____

    B. _____

16. List three chest pathologic conditions that may result from a rib injury and may require that a PA and lateral chest projections be included with the rib routine.

A. _____

B. _____

C. _____

17. A. What is the range of body rotation for an RAO position of the sternum?

_____

B. Does an asthenic patient require a little more or a little less obliquity than a hypersthenic patient?

_____

18. Nuclear medicine bone scans are not normally performed for which of the following conditions of the bony thorax?

A. Possible fractures

B. Osteoporosis

C. History of multiple myeloma

D. Osteomyelitis

19. Pathology of the sternum is most commonly caused by:

A. Metastases

B. Osteoporosis

C. Infection

D. Blunt trauma

20. The most common cause of osteomyelitis is _____.

21. What other position can be used for the sternum if the patient cannot assume the recumbent RAO position?

A. LAO

B. RPO

C. LPO

D. Left lateral decubitus

22. How should the arms be positioned for an erect lateral projection of the sternum?

A. Raised over the head

B. Drawn back

C. Depressed by holding 5–10 lb (2–4 kg) minimum in each hand

D. Extended in front of the thorax

23. Which radiographic sign can be evaluated to determine whether rotation is present on a PA projection of the sternoclavicular joints? _____

24. How much rotation of the thorax is required for the anterior oblique projection of the sternoclavicular joints?

_____

25. Where is the central ray centered for an AP, bilateral projection of the posterior ribs below the diaphragm?

_____

26. What range of kVp for imaging should be used for ribs below the diaphragm?

A. 55–65 kVp

B. 75–85 kVp

C. 100–110 kVp

D. 90–100 kVp

27. Which of the following positions or projections will best demonstrate the right axillary ribs?

    A. LAO   C. RAO

    B. LPO   D. PA

28. A radiograph of an RAO projection of the sternum shows the width of the sternum is foreshortened and the sternum is shifted away from the spine and out of the heart shadow. The patient has a broad "barrel" chest. The technologist performed the RAO with 20–25 degrees of rotation and used a breathing technique. Which positioning error led to this radiographic outcome?

    _____

29. A radiograph of a lateral sternum shows that anterior ribs are superimposed over the sternum. Which specific positioning error led to this radiographic outcome?

    _____

30. **Situation:** A patient with an injury to the right lower posterior ribs comes to the emergency room. She is unable to stand. List the positioning routine that would be performed for this patient. Include breathing instructions.

    A. Positions performed: _____

    B. Breathing instructions: _____

31. **Situation:** A patient with an injury to the left upper anterior ribs comes to the ER. He is unable to stand but can lie on his abdomen. List the positioning routine that would be used for this patient. Include breathing instructions.

    A. Positions performed: _____

    B. Breathing instructions: _____

32. **Situation:** A routine chest study shows a possible lesion near the right sternoclavicular joint. A PA projection of the sternoclavicular joints is taken, but the area of interest is superimposed over the spine. What specific position can be used to better demonstrate this region?

    _____

33. **Situation:** A patient is brought to the ER with multiple injuries because of a motor vehicle accident. The patient can roll side-to-side but cannot stand or lie prone because of his injuries. A sternum study is ordered. What positions should be performed for this patient?

    _____

34. **Situation:** A patient comes to the ER with multiple rib fractures. The ER physician suspects a flail chest. The patient is able to stand and move. Beyond a rib series, what projections should be taken for this patient?

    _____

35. True/False: The automatic exposure control system is recommended for the RAO sternum projection if the center chamber is used.

36. True/False: An orthostatic-breathing technique is recommended for studies of the sternoclavicular joints.

37. **Situation:** A patient comes to the ER with a right, upper, anterior rib injury. A unilateral rib study is ordered. What are the basic projections taken for this patient?

    _____

38. **Situation:** A patient comes to the ER with a left, lower posterior rib injury. A unilateral rib study is ordered. The patient is unable to stand because of multiple injuries. What are the basic projections taken for this patient?

_____

39. **Situation:** A patient comes to radiology with a clinical history of pectus excavatum. What positioning routine would best demonstrate the condition?

_____

40. **Situation:** A patient comes to radiology with widespread metastases involving the bony thorax. Beyond radiographic studies, what other imaging modality demonstrates the extent of this condition?

_____

10 Bony Thorax—Sternum and Ribs

1. A. Manubrium
   B. Body
   C. Xiphoid process
2. Xiphoid process
3. Sternal angle
4. D. Manubrium
5. A. A true rib attaches directly to the sternum with its own costal cartilage.
6. D. A floating rib does not possess costal cartilage.
7. True rib
8. D. Sternal angle
9. D. All of the above
10. 1. A
    2. A
    3. B
    4. A
    5. B
11. A. Left clavicle
    B. Left sternoclavicular (SC) joint
    C. First rib (sternal end)
    D. Manubrium
    E. Sternal angle
    F. Body
    G. Xiphoid process
    H. Jugular (suprasternal or manubrial) notch
    I. Manubrium
    J. Sternal angle
    K. Body of sternum
    L. Xiphoid process
12. A. Suspended inspiration
    B. Medium kVp range (70–85 kVp)

C. Erect (if patient is able to sit or stand upright)
13. 40 inches (100 cm). There must be a minimum of 15 inches (40 cm) between the patient's skin and the collimator.
14. B. Orthostatic-breathing technique (if patient is cooperative)
15. A. Place the area of interest closest to IR.
    B. Rotate the spine away from the area of interest for axillary ribs.
16. A. Pneumothorax
    B. Hemothorax
    C. Pulmonary contusion
17. A. 15 degrees to 20 degrees
    B. More
18. C. For patients with a history of multiple myeloma
19. D. Blunt trauma
20. Bacterial infection
21. C. LPO
22. B. Drawn back
23. The SC joints are in equal distance from the midline of the spine.
24. 10 degrees to 15 degrees
25. Midway between the xiphoid process and the lower rib cage
26. B. 75–85 kVp
27. A. LAO
28. Over-rotation of the sternum. A large-chested patient only requires approximately 15 degrees of rotation. Over-rotation leads to foreshortening along the width of the

sternum and shifts the sternum away excessively from the spine.
29. Rotation of the upper body from a true lateral will cause the ribs to be superimposed over the sternum.
30. A. AP and RPO performed recumbent
    B. Suspend on expiration
31. A. PA and RAO performed recumbent
    B. Expose on inspiration
32. A 10-degree to 15-degree RAO will project the right SC joint adjacent to the spine.
33. LPO and horizontal beam lateral positions.
34. PA and lateral chest projections (chest study).
35. False. (AEC is generally not recommended for the RAO sternum projection because of the need for high-contrast (short-scale), optimum-detail exposures, which can generally be better achieved manually using an orthostatic-breathing technique.)
36. False. Exposure is made with suspended respiration on expiration.
37. PA and LAO positions are taken erect if possible.
38. Recumbent AP and LPO positions
39. RAO and lateral sternum (possibly a chest examination)
40. Nuclear medicine bone scan

A1

11 Skull and Cranial Bones

CHAPTER OBJECTIVES

Cranium

After you have successfully completed the activities in this chapter, you will be able to:

_____ 1. List the eight cranial bones and describe their features, related structures, location, and function.

_____ 2. Using drawings and/or radiographs, identify specific structures of the eight cranial bones.

_____ 3. Define specific terminology, reference points, positioning lines, and topographic landmarks of the cranium.

_____ 4. Identify specific radiographic and topographic landmarks of the cranium.

_____ 5. List the location, joint classification, and related terminology for the sutures and joints of the cranium.

_____ 6. List the differences among the three shape and size (morphology) classifications of the skull and their implications for radiography of the cranium.

_____ 7. Identify alternative imaging modalities that best demonstrate specific conditions or disease processes of the cranium and brain.

_____ 8. Match specific clinical indications of the cranium to the correct definition or statements.

_____ 9. List the three main portions of the temporal bones.

_____ 10. Identify specific structures of the external, middle, and internal ear.

_____ 11. Using drawings, identify the three divisions of the ear and the structures found in each division.

_____ 12. List the specific features, characteristics, location, and functions of the 14 facial bones.

_____ 13. List the seven cranial and facial bones that make up the bony orbit.

_____ 14. Using drawings and/or radiographs, identify specific structures of the facial bone region.

_____ 15. Match specific clinical indications of the temporal bone to the correct definition.

_____ 16. Using radiographs, identify specific structures of the temporal bone.

_____ 17. List the location, function, and characteristics of the four groups of paranasal sinuses.

_____ 18. Using drawings and radiographs, identify specific paranasal sinuses.

_____ 19. Match specific clinical indications of the paranasal sinuses to the correct definition.

_____ 20. Identify the correct field size and central ray (CR) location, direction, and angle for routine and special projections of the cranium.

_____ 21. Identify the structures that are best seen with specific projections of the cranium.

_____ 22. Given various hypothetic situations, identify the correct modification of a position and/or exposure factors to improve the radiographic image.

Facial Bones and Paranasal Sinuses

After you have successfully completed the activities in this chapter, you will be able to:

_____ 1. Explain the technical and positioning considerations for facial bone routines.

_____ 2. Identify alternative imaging modalities that best demonstrate specific facial bone and paranasal sinus pathology.

_____ 3. Identify specific types of fractures of the facial bone region.

_____ 4. Identify routine and special projections of the facial bones and list the correct field size, as well as the location, direction, and angulation of the central ray for each projection.

_____ 5. List the structures that are best seen with basic and special projections of the facial bones.

_____ 6. List technical and positioning considerations when performing a mandible study using the orthopantomography (panoramic tomography) imaging system.

_____ 7. Identify routine and special projections of the paranasal sinuses and list the correct field size, as well as the location, direction, and angulation of the central ray for each position.

_____ 8. Given various hypothetic situations, identify the correct modification of a position and/or exposure factors to improve the radiographic image.

_____ 9. Given radiographs of specific facial and paranasal sinus projections/positions, identify specific errors in positioning and exposure factors.

POSITIONING AND RADIOGRAPHIC CRITIQUE

_____ 1. Using a peer, position for routine and special projections of the cranium, facial bones, and paranasal sinuses.

_____ 2. Using a cranial radiographic phantom, produce satisfactory radiographs of specific positions (if equipment is available).

_____ 3. Critique and evaluate cranial radiographs based on the five divisions of radiographic criteria: (1) anatomy demonstrated, (2) position, (3) collimation field size and central ray, (4) exposure, and (5) anatomic side markers.

_____ 4. Distinguish between acceptable and unacceptable cranial radiographs based on exposure factors, motion, collimation, positioning, or other errors.

LEARNING EXERCISES

Complete the following review exercises after reading the associated pages in the textbook as indicated by each exercise. Answers to each review exercise are given at the end of the review exercises.

REVIEW EXERCISE A: Radiographic Anatomy of the Cranium (see textbook pp. 386–388)

1. Fill in the total number of bones.

   A. Cranium _____

   B. Facial bones _____

2. List the four cranial bones that form the calvaria (skull cap).

   A. _____

   C. _____

   B. _____

   D. _____

3. List the four cranial bones that form the floor of the cranium.

   A. _____

   C. _____

   B. _____

   D. _____

4. Identify the cranial bones labeled in Figs. 11.1 and 11.2. (Note: All eight cranial bones, including each paired bone, are visible in at least one of the following drawings.)

   A. _____

   B. _____

   C. _____

   D. _____

   E. _____

   F. _____

   G. _____

   H. _____

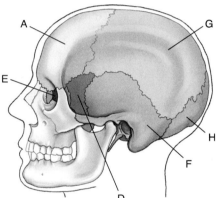

Fig. 11.1 Frontal view.   **Fig. 11.2** Lateral view.

5. Identify all eight cranial bones on the two superior-view drawings (Figs. 11.3 and 11.4).

A. _____

B. _____

C. _____

D. _____

E. _____

F. _____

G. _____

H. _____

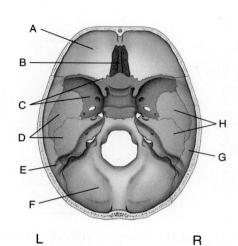

Fig. 11.3 Superior, cutaway view.

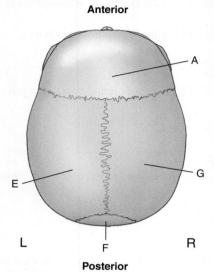

Fig. 11.4 Superior view.

6. Identify the labeled parts on the three views of the ethmoid bone (Figs. 11.5 and 11.6).

A. _____

B. _____

C. _____

D. _____

E. _____

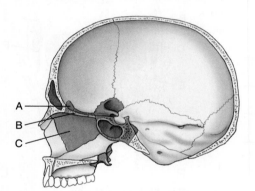

Fig. 11.5 Medial sectional view.

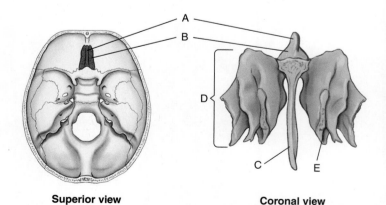

Superior view   Coronal view

Fig. 11.6 Superior (left) and coronal sectional (right) views.

249

7. The small horizontal plate of the ethmoid, seen on Fig. 11.6, is called the

   _____.

8. The vertical plate of the ethmoid bone forming the upper portion of the bony nasal septum is the

   _____.

9. Identify the labeled parts on the four views of the sphenoid in Figs. 11.7 through 11.10. (Note: Most of the parts are identified on more than one drawing.)

A. _____

B. _____

C. _____

D. _____

E. _____

F. _____

G. _____

Foramina (H–L)

H. _____

I. _____

J. _____

K. _____

L. _____

M. _____

N. _____

O. _____

P. _____

Q. _____

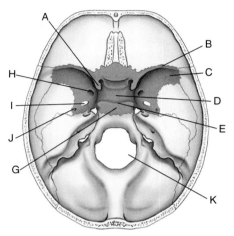

Fig. 11.7 Sphenoid, superior view.

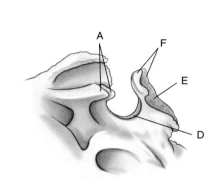

Fig. 11.8 Sphenoid, lateral view.

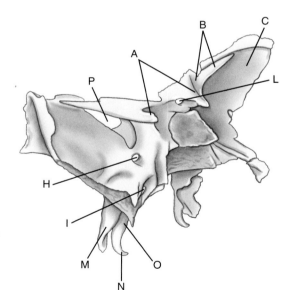

Fig. 11.9 Sphenoid, oblique view.

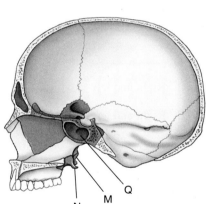

Fig. 11.10 Sphenoid, medial sectional view.

10. A structure found in the middle of the sphenoid bone that surrounds the pituitary gland is the

_____

11. The posterior aspect of the sella turcica is called the _____

12. Which structure of the sphenoid bone allows for the passage of the optic nerve and is the actual opening into the orbit? _____

13. Which structures of the sphenoid bone help to form part of the lateral walls of the nasal cavities?

_____

14. Which radiographic projection best demonstrates the sella turcica and dorsum sellae?

_____

15. Which aspect of the frontal bone forms the superior aspect of the orbit? _____

16. Identify the four major sutures and the six associated asterions and fontanels labeled on these drawings of an adult cranium and an infant cranium (Figs. 11.11 to 11.14).

Sutures

    A. _____

    B. _____

    C. _____

    D. _____

Suture Junctions

    E. _____

    F. _____

    G. Right and left _____

    H. Right and left _____

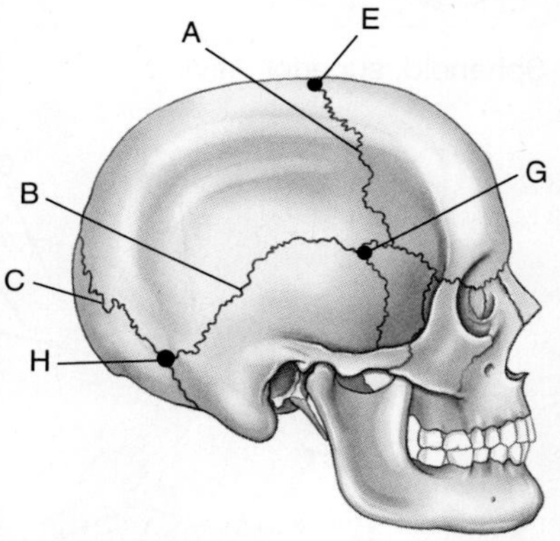

Fig. 11.11 Adult cranium, lateral view.

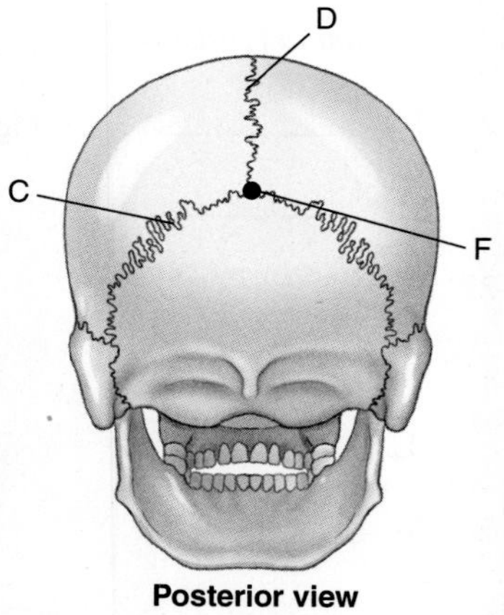

Posterior view

Fig. 11.12 Posterior view.

Fontanels

    I. _____

    J. _____

    K. Right and left _____

    L. Right and left _____

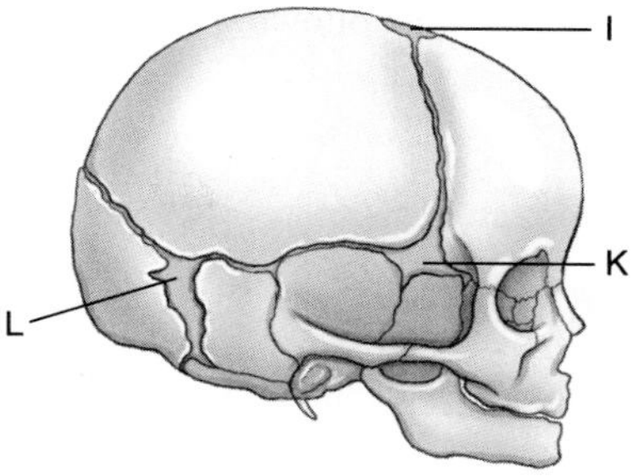

17. Cranial sutures are classified as being _____ joints.

Fig. 11.13 Infant cranium, lateral view.

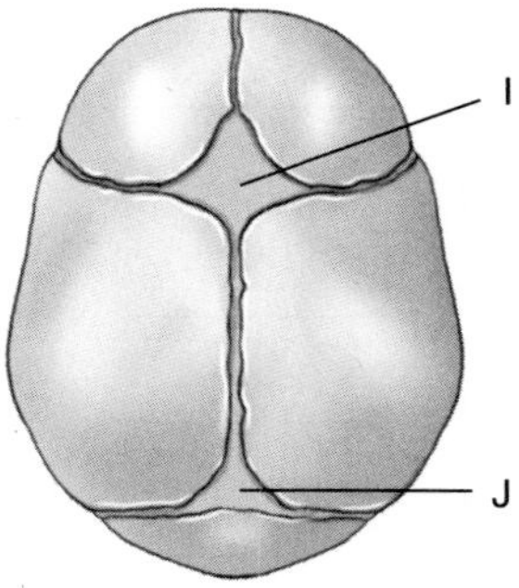

18. Small, irregular bones that sometimes develop in adult skull sutures are

called _____ or _____ bones

and are most frequently found in the _____ suture.

19. Which term describes the superior rim of the orbit? (Include the abbreviation also.)

_____

20. What is the name of the notch that separates the orbital plates from each other?

_____

Fig. 11.14 Infant cranium, superior view.

21. Which cranial bones form the upper lateral walls of the calvarium?

_____

22. Which cranial bone contains the foramen magnum? _____

23. A small prominence located on the squamous portion of the occipital bone is called the

_____.

24. What is the name of the oval processes found on the occipital bone that help form the atlanto-occipital joint?

_____

25. List the three aspects of the temporal bones.

    A. _____   B. _____   C. _____

26. True/False: The mastoid portion of the temporal bone is the densest of the three aspects of the temporal bone.

27. Which external landmark corresponds with the level of the petrous ridge?

_____

28. Which opening in the temporal bone serves as a passageway for nerves of hearing and equilibrium?

_____

29. Identify the following cranial structures labeled on Figs. 11.15 and 11.16.

Fig. 11.15

A. _____

B. _____

C. _____ (suture)

D. _____ (suture)

E. _____

F. _____

Fig. 11.16

A. _____

B. _____

C. _____

D. _____ (suture)

E. _____

F. _____

G. _____

H. _____ (suture)

I. _____

J. _____

K. _____

L. _____

M. _____

N. _____

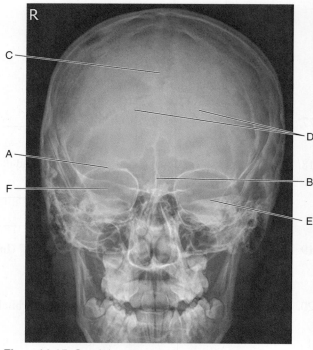

Fig. 11.15 Cranial structures, posteroanterior axial (Caldwell) projection.

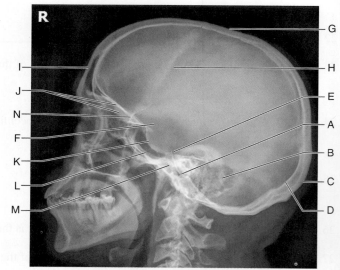

Fig. 11.16 Cranial structures, lateral projection.

REVIEW EXERCISE B: Specific Anatomy and Pathology of the Temporal Bone (see textbook pp. 389–397)

1. List the three aspects of the temporal bone.

   A. _____　　　B. _____　　　C. _____

2. Which aspect of the temporal bone is considered the densest? _____

3. Which structure makes up the cartilaginous external ear? _____

4. How long is the average external acoustic meatus (EAM)? _____

5. Which small membrane marks the beginning of the middle ear? _____

6. What is the collective term for the small bones of the middle ear? _____

7. Which structure allows for communication between the nasopharynx and middle ear?

   _____

8. What is the major function of the structure described in Question 7? _____

9. Which structure serves as an opening between the mastoid portion of the temporal bone and the middle ear?

   _____

10. What is the name of the thin plate of bone that separates the mastoid air cells from the brain?

    _____

11. Which of the auditory ossicles picks up sound vibrations from the tympanic membrane?

    _____

12. Which of the auditory ossicles is considered the smallest? _____

13. Which of the auditory ossicles resembles a premolar tooth? _____

14. What is the name of the small membrane that connects the middle to the inner ear?

    _____

15. Which two sensory functions occur within the inner ear?

    A. _____　　　　　　　　　　B. _____

16. What is the name of the small membrane found at the base of the cochlea (two terms possible)?

17. True/False: The semicircular canals include a closed system specific to the sense of hearing.

254

Chapter **11** **Skull and Cranial Bones**

Copyright © 2025 by Elsevier Inc.
All rights are reserved, including those for text and data mining, AI training, and similar technologies.

18. Identify the structures labeled in Fig. 11.17.

A. _____

B. _____

C. _____

D. _____

E. _____

F. _____

G. _____

H. _____

I. _____

J. _____

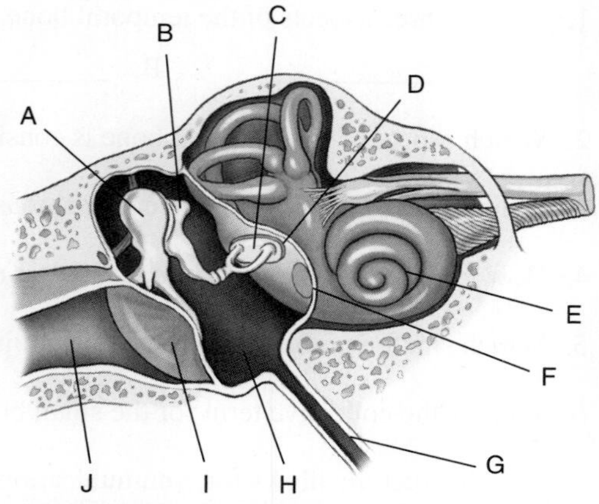

Fig. 11.17 Structures of the middle and internal ear.

19. Match each of the following clinical indications for the temporal bone to the correct definition or description. (Use each choice only once. See Temporal Bone Pathology found on p. 412 in text)

A. Neoplasia

B. Otosclerosis

C. Mastoiditis

D. Acoustic neuroma

E. Polyp

F. Cholesteatoma

1. Bacterial infection of the mastoid process

2. Growth arising from a mucous membrane

3. Hereditary disease involving excessive bone formation of middle ear

4. Benign, cystic mass or tumor of the middle ear

5. New and abnormal growth

6. Benign tumor of the auditory nerve sheath

20. Which of the following radiographic appearances pertains to an acoustic neuroma?

A. Expansion of the internal acoustic canal

B. Bone destruction within the middle ear

C. Increased opacification in the sinus

D. Sinus mucosal thickening

21. Which of the following imaging modalities best demonstrates otosclerosis?

A. Nuclear medicine

B. Computed tomography (CT)

C. Conventional radiography

D. Diagnostic medical sonography (DMS)

REVIEW EXERCISE C: Radiographic Anatomy of the Facial Bones (see textbook pp. 398–403)

1. Which of the following bones is not a facial bone?

    A. Middle nasal conchae

    B. Vomer

    C. Lacrimal bone

    D. Mandible

2. What is the largest immovable bone of the face? _____

3. List the four processes of the maxilla.

    A. _____

    B. _____

    C. _____

    D. _____

4. Which of the processes mentioned in Question 3 is considered most superior? _____

5. Which soft tissue landmark is found at the base of the anterior nasal spine? _____

6. Which facial bones form the posterior aspect of the hard palate? _____

7. Which two cranial bones articulate with the maxilla? _____

8. Which facial bones are sometimes called the "cheek bones"? _____

9. Which of the following bones does not articulate with the zygomatic bone?

    A. Temporal

    B. Mandible

    C. Frontal

    D. Sphenoid

10. Which facial bone is associated with the tear ducts? _____

11. The purpose of the _____, or _____, is to divide the nasal cavity into compartments and to circulate air coming into the nasal cavities. (Include both terms for these bones.)

12. True/False: The right and left nasal bones form the largest part of the nose.

13. A deviated nasal septum is most likely to occur at the junction between _____ and _____.

14. Match each of the following mandibular terms to the correct definition or description. (Use each choice only once.)

    A. Gonion

    B. Mandibular notch

    C. Body

    D. Condyloid process

    E. Coronoid process

    F. Ramus

    G. Mentum

    H. Symphysis menti

    1. Vertical portion of mandible

    2. Chin

    3. Mandibular angle

    4. Point of union between both halves of the mandible

    5. Bony process located anterior to mandibular notch

    6. Horizontal portion of mandible

    7. Posterior process of the upper ramus

    8. U-shaped notch

Identify the labeled facial bones visible in Figs. 11.18 and 11.19.

Paired Bones

A. _____

B. _____

C. _____

D. _____

E. _____

Single Bone

F. _____

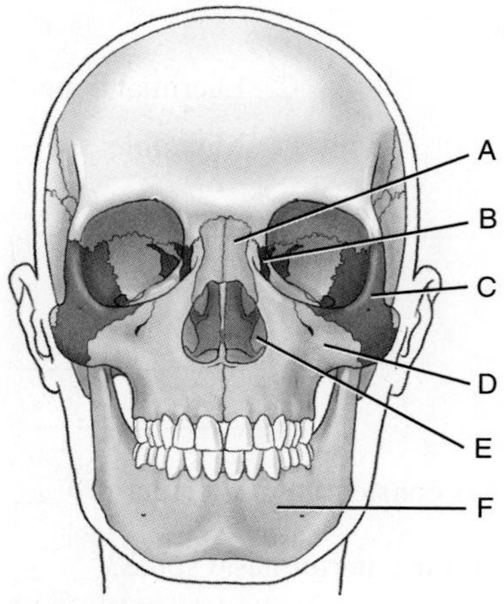

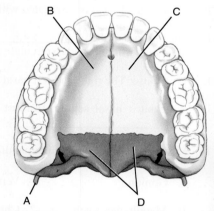

Fig. 11.18 Frontal view.

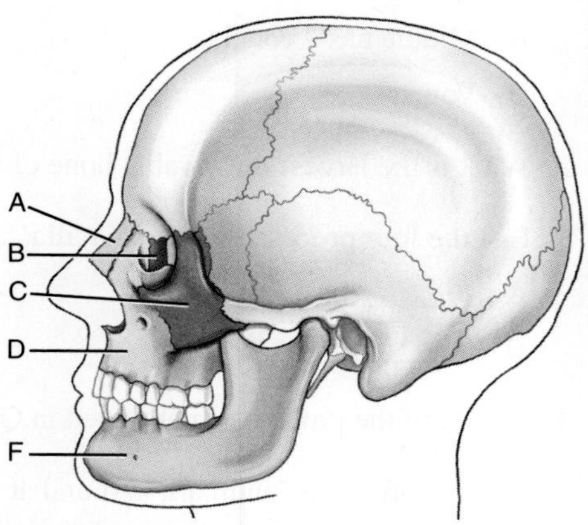

Fig. 11.19 Side view.

15. The single facial bone and the one pair of facial bones not visible from the exterior and not demonstrated in

Figs. 11.18 and 11.19 are the _____ and the _____, respectively. (These are demonstrated in special-view drawings in the following questions.)

Identify the labeled structures (and the facial bones of which they are a part of) on this inferior surface view of the maxillae (Fig. 11.20).

Structure	Bone(s)
A. _____	(_____)
B. _____	(_____)
C. _____	(_____)
D. _____	(_____)

Fig. 11.20 Inferior surface view of the maxillae.

16. List the three structures that form the nasal septum as shown in Fig. 11.21.

A. _____

B. _____

C. _____

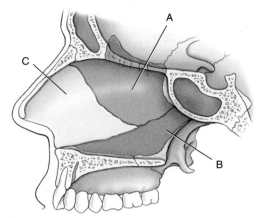

Fig. 11.21 Nasal septum.

17. Identify the parts of the mandible and skull as labeled in Figs. 11.22 and 11.23.

A. _____

B. _____

C. _____

D. _____

E. _____

F. _____

G. _____

H. _____

I. _____

J. _____

K. (Cranial bone) _____

L. (Joint) _____

M. (Key landmark) _____

N. (Landmark) _____

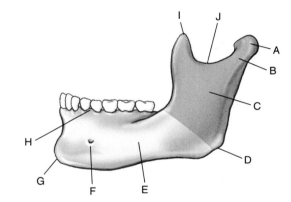

Fig. 11.22 Mandible.

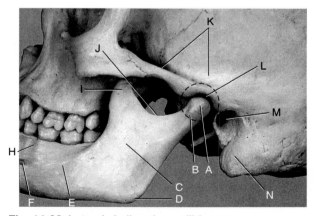

Fig. 11.23 Lateral skull and mandible.

18. Identify the seven bones that form the orbit and indicate whether they are cranial or facial bones (Fig. 11.24). (See pp. 408–409)

Bone   **Cranial or Facial?**

A. _____   (_____)

B. _____   (_____)

C. _____   (_____)

D. _____   (_____)

E. _____   (_____)

F. _____   (_____)

G. _____   (_____)

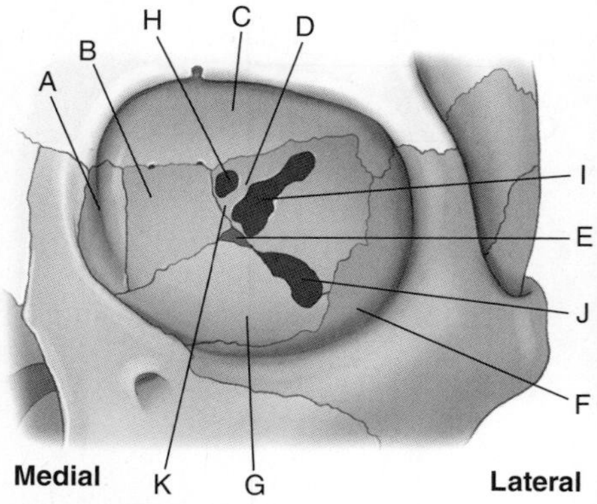

Fig. 11.24 Slightly oblique frontal view of orbit, A–K.

19. Identify the three foramina found within the orbits as labeled in Fig. 11.24.

H. _____

I. _____

J. _____

Small section of bone:

K. _____

20. From anterior to posterior, the cone-shaped orbits project upward at an angle of _____

____° and toward the midsagittal plane at an angle of _____°.

21. Which facial bone opening has the maxillary branch of the fifth cranial nerve passing through it?

_____

22. Which of the facial bone openings is formed by a cleft between the greater and lesser wings of the sphenoid bone?

A. Superior orbital fissure   C. Inferior orbital fissure

B. Optic foramen   D. Optic canal

23. What is another term for the second cranial nerve?

A. Olfactory nerve   C. Maxillary nerve

B. Optic nerve   D. Trigeminal nerve

REVIEW EXERCISE D: Radiographic Anatomy of the Paranasal Sinuses (see textbook pp. 404–407)

1. What is the older term for the maxillary sinuses? _____

2. An infection of the teeth may travel upward and involve the _____ sinus.

3. Specifically, where are the frontal sinuses located? _____

4. The frontal sinuses rarely become aerated before the age of _____.

5. Which specific aspect of the ethmoid bone contains the ethmoid sinuses? _____

6. The drainage pathway for the paranasal sinuses is called the:

   A. Uncinate process   C. Paranasal meatus

   B. Osteomeatal complex   D. Lateral masses

7. Which sinus is projected through the open mouth with a posteroanterior (PA) axial transoral projection?

   _____

8. Identify the paranasal sinuses, structures, or bones labeled in Fig. 11.25.

   A. _____

   B. _____

   C. _____

   D. _____

   E. _____

   F. _____

   G. _____

   H. _____

   I. _____

   J. _____

   K. _____

   L. _____

   M. _____

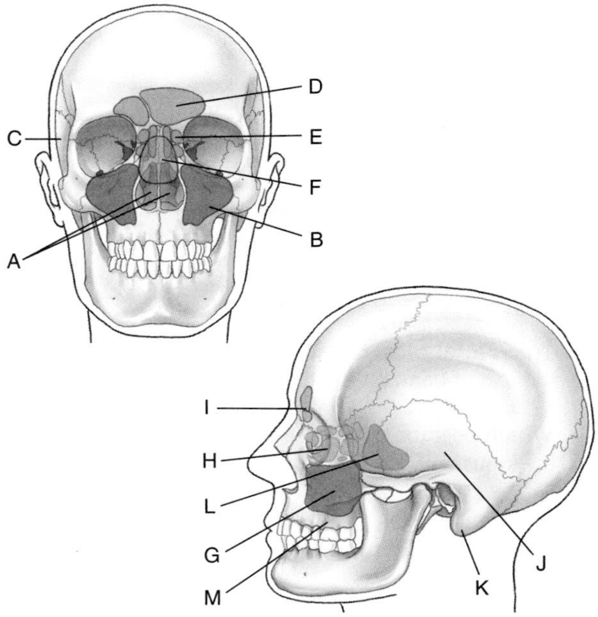

Fig. 11.25 Frontal and lateral views.

9. Identify the following paranasal sinuses labeled in Figs. 11.26 and 11.27.

Fig. 11.26

    A. _____

    B. _____

    C. _____

    D. _____

Fig. 11.27

    E. _____

    F. _____

    G. _____

    H. _____

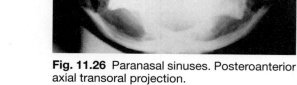

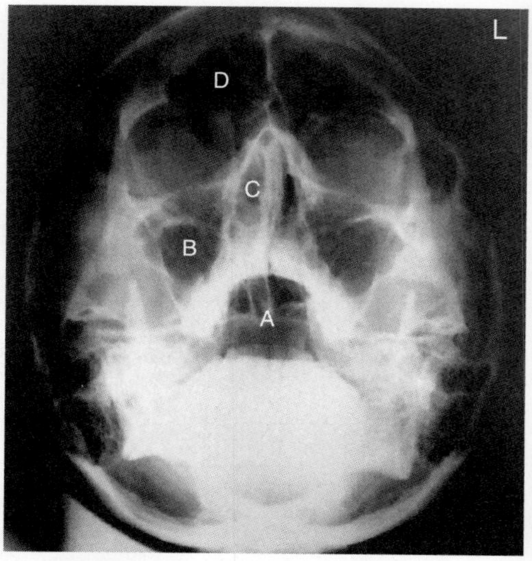

Fig. 11.26 Paranasal sinuses. Posteroanterior axial transoral projection.

10. What is the name of the passageway between the maxillary sinuses and the middle nasal meatus?

    _____

11. True/False: Most CT studies of the paranasal sinuses do not require the use of contrast media.

12. Which position is most often used when performing a CT study of the sinuses?

    A. Supine

    B. Prone

    C. Erect

    D. Supine with 20° oblique of skull from anteroposterior (AP) position

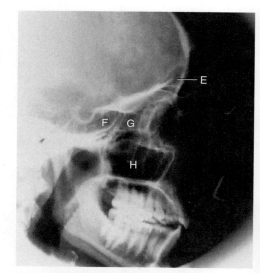

Fig. 11.27 Paranasal sinuses. Lateral projection.

PART II: RADIOGRAPHIC POSITIONING OF CRANIUM

REVIEW EXERCISE A: Skull Morphology, Topography, Pathology, and Positioning of the Cranium (see textbook pp. 412–419 and 422–428)

1. List the three classifications of the skull; then match them with the correct shape description listed on the right.

    Classification

    A. _____

    B. _____

    C. _____

    Shape Description

    a. Width <75% of length

    b. Width ≥80% of length

    c. Width between 75% and 80% of length

261

2. Central ray angles and degree of rotation stated for basic skull positions are based on the

_____ (average) skull, which has an approximate angle of

_____ between the midsagittal plane and the long axis of the petrous bone.

3. The long, narrow-shaped skull has an angle of approximately _____° between the midsagittal plane and the long axis of the petrous bone.

4. True/False: Skull morphology has no impact on positioning considerations.

5. There is a _____° difference between the orbitomeatal and infraorbitomeatal

lines, and _____° between the orbitomeatal and glabellomeatal lines.

6. Match each of the following cranial landmarks and positioning lines with the correct definition. (Use each choice only once.)

_____ 1. Lateral junction of the eyelid

_____ 2. Posterior angle of the jaw

_____ 3. A line between the infraorbital margin and the EAM

_____ 4. Corresponds to the highest "nuchal" line of the occipital bone

_____ 5. A line between the glabella and alveolar process of the maxilla

_____ 6. A line between the mental point and the EAM

_____ 7. Located at the junction of the two nasal bones and the frontal bone

_____ 8. The small cartilaginous flap covering the ear opening

_____ 9. Corresponds to the highest level of the facial bone mass

_____ 10. A line between the midlateral orbital margin and the EAM

_____ 11. The center point of the EAM

_____ 12. A positioning line that is primarily used for the modified Waters projection

_____ 13. A line used in positioning to ensure that the skull is in a true lateral position

_____ 14. Corresponds to the level of the petrous ridge

_____ 15. A smooth, slightly depressed area between the eyebrows

A. Top of the ear attachment (TEA)

B. Supraorbital groove

C. Interpupillary line

D. Nasion

E. Gonion

F. Tragus

G. Outer canthus

H. Glabelloalveolar line (GAL)

I. OML

J. Infraorbitomeatal line (IOML)

K. Mentomeatal line

L. Lips-meatal line

M. Glabella

N. Inion

O. Auricular point

7. What is the average kVp range for skull radiography?

_____

8. List the five most common errors made during skull radiography.

   A. _____   C. _____   E. _____

   B. _____   D. _____

9. Of the five causes listed in the previous question, which two are the most common?

   A. _____   B. _____

10. Bilateral horizontal fractures of the maxillae describe a _____ fracture.

    A. Le Fort   C. Tripod

    B. Blowout   D. Contrecoup

11. Which of the following imaging modalities is the most common neuroimaging procedure performed for the cranium?

    A. CT   C. Magnetic resonance imaging (MR)

    B. Diagnostic medical sonography   D. Nuclear medicine

12. Which of the following imaging modalities is commonly performed on neonates with a possible intracranial hemorrhage?

    A. CT   C. MR

    B. Diagnostic medical sonography (DMS) D. Nuclear medicine (NM)

13. Which of the following imaging modalities is most commonly performed to evaluate patients for Alzheimer disease?

    A. CT   C. MR

    B. Diagnostic medical sonography (DMS) D. Nuclear medicine (NM)

14. Match each of the following clinical indications to the correct definition or statement. (Use each choice only once.)

    A. Fracture that may produce an air-fluid level in the sphenoid sinus   1. Osteoblastic neoplasm

    B. Destructive lesion with irregular margins   2. Pituitary adenoma

    C. Also called a "ping-pong" fracture   3. Basal skull fracture

    D. Proliferative bony lesion of increased opacification   4. Paget disease

    E. A tumor that may produce erosion of the sella turcica   5. Osteolytic neoplasm

    F. Also known as osteitis deformans   6. Depressed skull fracture

    G. A bone tumor that originates in the bone marrow   7. Multiple myeloma

15. Which of the following clinical indications may require an increase in manual exposure factors?

    A. Advanced Paget disease   C. Multiple myeloma

    B. Metastatic neoplasm   D. Basal skull fracture

16. Which cranial bone is best demonstrated with an AP axial (Towne method) projection of the skull?

    _____

17. When using a 30° caudad angle for the AP axial (Towne method) projection of the skull, which positioning line should be perpendicular to the IR?

A. OML

B. IOML

C. GAL

D. Acanthiomeatal line (AML)

18. A properly positioned AP axial (Towne method) projection should place the dorsum sellae into the middle aspect of the:

A. Orbits

B. Clivus

C. Foramen magnum

D. Anterior arch of C1

19. A lack of symmetry of the petrous ridges indicates which of the following problems with a radiograph of an AP axial projection?

A. Tilt

B. Central ray angle

C. Flexion or extension

D. Rotation

20. If the patient cannot flex the head adequately for the AP axial (Towne method) projection, the technologist could

place the _____ perpendicular to the IR and angle the central ray

_____° caudad.

21. What evidence on an AP axial (Towne method) radiograph indicates whether the correct central ray angle and

correct head flexion were used? _____

22. What central ray angle should be used for the PA axial (Haas method) projection for the cranium?

_____

23. Where is the central ray centered for a lateral projection of the skull? _____

24. Which specific positioning error is present if the mandibular rami are not superimposed on a lateral skull radiograph?

A. Tilt

B. Rotation

C. Hyperflexion of head and neck

D. Incorrect central ray angle

25. Where will the petrous ridges be projected with a 15° PA axial (Caldwell) projection of the cranium?

_____

26. Which specific positioning error is present if the petrous ridges are projected higher in the orbits than expected for

a 15° PA axial projection? _____

27. Which projection of the cranium produces an image of the frontal bone with little or no distortion?

_____

28. For a patient with possible trauma, what must be determined before performing the submentovertical (SMV)

projection of the skull? _____

29. What positioning error has been committed if the EAMs are not superimposed with one of them more superior

than the other on a lateral projection of the cranium? _____

264

30. Which skull positioning line is placed parallel to the plane of the IR for the SMV projection?

A. OML

B. IOML

C. AML

D. Glabellomeatal line (GML)

31. Which of the following projections best demonstrates the sella turcica in profile?

A. AP axial

B. SMV

C. 15° PA axial

D. Lateral

32. Which of the following projections best demonstrates the foramen rotundum?

A. SMV

B. 25° to 30° AP axial

C. 25° to 30° PA axial

D. Lateral

33. Which of the following projections best demonstrates the clivus in profile?

A. AP axial

B. 15° PA

C. Lateral

D. SMV

34. Where does the CR exit for a PA axial (Haas method) projection of the skull?

A. 1.5 inches (4 cm) superior to the nasion

B. 0.75 inch (2 cm) anterior to the EAM

C. 2.5 inches (6.5 cm) above the glabella

D. Level of nasion

35. Which imaging modality is best to differentiate between an epidural and a subdural hemorrhage?

A. CT

B. MR

C. Nuclear medicine (NM)

D. Positron emission tomography (PET)

REVIEW EXERCISE B: Problem Solving for Technical and Positioning Errors of the Cranium

1. A radiograph of an AP axial (Towne method) projection of the cranium shows the right petrous ridge is wider than the left side. Which specific positioning error is present on this radiograph?

_____

2. A radiograph of a 15° PA axial (Caldwell) projection of the cranium demonstrates the petrous ridges are projected at the inferior orbital margin. Which positioning error(s) led to this radiographic outcome?

_____

3. A radiograph of a 15° PA axial (Caldwell) projection demonstrates the distance between the right midlateral orbital borders and lateral margin of the skull cortex is greater than the left side. Which positioning error led to this radiographic outcome?

_____

4. A radiograph of an SMV projection of the skull shows the mandibular condyles are within the petrous bone. Which specific positioning error led to this problem?

_____

5. A radiograph of a lateral projection of the skull shows the orbital plates are not superimposed. (One orbital plate is slightly superior to the other.) Which specific positioning error led to this radiographic outcome?

_____

6. A lateral skull radiograph demonstrates one mandibular ramus about 0.5 cm more anterior than the other. Which positioning error occurred?

_____

7. An AP axial (Towne method) radiograph for the cranium demonstrates the dorsum sellae projected above, or superior to, the foramen magnum. The foramen magnum is distorted. Which positioning error(s) occurred?

_____

8. **Situation:** A patient comes to the radiology department with a possible tumor of the pituitary gland. Which radiographic projection of the cranium best demonstrates any bony involvement of the sella turcica?

_____

9. **Situation:** A patient with a possible linear fracture of the right parietal bone enters the emergency room. Which single radiographic projection of the skull best demonstrates this fracture?

_____

10. **Situation:** A patient comes to the radiology department for a skull series, but the patient cannot assume the correct position for either version of the AP axial (Towne method) projection because of a very short neck and severe spinal kyphosis. What can the technologist do to demonstrate the occipital bone?

_____

11. **Situation:** A patient with a possible basal skull fracture enters the emergency room. No CT scanner is available. Which specific position may provide radiographic evidence of this fracture?

_____

12. **Situation:** A neonate has a clinical history of craniosynostosis. Because of the age of the patient, the physician does not order a radiographic procedure of the cranium. What other imaging modality can be performed to evaluate the patient for this condition?

_____

13. **Situation:** A patient with a clinical history of acoustic neuroma comes to the radiology department. Which imaging modality or modalities can be performed for this type of pathology?

_____

14. A radiograph of an AP axial (Towne method) projection for the cranium shows that the posterior arch of C1 is projected within the foramen magnum. The dorsum sellae is superimposed on the posterior arch as well. What is (are) the positioning error(s)?

_____

15. A radiograph of an AP axial (Towne method) projection for the cranium shows the mid- to lower mandible is cut off and not demonstrated. What should the technologist do?

_____

PART III: RADIOGRAPHIC POSITIONING OF FACIAL BONES, MANDIBLE, AND PARANASAL SINUSES

REVIEW EXERCISE A: Positioning of the Facial Bones (see textbook pp. 420–422 and 429–434)

1. True/False: Facial bone studies should always be performed recumbent whenever possible.

2. True/False: The common basic PA axial projection for facial bones requires a 15° caudad angle of the central ray, which projects the dense petrous ridges into the lower one-third of the orbits.

3. True/False: An increase in kVp of 25%–30% (using manual techniques) is often required for the geriatric patient with advanced osteoporosis.

4. True/False: CT is ideal for facial bone studies because it allows for the visualization of bony structures as well as related soft tissues of the facial bones.

5. True/False: Nuclear medicine is not helpful in diagnosing occult facial bone fractures.

6. True/False: MR is an excellent imaging modality for the detection of small metal foreign bodies in the eye.

7. What is the name of the fracture that results from a direct blow to the orbit leading to a disruption of the inferior

   orbital margin? _____

8. A "free-floating" zygomatic bone is the frequent result of a _____ fracture.

9. What is the major disadvantage of performing a straight PA projection for facial bones, with no CR angulation or neck extension, as compared with other PA facial bone projections?

   _____

10. Where is the CR centered for a lateral position for the facial bones?
    A. Outer canthus   C. Zygoma
    B. Acanthion   D. Nasion

11. What is the proper method name for the parietoacanthial projection of the facial bones?

    _____

12. Which facial bone structures are best seen with a parietoacanthial projection?

    _____

13. What CR angle must be used to project the petrous ridges just below the orbital floor with the PA axial (Caldwell method) projection?
    A. None. CR is perpendicular.   C. 20°
    B. 30°   D. 45°

14. Which structures specifically are better visualized on the modified parietoacanthial projection as compared with the basic parietoacanthial projection?

    _____

15. Give two reasons why projections of the facial bones are performed PA rather than AP when possible.

    A. _____   B. _____

16. What are two differences between the lateral projection of the cranium and the lateral projection for the facial bones?

    A. _____   B. _____

17. The parietoacanthial projection for the facial bones has the _____ line perpendicular to the IR, which places the OML at a

    _____° angle to the tabletop and IR.

18. Where does the CR exit for a parietoacanthial projection of the facial bones?

    _____

19. Where does the CR exit for a 15° PA axial (Caldwell) projection for the facial bones?

    _____

20. The modified parietoacanthial projection requires that the _____ line

    is perpendicular to the IR, which places the OML at a _____° angle to the tabletop and IR.

21. True/False: Lateral projections for nasal bones generally are taken bilaterally for comparison.

22. True/False: The oblique inferosuperior (tangential) projection for the zygomatic arch requires that the skull be rotated and tilted 15° *away from* the affected side.

23. True/False: Both oblique inferosuperior (tangential) projections for the zygomatic arch are generally taken for comparison.

24. For a parietoacanthial (PA Waters) projection, the petrous ridges should be projected directly below the

    _____ and projected into the lower half of the maxillary sinuses or below the

    _____ for a modified Waters projection.

25. For the superoinferior projection of the nasal bones, the IR is placed perpendicular to the

    _____ line. (Include the full term and abbreviation.)

26. Which specific facial bone structures (other than the mandible) are best demonstrated with the SMV projection if the correct exposure factors are used (soft tissue technique)?

    _____

27. Where is the CR centered for an AP axial projection for the zygomatic arches?

    _____

28. List the proper method name and the common descriptive name for the parieto-orbital oblique projection for the optic foramen.

    A. _____   B. _____

29. The three aspects of the face that should be in contact with the head unit or tabletop when beginning positioning for the parieto-orbital oblique projection are the (A) _____, _____, and _____. The final angle between the midsagittal plane and the IR should be (B) _____, with the (C) _____ line perpendicular to the IR. This places the optic foramen in the (D) _____ quadrant of the orbit.

30. Match each of the following structures to the facial bone projection that best demonstrates the structure(s). (Use each choice only once.)

    _____ 1. Floor of orbits (blowout fractures)   A. Lateral (nasal bones)

    _____ 2. Optic foramen   B. Parietoacanthial projection

    _____ 3. View of single zygomatic arch   C. Parieto-orbital oblique projection

    _____ 4. Profile image of nasal bones and nasal septum   D. SMV projection

    _____ 5. Bilateral zygomatic arches   E. Modified parietoacanthial method

    _____ 6. Inferior orbital rim, maxillae, nasal septum, nasal spine, F. Oblique inferosuperior projection
                  zygomatic bone, and arches

REVIEW EXERCISE B: Positioning of the Mandible and Temporomandibular Joints (TMJ) (see textbook pp. 439–448)

1. True/False: The PA axial projection of the mandible produces an elongated view of the condyloid processes.

    _____

2. Which projection of the mandible projects the opposite half of the mandible away from the side of interest?

    _____

3. What must be done to prevent the ramus of the mandible from being superimposed over the cervical spine with an axiolateral oblique projection of the mandible?

    _____

4. How much skull rotation (from the lateral skull position) toward the IR is required with an axiolateral oblique projection for demonstrating each of the following?

    A. Body of the mandible: _____

    B. Mentum region: _____

    C. Ramus region: _____

    D. General survey of the mandible: _____

    E. What is the maximum CR angle needed for all of these projections? _____

269

5. What specific positioning error has been committed if both sides of the mandible are superimposed with an axiolateral oblique projection?

_____

6. Where should the CR exit for a PA axial projection of the mandible?

_____

7. Which cranial positioning line is placed perpendicular to the IR for a PA or PA axial projection of the mandible?

_____

8. True/False: For a true PA projection of the mandibular body (if this is the area of interest), the AML should be perpendicular to the IR.

9. True/False: The CR should be angled 20°–25° caudad for the PA axial projection of the mandible.

10. Which aspect of the mandible is best visualized with an AP axial projection?

_____

11. A. What CR angle is required for the AP axial projection of the mandible if the OML is placed perpendicular to

the IR? _____

B. If the IOML is perpendicular to IR, what CR angle is needed?_____

12. Where is the CR centered for an AP axial projection of the mandible?

_____

13. Which projection of the mandible demonstrates the entire mandible, including the coronoid and condyloid processes?

_____

14. Which imaging system provides a single, frontal perspective of the entire mandible?

_____

15. What device provides inherent collimation during an orthopantomographic procedure?

_____

16. Which cranial line is placed parallel to the floor for orthopantomography of the mandible?

_____

17. What type of IR must be used with digital orthopantomography?

_____

18. True/False: The modified Law method provides a bilateral and functional study of the TMJ.

19. True/False: The mandibular condyles move anteriorly as the mouth is opened.

20. Which projection/method of the TMJ requires that the skull be kept in a true lateral position?

    A. Modified law   C. Axiolateral oblique projection

    B. Schuller   D. Modified Towne

21. The axiolateral (Schuller method) projection for the TMJ requires a CR angle of _____°
    (caudad or cephalad).

22. The axiolateral oblique projection of the TMJ is commonly referred to as the (A) _____

    method, which requires a (B) _____° head rotation from lateral and a (C)

    _____° caudad CR angle.

23. If the area of interest is the temporomandibular fossae, angle the CR _____ to the OML for
    the AP axial (modified Towne) projection to reduce superimposition of the temporomandibular fossae and mastoid
    portions of the temporal bone.

24. Aligning the _____ plane perpendicular to the IR prevents rotation of either a PA or an AP
    axial mandible.

REVIEW EXERCISE C: Positioning of the Paranasal Sinuses (see textbook pp. 449–453)

1. What kVp range should be used for paranasal sinus radiography? _____

2. To demonstrate any possible air or fluid levels within the paranasal sinuses, it is important to:

    A. _____

    B. _____

3. True/False: Diagnostic medical sonography exams of the maxillary sinuses to rule out sinusitis are possible.

4. True/False: MR is the preferred modality to study soft tissue changes and masses within the paranasal sinuses.

5. True/False: Secondary osteomyelitis is often caused by tumor invasion.

6. List the four most commonly performed routine projections for paranasal sinuses.

    A. _____   C. _____

    B. _____   D. _____

7. Which single projection for a paranasal sinus routine provides an image of all four sinus groups?

    _____

8. If the patient cannot stand for the lateral projection of the paranasal sinuses, the projection should be taken with:

    _____

9. Which paranasal sinuses are best demonstrated with a PA (Caldwell) projection?

    _____

10. To avoid angling the CR for the erect PA (axial) Caldwell sinus projection, the head should be adjusted so that the OML is _____ ° from horizontal.

11. A. Which group of paranasal sinuses is best demonstrated with a parietoacanthial projection?

_____

   B. The OML forms a _____° angle with the IR with this projection.

12. Which positioning line is placed perpendicular to the IR for a parietoacanthial projection?

_____

13. Where are the petrous ridges located on a well-positioned parietoacanthial projection?

_____

14. Which paranasal sinuses are demonstrated with an SMV projection of the paranasal sinuses?

_____

15. Where should the CR exit for both the PA parietoacanthial (Waters) and the PA transoral (open-mouth Waters) projections? _____

16. What is the one major difference in positioning between the parietoacanthial and PA axial transoral projections?

_____

17. Which paranasal sinuses are projected through the oral cavity with the PA axial transoral projection?

_____

18. Match each of the following sinus projections with the anatomy best seen. (Use each choice only once.)

   _____ 1. Lateral   A. Sphenoid sinus in oral cavity

   _____ 2. Parietoacanthial   B. Inferosuperior view of sphenoid and ethmoid sinus

   _____ 3. PA (axial) Caldwell   C. All four paranasal sinuses demonstrated

   _____ 4. PA transoral   D. Best view of maxillary sinuses

   _____ 5. SMV for sinuses   E. Best view of frontal and ethmoid sinuses

REVIEW EXERCISE D: Problem Solving for Technical and Positioning Errors for Facial Bones, Mandible, and Paranasal Sinuses

1. **Situation**: A radiograph of a lateral projection of the facial bones shows the mandibular rami are not superimposed. What positioning error led to this radiographic outcome?

_____

2. **Situation:** A radiograph of a parietoacanthial (Waters) projection shows the petrous ridges are projected within the maxillary sinuses. Is this an acceptable image? If not, what must be done to improve the image during the repeat exposure?

   _____

3. **Situation**: A radiograph of a parietoacanthial projection shows the distance between the lateral margins of the orbits and the lateral aspect of the cranial cortex is not equal. What type of positioning error led to this radiographic outcome?

   _____

4. **Situation:** A radiograph of a 30° PA axial projection of the facial bones shows the petrous ridges are projected at the level of the inferior orbital margins. Is this an acceptable image for this projection? If not, what must be done to improve the quality of the image during the repeat exposure?

   _____

5. **Situation:** A radiograph of a superoinferior projection of the nasal bones shows the glabella are superimposed over the nasal bones. What positioning error led to this radiographic outcome, and how can it be corrected during the repeat exposure?

   _____

6. **Situation:** A lateral radiograph of the facial bones demonstrates the bodies of the mandible are not superimposed; one is about 1 cm superior to the other. How would this be corrected on a repeat exposure?

   _____

7. **Situation:** A radiograph of a parieto-orbital oblique (Rhese) projection shows the optic foramen is located in the upper outer quadrant of the orbit. Is this an acceptable image for this projection? If not, what must be done to correct this problem during the repeat exposure?

   _____

8. **Situation:** A radiograph of an axiolateral oblique projection of the mandible shows the body of the mandible is severely foreshortened. The body of the mandible is the area of interest. What positioning error led to this radiographic outcome?

   _____

9. **Situation:** A patient with a possible fracture of the nasal bones enters the emergency room. The physician is concerned about deviation of the bony nasal septum along with possible fracture of nasal bones. What radiographic routine would be best for this situation?

   _____

10. **Situation:** A patient with a possible blowout fracture of the right orbit enters the emergency room. In addition to the basic facial bone routine, what single projection would best demonstrate this type of injury?

    _____

11. **Situation:** A patient with a possible fracture of the left zygomatic arch enters the emergency room. Neither the AP axial nor the SMV projection demonstrates the left side well. The radiologist is indecisive as to whether this zygomatic arch is fractured. What other projections can the technologist provide to better define this area?

    _____

12. **Situation:** As part of a study of the zygomatic arches, the technologist attempts to perform the SMV position. Because of the size of the patient's shoulders, he is unable to flex his neck adequately to place the IOML parallel to the IR. What other options does the technologist have to produce an acceptable SMV projection?

_____

13. **Situation:** A radiograph of a PA (Caldwell) projection for paranasal sinuses shows the petrous ridges are projected into the lower half of the orbits and are obscuring the ethmoid sinuses. The technologist used a horizontal x-ray beam for the projection. The skull was positioned to place the OML at a 15° angle from the horizontal plane. What positioning modification is needed to correct this problem during the repeat exposure?

_____

14. **Situation:** A radiograph of a parietoacanthial projection shows the distance between the midsagittal plane and the outer orbital margin is not equal. What positioning error is present on this radiograph?

_____

15. **Situation:** A radiograph of an SMV projection for paranasal sinuses shows the distance between the mandibular condyles and lateral border of the skull is not equal. What specific positioning error is present on this radiograph?

_____

16. **Situation:** A radiograph of a PA transoral projection shows the sphenoid sinus is superimposed over the upper teeth and the nasal cavity. How must the position be modified to avoid this problem during the repeat exposure?

_____

17. **Situation:** A radiograph of a parietoacanthial projection (Waters method) shows the petrous ridges are projected just below the maxillary sinuses. What positioning error (if any) is present?

_____

18. **Situation:** A patient with a clinical history of sinusitis comes to the radiology department for a sinus study. The patient is quadriplegic and cannot be placed erect. Which single projection demonstrates any possible air-fluid levels in the paranasal sinuses?

_____

19. **Situation:** A patient comes to the radiology department to rule out a possible polyp within the sphenoid sinus. What routine and/or special projection provides the best overall assessment of the paranasal sinuses for this patient?

_____

20. **Situation:** A patient comes to the radiology department with a clinical history of a deviated bony nasal septum. Which facial bone projections best demonstrate the degree of deviation? (More than one correct answer is possible.)

_____

_____

The following review exercises should be completed only after careful study of the associated pages in the textbook as indicated by each exercise. Answers to each review exercise are given at the end of the review exercises.

REVIEW EXERCISE A: Critique Radiographs of the Cranium

The following questions relate to the radiographs in this exercise. Evaluate these radiographs for the radiographic criteria categories (1–5) that follow. Describe the corrections needed to improve the overall image. The major, or "repeatable," errors are specific errors that indicate the need for a repeat exposure, regardless of the nature of the other errors.

A. Lateral skull: 4-year old (Fig. 11.28)

1. Anatomy demonstrated:

   _____

2. Part positioning:

   _____

3. Collimation field size and central ray:

   _____

4. Exposure:

   _____

5. Anatomic side markers:

   _____

Repeatable error(s):

   _____

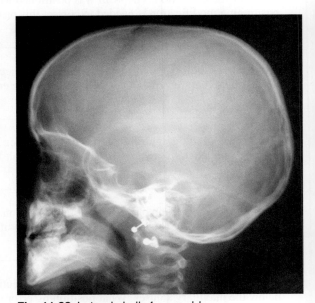

Fig. 11.28 Lateral skull: 4-year old.

B. Lateral skull: 54 year old, posttraumatic injury (Fig. 11.29)

1. Anatomy demonstrated:

   _____

2. Part positioning:

   _____

3. Collimation field size and central ray:

   _____

4. Exposure:

   _____

5. Anatomic side markers:

   _____

Repeatable error(s):

   _____

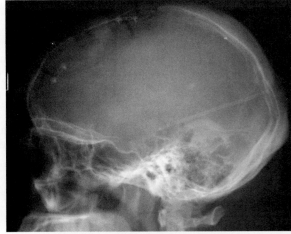

Fig. 11.29 Lateral skull: 54-year old, posttraumatic injury.

C. AP axial skull (Towne) (Fig. 11.30)

   1. Anatomy demonstrated:

      _____

   2. Part positioning:

      _____

   3. Collimation field size and central ray:

      _____

   4. Exposure:

      _____

   5. Anatomic side markers:

      _____

Repeatable error(s):

_____

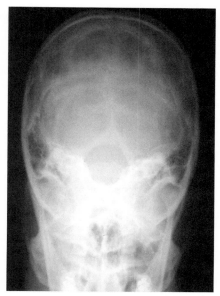

Fig. 11.30 Anteroposterior axial skull (Towne).

D. AP or PA skull (Fig. 11.31)

How can you determine whether this was a PA or an AP projection?

   1. Anatomy demonstrated:

      _____

   2. Part positioning:

      _____

   3. Collimation field size and central ray:

      _____

   4. Exposure:

      _____

   5. Anatomic side markers:

      _____

Repeatable error(s):

_____

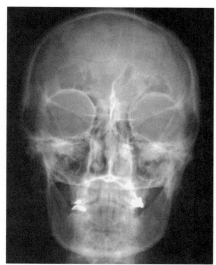

Fig. 11.31 Anteroposterior or posteroanterior skull.

E. AP or PA skull (Fig. 11.32)

Is this an AP or a PA skull? (Compare with Fig. 11.31, looking at the size of the orbits.)

1. Anatomy demonstrated:

   _____

2. Part positioning:

   _____

3. Collimation field size and central ray:

   _____

4. Exposure:

   _____

5. Anatomic side markers:

   _____

Repeatable error(s): _____

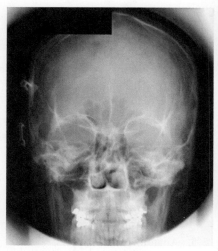

Fig. 11.32 Anteroposterior or posteroanterior skull.

REVIEW EXERCISE B: Critique Radiographs of the Facial Bones

The following questions relate to the radiographs found in this exercise. Evaluate these radiographs for the radiographic criteria categories (1–5) that follow. Describe the corrections needed to improve the overall image. The major, or "repeatable," error(s) are specific errors that indicate the need for a repeat exposure, regardless of the nature or degree of the other errors.

A. Parietoacanthial (Waters method) projection (Fig. 11.33)

Description of possible error:

1. Anatomy demonstrated:

   _____

2. Part positioning:

   _____

3. Collimation field size and central ray:

   _____

4. Exposure:

   _____

5. Anatomic side markers:

Repeatable error(s):

   _____

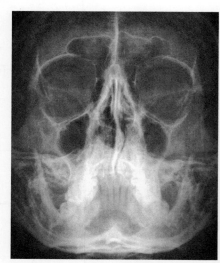

Fig. 11.33 Parietoacanthial (Waters method) projection.

B. SMV mandible (Fig.11.34)

Description of possible error:

1. Anatomy demonstrated:

   _____

2. Part positioning:

   _____

3. Collimation field size and central ray:

   _____

4. Exposure:

   _____

5. Anatomic side markers:

   _____

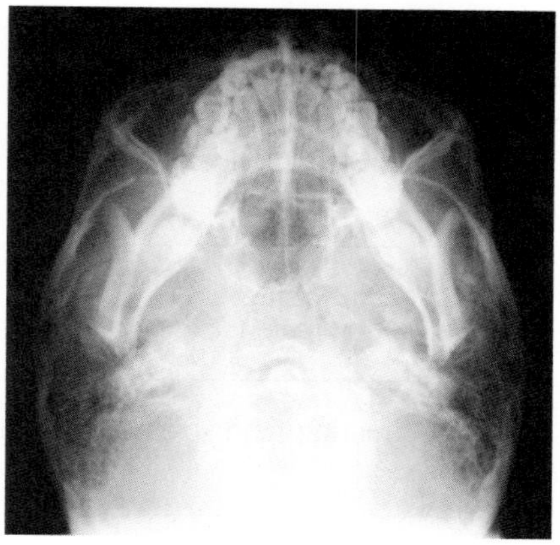

Fig. 11.34 Submentovertical mandible.

Repeatable error(s): _____

C. Optic foramina, parieto-orbital oblique (Rhese method) (Fig. 11.35)

Description of possible error:

1. Anatomy demonstrated:

   _____

2. Part positioning:

   _____

3. Collimation field size and central ray:

   _____

4. Exposure:

   _____

5. Anatomic side markers:

   _____

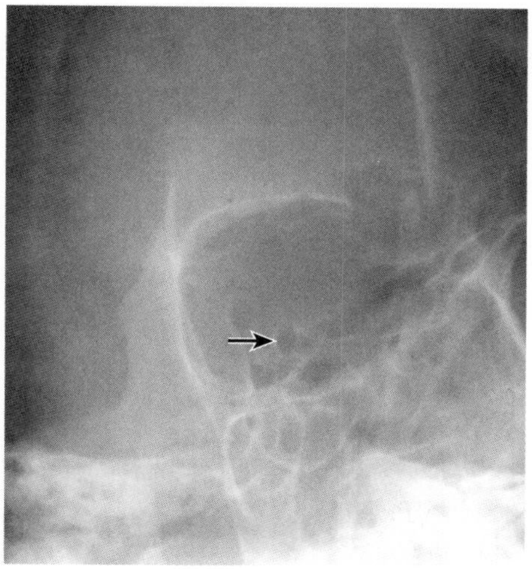

Fig. 11.35 Optic foramina, parieto-orbital oblique (Rhese method).

Repeatable error(s):

   _____

D. Optic foramina, parieto-orbital oblique (Rhese method) (Fig. 11.36)

Description of possible error:

   1. Anatomy demonstrated:

   _____

   2. Part positioning:

   _____

   3. Collimation field size and central ray:

   _____

   4. Exposure:

   _____

   5. Anatomic side markers:

   _____

Repeatable error(s):

_____

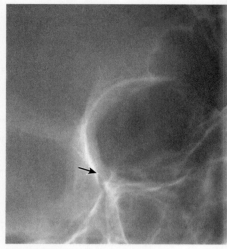

Fig. 11.36 Optic foramina, parieto-orbital oblique (Rhese method).

E. Lateral facial bones (Fig. 11.37)

Description of possible error:

   1. Anatomy demonstrated:

   _____

   2. Part positioning:

   _____

   3. Collimation field size and central ray:

   _____

   4. Exposure:

   _____

   5. Anatomic side markers:

   _____

Repeatable error(s):

_____

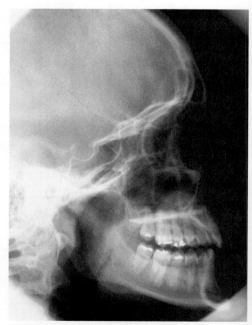

Fig. 11.37 Lateral facial bones.

REVIEW EXERCISE C: Critique Radiographs of the Paranasal Sinuses

The following questions relate to the radiographs found in this exercise. Evaluate these radiographs for positioning accuracy as well as exposure factors, collimation, and correct use of anatomic markers. Describe the corrections needed to improve the overall image. The major, or "repeatable," error(s) imply that these specific errors require that a repeat exposure be taken regardless of the nature or degree of the other errors. Answers to each critique are provided at the end of the laboratory activities.

A. Parietoacanthial transoral (open-mouth Waters method) (Fig. 11.38)

Description of possible error:

    1. Anatomy demonstrated:

    _____

    2. Part positioning:

    _____

    3. Collimation field size and central ray:

    _____

    4. Exposure:

    _____

    5. Anatomic side markers:

    _____

Repeatable error(s):

_____

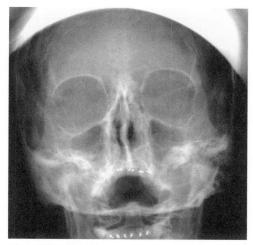

Fig. 11.38 Parietoacanthial transoral (open-mouth Waters method).

B. Parietoacanthial (Waters) (Fig. 11.39)

Description of possible error:

    1. Anatomy demonstrated:

    _____

    2. Part positioning:

    _____

    3. Collimation field size and central ray:

    _____

    4. Exposure:

    _____

    5. Anatomic side markers:

    _____

Repeatable error(s):

_____

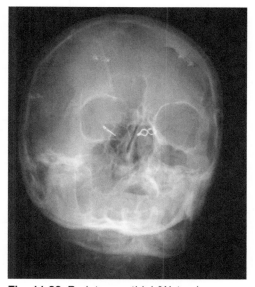

Fig. 11.39 Parietoacanthial (Waters).

C. SMV (Fig. 11.40)

Description of possible error:

1. Anatomy demonstrated:

   _____

2. Part positioning:

   _____

3. Collimation field size and central ray:

   _____

4. Exposure:

   _____

5. Anatomic side markers:

   _____

Repeatable error(s):

_____

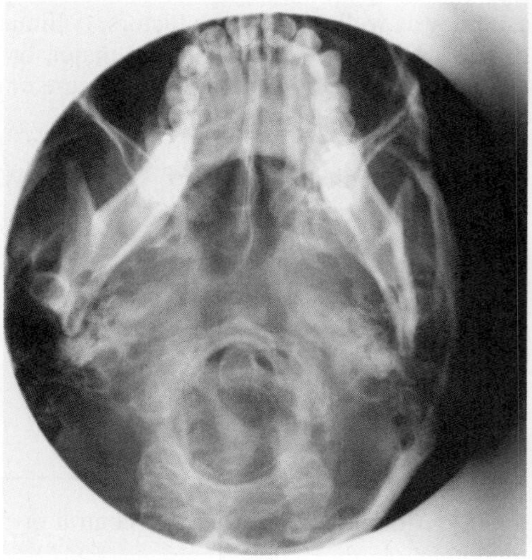

Fig. 11.40 Submentovertical.

D. Lateral projection (Fig. 11.41)

Description of possible error:

1. Anatomy demonstrated:

   _____

2. Part positioning:

   _____

3. Collimation field size and central ray:

   _____

4. Exposure:

   _____

5. Anatomic side markers:

   _____

Repeatable error(s):

_____

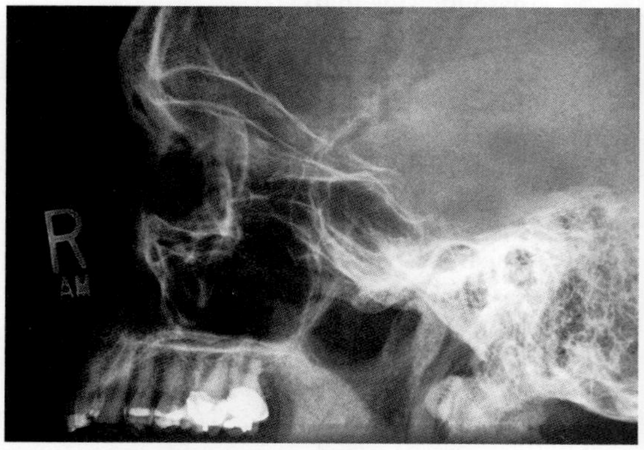

Fig. 11.41 Lateral projection.

PART V: LABORATORY EXERCISES OF CRANIUM

You must gain experience in positioning each part of the cranium before performing the following exams on actual patients. You can obtain experience in positioning and radiographic evaluation of these projections by performing exercises using radiographic phantoms and by practicing on other students (although you will not be taking actual exposures).

The following suggested activities assume that your teaching institution has an energized lab and radiographic phantoms. If not, perform the laboratory exercises, the radiographic evaluation, and the physical positioning exercises. (Check off each step and projection as you complete it.)

Laboratory Exercise A: Energized Laboratory

1. Using the skull radiographic phantom, produce radiographs of the following basic routines:

_____ 15° PA axial (Caldwell) skull

_____ Lateral skull

_____ AP axial skull

_____ PA axial (Haas)

_____ SMV

Laboratory Exercise B: Radiographic Evaluation

1. Evaluate and critique the radiographs produced in the preceding, additional radiographs provided by your instructor, or both. Evaluate each radiograph for the following points.

_____ Evaluate the completeness of the study. (Are all the pertinent anatomic structures included on the radiograph?)

_____ Evaluate for positioning or centering errors (e.g., rotation, off centering).

_____ Evaluate for correct exposure factors and possible motion. (Is the image receptor exposure and contrast of the images acceptable?)

_____ Determine whether anatomic side markers and an acceptable degree of collimation are visible on the images.

Laboratory Exercise C: Physical Positioning

On another person, simulate performing all basic and special projections of the cranium as follows. Include the six steps listed in the following and described in the textbook. (Check off each step when completed satisfactorily.)

Step 1. Appropriate field size with correct markers

Step 2. Correct central ray placement and centering of part to central ray and/or IR

Step 3. Accurate collimation

Step 4. Area shielding of patient when required

Step 5. Use of proper immobilizing devices when needed

Step 6. Approximate correct exposure factors, breathing instructions where applicable, and initiating exposure

Projections	Step 1	Step 2	Step 3	Step 4	Step 5	Step 6
Skull series: routine						
• AP axial (Towne)	_____	_____	_____	_____	_____	_____
• Lateral skull	_____	_____	_____	_____	_____	_____
• PA 15° axial (Caldwell)	_____	_____	_____	_____	_____	_____
Skull series: special	_____	_____	_____	_____	_____	_____
• PA axial (Haas)	_____	_____	_____	_____	_____	_____
• SMV	_____	_____	_____	_____	_____	_____

PART VI: LABORATORY EXERCISES FOR FACIAL BONES, MANDIBLE, AND PARANASAL SINUSES

You must gain experience in positioning each part of the facial bones before performing the following exams on actual patients. You can obtain experience in positioning and radiographic evaluation of these projections by performing exercises using radiographic phantoms and by practicing on other students (although you will not be taking actual exposures).

The following suggested activities assume that your teaching institution has an energized lab and radiographic phantoms. If not, perform the laboratory exercises, the radiographic evaluation, and the physical positioning activities. (Check off each step and projection as you complete it.)

Laboratory Exercise A: Energized Laboratory

1. Using the skull radiographic phantom, produce radiographs of the following routine facial bone studies:

Facial bones	*Zygomatic arches*	*Temporomandibular joints*
_____ Parietoacanthial (Waters)	_____ SMV	_____ Modified Law
_____ Modified Waters	_____ Oblique inferosuperior (tangential)	_____ Schuller method
_____ Lateral	_____ AP axial	_____ AP axial
_____ 15° PA axial (Caldwell)		

Nasal bones	*Mandible*	*Optic foramina*
_____ Lateral	_____ Axiolateral oblique	_____ Parieto-orbital oblique (Rhese)
_____ Superoinferior (tangential)	_____ PA	
_____ SMV	_____ AP axial	

2. Using the skull radiographic phantom, produce radiographs of the following basic routines:

Paranasal sinuses

_____ Parietoacanthial (Waters)   _____ PA

_____ Lateral   _____ SMV

Laboratory Exercise B: Radiographic Evaluation

1. Evaluate and critique the radiographs produced during the previous experiments, additional radiographs provided by your instructor, or both. Evaluate each radiograph for the following points.

_____ Evaluate the completeness of the study. (Are all pertinent anatomic structures included on the radiograph?)

_____ Evaluate for positioning or centering errors (e.g., rotation, off- centering).

_____ Evaluate for correct exposure factors and possible motion. (Is the image receptor exposure and contrast of the images acceptable?)

_____ Determine whether anatomic side markers and an acceptable degree of collimation are visible on the images.

Laboratory Exercise C: Physical Positioning

On another person, simulate performing all basic and special projections of the facial bones as follows. Include the six steps listed in the following and described in the textbook. (Check off each step when completed satisfactorily.)

Step 1. Appropriate field size with correct markers

Step 2. Correct CR placement and centering of part to CR and/or IR

Step 3. Accurate collimation

Step 4. Area shielding of patient when required

Step 5. Use of proper immobilizing devices when needed

Step 6. Approximate correct exposure factors, breathing instructions where applicable, and initiating exposure

Projections	Step 1	Step 2	Step 3	Step 4	Step 5	Step 6
Facial bones						
• Parietoacanthial (Waters)	___	___	___	___	___	___
• Modified parietoacanthial	___	___	___	___	___	___
• Lateral facial bones	___	___	___	___	___	___
• 15° PA axial (Caldwell)	___	___	___	___	___	___
Nasal bones						
• Laterals	___	___	___	___	___	___
• Superoinferior nasal bones	___	___	___	___	___	___
Zygomatic arches						
• SMV	___	___	___	___	___	___
• Oblique inferosuperior (tangential)	___	___	___	___	___	___
• AP axial	___	___	___	___	___	___
Optic foramina						
• Parieto-orbital oblique (Rhese)	___	___	___	___	___	___
Mandible						
• PA	___	___	___	___	___	___
• AP axial	___	___	___	___	___	___
• Axiolateral oblique (general survey)	___	___	___	___	___	___
Temporomandibular joints						
• Modified Law	___	___	___	___	___	___
• Schuller method	___	___	___	___	___	___
• AP axial	___	___	___	___	___	___
Paranasal sinus projections						
• Parietoacanthial (Waters)	___	___	___	___	___	___
• Lateral	___	___	___	___	___	___
• PA	___	___	___	___	___	___
• SMV	___	___	___	___	___	___
• Parietoacanthial transoral (open-mouth Waters)	___	___	___	___	___	___

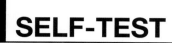

SELF-TEST

MY SCORE = _____ %

This self-test should be taken only after completing all of the readings, review exercises, and laboratory activities for a particular section. The purpose of this test is not only to provide a good learning exercise but also to serve as a strong indicator of what your final evaluation exam for this chapter will cover. It is strongly suggested that if you do not get at least a 90%–95% grade on each self-test, you should review those areas in which you missed questions before going to your instructor for the final evaluation exam. The self-test is divided into two regions of study: cranium and facial bones/paranasal sinuses.

ANATOMY AND POSITIONING OF CRANIUM

1. Which of the following bones is not part of the floor of the cranium?

   A. Temporal   B. Ethmoid   C. Occipital   D. Sphenoid

2. Which aspect of the frontal bone is thin-walled and forms the forehead?

   A. Orbital   B. Horizontal   C. Squamous   D. Superciliary margin

3. Which four cranial bones articulate with the frontal bone?

   A. _____

   B. _____

   C. _____

   D. _____

4. Which structures are found at the widest aspect of the skull? _____

5. What is the name of a prominent landmark (or "bump") found on the external surface of the occipital bone?

   _____

6. List the number of individual bones that articulate with the following cranial bones.

   A. Parietal bone: _____

   B. Occipital bone: _____

   C. Temporal bone: _____

   D. Sphenoid: _____

   E. Ethmoid: _____

7. What is the thickest and densest structure in the cranium? _____

8. True/False: The hypophysis cerebri is another term for the pituitary gland.

9. True/False: The sphenoid bone articulates with all the other cranial bones.

10. The shallow depression just posterior to the base of the dorsum sellae and anterior to the foramen magnum is the

    _____.

11. What is the name of the paired collections of bone found inferior to the cribriform plate that contain numerous air cells and help form the lateral walls of the nasal cavity?

    _____

12. Which small section of bone is located superior to the cribriform plate?

    _____

13. What is the formal term for the left sphenoid fontanel in the adult?

    _____

14. What is the name of the cranial suture formed by the inferior junction of the parietals to the temporal bones?

    _____

15. What are the two terms for the small, irregular bones found in the adult skull sutures?

    _____

16. Match each of the following structures to its related cranial bone.

    _____   1. Pterygoid hamulus   A. Occipital

    _____   2. Anterior clinoid processes   B. Frontal

    _____   3. Glabella   C. Sphenoid

    _____   4. Foramen ovale   D. Ethmoid

    _____   5. Perpendicular plate   E. Temporal

    _____   6. Superior nasal conchae   F. Parietal

    _____   7. Foramen magnum

    _____   8. Cribriform plate

    _____   9. Zygomatic process

    _____   10. Lateral condylar portions

    _____   11. Superciliary arch

    _____   12. EAM

    _____   13. Inion

    _____   14. Sella turcica

    _____   15. Petrous ridge

17. Identify the cranial structures, sutures, and regions labeled on the following radiographs (Figs. 11.42 and 11.43):

Structure	*Bone(s)*
A. _____	_____
B. _____	_____
C. _____	_____
D. _____ (suture)	_____
E. _____	_____
F. _____	_____
G. _____	_____
H. _____	_____
I. _____	_____
J. _____	_____
K. _____	_____
L. _____	_____
M. _____	_____

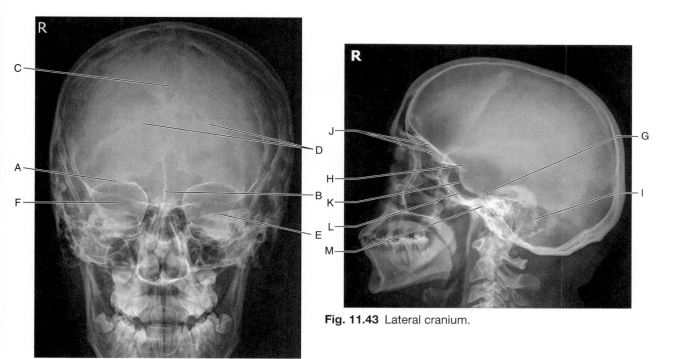

Fig. 11.42 Posteroanterior axial (Caldwell) projection of the cranium.

Fig. 11.43 Lateral cranium.

18. Which of the following skull classifications applies to a skull with an angle of 54° between the midsagittal plane and the long axis of the pars petrosa?

    A. Mesocephalic
    B. Dolichocephalic
    C. Brachycephalic
    D. None of these

19. Which of the classifications in the preceding question is considered an average-shaped skull?

20. Identify the labeled landmarks and positioning lines used in skull and facial bone positioning, as shown in Fig. 11.44 (including abbreviations, if they apply).

    A. _____
    B. _____
    C. _____
    D. _____
    E. _____
    F. _____
    G. _____
    H. _____
    I. _____
    J. _____
    K. _____
    L. _____

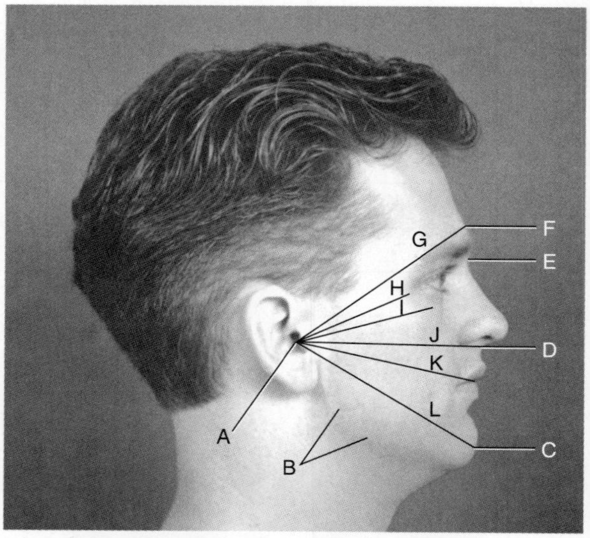

Fig. 11.44 Skull and facial bone landmarks and positioning lines.

21. Which of the following landmarks corresponds to the highest level of the petrous ridge?

    A. EAM
    B. TEA
    C. Outer canthus
    D. Acanthion

22. Which of the following terms is defined as the large cartilaginous aspect of the external ear?

    A. Pinna
    B. Tragus
    C. Glabella
    D. Acanthion

23. Which of the following is defined as the small cartilaginous flap that covers the opening of the ear?

    A. Pinna
    B. Tragus
    C. Glabella
    D. Acanthion

24. How much difference in degrees is there between the OML and the IOML?

    A. 10°
    B. 7°
    C. 3°
    D. None. (They represent the same positioning line.)

25. Which of the following positioning errors frequently results in a repeat exposure of a cranial position?

    A. Rotation
    B. Incorrect central ray placement
    C. Flexion
    D. Extension

26. Match each of the following pathologic indications to the correct definition or description. (Use each choice only once.)

    _____ A. Bone tumor originating in the bone marrow

    _____ B. Fracture evident by sphenoid sinus effusion

    _____ C. Condition that begins with bony destruction followed by bony repair

    _____ D. Destructive lesion with irregular margins

    _____ E. Fracture of the skull with jagged or irregular lucent line that lies at an angle to the axis of the bone

    _____ F. Tangential view may help in determining extent or degree of this fracture

    1. Linear fracture
    2. Paget disease
    3. Depressed fracture
    4. Osteolytic neoplasm
    5. Multiple myeloma right
    6. Basal fracture

27. Which of the following clinical indications may require a decrease in manual exposure factors?

    A. Pituitary adenoma
    B. Linear skull fracture
    C. Paget disease
    D. Multiple myeloma

28. Which of the following imaging modalities may be used to examine a possible cranial bleed caused by trauma?

    A. CT
    B. MR
    C. Diagnostic medical sonography
    D. Nuclear medicine (NM)

29. Which of the following imaging modalities provides an excellent distinction between normal and abnormal brain tissue?

    A. CT
    B. MR
    C. DMS
    D. Nuclear medicine (NM)

30. Which aspect of the temporal bone is considered the thinnest?

    _____

31. Which aspect of the temporal bone contains the organs of hearing and balance?

    _____

32. The correct term for the eardrum is the _____.

33. Which of the following middle ear structures is considered the most lateral?

    A. Malleus
    B. Incus
    C. Stapes
    D. Oval window

34. Which structure helps equalize atmospheric pressure in the middle ear? _____

35. What passes through the internal acoustic meatus? _____

36. The aditus is an opening between the _____ and the _____ portion of the temporal bone.

37. An infection of the mastoid air cells, if untreated, can lead to a serious infection of the brain that is called

    _____.

38. Which auditory ossicle attaches to the oval window?

    A. Malleus   C. Stapes

    B. Incus   D. None

39. The internal ear is divided into the osseous or bony labyrinth and the _____ labyrinth.

40. List the three divisions of the bony labyrinth of the inner ear.

    A. _____   B. _____   C. _____

41. Identify the structures labeled in Fig. 11.45.

    A. _____

    B. _____

    C. _____

    D. _____

    E. _____

    F. _____

    G. _____

    H. _____

    I. _____

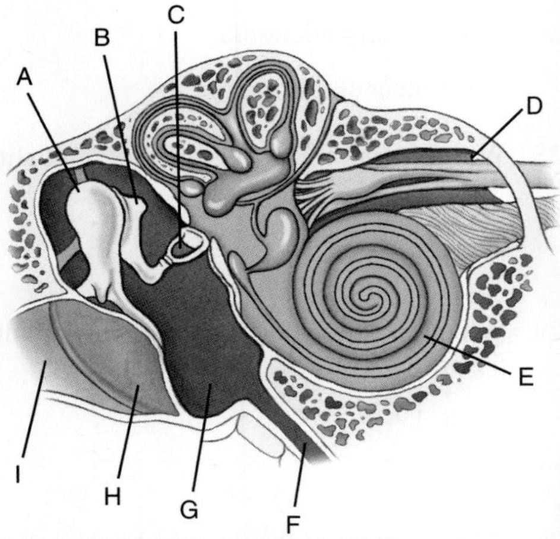

Fig. 11.45 Three divisions of the ear.

42. A benign, cystic mass of the middle ear is a(n):

    A. Acoustic neuroma   C. Cholesteatoma

    B. Osteomyelitis   D. Acoustic sarcoma

43. True/False: Otosclerosis is a hereditary disease.

44. Which two projections of the cranium project the dorsum sellae within the foramen magnum?

    A. _____   B. _____

45. A. How much central ray angle is required for the AP axial projection (Towne method) for a skull with the IOML perpendicular to the IR?

_____

   B. What is the central ray angle for this same projection with a perpendicular OML?

_____

46. Where is the central ray centered for a lateral projection of the cranium?

_____

47. To prevent tilting of the skull for the lateral projection of the cranium, the _____ line is placed perpendicular to the IR.

48. Where should the petrous ridges be located (on the image) for a well-positioned, 25° caudad PA axial (Haas

   method) projection? _____

49. Where is the central ray centered for an SMV projection of the skull?

_____

50. Which positioning line is parallel to the IR for the SMV projection of the skull?

_____

51. **Situation:** A radiograph of an AP axial projection for the cranium shows the dorsum sellae is projected superior to the foramen magnum. What must be modified during the repeat exposure to correct this problem?

_____

52. **Situation:** A radiograph of a lateral projection of the cranium shows the greater wings of the sphenoid are not superimposed. What type of positioning error is present on this radiograph?

_____

53. **Situation:** A radiograph of a 15° caudad PA axial projection of the cranium shows the petrous ridges are at the level of the supraorbital margin. Without changing the central ray angle, how must the head position be modified during the repeat exposure to produce a more acceptable image?

_____

54. **Situation:** A patient with a possible basilar skull fracture enters the emergency room. The physician wants a projection to demonstrate a possible sphenoid sinus effusion. Which projection of the cranium is best for this situation?

_____

55. **Situation:** The same patient as in the previous situation also requires a frontal projection of the skull. The physician wants the projection to demonstrate the frontal bone and to place the petrous ridges in the lower one-third of the orbits, but it has not been determined whether the patient's cervical spine has been fractured, so the patient cannot be moved from a supine position. What should the technologist do to obtain this image?

_____

56. **Situation:** A patient comes to the radiology department for a skull series. Because of the size of the patient's shoulders, he is unable to flex his neck sufficiently to place the OML perpendicular to the IR for the AP axial projection. His head cannot be raised because of possible cervical trauma. What other options does the technologist have to obtain an acceptable AP axial projection?

_____

57. **Situation:** A radiograph of an AP axial (Towne method) projection for the cranium shows the posterior arch of C1 and the dorsum sellae are superimposed. Both are projected into the foramen magnum. What modification is needed to correct this error that is present on the initial radiograph?

_____

58. **Situation:** A radiograph of a lateral skull demonstrates the orbital plates (roof) of the frontal bone are not superimposed. What is the positioning error present on this radiograph?

_____

59. **Situation:** A radiograph of an AP axial (Towne method) for cranium shows the left petrous portion of the temporal bone is wider than the right. What is the specific positioning error present on this radiograph?

_____

60. **Situation:** A radiograph of an SMV projection of the cranium demonstrates mandibular condyles are projected into the petrous portion (pyramids) of the temporal bone. How must the position be altered during the repeat exposure to correct this error?

_____

ANATOMY AND POSITIONING OF FACIAL BONES, MANDIBLE, AND PARANASAL SINUSES

1. The majority of the hard palate is formed by:

   A. Maxilla

   B. Palatine bones

   C. Zygomatic bone

   D. Mandible

2. Which of the following is *not* an aspect of the maxilla?

   A. Frontal process

   B. Body

   C. Zygomatic process

   D. Ramus

3. Match each of the following definitions or characteristics to the correct facial bone. (Use each choice only once.)

   _____ A. Mandible

   _____ B. Lacrimal bones

   _____ C. Palatine bones

   _____ D. Inferior nasal conchae

   _____ E. Nasal bones

   _____ F. Maxilla

   _____ G. Zygomatic bone

   1. Contains four processes

   2. Forms lower, outer aspect of orbit

   3. Lie just anterior and medial to the frontal process of maxilla

   4. Unpaired bone in the adult

   5. Located anteriorly in medial aspect of orbit

   6. Help to mix air drawn into nasal cavity

   7. Possesses a vertical and horizontal portion

4. Identify the seven (cranial and facial) bones that form the bony orbit (Fig. 11.46).

A. _____

B. _____

C. _____

D. _____

E. _____

F. _____

G. _____

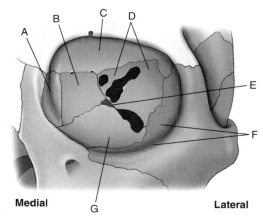

Fig. 11.46 Slightly oblique frontal view of orbit, A–G.

5. On average, how many separate cavities make up the frontal sinus? _____

6. True/False: All of the paranasal sinuses are contained within cranial bones, except the maxillary sinuses.

7. True/False: All of the paranasal sinuses except the sphenoid communicate with the nasal cavity.

8. True/False: In general, all of the paranasal sinuses are fully developed by the age of 6 or 7 years.

9. True/False: The frontal sinuses are usually larger in men than in women.

10. Identify the labeled structures on these radiographs of the paranasal sinuses (Figs. 11.47, 11.48, and 11.49).

A. _____

B. _____

C. _____

D. _____

E. _____

F. _____

G. _____

H. _____

I. _____

J. _____

K. _____

L. _____

M. _____

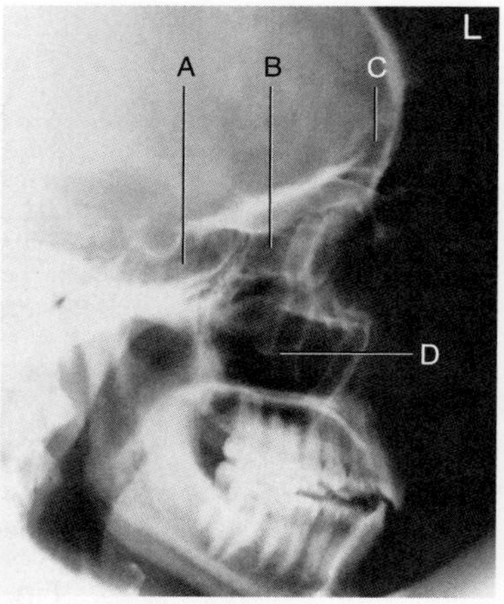

Fig. 11.47 Paranasal sinuses, A–D.

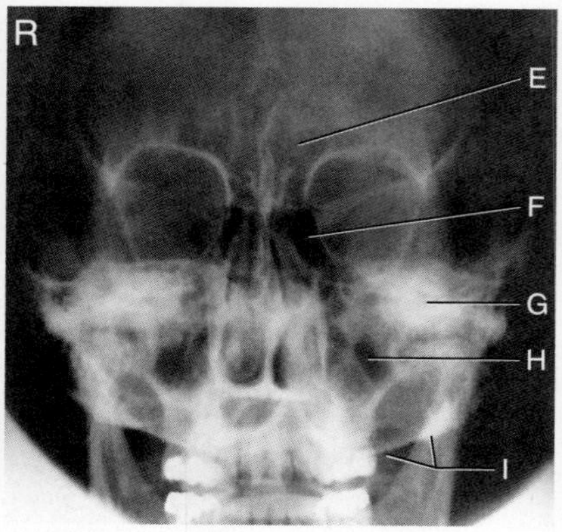

Fig. 11.48 Paranasal sinuses, E–I.

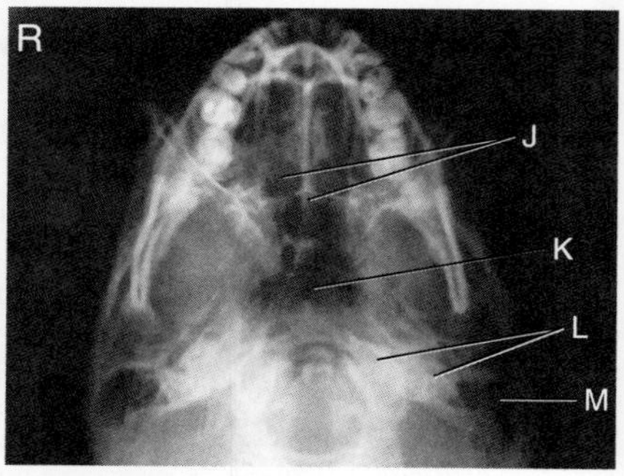

Fig. 11.49 Paranasal sinuses, J–M.

11. Which aspect of the ethmoid bone contains the ethmoid air cells?

_____

12. The sphenoid sinus lies directly inferior to the _____.

13. True/False: Ultrasound of the sphenoid sinus can be performed to rule out sinusitis.

14. Which of the following imaging modalities best demonstrates bony erosion of the maxillary sinus resulting from acute sinusitis?

A. CT

B. MR

C. Diagnostic medical sonography (DMS)

D. Conventional radiography

15. True/False: Facial bone studies should be performed erect whenever possible.

16. True/False: A Le Fort fracture produces a "free-floating" zygomatic bone.

17. Which frontal projection of the facial bones best visualizes the region of the maxilla and orbits?

_____

18. Which single projection of the facial bones best demonstrates any possible air-fluid levels in the paranasal sinuses if the patient cannot stand or sit erect?

_____

19. Which plane is placed parallel to the IR with a true lateral projection of the facial bones?

_____

20. A. What is the angle between the OML and plane of IR with a parietoacanthial (Waters method) projection?

_____

B. This places the _____ positioning perpendicular to the IR.

21. The CR is centered to exit at the level of the _____ for a well-positioned parietoacanthial projection.

    A. Nasion   C. Inner canthus

    B. Glabella   D. Acanthion

22. The CR is centered to exit at the level of the _____ for a well-positioned 15° PA axial projection of the facial bones.

    A. Nasion   C. Midorbits

    B. Glabella   D. Acanthion

23. Where are the petrous ridges projected for a properly positioned modified parietoacanthial projection? _____

_____

24. True/False: The lateral projection of the nasal bones should be performed using a small focal spot, 65–80 kVp, and close collimation.

25. True/False: The CR should be angled as needed to be parallel to the GML for the superoinferior tangential projection of the nasal bones.

26. Which positioning line is placed perpendicular to the IR for a modified parietoacanthial projection?

_____

27. Where is the CR centered for a lateral projection of the nasal bones?

_____

28. Which positioning line, if placed parallel to the IR, ensures adequate extension of the head for the SMV projection for zygomatic arches?

_____

29. How much skull tilt and rotation are required for the oblique inferosuperior (tangential) projection for zygomatic arches? _____

30. How much CR angle is required for the AP axial projection of the zygomatic arches if the IOML is placed perpendicular to the IR? (Hint: This is the same as for an AP axial skull.)

_____

296

31. The proper method and projection name for the "three-point landing" projection for the optic foramen is the

_____

32. Where should the optic foramen be located with a well-positioned three-point landing projection?

_____

33. What is the maximum amount of CR angulation that should be used for an axiolateral oblique projection of the mandible?

34. Which of the following factors prevents superimposition of the ramus on the cervical spine for the axiolateral oblique mandible projection?

   A. Angle CR 10°–15° cephalad   C. Extend chin

   B. Have patient open mouth during exposure   D. Rotate head toward IR

35. How much skull rotation (from the lateral position) toward the IR is required for the axiolateral oblique projection specifically for the mentum?

   A. 10° to 15°   C. 45°

   B. 30°   D. None. Keep the skull in the true lateral position.

36. What type of CR angulation should be used for a PA axial projection of the mandible?

   A. None   C. 20°–25° cephalad

   B. 10°–15° cephalad   D. 5° cephalad

37. What structures are better defined when the CR angulation is increased from 35° to 40° caudad for the AP axial projection of the mandible?

_____

38. Where is the CR centered for an SMV projection of the mandible?

_____

39. During an orthopantomographic procedure, it is important to keep the _____ positioning line parallel to the floor.

   A. OML   C. IOML

   B. AML   D. GAL

40. What CR angulation is used for the AP axial projection of the TMJ with the OML perpendicular to the IR?

_____

41. True/False: The modified Law method requires a tube angulation of 25° caudad.

42. True/False: The Schuller method requires that the skull be placed in a true lateral position.

43. True/False: A grid is not required for the lateral projection of the nasal bones.

44. Where is the CR centered for a lateral projection of the paranasal sinuses?

_____

45. Why should a patient remain in an erect position for at least 5 minutes before sinus radiography?

_____

46. Which routine projection is best for demonstrating the maxillary sinuses?

_____

47. Why should a horizontal CR be used for the erect PA (Caldwell) projection for paranasal sinuses rather than the usual

15° caudad angle? _____

48. A radiograph of a 15° PA projection of the facial bones shows the petrous ridges are projected at the level of the midorbital rims. What specific positioning or CR angling error led to this radiographic outcome?

_____

49. Which positioning line should be perpendicular to the IR for the parieto-orbital oblique (Rhese method) projections for optic foramina?

   A. Acanthomeatal line (AML)   C. Infraorbitomeatal line (IOML)

   B. Mentomeatal line (MML)   D. Glabellomeatal line (GML)

50. A radiograph of lateral position for paranasal sinuses shows the greater wings of the sphenoid bone are not superimposed. What specific positioning error is present?

_____

51. **Situation:** A patient with severe facial bone injuries comes into the emergency room. The patient is wearing a cervical collar and cannot be moved. What type of positioning routine should be performed for this situation?

_____

52. **Situation:** A superoinferior, tangential projection for the nasal bones was taken with the following exposure factors: 8- × 10-inch (18- × 24-cm) recommended field size, 90 kVp, 13 mAs, 40-inch (100-cm) SID. The resultant radiograph was unsatisfactory because of poor visibility of the nasal bones. Which technical factors should be changed for the repeat exposure?

_____

53. **Situation:** A patient with possible facial fractures, including a possible "blowout" fracture to the right orbit, was brought from the emergency room to the radiology department. What special facial bone projection should be included with the basic facial bone routine of a lateral, parietoacanthial (Waters), and PA axial (Caldwell)?

_____

54. **Situation:** A patient with a clinical history of secondary osteomyelitis comes to the radiology department. Which imaging modalities or procedures can be performed to demonstrate the extent of damage to the paranasal sinuses?

_____

11 Skull and Cranial Bones

ANATOMY AND POSITIONING OF CRANIUM

1. C. Occipital
2. C. Squamous
3. A. Right parietal
   B. Left parietal
   C. Sphenoid
   D. Ethmoid
4. Parietal tubercles or eminences
5. External occipital protuberance or inion
6. A. 5
   B. 6
   C. 3
   D. 7
   E. 2
7. Petrous portion or petrous pyramids
8. True
9. True
10. Clivus
11. Lateral masses or labyrinth
12. Crista galli
13. Left pterion
14. Squamosal suture
15. Sutural or wormian bones
16. 1. C
    2. C
    3. B
    4. C
    5. D
    6. D
    7. A
    8. D
    9. E
    10. A
    11. B
    12. E
    13. A
    14. C
    15. E
17. A. Supraorbital margin (SOM), frontal
    B. Crista galli, ethmoid
    C. Sagittal suture, parietal
    D. Coronal suture, frontal and parietal

E. Petrous ridge, temporal
F. Orbital or horizontal portion, frontal
G. Dorsum sellae, sphenoid
H. Anterior clinoid process, sphenoid
I. Mastoid portion, temporal bone
J. Orbital plates, frontal bone
K. Sella turcica (body), sphenoid
L. Sphenoid sinus, sphenoid
M. Petrous portion, temporal bone
18. C. Brachycephalic
19. A. Mesocephalic
20. A. External acoustic meatus (EAM)
    B. Angle (gonion) of mandible
    C. Mental point (mentum)
    D. Acanthion
    E. Nasion
    F. Glabella
    G. Glabellomeatal line (GML)
    H. Orbitomeatal line (OML)
    I. Infraorbitomeatal line (IOML)
    J. Acanthomeatal line (AML)
    K. Lips-meatal line (LML)
    L. Mentomeatal line (MML)
21. B. TEA
22. A. Pinna
23. B. Tragus
24. B. 7°
25. A. Rotation
26. A. 5
    B. 6
    C. 2
    D. 4
    E. 1
    F. 3
27. D. Multiple myeloma
28. A. CT
29. B. MR
30. Squamous portion
31. Petrous portion
32. Tympanic membrane
33. A. Malleus
34. Eustachian or auditory tube
35. Auditory nerve and blood vessels
36. Epitympanic recess; mastoid

37. Encephalitis
38. C. Stapes
39. Membranous
40. Cochlea, vestibule, semicircular canals
41. A. Malleus
    B. Incus
    C. Stapes
    D. Internal acoustic meatus— for auditory nerve and blood vessels
    E. Cochlea
    F. Eustachian or auditory tube
    G. Tympanic cavity
    H. Tympanic membrane or eardrum
    I. External acoustic meatus (EAM)
42. C. Cholesteatoma
43. True
44. A. AP axial projection (Towne method)
    B. PA axial projection (Haas method)
45. A. 37° caudad
    B. 30° caudad
46. 2 inches (5 cm) superior to the EAM
47. Interpupillary
48. Superior to the mastoid processes and symmetrical
49. 1½ inch (4 cm) inferior to the mandibular symphysis, midway between the gonions
50. IOML
51. Increase CR angle approximately 7° caudad.
52. Rotation
53. Increase extension of the skull to place the OML perpendicular to the IR (this will project the petrous ridges into the lower one-third of the orbits).
54. A horizontal beam (dorsal decubitus) lateral skull projection will demonstrate any possible air-fluid levels in the sphenoid sinus.
55. Perform the AP projection with a 15° cephalad CR angle to the OML.

A1

56. Use the IOML instead of OML and increase CR angle an additional 7° caudad for a total of 37°.
57. Decrease CR angle based on the cranial line used (OML = 30°; IOML = 37°). Another option is to decrease the flexion of the neck.
58. Tilt of the skull
59. Rotation of the skull, positioning the patient's face to the right
60. Extend the skull further to place the IOML parallel to the IR.

ANATOMY AND POSITIONING OF FACIAL BONES AND PARANASAL SINUSES

1. A. Maxilla
2. D. Ramus
3. A. 4
   B. 5
   C. 7
   D. 6
   E. 3
   F. 1
   G. 2
4. A. Lacrimal
   B. Ethmoid
   C. Frontal
   D. Sphenoid
   E. Palatine
   F. Zygomatic
   G. Maxilla
5. 1 to 2 sinuses
6. True
7. False
8. False
9. True
10. A. Sphenoid sinuses
    B. Ethmoid sinuses
    C. Frontal sinuses
    D. Maxillary sinuses
    E. Frontal sinuses
    F. Ethmoid and sphenoid sinuses superimposed

G. Petrous portion of temporal bone
H. Maxillary sinuses
I. Base of skull
J. Ethmoid sinuses
K. Sphenoid sinus
L. Petrous portion of temporal bone
M. Mastoid portion of temporal bone
11. Lateral masses or labyrinth
12. Sella turcica
13. True
14. A. CT
15. True
16. False (the tripod fracture)
17. Parietoacanthial (Waters method) projection (dense petrous pyramids are projected below the maxillary sinuses)
18. Horizontal beam (cross-table) lateral projection
19. Midsagittal plane
20. A. 37°
    B. Mentomeatal line (MML)
21. D. Acanthion
22. A. Nasion
23. Lower half of the maxillary sinuses
24. True
25. False (glabelloalveolar, GAL)
26. Lips-meatal line (LML)
27. ½ inch (1.25 cm) inferior to nasion
28. Infraorbitomeatal line (IOML)
29. 15° rotation and 15° tilt toward the affected side
30. 37° caudad
31. Parieto-orbital oblique projection or Rhese method
32. Lower outer quadrant of the orbit
33. 25° cephalad
34. C. Extend chin
35. C. 45°
36. C. 20°–25° cephalad
37. Temporomandibular fossae

38. 1½ inches (4 cm) inferior to mandibular symphysis (or midway between angles of the mandible)
39. C. IOML
40. 35° caudad
41. False (15° caudad)
42. True
43. True
44. Midway between outer canthus and EAM
45. To allow any fluid in the sinuses to settle
46. Parietoacanthial (Waters method) projection
47. To demonstrate any air-fluid levels without distortion
48. Excessive flexion of the head, or insufficient caudal CR angle
49. A. Acanthomeatal (AML)
50. Rotation of the skull
51. Reverse parietoacanthial (Waters method) projection with the use of cephalic CR angle to keep CR parallel to MML. In addition, horizontal beam lateral projection must be included as part of the positioning routine.
52. Reduce kVp to the 60–85 range and increase mAs accordingly.
53. Modified parietoacanthial (modified Waters method) or a PA axial projection with a 30° caudad angle will best demonstrate the floor of the orbit. Note that the modified Waters is more commonly performed for possible blowout fractures over the standard parietoacanthial (Waters method) projection.
54. Routine radiographic sinus series can be performed, but CT of the sinuses may best demonstrate bony erosion.

12 Biliary Tract and Upper Gastrointestinal System

Radiographic procedures involving the administration of some form of contrast media are described in the next four chapters. You will likely be performing these examinations early in your clinical training. If you learn and understand the fundamentals provided in these next four chapters, combined with clinical experience, you will soon become a proficient technologist of these organ systems.

CHAPTER OBJECTIVES

After you have successfully completed the activities in this chapter, you will be able to:

_____ 1. Identify specific anatomy and functions of the liver, gallbladder, and biliary ductal system.

_____ 2. Describe the production, storage, and purpose of bile.

_____ 3. On drawings and radiographs, identify specific anatomy of the biliary system.

_____ 4. Describe the effect of body habitus on the location of the gallbladder.

_____ 5. Define specific terms related to conditions and procedures of the biliary system.

_____ 6. Define specific pathologies of the biliary system.

_____ 7. Match specific biliary pathologies to the correct radiographic appearances and signs.

_____ 8. List the major organs of the upper gastrointestinal (GI) system and specific accessory organs.

_____ 9. List the three primary functions of the digestive system.

_____ 10. List three divisions of the pharynx.

_____ 11. Identify the anatomic location, function, and features of the esophagus, stomach, and duodenum.

_____ 12. Identify the effect of body position on the distribution of air and contrast media in the stomach.

_____ 13. Describe the effect of body habitus on the position and shape of the stomach.

_____ 14. Using drawings and radiographs, identify specific anatomy of the upper GI system.

_____ 15. Identify differences between mechanical digestion and chemical digestion.

_____ 16. Identify the contrast media, patient preparation, room preparation, and fluoroscopic procedure for esophagography and an upper GI series.

_____ 17. List and define the specific clinical indications and contraindications for esophagography and an upper GI series.

_____ 18. Match specific types of pathology to the correct radiographic appearances and signs.

_____ 19. Describe specific breathing maneuvers and positioning techniques used to detect esophageal reflux.

_____ 20. List the routine and special positions or projections for esophagography and an upper GI series to include collimation field size and central ray (CR) location, direction and angulation of the central ray, and anatomy best demonstrated.

_____ 21. Identify the anatomy that is best demonstrated with specific projections of esophagography and an upper GI series.

_____ 22. Given various hypothetic situations, identify the correct modification of a position and/or exposure factors to improve the radiographic image.

POSITIONING AND RADIOGRAPHIC TECHNIQUE

_____ 1. Using a peer, position for routine and special projections for esophagography and an upper GI series.

_____ 2. Critique and evaluate esophagography and upper GI series radiographs based on the five divisions of radiographic criteria: (1) anatomy demonstrated, (2) position, (3) collimation field size and CR, (4) exposure, and (5) anatomic side markers.

_____ 3. Distinguish between acceptable and unacceptable esophagography and upper GI series radiographs that result from exposure factors, motion, collimation, positioning, or other errors.

LEARNING EXERCISES

Complete the following review exercises after reading the associated pages in the textbook as indicated by each exercise. Answers to each review exercise are given at the end of the review exercises.

PART I: RADIOGRAPHIC ANATOMY

REVIEW EXERCISE A: Radiographic Anatomy and Clinical Indications of the Gallbladder and Biliary System (see textbook pp. 458–460)

1. What is the average weight of the adult human liver? _____

2. Which abdominal quadrant contains the gallbladder? _____

3. What is the name of the soft tissue structure that separates the right from the left lobe of the liver? _____

4. Which lobe of the liver is larger, the right or the left? _____

5. List the minor lobes of the liver (the right and left lobes are the major lobes).

   A. _____   B. _____

6. True/False: The liver performs more than 100 functions.

7. True/False: The average healthy adult liver produces 1 gallon, or 3000–4000 mL, of bile per day.

8. List the three primary functions of the gallbladder.

   A. _____

   B. _____

   C. _____

9. True/False: Concentrated levels of cholesterol in bile may lead to gallstones.

300

10. What is a common site for impaction, or lodging, of gallstones? _____

11. True/False: In about 40% of individuals, the end of the common bile duct and the end of the pancreatic duct are totally separated into two ducts rather than combining into one single passageway into the duodenum.

12. True/False: Older terminology for the main pancreatic duct is the duct of Vater.

13. The gallbladder is located more _____ (posteriorly or anteriorly) within the abdomen.

14. Match the following structures to their primary location within the abdomen.

_____ 1. Liver

_____ 2. Gallbladder on asthenic patient

_____ 3. Gallbladder on hypersthenic patient

_____ 4. Gallbladder on hyposthenic patient

A. Near the midsagittal plane

B. To the left of the midsagittal plane

C. To the right of the midsagittal plane

15. Identify the major components of the gallbladder and biliary system labeled in Fig. 12.1.

A. _____

B. _____

C. _____

D. _____

E. _____

F. _____

G. _____

H. _____

I. _____

J. _____

K. _____

L. _____

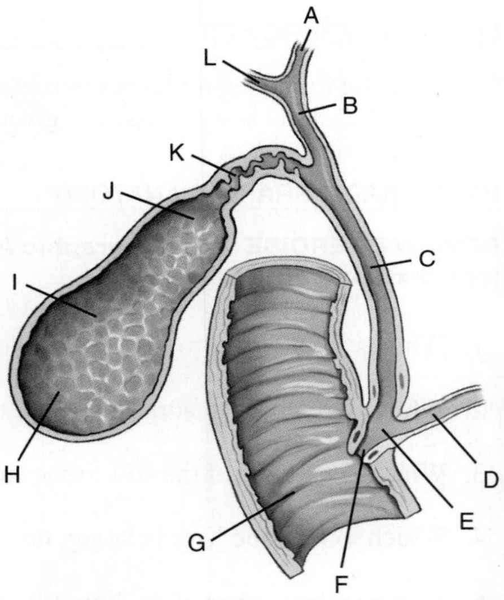

Fig. 12.1 Components of the gallbladder and biliary system.

16. List four advantages of diagnostic medical sonography (DMS) as a noninvasive means to study the gallbladder and biliary ducts.

A. _____

B. _____

C. _____

D. _____

17. A cholecystocholangiogram is a radiographic examination of _____.

18. Which imaging modality produces cholescintigraphy?

   A. Computed tomography (CT)

   B. Magnetic resonance imaging (MR)

   C. Radiography

   D. Nuclear medicine (NM)

19. True/False: Acute cholecystitis may produce a thickened gallbladder wall.

20. Match each of the following clinical indications with its correct definition.

   _____ 1. Cholelithiasis

   _____ 2. Cholecystitis

   _____ 3. Biliary stenosis

   _____ 4. Cholecystectomy

   _____ 5. Neoplasm

   _____ 6. Choledocholithiasis

   A. Surgical removal of the gallbladder

   B. Enlargement or narrowing of the biliary ducts because of the presence of stones

   C. Condition of having gallstones

   D. Inflammation of the gallbladder

   E. Benign or malignant tumors

   F. Narrowing of the biliary ducts

REVIEW EXERCISE B: Specific Anatomy of the Upper Gastrointestinal System (see textbook pp. 461–468)

1. List the seven major components of the alimentary canal.

   A. _____

   B. _____

   C. _____

   D. _____

   E. _____

   F. _____

   G. _____

2. List the four accessory organs of digestion.

   A. _____

   B. _____

   C. _____

   D. _____

3. What are the three primary functions of the digestive system?

   A. _____

   B. _____

   C. _____

4. What two terms refer to a radiographic examination of the pharynx and esophagus?

   _____ or _____

5. Which term describes the radiographic study of the distal esophagus, stomach, and duodenum?

   _____ or _____

6. Which three pairs of salivary glands are accessory organs of digestion associated with the mouth?

   A. _____

   B. _____

   C. _____

7. The act of swallowing is called _____.

8. List the three divisions of the pharynx.

   A. _____   B. _____   C. _____

9. What structures create the two indentations seen along the lateral border of the esophagus?

   A. _____   B. _____

10. List the three structures that pass through the diaphragm.

    A. _____   B. _____   C. _____

11. What part of the upper GI tract is a common site for ulcer disease? _____

12. What term describes the junction between the duodenum and jejunum? _____ (This is a significant reference point in small-bowel studies.)

13. The C-loop of the duodenum and pancreas are _____ (intraperitoneal or retroperitoneal) structures.

14. Name the structures of the mouth and pharynx (Fig. 12.2).

    A. _____

    B. _____

    C. _____

    D. _____

    E. _____

    F. _____

    G. _____

    H. _____

    I. _____

    J. _____

    K. _____

    L. _____

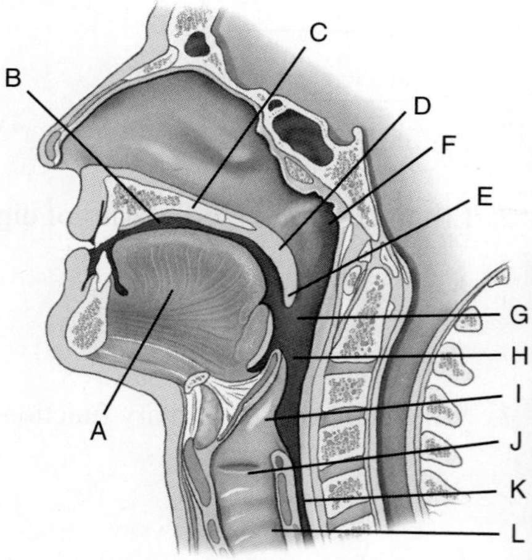

Fig. 12.2 Structures of the mouth and pharynx.

15. True/False: The body of the stomach curves inferiorly and posteriorly from the fundus.

16. Identify the parts labeled in Fig. 12.3.

   A. _____

   B. _____

   C. _____

   D. _____ (formed by rugae along the lesser curvature)

   E. _____

   F. _____

   G. _____

   H. _____

   I. _____

   J. _____ (abdominal segment of the esophagus)

   K. _____

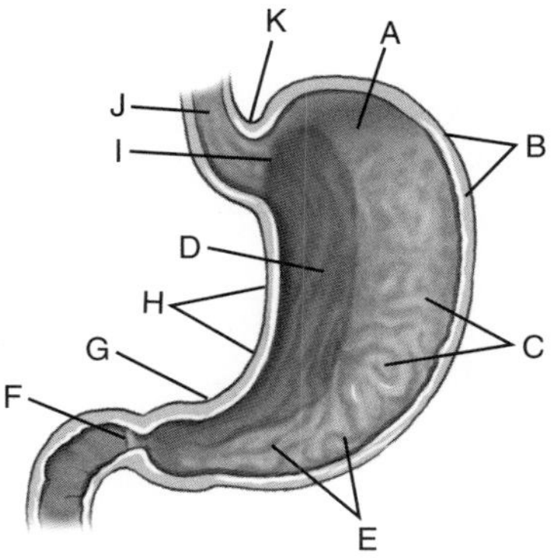

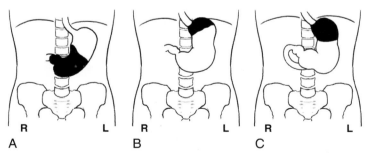

Fig. 12.3 Sectional anatomy of the stomach.

17. The three main subdivisions of the stomach are:

   A. _____   B. _____   C. _____

18. The division of the stomach labeled E in Fig. 12.3 is divided into two parts: _____ and

   _____.

19. Another term for mucosal folds of the stomach is _____.

20. Identify the correct body position (erect, prone, or supine) for each of the drawings of the stomach filled with air and barium (Fig. 12.4). (Barium = white; air = black)

   A. _____   B. _____   C. _____

Fig. 12.4 Body position identification based on a stomach filled with air or barium.

21. Identify the parts labeled in Fig. 12.5.

A. _____

B. _____

C. _____

D. _____

E. _____

F. _____

G. _____

H. _____

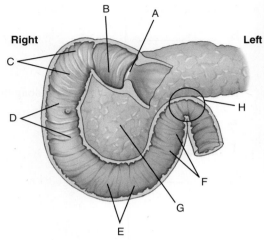

Fig. 12.5 Anatomy of the duodenum and pancreas.

22. Name the two anatomic structures implicated in the phrase "romance of the abdomen" illustrated in Fig. 12.5.

A. _____   B. _____

23. Identify the GI structures labeled in Fig. 12.6.

A. _____

B. _____

C. _____

D. _____

E. _____

F. _____

G. _____

H. _____

I. _____

J. _____

K. _____

L. _____

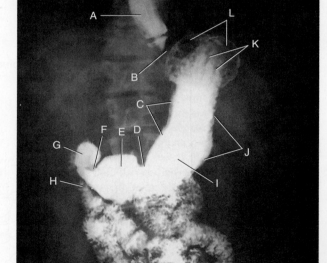

Fig. 12.6 Radiograph of gastrointestinal structures.

REVIEW EXERCISE C: Mechanical and Chemical Digestion and Body Habitus (see textbook pp. 469–471)

1. True/False: Mechanical digestion includes movements of the entire GI tract.

2. Peristaltic activity is *not* found in which of the following structures?

   A. Pharynx

   B. Esophagus

   C. Stomach

   D. Small intestine

3. Stomach contents are churned into a semifluid mass called _____.

4. A churning or mixing activity that is present in the small bowel is called _____.

5. List the three groups of food that are ingested and must be chemically digested.

   A. _____   B. _____   C. _____

6. Biologic catalysts that speed up the process of digestion are called _____.

7. List the end products of digestion for the following classes of food.

   A. Carbohydrates: _____

   B. Lipids: _____

   C. Proteins: _____

8. What is the name of the liquid substance that aids in digestion, is manufactured in the liver, and is stored in the

   gallbladder? _____

9. How does the material from Question 8 assist in emulsification in fat? _____

10. Absorption of nutrients primarily takes place in the (A) _____, although some substances are absorbed through the lining of the (B) _____.

11. Digestion of which of the three primary food classifications listed in Question 7 begins in the mouth?

    _____

12. Any residues of digestion or unabsorbed digestive products are eliminated from the

    _____ as a component of feces.

13. Peristalsis is an example of which type of digestion? _____

14. Which term describes food after it is mixed with gastric secretions in the stomach?

    _____

15. A high and transverse stomach would be found in a(n) _____ patient.

    A. Hypersthenic

    B. Sthenic

    C. Hyposthenic

    D. Asthenic

16. A J-shaped stomach that is more vertical and lower in the abdomen, with the duodenal bulb at the level of L3–L4,

    would be found in a(n) _____ patient.

    A. Hypersthenic   C. Hyposthenic/asthenic

    B. Sthenic   D. None of the above

17. In the erect position, how much will abdominal organs drop on average? _____

18. Name the two GI organs most dramatically affected, in relation to location, by body habitus.

    A. _____   B. _____

19. Would the fundus of the stomach be more superior or more inferior during deep inhalation?

    _____ Why? _____

20. Match the types of mechanical digestion and/or movement that occur in each of the following anatomic sites. (Each anatomic site may have more than one type of digestion.)

    Anatomic sites   *Types of mechanical digestion*

    _____ 1. Oral cavity   A. Mastication

    _____ 2. Pharynx   B. Deglutition

    _____ 3. Esophagus   C. Peristalsis

    _____ 4. Stomach   D. Mixing

    _____ 5. Small intestine   E. Rhythmic segmentation

PART II: RADIOGRAPHIC POSITIONING

REVIEW EXERCISE D: Contrast Media, Fluoroscopy, and Clinical Indications and Contraindications for Upper Gastrointestinal Studies (see textbook pp. 472–480)

1. True/False: With the use of digital fluoroscopy, the number of postfluoroscopy radiographs ordered has greatly diminished.

2. Another term for a negative contrast medium is _____.

3. What substance is most commonly ingested to produce carbon dioxide gas as a negative contrast medium for GI studies?

    _____

4. What is the most common form of positive contrast medium used for studies of the GI system?

    _____

5. Is a mixture of barium sulfate a suspension or a solution? _____

6. True/False: Barium sulfate never dissolves in water.

7. True/False: Certain salts of barium are poisonous to humans, so barium contrast studies require a pure sulfate salt of barium for human consumption during GI studies.

8. What is the ratio of water to barium for a thin mixture of barium sulfate?

   _____

9. What is the chemical symbol for barium sulfate? _____

10. When is the use of barium sulfate contraindicated? _____

11. What patient condition prevents the use of a water-soluble contrast medium for an upper GI series?

   _____

12. What is the major advantage for using a double-contrast medium technique for esophagography and upper GI series?

   _____

13. The speed with which barium sulfate passes through the GI tract is called gastric _____

14. What is the purpose of the gas with a double-contrast media technique?

   _____

15. Which of the following devices on a digital fluoroscopy system converts the analog into a digital signal?

   A. Picture archiving and communication system (PACS)   C. Charge-coupled device (CCD)

   B. Light converter   D. Optical tracking system (OTS)

16. What device (found beneath the radiographic table when correctly positioned) greatly reduces exposure to the technologist from the fluoroscopic x-ray tube?

   A. Lead skirt   C. Bucky slot shield

   B. Lead drape   D. Fluoroscopy tube shield

17. How is the device referred to in Question 16 activated or placed in its correct position for fluoroscopy?

   _____

18. What is the *minimum* level of protective apron worn during fluoroscopy?

   A. 0.25 mm Pb/Eq apron   C. 1.0 mm Pb/Eq apron

   B. 0.5 mm Pb/Eq apron   D. 1.5 mm Pb/Eq apron

19. What is the major benefit of using a compression paddle during an upper GI study?

   A. Reduces exposure to the patient

   B. Reduces exposure to the eyes of the fluoroscopist

   C. Reduces exposure to arms and hands of the fluoroscopist

   D. Reduces exposure to the torso of the fluoroscopist

20. If a compression paddle is unavailable, what should the fluoroscopist or technologist wear before placing their hands into the fluoroscopic beam? _____

21. List the three cardinal principles of radiation protection.

    A. _____   B. _____   C. _____

22. Which of the three cardinal principles is most effective in reducing exposure to the technologist during a fluoroscopic procedure?

    _____

23. List the four advantages or unique features and capabilities of digital fluoroscopy over conventional fluoroscopic recording systems.

    A. _____   C. _____

    B. _____   D. _____

24. Which capability on most digital fluoroscopy systems demonstrates a dynamic flow of contrast media through the

    GI tract? _____

25. Match the following definitions or descriptions to the correct pathologic condition for esophagography.

    _____ A. Difficulty in swallowing   1. Achalasia

    _____ B. Replacement of normal squamous epithelium with   2. Zenker diverticulum
              columnar epithelium
                                                                             3. Esophageal varices
    _____ C. May lead to esophagitis
                                                                             4. Carcinoma of esophagus
    _____ D. May be secondary to cirrhosis of the liver
                                                                             5. Barrett esophagus
    _____ E. Large outpouching of the esophagus
                                                                             6. Gastroesophageal reflux disease (GERD)
    _____ F. Also called cardiospasm
                                                                             7. Dysphagia
    _____ G. Most common form is adenocarcinoma

26. Match the following definitions or descriptions to the correct pathology for the upper GI series.

    _____ A. Blood in vomit   1. Hiatal hernia

    _____ B. Inflammation of lining of stomach   2. Gastric carcinoma

    _____ C. Blind outpouching of the mucosal wall   3. Bezoar

    _____ D. Undigested material trapped in stomach   4. Hematemesis

    _____ E. Synonymous with gastric or duodenal ulcer   5. Gastritis

    _____ F. Portion of stomach protruding through the diaphragmatic opening   6. Perforating ulcer

    _____ G. Only 5% of ulcers lead to this condition   7. Peptic ulcer

    _____ H. Double-contrast upper GI is recommended for this type of tumor   8. Diverticula

309

27. Match the following pathologic conditions or diseases to the correct radiographic appearance.

_____ A. Its presence indicates a possible sliding hiatal hernia   1. Ulcers

_____ B. Speckled appearance of gastric mucus   2. Hiatal hernia

_____ C. "Wormlike" appearance of esophagus   3. Achalasia

_____ D. Stricture of esophagus   4. Zenker diverticulum

_____ E. Gastric bubble above diaphragm   5. Schatzki ring

_____ F. Irregular filling defect within stomach   6. Gastritis

_____ G. Enlarged recess in proximal esophagus   7. Esophageal varices

_____ H. "Lucent-halo" sign during upper GI   8. Gastric carcinoma

28. Which procedure is often performed to detect early signs of GERD?

_____

29. Which specific structure of the GI system is affected by hypertrophic pyloric stenosis (HPS)?

_____

30. Which imaging modality is most effective in diagnosing HPS while reducing dose to the patient?

_____

REVIEW EXERCISE E: Patient Preparation and Positioning for Esophagography and Upper Gastrointestinal Study (see textbook pp. 481–498)

1. What does the acronym *NPO* stand for, and what does it mean? _____

2. True/False: The patient must be NPO 4–6 hours before esophagography.

3. True/False: Esophagography usually begins with fluoroscopy with the patient in the erect position.

4. What materials may be used for swallowing to aid in the diagnosis of radiolucent foreign bodies in the esophagus?

_____

5. List the four radiographic tests that may be performed to detect signs of GERD.

    A. _____   C. _____

    B. _____   D. _____

6. A breathing technique in which the patient takes in a deep breath and bears down is called the _____.

7. In what position is the patient usually placed during the water test? _____

8. Which region of the GI tract is better visualized when the radiologist uses a compression paddle during

    esophagography? _____

310

9. What type of contrast medium should be used if the patient has a history of bowel perforation?

_____

10. What is the minimum amount of time that the patient should be NPO before an upper GI?

_____

11. Why should cigarette use and gum chewing be restricted before an upper GI?

_____

12. Why should the technologist review the patient's chart before the beginning of an upper GI?

    A. To identify any known allergies   C. To look for pertinent clinical history

    B. To ensure that the proper study has been ordered   D. All of the above

13. In which hand does the patient usually hold the barium cup during the start of an upper GI?

_____

14. List the suggested dosages of barium sulfate during an upper GI for each of the following pediatric age groups.

    Newborn to 1 year: _____

    1–3 years: _____

    3–10 years: _____

    More than 10 years: _____

15. What type of fluoroscopy generator is recommended for pediatric procedures?

_____

16. Which of the following modalities is an alternative to esophagography in detecting esophageal varices?

    A. Nuclear medicine   C. DMS

    B. CT   D. Endoscopy

17. Gastric emptying studies are performed using:

    A. Intraesophageal sonography   C. MR

    B. Radionuclides   D. CT

18. Why is the right anterior oblique (RAO) preferred rather than the left anterior oblique (LAO) for esophagography?

_____

19. How much rotation of the body should be used for the RAO projection of the esophagus?

_____

20. Which optional position should be performed to demonstrate the mid-to-upper esophagus located between the shoulders?

_____

21. The three most common routine projections for esophagography are:

A. _____   B. _____   C. _____

22. Which aspect of the GI tract is best demonstrated with an RAO position during an upper GI?

A. Fundus of stomach   C. Body of stomach

B. Pylorus of stomach and C-loop   D. Fourth (ascending) portion of duodenum

23. How much rotation of the body is required for the RAO position during an upper GI on a sthenic patient?

A. 30–35 degrees   C. 40–70 degrees

B. 15–20 degrees   D. 10–15 degrees

24. What is the average kVp range for esophagography and an upper GI when using barium sulfate (single-contrast study)?

_____

25. Which aspects of the upper GI tract will be filled with barium in the posteroanterior (PA) projection (prone position)?

_____

26. What is the purpose of the PA axial projection for the hypersthenic patient during an upper GI?

_____

27. What CR angle is required for the PA axial projection for a hypersthenic patient during an upper GI?

A. 10–15 degrees caudad   C. 35–45 degrees cephalad

B. 20–25 degrees cephalad   D. 60–70 degrees cephalad

28. Which projection taken during an upper GI will best demonstrate the retrogastric space?

A. RAO   C. LPO

B. Lateral   D. PA

29. What is the recommended kVp range for a double-contrast upper GI projection?

_____

30. The upper GI series usually begins with the table and patient in the _____ position.

31. The five most common routine projections for an upper GI series are:

A. _____   C. _____   E. _____

B. _____   D. _____

32. The major parts of the stomach on an average patient are usually confined to which abdominal quadrant?

_____

33. Most of the duodenum is usually found to the _____ (right or left) of the midline on a sthenic patient.

34. True/False: Respiration should be suspended during inspiration for upper GI radiographic projections.

312

Chapter **12 Biliary Tract and Upper Gastrointestinal System**

REVIEW EXERCISE F: Problem Solving for Technical and Positioning Errors

1. **Situation:** A radiograph of an RAO projection taken during esophagography demonstrates incomplete filling of the esophagus with barium. What can the technologist do to ensure better filling of the esophagus during the repeat exposure?

_____

_____

2. **Situation:** A series of radiographs taken during an upper GI shows that the stomach mucosa is not well visualized. The following factors were used during this positioning routine: Bucky, 40-inch (100-cm) SID, 80 kVp, 30 mAs, and 300 mL of barium sulfate ingested during the procedure. Which exposure factor should be changed to produce a more diagnostic study?

_____

_____

3. **Situation:** A radiograph taken during an upper GI (double-contrast study) shows that the anatomic side marker is missing. The technologist is unsure whether it is a recumbent anteroposterior (AP) or PA projection. The fundus of the stomach is filled with barium. Which position does this radiograph represent?

_____

_____

4. **Situation:** A radiograph of an RAO projection taken during an upper GI shows that the duodenal bulb is not well demonstrated and is not profiled. The RAO was a 45-degree oblique performed on a hypersthenic type of patient. What positioning modification needs to be made to produce a better image of the duodenal bulb?

_____

_____

5. **Situation:** A radiograph of an upper GI was taken, but the student technologist is unsure of the position. The radiograph demonstrates that the fundus is filled with barium, but the duodenal bulb is air filled and is seen in profile. Which position does this radiograph represent?

_____

_____

6. **Situation:** A patient with a clinical history of hiatal hernia comes to the radiology department. Which procedure should be performed on this patient to rule out this condition?

_____

_____

7. **Situation:** A patient with a possible lacerated duodenum enters the emergency room. The ER physician orders an upper GI to determine the extent of the injury. What type of contrast medium should be used for this examination?

_____

_____

8. **Situation:** A patient with a fish bone stuck in his esophagus enters the emergency room. What modification to standard esophagography may be needed to locate the foreign body?

_____

_____

9. **Situation:** An upper GI is being performed on a thin, asthenic-type patient. Because of room-scheduling conflicts, this patient was brought into your room for the overhead follow-up images following fluoroscopy. Where would you center the CR and the recommended field size of 11- × 14-inch (30- × 35-cm) to ensure that you included the stomach and the duodenal regions?

_____

_____

10. **Situation:** A patient with a clinical history of a possible bezoar comes to the radiology department. What is a bezoar, and what radiographic study should be performed to demonstrate this condition?

_____

_____

11. **Situation:** A radiograph of an RAO position taken during esophagography shows that the esophagus is superimposed over the vertebral column. What positioning error led to this radiographic outcome? What must be altered to eliminate this problem during the repeat exposure?

_____

_____

12. **Situation:** A PA projection taken during an upper GI series performed on an infant shows that the body and pylorus of the stomach are superimposed. What modification needs to be used during the repeat exposure to separate these two regions?

_____

_____

13. **Situation:** A patient comes to radiology with a clinical history of possible gastric diverticulum in the posterior aspect of the fundus. Which projection taken during the upper GI series best demonstrates this defect?

_____

_____

14. **Situation:** A patient comes to radiology with a clinical history of Barrett esophagus. In addition to esophagography, what other imaging modality is ideal in demonstrating this condition?

_____

_____

15. **Situation:** A patient has a clinical history of hemochromatosis. Which imaging modality is most effective in diagnosing this condition?

_____

_____

PART III: LABORATORY EXERCISES

You must gain experience in positioning each part of the esophagography and upper GI procedures before performing the following exams on actual patients. You can obtain experience in positioning and radiographic evaluation of these projections by performing exercises using radiographic phantoms and practicing on other students (although you will not be taking actual exposures).

Laboratory Exercise A: Radiographic Evaluation

1. Evaluate and critique the radiographs produced during the previous experiments, additional radiographs of esophagography and upper GI procedures provided by your instructor, or both. Evaluate each position for the following points (check off when completed).

_____ Evaluate the completeness of the study. (Are all the pertinent anatomic structures included on the radiograph?)

_____ Evaluate for positioning or centering errors (e.g., rotation, off-centering).

_____ Evaluate for correct exposure factors and possible motion. (Are the image receptor exposure and contrast of the images acceptable?)

_____ Determine whether anatomic side markers and an acceptable degree of collimation are visible on the images.

Laboratory Exercise B: Physical Positioning

On another person, simulate performing all routine and special projections of the upper GI as follows. Include the six steps listed in the following and described in the textbook. (Check off each step when it is completed satisfactorily.)

Step 1. Appropriate collimation field size with correct markers

Step 2. Correct CR placement and centering of part to central ray and/or IR

Step 3. Accurate collimation

Step 4. Area shielding of patient (when required)

Step 5. Use of proper immobilizing devices when needed

Step 6. Approximate correct exposure factors, breathing instructions where applicable, and initiating exposure

Projections	Step 1	Step 2	Step 3	Step 4	Step 5	Step 6
• RAO esophagography	_____	_____	_____	_____	_____	_____
• Left lateral esophagography	_____	_____	_____	_____	_____	_____
• AP (PA) esophagography	_____	_____	_____	_____	_____	_____
• LAO esophagography	_____	_____	_____	_____	_____	_____
• Soft tissue lateral esophagography	_____	_____	_____	_____	_____	_____
• RAO upper GI	_____	_____	_____	_____	_____	_____
• PA upper GI	_____	_____	_____	_____	_____	_____
• Right lateral upper GI	_____	_____	_____	_____	_____	_____
• LPO upper GI	_____	_____	_____	_____	_____	_____
• AP upper GI	_____	_____	_____	_____	_____	_____

SELF-TEST

MY SCORE = _____ %

This self-test should be taken only after completing all of the readings, review exercises, and laboratory activities for a particular section. The purpose of this test is not only to provide a good learning exercise but also to serve as a strong indicator of what your final evaluation exam for this chapter will cover. It is strongly suggested that if you do not get at least a 90%–95% grade on each self-test, you should review those areas in which you missed questions before going to your instructor for the final evaluation exam.

1. The gallbladder is located in the _____ margin of the liver.
    A. Posterior inferior
    B. Posterior superior
    C. Midaspect
    D. Anterior superior

2. Which of the following is not a recognized lobe of the liver?
    A. Caudate
    B. Quadrate
    C. Inferior
    D. Left

3. In which quadrant is the liver located in the sthenic patient?
    A. Right lower quadrant
    B. Left lower quadrant
    C. Left upper quadrant
    D. Right upper quadrant

4. What is the name of the soft tissue structure that divides the liver into left and right lobes?

5. What is the primary function of bile?

6. The union of the left and right hepatic ducts form which duct?

7. Which duct carries bile from the cystic duct to the duodenum?

8. What is the average capacity of the adult gallbladder?

9. Which process leads to a concentration of bile within the gallbladder?

10. Which hormone leads to contraction of the gallbladder to release bile?

11. Match each of the following biliary structures to its correct description or definition.

_____1.	Pancreatic duct	A.	Series of mucosal folds in cystic duct
_____2.	Fundus	B.	A protrusion into the duodenum
_____3.	Hepatopancreatic ampulla	C.	Middle aspect of gallbladder
_____4.	Spiral valve	D.	Duct connected directly to gallbladder
_____5.	Hepatopancreatic sphincter	E.	Narrowest portion of gallbladder
_____6.	Duodenal papilla	F.	Broadest portion of gallbladder
_____7.	Cystic duct	G.	Enlarged chamber in distal aspect of common bile duct
_____8.	Neck	H.	Duct of Wirsung
_____9.	Body	I.	Circular muscle fibers adjacent to duodenal papilla

12. Identify the labeled parts and/or structures on the radiograph of an oral cholecystogram (Fig. 12.7).

A. _____

B. _____

C. _____

D. _____

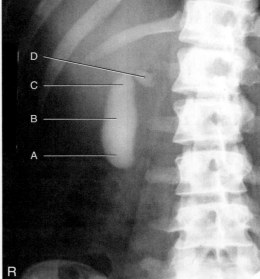

Fig. 12.7 Radiograph of an oral cholecystogram and of biliary ducts.

13. Which of the following terms describes the condition of having gallstones?

A. Cholecystitis

B. Cholelithiasis

C. Cholecystectomy

D. Choleliths

14. Which of the following is *not* a function of the GI system?

A. Intake and digestion of food

B. Absorption of nutrients

C. Production of hormones

D. Elimination of waste products

15. What is another term for esophagography?

_____

16. Which of the following is *not* a salivary gland?
   A. Parotid
   B. Sublingual
   C. Vallecula
   D. Submandibular

17. What is the name of the condition that results from a viral infection of the parotid gland?

_____

18. Which structure in the pharynx prevents aspiration of food and fluid into the larynx?
   A. Uvula
   B. Epiglottis
   C. Soft palate
   D. Laryngopharynx

19. The esophagus extends from C5–C6 to
   A. T9
   B. L1
   C. T10
   D. T11

20. Which of the following structures does not pass through the diaphragm?
   A. Trachea
   B. Esophagus
   C. Aorta
   D. Inferior vena cava

21. Wavelike involuntary contractions that help propel food down the esophagus are called

_____

22. The Greek term *gaster*, or *gastro*, means _____.

23. Which of the following aspects of the stomach is defined as an indentation between the body and pylorus?
   A. Cardiac antrum
   B. Pyloric antrum
   C. Cardiac notch (incisura cardiaca)
   D. Angular notch (incisura angularis)

24. True/False: The numerous mucosal folds found in the small bowel are called rugae.

25. Which aspect of the stomach fills with air when the patient is prone during a double-contrast upper gastrointestinal series?
   A. Fundus
   B. Body
   C. Duodenal bulb
   D. Pylorus

26. True/False: The lateral margin of the stomach is called the lesser curvature.

27. To which aspect of the stomach does barium gravitate when the patient is in the supine position?

_____

28. Which two structures create the romance of the abdomen?

_____

29. Match each of the following aspects of the upper GI with the correct definition.

_____ 1. Pyloric orifice   A. Middle aspect of stomach

_____ 2. Cardiac notch   B. Horizontal portion of duodenum

_____ 3. Fundus   C. Rugae

_____ 4. Fourth portion of duodenum   D. Opening between esophagus and stomach

_____ 5. Mucosal folds   E. Opening leaving the stomach

_____ 6. Body   F. Found along superior aspect of fundus

_____ 7. Esophagogastric junction   G. Indentation found along lesser curvature

_____ 8. Angular notch   H. Ascending portion of duodenum

_____ 9. Third portion of duodenum   I. Most posterior aspect of stomach

30. Identify the structures labeled in Fig. 12.8.

A. _____

B. _____

C. _____

D. _____

E. _____

F. _____

G. _____

H. _____

I. _____

J. _____

K. _____

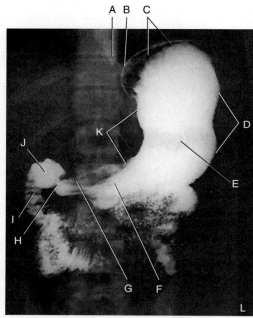

Fig. 12.8 Radiograph of gastrointestinal structures, demonstrating body position.

31. A. Which radiographic position does Fig. 12.8 represent? _____

B. How could you determine this? _____

32. Which radiographic position does Fig. 12.9 represent?

   _____

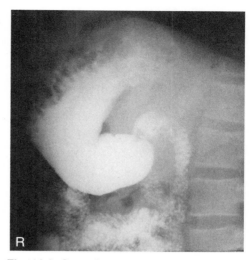

Fig. 12.9 Gastrointestinal radiograph demonstrating body position.

33. A.   Which radiographic position does Fig. 12.10 represent?

   _____

   B.   How could you determine this? _____

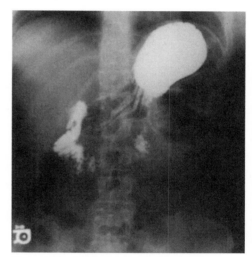

Fig. 12.10 Gastrointestinal radiograph demonstrating body position.

34. A. Fig. 12.11 represents a(n) _____ (anterior or posterior) oblique position.

    B. How could you determine this? _____

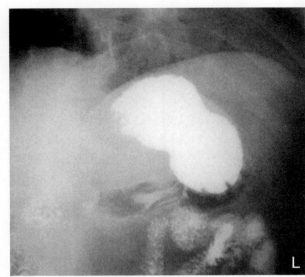

Fig. 12.11 Oblique radiograph of gastrointestinal structures.

    C. Which specific radiographic position does Fig. 12.12 represent? _____

    D. How could you determine this? _____

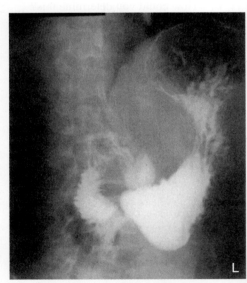

Fig. 12.12 Oblique radiograph of gastrointestinal structures.

35. The act of chewing is termed:

A. Mastication

B. Deglutition

C. Aspiration

D. Peristalsis

36. Which term describes food after it enters the stomach and is mixed with gastric secretions?

_____

37. The churning or mixing activity of chyme in the small intestine is called

A. Peristalsis

B. Deglutition

C. Rhythmic segmentation

D. Digestion

38. Which of the following nutrients is not digested?

A. Vitamins

B. Lipids

C. Carbohydrates

D. Proteins

39. A high and transverse stomach indicates a _____ body type with the duodenal bulb at

the vertebral level of _____.

40. A _____ or _____ type of body habitus usually includes

a low and vertical stomach with the duodenal bulb at the vertebral level of _____.

41. What is the most common radiopaque contrast media used in the GI system?

_____

42. What type of radiolucent contrast medium is most commonly used for double-contrast GI studies?

43. A. What is the ratio of barium to water for a thick mixture of barium sulfate? _____

B. What is the ratio for a thin barium mixture? _____

44. During an upper GI, when should a water-soluble contrast medium be used rather than barium sulfate?

_____

45. Which of the following conditions may prevent the use of water-soluble contrast agents for a geriatric patient?

A. Bowel obstruction

B. Pre-surgical imaging

C. Dehydration

D. Perforated ulcer

46. True/False: Water-soluble contrast agents pass through the GI tract faster than barium sulfate.

47. True/False: Digital fluoroscopy does not require the use of an IR.

48. Which of the cardinal principles of radiation protection is most effective in reducing exposure to the technologist

during fluoroscopy? _____

49. Protective aprons of what lead equivalency must be worn during fluoroscopy?

   A. 1.0 mm Pb/Eq
   B. 0.50 mm Pb/Eq
   C. 0.25 mm Pb/Eq
   D. 0.15 mm Pb/Eq

50. Which of the following is the older term for GERD?

   A. Esophageal reflux
   B. Barrett esophagus
   C. Esophageal varices
   D. Zenker diverticulum

51. A large outpouching of the mid-to-upper esophagus is termed

   A. Zenker diverticulum
   B. Achalasia
   C. Barrett esophagus
   D. Esophageal varices

52. A phytobezoar is

   A. An outpouching of the mucosal wall
   B. Trapped mass of hair in the stomach
   C. A rare tumor
   D. Trapped vegetable fiber in the stomach

53. What can be added to barium sulfate and swallowed to detect a radiolucent foreign body lodged in the esophagus?

   _____

54. What is the reason that the patient may be asked to swallow a mouthful of water drawn through a straw during esophagography?

   _____

55. How much rotation of the body should be used for an RAO esophagography projection?

   _____

56. Why is an RAO position preferred rather than an LAO during esophagography?

   _____

57. Why is the AP projection of the esophagus not a preferred projection for the esophagography series?

   _____

58. What criterion is used with ultrasound in determining whether a patient has HPS?

   A. Abnormally long pylorus
   B. Absence of rugae
   C. Presence of air-fluid level in the duodenum
   D. Antral muscle thickness exceeding 4 mm (0.15 inches)

59. Other than esophagography, what other imaging modality is performed to diagnose Barrett esophagus?

   A. CT
   B. Nuclear medicine
   C. MR
   D. Diagnostic medical sonography (DMS)

60. Which upper GI position best demonstrates a possible gastric diverticulum in the posterior wall of the fundus of the stomach?

   _____

61. **Situation:** An upper GI series is performed on an asthenic patient. A radiograph of the RAO position shows the duodenal bulb and the C-loop are not in profile. The technologist rotated the patient 70 degrees. What modification of the position is required during the repeat exposure?

_____

62. **Situation:** A radiograph taken during a double-contrast upper GI demonstrates the fundus is barium filled and the body is air filled. This was either an AP or a PA radiograph, which needs to be repeated. Which specific position does this radiograph represent?

_____

63. **Situation:** A patient with a clinical history of cirrhosis of the liver with acute GI bleeding comes to the radiology department. What may be the most likely reason that esophagography was ordered for this patient?

_____

64. **Situation:** During esophagography, the radiologist asks the patient to try to bear down as if having a bowel movement. What is this maneuver called, and why did the radiologist make such a request?

_____

65. **Situation:** During an upper GI, the radiologist reports that she sees a lucent-halo sign in the duodenum. What form of pathology did the radiologist observe?

_____

66. Which of the following technical/positioning factors does not apply to a water-soluble oral contrast media upper GI study?

   A. 125 kVp

   B. Exposure made on expiration

   C. 40-inch (100-cm) SID

   D. Erect and recumbent positions performed

67. **Situation:** A radiograph of an upper GI is not labeled correctly, but the technologist is unsure of the position that was performed. A double-contrast GI study was completed with all positions performed recumbent. The radiograph demonstrates barium in the fundus and air/gas in the body and pylorus and duodenal bulb in profile. Which position was performed?

_____

68. Which of the following shielding devices best reduces exposure to the lower torso of the fluoroscopist?

   A. Lead drape

   B. Bucky slot shield

   C. Lead gloves

   D. Grid

69. **Situation:** During esophagography, the radiologist remarks that Schatzki ring is present. Which condition or disease process is indicated by the presence of this radiographic sign?

_____

70. **Situation:** A patient comes to radiology with a clinical history of a possible trichobezoar. What is a trichobezoar and which radiographic procedure is best to diagnose it?

_____

324

12 Biliary Tract and Upper Gastrointestinal System

1. A. Posterior inferior
2. C. Inferior
3. D. Right upper quadrant
4. Falciform ligament
5. To break down or emulsify fats
6. Common hepatic duct
7. Common bile duct (CBD)
8. 30–40 mL
9. Hydrolysis
10. Cholecystokinin (CCK)
11. 1. H
    2. F
    3. G
    4. A
    5. I
    6. B
    7. D
    8. E
    9. C
12. A. Fundus
    B. Body
    C. Neck
    D. Cystic duct
13. B. Cholelithiasis
14. C. Production of hormones
15. Barium swallow
16. C. Vallecula
17. Mumps
18. B. Epiglottis
19. D. T11
20. A. Trachea
21. Peristalsis
22. Stomach
23. D. Angular notch (incisura angularis)
24. False (in the stomach)
25. A. Fundus
26. False (the greater curvature)
27. Fundus
28. Head of pancreas and C-loop of duodenum
29. 1. E
    2. F
    3. I

4. H
5. C
6. A
7. D
8. G
9. B
30. A. Distal esophagus (cardiac antrum)
    B. Region of esophagogastric junction (cardiac orifice)
    C. Fundus
    D. Greater curvature
    E. Body of stomach
    F. Pylorus (pyloric antrum)
    G. Pyloric canal
    H. Pyloric orifice (sphincter)
    I. Descending portion of duodenum
    J. Duodenal bulb
    K. Lesser curvature
31. A. Prone—PA projection
    B. Air in fundus with barium in the body of the stomach
32. Lateral
33. A. Supine—AP projection
    B. Barium-filled fundus (air in pylorus); also no spine rotation
34. A. Posterior—left posterior oblique position
    B. Air in pylorus with barium in the fundus indicates a semi-supine position
    C. RAO
    D. Spine rotation is indicating an oblique position. Air in fundus indicates a semiprone position, and duodenal bulb and C-loop in profile indicate an RAO and not an LAO.
35. A. Mastication
36. Chyme
37. C. Rhythmic segmentation
38. A. Vitamins
39. Hypersthenic, T11–T12
40. Hyposthenic or asthenic; L3–L4
41. Barium sulfate

42. Carbon dioxide (calcium or magnesium citrate)
43. A. Three or four parts barium to one part water
    B. One part barium to one part water
44. When there is a possibility that the contrast media may spill into the peritoneum (such as during presurgery or in the case of a perforated bowel)
45. C. Dehydration
46. True
47. True
48. Distance
49. B. 0.50 mm Pb/Eq
50. A. Esophageal reflux
51. A. Zenker diverticulum
52. D. Trapped vegetable fiber in the stomach
53. Cotton balls or marshmallows
54. To detect signs of esophageal reflux (GERD)
55. 35–40 degrees
56. The RAO places the esophagus between the heart and the vertebra better than an LAO.
57. Majority of esophagus is superimposed over the spine and is thus not well visualized.
58. D. Antral muscle thickness exceeding 4 mm (0.15 inches)
59. B. Nuclear medicine (NM)
60. Right lateral position
61. Reduce patient rotation to 40 degrees for an asthenic patient.
62. AP projection performed recumbent
63. To rule out esophageal varices (a condition of dilation of the veins, which in advanced stages may lead to internal bleeding). Endoscopy is often preferred rather than an esophagram.
64. The Valsalva maneuver, requested to rule out esophageal reflux (a condition wherein gastric

A1

contents return back through the gastric orifice into the esophagus, causing irritation of the esophageal lining).

65. An ulcer

66. A. 125 kVp (90–100 recommended)
67. Left posterior oblique (LPO) recumbent
68. B. Bucky slot shield
69. Sliding hiatal hernia

70. A mass of hair trapped in the stomach. An upper GI study may be performed to diagnose this condition.

13 Lower Gastrointestinal System

CHAPTER OBJECTIVES

After you have successfully completed the activities in this chapter, you will be able to:

_____ 1. List three divisions of the small intestine and the major parts of the large intestine.

_____ 2. Identify the function, location, and pertinent anatomy of the small and large intestine.

_____ 3. Differentiate between the terms *colon* and *large intestine*.

_____ 4. On drawings and radiographs, identify specific anatomy of the lower gastrointestinal (GI) canal from the duodenum through the anus.

_____ 5. Identify the sectional differences that differentiate the large intestine from the small intestine.

_____ 6. List specific clinical indications and contraindications for a small bowel series and a barium enema (BE) examination.

_____ 7. Match specific types of pathology to the correct radiographic appearances and signs.

_____ 8. Identify patient preparation for a small bowel series and BE.

_____ 9. List five safety concerns that must be followed during a BE procedure.

_____ 10. Identify the radiographic procedure and sequence for a small bowel series.

_____ 11. Identify the purpose, clinical indications, and methodology for the enteroclysis, computed tomography (CT) enteroclysis, CT colonography (CTC), and the intubation small bowel method procedures.

_____ 12. Identify the patient preparation, room preparation, and fluoroscopic procedure for a BE.

_____ 13. Identify the purpose, clinical indications, and methodology for an evacuative proctogram.

_____ 14. Identify the correct procedure for inserting a rectal enema tube.

_____ 15. List specific information related to the routine positions or projections of a small bowel series and BE examination to include recommended collimation field size, central ray (CR) location, direction and angulation of the central ray, and the anatomy best demonstrated.

_____ 16. Identify the advantages, procedure, and positioning for an air-contrast BE.

_____ 17. Given various hypothetic situations, identify the correct modification of a position and/or exposure considerations to improve the radiographic image.

POSITIONING AND RADIOGRAPHIC TECHNIQUE

_____ 1. Using a peer, position for routine and special projections for the small bowel and BE series.

_____ 2. Critique and evaluate small bowel and BE series radiographs based on the five divisions of radiographic criteria: (1) anatomy demonstrated, (2) position, (3) collimation field size and CR, (4) exposure, and (5) anatomic side markers.

_____ 3. Distinguish between acceptable and unacceptable small bowel and BE series radiographs resulting from exposure factors, motion, collimation, positioning, or other errors.

LEARNING EXERCISES

Complete the following review exercises after reading the associated pages in the textbook as indicated by each exercise. Answers to each review exercise are given at the end of the review exercises.

PART I: RADIOGRAPHIC ANATOMY

REVIEW EXERCISE A: Radiographic Anatomy of the Lower Gastrointestinal System (see textbook pp. 500–505)

1. A. How long is the average small bowel if removed and stretched out?

   _____

   B. In a person with good muscle tone, the length of the entire small intestine is _____.

   C. The average length of the large intestine is _____.

2. List the three divisions of the small intestine in descending order, starting with the widest division.

   A. _____   B. _____   C. _____

3. Which division of the small intestine is the shortest? _____

4. In which two abdominal quadrants would the majority of the jejunum be found?

   _____

5. Which division of the small intestine has a feathery or coiled-spring appearance during a small bowel series?

   _____

6. Which division of the small intestine is the longest? _____

7. Which two aspects of the large intestine are not considered part of the colon?

   _____

8. The colon is divided into _____ sections and has _____ flexures.

9. List the two functions of the ileocecal valve.

   A. _____   B. _____

10. What is another term for the appendix? _____

11. Match the following aspects of the small and large intestine to their characteristics:

_____ 1. Jejunum   A. Longest aspect of the large intestine

_____ 2. Duodenum   B. Widest portion of the large intestine

_____ 3. Ileum   C. A blind pouch inferior to the ileocecal valve

_____ 4. Cecum   D. Aspect of small intestine that is the smallest in diameter but longest in length

_____ 5. Appendix   E. Distal part; also called the iliac colon

_____ 6. Ascending colon   F. Shortest aspect of small intestine

_____ 7. Descending colon   G. Lies in pelvis but possesses a wide freedom of motion

_____ 8. Transverse colon   H. Makes up 40% of the small intestine

_____ 9. Sigmoid colon   I. Found between the cecum and transverse colon

12. A. What is the term for the three bands of muscle that pull the large intestine into pouches?

_____

B. These pouches, or sacculations, seen along the large intestine wall are called

_____.

13. What is an older term for the mucosal folds found within the jejunum? _____

14. Identify the structures labeled in Figs. 13.1 and 13.2. Include secondary names in parentheses where indicated.

Fig. 13.1

A. _____ (_____)

B. _____

C. _____

D. _____

E. _____ _____ (_____)

F. _____

G. _____ _____ (_____)

H. _____

I. _____

J. _____

K. _____

L. _____

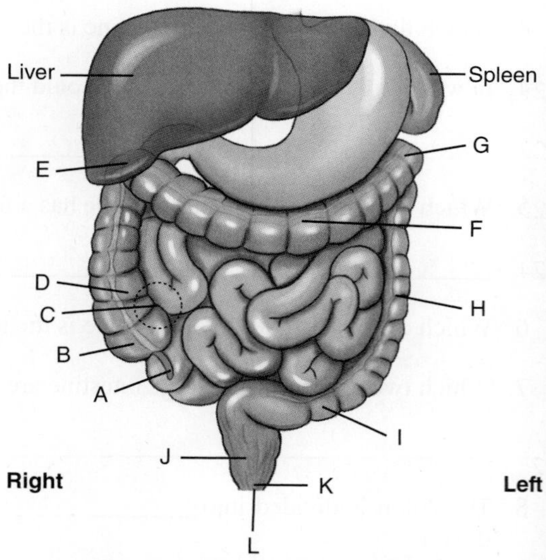

Fig. 13.1 Structures of the lower gastrointestinal tract, anterior view.

Fig. 13.2

M. _____

N. _____

O. _____

P. _____

Q. _____

R. _____

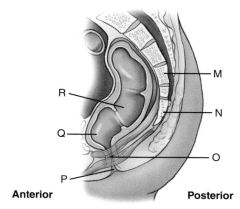

Fig. 13.2 Structures of the lower gastrointestinal tract, lateral view.

15. Which portion of the small intestine is located primarily to the left of the midline?

    _____

16. Which portion of the small intestine is located primarily in the right lower quadrant? _____

17. Which portion of the small intestine has the smoothest internal lining and does not present a feathery appearance when barium filled? _____

18. Which aspect of the small intestine is the most fixed in position? _____

19. In which quadrant does the terminal ileum connect with the large intestine? _____

20. Which muscular band marks the junction between the duodenum and the jejunum?

    _____

21. The widest portion of the large intestine is the _____.

22. Which flexure of the large intestine usually extends more superiorly? _____

23. Inflammation of the vermiform appendix is called _____.

24. Which of the following structures will fill with air during a double-contrast BE with the patient supine? (More than one answer may be correct.)

    A. Ascending colon   C. Rectum   E. Descending colon

    B. Transverse colon   D. Sigmoid colon

25. Which aspect of the GI tract is primarily responsible for digestion, absorption, and reabsorption?

    A. Small intestine   C. Large intestine

    B. Stomach   D. Colon

26. Which aspect of the GI tract is responsible for the synthesis and absorption of vitamins B and K and amino acids?

    A. Duodenum   C. Large intestine

    B. Jejunum   D. Stomach

27. Four types of digestive movements occurring in the large intestine are listed here. Which of these movement types also occurs in the small intestine?

    A. Peristalsis

    B. Haustral churning

    C. Mass peristalsis

    D. Defecation

28. Identify the GI structures labeled in Fig. 13.3.

    A. _____

    B. _____ (region)

    C. _____

    D. _____

    E. _____ (region)

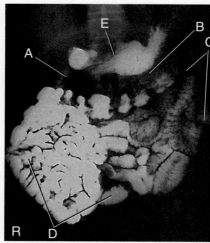

Fig. 13.3 Structure identification on a posteroanterior 30-min small bowel radiograph.

29. Identify the GI structures labeled in Fig. 13.4.

    A. _____

    B. _____

    C. _____

    D. _____

    E. _____

    F. _____

    G. _____

    H. _____

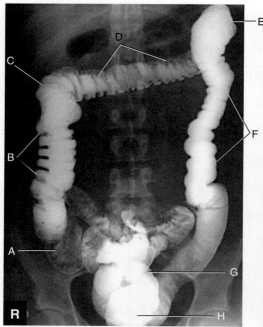

Fig. 13.4 Structure identification on an anteroposterior barium enema radiograph.

30. Classify the following structures as being intraperitoneal, retroperitoneal, or infraperitoneal.

_____ 1. Cecum   A. Intraperitoneal

_____ 2. Ascending colon   B. Retroperitoneal

_____ 3. Transverse colon   C. Infraperitoneal

_____ 4. Descending colon

_____ 5. Sigmoid colon

_____ 6. Upper rectum

_____ 7. Lower rectum

_____ 8. C-loop of duodenum

_____ 9. Jejunum

_____ 10. Ileum

REVIEW EXERCISE B: Clinical Indications and Radiographic Procedures for the Small Bowel Series and Barium Enema (see textbook pp. 506–524)

1. Which of the following conditions or factors pertains to a radiographic study of the small intestine?

    A. May perform as a double-contrast media study   C. Timing of the procedure is necessary

    B. May be performed as an enteroclysis procedure   D. All of the above

2. List the two conditions that may prevent the use of barium sulfate during a small bowel series.

    A. _____   B. _____

3. What type of patients should receive extra care when using a water-soluble contrast medium?

_____ and _____

4. Match the following definitions or statements to the correct clinical indications for the small bowel series.

_____ A. Common birth defect found in the ileum   1. Ileus

_____ B. Common parasitic infection of the small intestine   2. Neoplasm

_____ C. Obstruction of the small intestine   3. Meckel diverticulum

_____ D. Patient with lactose or sucrose sensitivities   4. Malabsorption syndrome

_____ E. New growth   5. Enteritis

_____ F. A form of sprue   6. Celiac disease

_____ G. Inflammation of the intestine   7. Regional enteritis

_____ H. Form of inflammatory disease of the GI tract   8. Giardiasis

5. Match the following pathologic conditions or diseases to the correct radiographic appearance.

_____ A. Circular staircase or herringbone sign		1. Adenocarcinoma
_____ B. Cobblestone appearance		2. Meckel diverticulum
_____ C. Apple core sign		3. Ileus
_____ D. Dilation of the intestine with thickening of circular folds		4. Giardiasis
_____ E. Large diverticulum of the ileum		5. Regional enteritis
_____ F. Beak sign		6. Volvulus

6. Giardiasis is a condition acquired through:
   A. Contaminated food
   B. Contaminated water
   C. Person-to-person contact
   D. All of the above

7. Meckel diverticulum is best diagnosed with which imaging modality?
   A. Small bowel series
   B. Enteroclysis
   C. Magnetic resonance imaging
   D. Nuclear medicine

8. Whipple disease is a rare disorder of the:
   A. Distal small intestine
   B. Proximal small intestine
   C. Proximal large intestine
   D. Distal large intestine

9. How much barium sulfate is generally given to an adult patient for a small-bowel-only series?

   _____

10. When is a small bowel series deemed complete? _____

11. How long does it usually take to complete an adult small bowel series? _____

12. When is the first radiograph generally taken during a small bowel series? _____

13. True/False: Fluoroscopy is sometimes used during a small bowel series to visualize the ileocecal valve.

14. The term *enteroclysis* describes what type of a small bowel study? _____

15. What two types of contrast media are used for an enteroclysis? _____

16. Which two pathologic conditions are best evaluated through an enteroclysis procedure?

   _____

17. True/False: It takes approximately 12 hours for barium sulfate in a healthy adult, given orally, to reach the rectum.

18. The tip of the catheter is advanced to the _____ during an enteroclysis.
   A. Duodenojejunal flexure (suspensory ligament)
   B. C-loop of duodenum
   C. Pyloric sphincter
   D. Ileocecal sphincter

19. What is the purpose of introducing methylcellulose during an enteroclysis? _____

20. A procedure to alleviate postoperative distention of a small intestine obstruction is called:

   A. Diagnostic intubation   C. Therapeutic intubation
   B. Enteroclysis   D. Small bowel series

21. What is the recommended patient preparation before a small bowel series? _____

22. Which position is recommended for small bowel radiographs? Why? _____

23. Match the following definitions or statements to the correct clinical indication for the BE procedure.

   _____ A. A twisting of a portion of the intestine on its own mesentery   1. Polyp

   _____ B. Outpouching of the mucosal wall   2. Diverticulum

   _____ C. Inflammatory condition of the large intestine   3. Intussusception

   _____ D. Severe form of colitis   4. Volvulus

   _____ E. Telescoping of one part of the intestine into another   5. Ulcerative colitis

   _____ F. Inward growth extending from the lumen of the intestinal wall   6. Colitis

24. Which type of patient most often experiences intussusception? _____

25. A condition of numerous herniations of the mucosal wall of the large intestine is called

   _____.

26. Which of the following pathologic conditions may produce a tapered or corkscrew radiographic sign during a BE?

   A. Diverticulosis   C. Volvulus
   B. Ulcerative colitis   D. Diverticulitis

27. Which of the following conditions may produce the cobblestone radiographic sign during a BE?

   A. Ulcerative colitis   C. Diverticulosis
   B. Appendicitis   D. Adenocarcinoma

28. What is one of the most common forms of malignant tumor found in the large intestine?

   A. Leiomyoma   C. Adenocarcinoma
   B. Basal cell carcinoma   D. Adenomas

29. True/False: Intestinal polyps and diverticula are very similar in structure.

30. True/False: Volvulus occurs more frequently in males than females.

31. True/False: The BE is a commonly recommended procedure for diagnosing possible acute appendicitis.

32. True/False: Any stool retained in the large intestine may require the postponement of a BE study.

33. Which four conditions would prevent the use of a laxative cathartic before a BE procedure?

    A. _____   C. _____

    B. _____   D. _____

34. True/False: An example of an irritant cathartic is magnesium citrate.

35. List the three types of enema tips commonly used (all are considered single-use and disposable).

    A. _____   C. _____

    B. _____

36. True/False: Synthetic latex enema tips or gloves do not cause problems for latex-sensitive patients.

37. What water temperature is recommended for BE mixtures? _____

38. To minimize spasm during a BE, _____ can be added to the contrast media mixture.
    A. Glucagon   C. Saline
    B. Lidocaine   D. Valium

39. Which patient position is recommended for insertion of the rectal enema tip?

    _____

40. The initial insertion of the rectal enema tip should be pointed toward the.
    A. Symphysis pubis   C. Umbilicus
    B. Bladder   D. Tip of coccyx

41. Which of the following procedures is most effective to demonstrate small polyps in the colon?
    A. Single-contrast BE   C. Enteroclysis
    B. Double-contrast BE   D. Evacuative proctogram

42. Which aspect of the large intestine must be demonstrated during evacuative proctography?
    A. Sigmoid colon   C. Anorectal angle
    B. Haustra   D. Rectal ligament

43. Which of the following clinical conditions is best demonstrated with evacuative proctography?
    A. Intussusception   C. Rectal prolapse
    B. Volvulus   D. Diverticulosis

44. Which of the following procedures uses the thickest mixture of barium sulfate?
    A. Single-contrast BE   C. Evacuative proctogram
    B. Double-contrast BE   D. Enteroclysis

45. Into which position is the patient placed for imaging during the evacuative proctogram?
    A. Anteroposterior (AP) spine   C. Ventral decubitus
    B. Left or right lateral decubitus   D. Lateral

46. True/False: A special tapered enema tip is inserted into the stoma before a colostomy BE.

47. True/False: The enema bag should not be more than 36 inches (90 cm) above the tabletop before the beginning of the procedure.

48. True/False: The technologist should review the patient's chart before a BE to determine whether a sigmoidoscopy or colonoscopy was performed recently.

49. True/False: Both CT and Diagnostic medical sonography (DMS) might be performed to aid in diagnosing appendicitis.

50. True/False: Because of the density and the amount of barium within the large intestine, computed radiography should not be used during a BE.

51. Which of the following statements is true regarding CT enteroclysis?

    A. A duodenojejunal tube does not have to be inserted for the procedure

    B. 0.1% barium sulfate suspension is often instilled before the procedure

    C. Does not detect obstructions of the small intestine

    D. Is rarely performed today

52. Another term for CT colonography (CTC) is _____.

53. True/False: A cleansing bowel prep is not required before a CTC.

54. Why is oral contrast media sometimes given during a CTC?

    A. To detect small polyps   C. To mark or "tag" fecal matter

    B. To detect bleeding outside the intestinal wall   D. Oral contrast never should be given before a CTC

55. What is the chief disadvantage of a CTC?

    A. Cannot remove polyps discovered during CTC

    B. Radiation dose to patient

    C. Inflating the large intestine with air may rupture the intestinal wall

    D. Procedure is painful for the patient

REVIEW EXERCISE C: Positioning of the Lower Gastrointestinal System (see textbook pp. 525–536)

1. True/False: Single-contrast BEs are performed commonly on patients who have a clinical history of diverticulosis.

2. Which of the following projections is recommended during a small bowel series?

    A. Supine AP   C. Erect AP

    B. Left lateral decubitus   D. Prone posteroanterior (PA)

3. True/False: A barium enema should not be performed on a pregnant patient unless absolutely necessary.

4. Because of faster transit time of barium from the stomach to the ileocecal valve in pediatric patients, how frequently should images be taken during a small bowel series to avoid overlooking critical anatomy and possible

   pathology? _____

5. True/False: If a retention-type enema tip is used, it should be removed after fluoroscopy is completed and before x-ray projections are taken to better visualize the rectal region.

6. The _____ position is a recommended alternative for the lateral rectum projection during a double-contrast BE procedure.

7. What kVp is recommended for a small bowel series (single-contrast study)? _____

8. Where is the CR centered for the 15-minute radiograph during a small bowel series?

   A. Iliac crest

   B. Xiphoid process

   C. 2 inches (5 cm) above iliac crest

   D. Anterior superior iliac spine

9. What are the breathing instructions for a projection taken during a small bowel series?

   _____

10. Generally, a small bowel series is complete after the contrast media reaches the _____.

11. Which type of patient habitus may require two recommended field sizes of 14- × 17-inch (35- × 43-cm) landscape alignment for an AP BE projection?

    A. Hypersthenic

    B. Sthenic

    C. Hyposthenic

    D. Asthenic

12. Which projection(s) taken during a BE best demonstrate(s) the right colic flexure?

    _____

13. How much body rotation is required for oblique BE projections?

    _____

14. Which position should be performed if the patient cannot lie prone on the table to visualize the left colic flexure?

    _____

15. Which projection, taken during a double-contrast BE, produces an air-filled image of the right colic flexure, ascending colon, and cecum? _____

16. Where is the CR centered for a lateral projection of the rectum? _____

17. Which projection during a double-contrast BE series best demonstrates the descending colon for possible polyps?

    _____

18. Which aspect of the large intestine is best demonstrated with an AP axial projection?

    _____

19. What is the advantage of performing an AP axial oblique projection rather than an AP axial?

    _____

20. A. What is another term describing the AP and PA axial projections? _____

    B. What CR angle is required for the AP axial? _____

    C. What CR angle is required for the PA axial? _____

21. Which position is recommended for the postevacuation projection taken following a BE?

    A. PA prone

    B. AP supine

    C. AP erect

    D. Left lateral decubitus

22. What kVp range is recommended for a postevacuation projection following a BE?

_____

23. A. What is the recommended kVp range for oblique projections taken during a single-contrast BE study?

    _____

    B. What is the recommended kVp range for oblique projections taken during a double-contrast study?

    _____

24. What medication can be given to minimize colonic spasm during a BE?

    _____

REVIEW EXERCISE D: Problem Solving for Technical and Positioning Errors

1. **Situation:** A radiograph of a double-contrast BE projection shows an obscured anatomic side marker. The technologist is unsure whether it is an AP or PA recumbent projection. The transverse colon is primarily filled with barium, with the ascending and descending colon containing a lesser amount. Which position does this radiograph represent?

_____

_____

2. **Situation:** A radiograph of a lateral decubitus projection taken during an air-contrast BE shows the upside aspect of the colon is overpenetrated. The following factors were used during this exposure: 120 kVp, 30 mAs, 40-inch (100-cm) SID, and compensating filter for the air-filled aspect of the large intestine. Which of these factors must be modified during the repeat exposure?

_____

_____

3. **Situation:** A radiograph of an AP axial BE projection of the rectosigmoid region shows there is considerable superimposition of the sigmoid colon and rectum. The following factors were used during this exposure: 120 kVp, 20 mAs, 40-inch (100-cm) SID, 35° caudad CR angle, and collimation. Which of these factors must be modified or corrected for the repeat exposure?

_____

_____

4. **Situation:** A BE study performed on a hypersthenic patient demonstrates that in the majority of the radiographs, the left colic flexure was cutoff. What can be done during the repeat exposures to avoid this problem?

_____

_____

5. **Situation:** A technologist has inserted an air-contrast retention tip for a double-contrast BE study. He is not sure how much to inflate the retention balloon. Should he inflate it as much as the patient can tolerate, or is there a better alternative?

_____

_____

6. **Situation:** A student technologist is asked to place the patient on the x-ray table in preparation for the tip insertion for a BE. Describe how the patient should be positioned.

_____

_____

7. **Situation:** A patient with a clinical history of regional enteritis arrives at the radiology department. What type of procedure would be most diagnostic for this condition?

_____

_____

8. **Situation:** A patient is referred to the radiology department for a presurgical small bowel series. What modification to the standard study needs to be made for this patient?

_____

_____

9. **Situation:** A patient comes to the radiology department for a small bowel series. However, because of a stroke, the patient is unable to swallow the contrast medium. What type of study should be performed for this patient?

_____

_____

10. **Situation:** An infant with a possible intussusception is brought to the emergency room. Which radiographic procedure may serve a therapeutic role in correcting this condition?

_____

_____

11. **Situation:** Before a BE, the technologist experienced difficulty inserting the enema rectal tip (without causing significant pain for the patient). What should the technologist do to complete this task?

_____

_____

12. **Situation:** During the fluoroscopy aspect of a BE, the fluoroscopist detects an unusual defect within the right colic flexure. She asks the technologist to provide the best images possible of this region. Which two projections will best demonstrate the right colic flexure?

_____

_____

13. **Situation:** A patient with a clinical history of possible enteritis comes to the radiology department. Which type of radiographic GI study would most likely be indicated for this condition? (Of course, this would have to be requested by the referring physician.)

_____

_____

14. **Situation:** A patient's clinical history includes possible giardiasis. What radiographic procedures would likely be indicated for this condition?

_____

_____

15. **Situation:** A patient is scheduled for a CTC. What is the recommended patient preparation for this procedure?

_____

_____

PART II: LABORATORY EXERCISES

You must gain experience in positioning each part of the lower GI before performing the following exams on actual patients. You can get experience in positioning and radiographic evaluation of these projections by performing exercises using radiographic phantoms and by practicing on other students (although you will not be taking actual exposures).

Laboratory Exercise A: Radiographic Evaluation

1. Evaluate and critique the radiographs produced during the previous experiments, additional esophagography and radiographs of lower GI procedures provided by your instructor, or both. Evaluate each projection for the following points (check off when completed).

_____ Evaluate the completeness of the study. (Are all of the pertinent anatomic structures included on the radiograph?)

_____ Evaluate for positioning or centering errors (e.g., rotation, off-centering).

_____ Evaluate for correct exposure considerations and possible motion. (Are the image receptor exposure and contrast of the images acceptable?)

_____ Determine whether markers and an acceptable degree of collimation is visible on the images.

338

Laboratory Exercise B: Physical Positioning

On another person, simulate performing all routine and special projections of the lower GI as follows. Include the six steps listed below and described in the textbook. (Check off each when completed satisfactorily.)

Step 1. Appropriate collimation field size with correct side markers

Step 2. Correct CR placement and centering of part to CR and/or IR

Step 3. Accurate collimation

Step 4. Area shielding of patient (when required)

Step 5. Use of proper immobilizing devices when needed

Step 6. Approximate correct exposure factors, breathing instructions where applicable, and initiating exposure

Projections	Step 1	Step 2	Step 3	Step 4	Step 5	Step 6
• PA 15- or 30-minute small bowel	____	____	____	____	____	____
• PA 1- or 2-hour small bowel	____	____	____	____	____	____
• PA or AP BE	____	____	____	____	____	____
• Right anterior oblique (RAO) and left anterior oblique (LAO) BE	____	____	____	____	____	____
• Left posterior oblique (LPO) and right posterior oblique (RPO) BE	____	____	____	____	____	____
• Right and left lateral decubitus	____	____	____	____	____	____
• AP and LPO axial	____	____	____	____	____	____
• PA and RAO axial	____	____	____	____	____	____
• Lateral rectum	____	____	____	____	____	____
• Ventral decubitus lateral rectum	____	____	____	____	____	____

This self-test should be taken only after completing all of the readings, review exercises, and laboratory activities for a particular section. The purpose of this test is not only to provide a good learning exercise but also to serve as a strong indicator of what your final evaluation exam for this chapter will cover. It is strongly suggested that if you do not get at least a 90%–95% grade on each self-test, you should review those areas in which you missed questions before going to your instructor for the final evaluation exam.

1. How long is the entire small intestine in the adult?

   A. 15–18 feet (4.5–5.5 m)

   B. 20–25 feet (6–7.5 m)

   C. 5–10 feet (1.5–3 m)

   D. 30–40 feet (9–12 m)

2. Which aspect of the small intestine is considered the longest?

   A. Duodenum

   B. Jejunum

   C. Ileum

   D. Cecum

3. Which aspect of the small intestine possesses the smallest diameter?

   A. Ileum

   B. Duodenum

   C. Cecum

   D. Jejunum

4. The part of the intestine with a feathery and coiled-spring appearance when filled with barium is the

   A. Ileum

   B. Duodenum

   C. Jejunum

   D. Cecum

5. List the two aspects of the large intestine not considered part of the colon.

   A. _____

   B. _____

6. What is the correct term for the appendix? _____

7. True/False: The rectum possesses two AP curves that have a direct impact on rectal enema tip insertions.

8. True/False: The small sacculations found within the jejunum are called haustra.

9. Which colic flexure (right or left) is located 1–2 inches (2.5–5 cm) higher or more superior in the abdomen?
   _____

10. What is the name for the band of muscular tissue found at the junction of the duodenum and jejunum?

    A. Valvulae conniventes

    B. Haustra

    C. Duodenal flexure

    D. Suspensory ligament of the duodenum

11. Identify the labeled structures on the following radiographs (Figs. 13.5 and 13.6). Include secondary names when indicated by parentheses.

Fig. 13.5:

A. _____

B. _____

C. _____

D. _____

E. _____

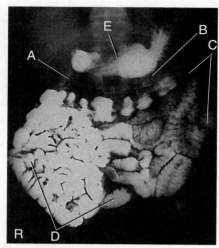

Fig. 13.5 Structure identification on a gastrointestinal radiograph.

Fig. 13.6

F. _____ _____ (_____)

G. _____

H. _____

I. _____

J. _____

K. _____

L. _____ _____ (_____)

M. _____

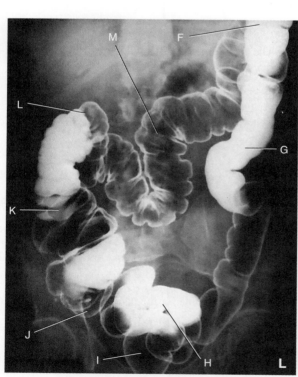

Fig. 13.6 Structure identification on a barium enema radiograph.

12. Which of the following structures is intraperitoneal?

    A. Descending colon

    B. Rectum

    C. Transverse colon

    D. Ascending colon

13. Where does the reabsorption of inorganic salts occur in the GI tract?

    A. Duodenum

    B. Large intestine

    C. Stomach

    D. Jejunum

14. Which of the following digestive movements occurs in the small intestine?

    A. Haustral churning

    B. Rhythmic segmentation

    C. Mass peristalsis

    D. Mastication

15. Match each of the following pathologic conditions to its correct definition.

_____ 1. Meckel diverticulum	A. Telescoping of the bowel into another aspect of it
_____ 2. Diverticulosis	B. A new growth extending from mucosal wall
_____ 3. Enteritis	C. A twisting of the intestine on its own mesentery
_____ 4. Whipple disease	D. Condition of small herniations present along the intestinal wall
_____ 5. Polyp	E. Chronic inflammatory condition of small intestine
_____ 6. Malabsorption syndrome	F. Outpouchings located in distal ileum
_____ 7. Diverticulitis	G. Unable to process certain nutrients
_____ 8. Volvulus	H. May be caused by cutting off blood supply to it or by infection
_____ 9. Intussusception	I. Inflammation of the small intestine
_____ 10. Crohn disease	J. Inflammation of small herniations in the intestinal wall
_____ 11. Ulcerative colitis	K. Caused by a flagellate protozoan
_____ 12. Giardiasis	L. Disorder of proximal small intestine
_____ 13. Appendicitis	M. Chronic inflammatory condition of the large intestine

16. Match the following radiographic appearances to the correct pathologic conditions.

_____ 1. A tapered or corkscrew appearance seen during a BE   A. Ulcerative colitis

_____ 2. Apple core lesion   B. Diverticulosis

_____ 3. String sign   C. Intussusception

_____ 4. Dilation of the intestine with thickening of the circular folds   D. Volvulus

_____ 5. Stovepipe appearance of colon   E. Regional enteritis

_____ 6. Mushroom-shaped dilation with a small amount of barium extending beyond it   F. Polyp

     G. Neoplasm

_____ 7. Jagged or sawtooth appearance of the intestinal wall   H. Giardiasis

_____ 8. Inward growth from intestinal wall

17. _____ is a group of intestinal malabsorption diseases involving the inability of absorbing certain proteins and dietary fat.

18. Which of the following imaging modalities/procedures is often performed to diagnose, and possibly treat, an intussusception?

A. BE   C. Nuclear medicine

B. Enteroclysis   D. CT

19. True/False: The BE is recommended to diagnose acute appendicitis.

20. Why is the PA rather than AP recumbent position recommended for a small bowel series?

_____

21. What is the minimum amount of time a patient needs to remain NPO before a small bowel series?

_____

22. What is another term for a laxative? _____

23. Which type of rectal enema tip is ideal for the patient with a relaxed anal sphincter?

_____

24. True/False: Natural latex–based gloves are safe to be worn by all technologists.

25. What drug can be added to the barium sulfate mixture to minimize intestinal spasm during a BE?

_____

26. What breathing instructions should be given to the patient during insertion of the enema tip?

_____

27. Which of the following disorders is best diagnosed during an evacuative proctogram?

    A. Regional enteritis

    B. Diverticulosis

    C. Volvulus

    D. Prolapse of rectum

28. Which type of health condition may restrict the use of glucagon during a BE?

29. Which region of the large intestine must be visualized during an evacuative proctogram study?

    A. Cecum

    B. Anorectal angle

    C. Ileocecal valve

    D. Left colic flexure

30. True/False: A small balloon retention catheter may be placed within the stoma of the colostomy to deliver contrast media during a BE.

31. Which oblique position, the LAO or the RAO, best demonstrates the ascending colon and right colic flexure?

    _____

32. What is the average length of time in a routine small bowel series for the barium to pass through the ileocecal sphincter (healthy adult)? _____

33. Which of the following commercial contrast media would be used during an evaluative proctogram?

    A. Hypaque

    B. Gastrografin

    C. MD-Gastroview

    D. Anatrast

34. How much rotation of the body is required for the LAO position during a BE? _____

35. The CR and IR should be centered approximately _____ higher for the 15- or 30-minute small bowel image than for the later images.

36. The term *evacuative proctography* is sometimes used for a lower GI tract procedure. This procedure is also

    commonly called _____.

37. **Situation:** A patient is unable to lie prone on the radiographic table during a BE. Which specific projection best

    demonstrates the right colic flexure? _____

38. **Situation:** A patient is scheduled for a double-contrast BE. During the fluoroscopy phase of the study, the fluoroscopist detects a possible polyp in the lower descending colon. Which specific projection best demonstrates this region of the colon?

    _____

    _____

39. **Situation:** A patient with a clinical history of a rectocele comes to the radiology department. Which radiographic procedure will best diagnose this condition?

    _____

344

40. True/False: A PA axial oblique (RAO) BE projection is an optional projection to demonstrate the right colic flexure.

41. True/False: For a hypersthenic type of patient, a field size of 14- × 17-inch (35- × 43-cm) in a portrait orientation and centered correctly generally includes the entire barium-filled large intestine on one IR.

42. What are the recommendations for performing a small bowel series or barium enema on a pregnant patient?

_____

43. A. The RAO projection best demonstrates the _____ (right or left) colic flexure with

the CR and IR centered to the level of _____.

B. The LAO projection best demonstrates the (right or left) colic flexure with the CR and IR centered to the level of

_____.

44. **Situation:** During a BE, a possible polyp is seen in the left colic flexure. Which of the following projections will best demonstrate it?

A. RPO   C. RAO

B. AP axial   D. PA

45. **Situation:** A patient has a clinical history of regional enteritis. Which of the following procedures is most often performed for this condition?

A. Intubation small bowel series   C. Enteroclysis

B. Single-contrast BE   D. Double-contrast BE

46. **Situation:** A patient comes to the radiology department with a clinical history of Meckel diverticulum. Which imaging modality is most often performed for this condition?

_____

47. **Situation:** A patient comes to the radiology department with a clinical history of giardiasis. She is scheduled for a BE procedure. Which of the following precautions must be followed during the procedure?

A. Wear gloves   C. Wear eye protection

B. Wear surgical mask   D. All of the above

48. True/False: The transit time of barium through the small intestine of the pediatric patient is usually less than that required for an adult.

13 Lower Gastrointestinal System

1. A. 15–18 feet (4.5–5.5 m)
2. C. Ileum
3. A. Ileum
4. C. Jejunum
5. A. Cecum
   B. Rectum
6. Vermiform appendix
7. True
8. False (in large inteswtine)
9. Left
10. D. Suspensory ligament of the duodenum
11. A. Duodenum
    B. Region of the ligament of Treitz
    C. Jejunum
    D. Ileum
    E. Pyloric portion of stomach
    F. Left colic (splenic) flexure
    G. Descending colon
    H. Sigmoid colon
    I. Rectum
    J. Cecum
    K. Ascending colon
    L. Right colic (hepatic) flexure
    M. Transverse colon
12. C. Transverse colon
13. B. Large intestine
14. B. Rhythmic segmentation

15. 1. F
    2. D
    3. I
    4. L
    5. B
    6. G
    7. J
    8. C
    9. A
    10. E
    11. M
    12. K
    13. H
16. 1. D
    2. G
    3. E
    4. H
    5. A
    6. C
    7. B
    8. F
17. Sprue
18. A. BE
19. False
20. Produces compression of the abdomen that leads to separation of the loops of the small intestine.
21. 8 hours
22. Cathartic
23. Rectal retention enema tip
24. False

25. Lidocaine
26. Hold breath on expiration
27. D. Prolapse of rectum
28. Diabetes
29. B. Anorectal angle
30. True
31. RAO position
32. 2 hours
33. D. Anatrast
34. 35–45°
35. 2 inches (5 cm)
36. Defecography
37. LPO position
38. Right lateral decubitus will drain excess barium from the descending colon, allowing for the detection of small polyps.
39. Evacuative proctography
40. False
41. False
42. Do not perform unless absolutely necessary
43. A. Right; iliac crest
    B. Left; 1–2 inches (2.5–5 cm) above the iliac crest
44. A. RPO
45. C. Enteroclysis
46. Nuclear medicine
47. A. Wear gloves
48. True

A1

14 Urinary System and Venipuncture

CHAPTER OBJECTIVES

After you have successfully completed the activities in this chapter, you will be able to:

_____ 1. Identify the location and pertinent anatomy of the urinary system to include the adrenal glands.

_____ 2. Identify specific structures of the macroscopic and microscopic anatomy and physiology of the kidney.

_____ 3. Identify the orientation of the kidneys, ureters, and urinary bladder with respect to the peritoneum and other structures of the abdomen.

_____ 4. List the primary functions of the urinary system.

_____ 5. Describe the spatial relationship between the male and female reproductive system and the urinary system.

_____ 6. On drawings and radiographs, identify specific anatomy of the urinary system.

_____ 7. Identify key lab values and drug concerns that must be verified before intravenous injections of contrast media.

_____ 8. Identify characteristics specific to either ionic or nonionic contrast media.

_____ 9. Describe the two categories of contrast media reactions and the symptoms specific to each type of reaction.

_____ 10. Differentiate among mild, moderate, and severe levels of systemic contrast media reactions.

_____ 11. Identify the steps and safety measures to follow during a venipuncture procedure.

_____ 12. List safety measures to follow before and during the injection of an iodinated contrast media.

_____ 13. Define specific urinary pathologic terminology and indicators.

_____ 14. Match specific types of urinary pathology to the correct radiographic appearances and signs.

_____ 15. List the purpose, contraindications, and high-risk patient conditions for intravenous urography.

_____ 16. Identify two methods used to enhance pelvicalyceal filling during intravenous urography and contraindications for their use.

_____ 17. Define a nephrogram.

_____ 18. Identify specific aspects related to the retrograde urogram and how this procedure differs from an intravenous urogram (IVU).

_____ 19. Identify specific aspects related to the retrograde cystogram.

_____20. Identify specific aspects related to the retrograde urethrogram.

_____21. List specific information related to the routine and special projections for excretory urography, retrograde urography, cystography, urethrography, and voiding cystourethrography to include collimation field size, central ray (CR) location, direction and angulation of central ray, and best visualization of anatomy.

_____22. Given various hypothetic situations, identify the correct modification of a position and/or exposure factors to improve the radiographic image.

POSITIONING AND RADIOGRAPHIC TECHNIQUE

_____ 1. Using a peer, position for routine and special projections for an IVU procedure.

_____ 2. Critique and evaluate urinary study radiographs based on the five divisions of radiographic criteria: (1) anatomy demonstrated, (2) position, (3) collimation field size and CR, (4) exposure, and (5) anatomic side markers.

_____ 3. Distinguish between acceptable and unacceptable urinary study radiographs based on exposure considerations, motion, collimation, positioning, or other errors.

LEARNING EXERCISES

Complete the following review exercises after reading the associated pages in the textbook as indicated by each exercise. Answers to each review exercise are provided at the end of the review exercises.

PART I: RADIOGRAPHIC ANATOMY

REVIEW EXERCISE A: Radiographic Anatomy of the Urinary System (see textbook pp. 538–544)

1. The kidneys and ureters are located in the _____ space.

    A. Intraperitoneal

    B. Infraperitoneal

    C. Extraperitoneal

    D. Retroperitoneal

2. The _____ glands are located directly superior to the kidneys.

3. Which structures create a 20° angle between the upper pole and the lower pole of the kidney?

    _____

4. What is the specific name for the mass of fat that surrounds each kidney? _____

5. What degree of rotation from supine is required to place the kidneys parallel to the IR?

    _____

6. Which two landmarks can be palpated to locate the kidneys? _____

7. Which term describes an abnormal drop of the kidneys when the patient is placed erect?

    _____

8. List the three functions of the urinary system:

   A. _____   C. _____

   B. _____

9. A buildup of nitrogenous waste in the blood is called:

   A. Hemotoxicity   C. Sepsis

   B. Uremia   D. Renotoxicity

10. The longitudinal fissure found along the central medial border of the kidney is called the _____.

11. The peripheral or outer portion of the kidney is called the _____.

12. The term that describes the total functioning portion of the kidney is _____.

13. The microscopic functional and structural unit of the kidney is the _____.

14. True/False: The efferent arterioles carry blood to the glomeruli.

15. What is another (older) name for the glomerular capsule? _____

16. True/False: The glomerular capsule and proximal and distal convoluted tubules are located in the medulla of the kidney.

17. Which structure of the medulla is made up of a collection of tubules that drain into the minor calyx? _____

18. Identify the renal structures labeled in Fig. 14.1.

    A. _____

    B. _____

    C. _____

    D. _____

    E. _____ (region)

    F. _____ (region)

    G. _____

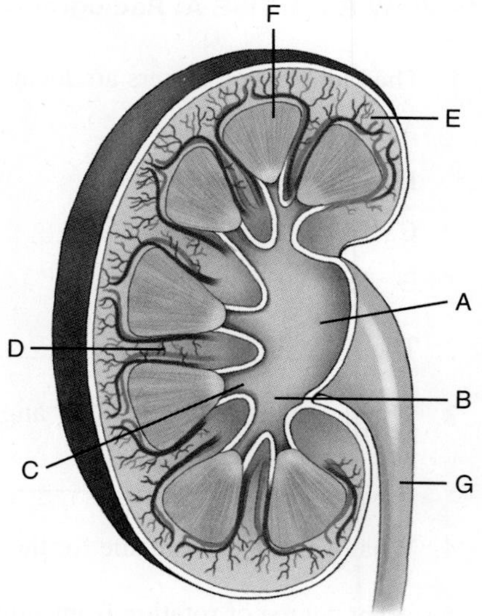

Fig. 14.1 Cross section of a kidney.

19. Identify the structures making up a nephron and collecting duct (Fig. 14.2). For each structure, indicate with a check mark whether it is located in the cortex or medulla portion of the kidney.

Structure	Cortex	Medulla
A. _____	_____	_____
B. _____	_____	_____
C. _____	_____	_____
D. _____	_____	_____
E. _____	_____	_____
F. _____	_____	_____
G. _____	_____	_____
H. _____	_____	_____
I. _____	_____	_____

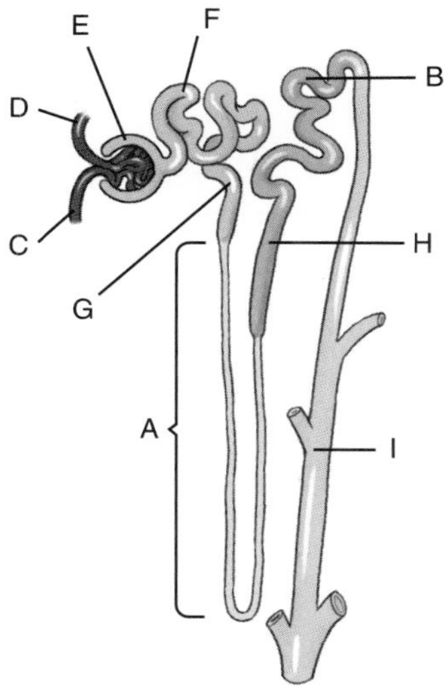

Fig. 14.2 Structures of a nephron and collecting duct.

20. Which two processes move urine through the ureters to the bladder?

A. _____   B. _____

21. Which of the following structures is located most anterior as compared with the others?

A. Proximal ureters   C. Urinary bladder

B. Kidneys   D. Suprarenal glands

22. What is the name of the junction found between the distal ureters and the urinary bladder?

_____

23. What is the name of the inner, posterior region of the bladder formed by the two ureters entering and the urethra exiting? _____

24. What is the name of the small gland found just inferior to the male bladder? _____

25. The total capacity for the average adult bladder is:

A. 100–200 mL   C. 350–500 mL

B. 200–300 mL   D. 500–700 mL

26. Which of the following structures is considered most posterior?

A. Ovaries   C. Vagina

B. Urethra   D. Kidneys

349

27. Identify the urinary structures labeled in Fig. 14.3.

A. _____

B. _____

C. _____

D. _____

E. _____

F. _____

G. _____

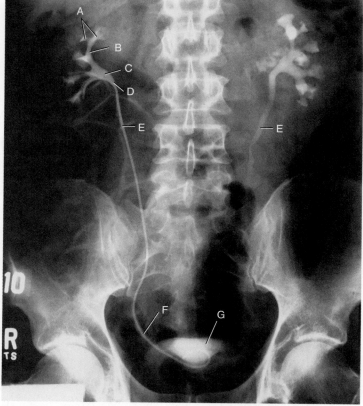

Fig. 14.3 Anteroposterior retrograde urogram radiograph.

PART II: RADIOGRAPHIC POSITIONING, CONTRAST MEDIA, AND PATHOLOGY

REVIEW EXERCISE B: Venipuncture (see textbook pp. 545–549)

1. Intravenous contrast media may be administered either by:

   A. _____ or _____

   B. _____

2. True/False: The parent (or legal guardian) must sign an informed consent form before a venipuncture procedure is performed on a pediatric patient.

3. For most IVUs, veins in the _____ are recommended for venipuncture.

   A. Iliac fossa

   B. Anterior, carpal region

   C. Axillary fossa

   D. Antecubital fossa

4. The most common size of needle used for bolus injections on adults is:

   A. 23–25 gauge

   B. 14–16 gauge

   C. 18–22 gauge

   D. 28 gauge

5. The two most common types of needles used for bolus injection of contrast media are

   _____ and _____.

6. In the correct order, list the six steps followed during a venipuncture procedure as listed and described in the textbook (pp. 547–549).

   1. _____

   2. _____

   3. _____

   4. _____

   5. _____

   6. _____

7. True/False: The bevel of the needle must face downward during the actual puncture into a vein.

8. True/False: If extravasation occurs during the puncture, the technologist should slightly retract the needle and then push it forward again.

9. True/False: If unsuccessful during the initial puncture, a new needle should be used during the second attempt.

10. True/False: The radiologist is responsible for documenting all aspects of the venipuncture procedure in the patient's chart.

REVIEW EXERCISE C: Contrast Media and Urography (see textbook pp. 550–554)

1. The two major types of iodinated contrast media used for urography are ionic and nonionic. Indicate whether each of the following characteristics applies to ionic (I) or nonionic (N) contrast media:

   _____A. Is a low osmolar contrast media (LOCM)

   _____B. Will not significantly increase the osmolality of the blood plasma

   _____C. Incorporates sodium or meglumine to increase solubility of the contrast media

   _____D. Creates a hypertonic condition in the blood plasma

   _____E. Is a high osmolar contrast media (HOCM)

   _____F. Produces less severe reactions

   _____G. Is a near-isotonic solution

   _____H. Poses a greater risk for disrupting homeostasis

   _____I. Uses a parent compound of an amide or glucose group

   _____J. May increase the severity of side effects

2. Which of the following compounds is a common anion found in ionic contrast media?

A. Diatrizoate or iothalamate

C. Benzoic acid

B. Sodium or meglumine

D. None of the above

3. Any disruption in the physiologic functions of the body that may lead to a contrast media reaction is the basis for the:

A. Homeostasis theory

C. Vasovagal theory

B. Anaphylactoid theory

D. Chemotoxic theory

4. The normal eGFR for adults is _____.

5. The normal creatinine level for an adult should range between _____ and

_____.

6. Normal blood urea nitrogen (BUN) levels for an adult should range between _____ and

_____.

7. A. Metformin hydrochloride is a drug that is taken for the management of _____.

B. The American College of Radiology recommends that metformin be withheld for _____
hours after a contrast medium procedure in patients with known acute renal injury, stage IV or V renal disease,
or an estimated glomerular filtration rate of <30 and resumed only if kidney function is again determined to be
within normal limits.

8. The leakage of contrast media from a vessel into the surrounding soft tissues is called

_____.

9. List the two general categories of contrast media reactions.

A. _____

B. _____

10. Which type of reaction is a true allergic response to iodinated contrast media? _____

11. Which type of reaction is caused by the stimulation of the vagus nerve by the introduction of a contrast medium,

which causes heart rate and blood pressure to fall? _____

12. True/False: Vasovagal reactions are not considered to be life threatening.

13. Matching: Match the following symptoms to the correct category of systemic contrast media reaction. (More than one symptom may apply to a type of reaction.)

_____ A. Brachycardia (<50 beats/min)

_____ B. Tachycardia (>100 beats/min)

_____ C. Angioedema

_____ D. Lightheadedness

_____ E. Hypotension (systolic blood pressure <80 mm Hg)

_____ F. Temporary renal failure

_____ G. Laryngeal swelling

_____ H. Cardiac arrest

_____ I. Mild hives

1. Mild

2. Moderate

3. Severe

14. True/False: Mild-level contrast media reactions do not usually require medication or medical assistance.

15. True/False: Urticaria is the formal term for excessive vomiting.

16. A temporary failure of the renal system is an example of a(n) _____ reaction.
    A. Mild
    B. Moderate
    C. Severe
    D. Local

17. Matching: For each of the following symptoms, identify the type (1–5) of contrast media reactions (responses may be used more than once).

_____ A. Convulsions

_____ B. Metallic taste

_____ C. Angioedema

_____ D. Bradycardia

_____ E. Itching

_____ F. Vomiting

_____ G. Temporary hot flash

_____ H. Respiratory arrest

_____ I. Pulmonary edema

_____ J. Extravasation

_____ K. Severe urticaria

1. Side effect

2. Mild systemic

3. Moderate systemic

4. Severe systemic

5. Local

18. What should the technologist do first when a patient is experiencing either a moderate- or a severe-level contrast media reaction? _____

19. What is the primary purpose of the premedication procedure before an iodinated contrast media procedure?

    _____

20. Which of the following drugs is often given to the patient as part of the premedication procedure?

    A. Epinephrine   C. Combination of Benadryl and prednisone

    B. Valium   D. Lasix

21. Which type of patient is a likely candidate for the premedication procedure before a contrast media study?

    A. Elderly patient   C. Pediatric patient

    B. Asthmatic patient   D. Patient with hypertension

22. In addition to notifying a nurse or physician when contrast media have extravasated into the soft tissues, what should the technologist first do to increase reabsorption?

    _____

23. True/False: Tissue inflammation from extravasated contrast media peaks 1–2 hours after the incident.

24. True/False: Acute renal failure may occur 48 hours after an iodinated contrast media procedure.

25. List 10 contraindications that may prevent a patient from having a contrast media procedure performed.

    A. _____   F. _____

    B. _____   G. _____

    C. _____   H. _____

    D. _____   I. _____

    E. _____   J. _____

REVIEW EXERCISE D: Radiographic Procedures, Pathologic Terms, and Clinical Indications (see textbook pp. 554–558)

1. A trademark name for a diuretic drug is _____.

2. A. Why is the term IVP incorrect when describing a radiographic examination of the kidneys, ureters, and bladder after the intravenous injection of contrast media?

    _____

    B. What is the correct term and correct abbreviation for the exam described in question A?

    _____

3. Which specific aspect of the kidney is visualized during an IVU? _____

4. Which of the following conditions is a common pathologic indication for an IVU?

    A. Sickle cell anemia   C. Hematuria

    B. Multiple myeloma   D. Anuria

5. Which of the following conditions is described as a rare tumor of the adrenal gland?

    A. Pheochromocytoma   C. Melanoma

    B. Multiple myeloma   D. Renal cell carcinoma

6. Matching: Match each of the following urinary pathologic terms to its correct definition.

_____ A. Pneumouria	1. Passage of a large volume of urine
_____ B. Urinary reflux	2. Presence of glucose in urine
_____ C. Uremia	3. Excess urea and creatinine in the blood
_____ D. Anuria	4. Diminished amount of urine being excreted
_____ E. Polyuria	5. Presence of gas in urine
_____ F. Micturition	6. Indicated by the presence of uremia, oliguria, or anuria
_____ G. Retention	7. Constant or frequent involuntary passage of urine
_____ H. Oliguria	8. Backward return flow of urine
_____ I. Glucosuria	9. Absence of a functioning kidney
_____ J. Urinary incontinence	10. Complete cessation of urinary secretion
_____ K. Renal agenesis	11. Act of voiding
_____ L. Acute renal failure	12. Inability to void

7. Match each of the following descriptions to the correct disorder.

_____ A. Enlargement of the prostate gland

_____ B. Fusion of the lower poles of kidneys during the development of the fetus

_____ C. Inflammation of the capillary loops of the glomeruli of the kidneys

_____ D. Artificial opening between the urinary bladder and aspects of the large intestine

_____ E. A large stone that grows and completely fills the renal pelvis

_____ F. Increased blood pressure to the kidneys resulting from atherosclerosis

_____ G. Normal kidney that fails to ascend into the abdomen but remains in the pelvis

_____ H. Multiple cysts in one or both kidneys

1. Vesicorectal fistula

2. Renal hypertension

3. Ectopic kidney

4. Horseshoe kidney

5. Staghorn calculus

6. Polycystic kidney disease

7. Benign prostatic hyperplasia (BPH)

8. Glomerulonephritis

8. Match each of the following radiographic appearances to the correct disorder.

_____ A. Rapid excretion of contrast media

_____ B. Mucosal changes within bladder

_____ C. Bilateral, small kidneys with blunted calyces

_____ D. Irregular appearance of renal parenchyma or collecting system

_____ E. Signs of abnormal fluid collections

_____ F. Abnormal rotation of the kidney

_____ G. Elevated or indented floor of bladder

_____ H. Signs of obstruction of urinary system

1. Malrotation

2. Vesicorectal fistula

3. Renal cell carcinoma

4. BPH

5. Renal hypertension

6. Renal calculi

7. Cystitis

8. Chronic Bright disease

9. A condition characterized by regions or areas of subcutaneous swelling caused by an allergic reaction to food or drugs is termed _____.

10. Contraction of the muscles within the walls of the bronchi and bronchioles, producing a restriction of air passing through them, is a condition called _____.

11. Loss of consciousness resulting from reduced cerebral blood flow is termed _____.

12. An eruption of wheals (hives), often caused by a hypersensitivity to food or drugs, is a condition termed _____.

13. What type of renal calculi is often associated with chronic urinary tract infections?

_____

14. True/False: The patient should void before an IVU to prevent possible rupture of the bladder if compression is applied.

15. What is the primary purpose of ureteric compression? _____

16. List the six conditions that could contraindicate the use of ureteric compression.

    A. _____   D. _____

    B. _____   E. _____

    C. _____   F. _____

17. When does the timing for an IVU exam start? _____

18. List the five-step imaging sequence for a routine IVU.

    A. _____   D. _____

    B. _____   E. _____

    C. _____

19. What is the primary difference between a standard IVU and a retrograde urography? _____

20. In which department are most retrograde urograms performed? _____

21. True/False: A retrograde urogram examines the anatomy and function of the pelvicalyceal system.

22. True/False: The Brodney clamp is used for male and female retrograde cystourethrograms.

23. Which of the following involves a direct introduction of the contrast media into the structure being studied?

    A. Retrograde urogram   C. Retrograde urethrogram

    B. Retrograde cystogram   D. All of the above

24. Which of the following alternative imaging modalities is *not* routinely used to diagnose renal calculi?

    A. Nuclear medicine (NM)   C. Magnetic resonance imaging (MR)

    B. Diagnostic medical sonography (DMS)   D. Computed tomography (CT)

25. True/False: Urinary studies on pediatric patients should be scheduled early in the morning to minimize the risk for dehydration.

26. True/False: The number of retrograde urography procedures for urethral calculi has been reduced as a result of the increased use of CT.

27. Exposure factors used during a CT procedure can be adjusted to compensate for a decrease or increase in body size

    according to _____ and _____.

28. True/False: A patient does not require extensive bowel preparation before a CT scan for renal calculi.

29. Which imaging modality is used to detect subtle tissue changes following a renal transplant?

    A. MR

    B. CT

    C. Radiography-IVU

    D. Nuclear medicine

30. True/False: Nuclear medicine is highly effective in demonstrating signs of vesicoureteral reflux.

REVIEW EXERCISE E: Radiographic Positioning of the Urinary System (see textbook pp. 559–573)

1. How will an enlarged prostate gland appear on a postvoid radiograph taken during an IVU?

   _____

2. Where should the pneumatic paddle be placed for the ureteric compression phase of an IVU?

   _____

3. What can be done to enhance filling of the calyces of the kidney if ureteric compression is contraindicated?

   _____

4. A retrograde pyelogram is primarily a nonfunctional study of the _____.

5. What are the four reasons a scout projection is taken before the injection of contrast media for an IVU?

   A. _____   C. _____

   B. _____   D. _____

6. What specific anatomy is examined during a retrograde ureterogram?

   A. Primarily the ureters

   B. Primarily the renal pelvis and calyces

   C. Entire urinary system

   D. Urinary bladder

7. Which specific position is recommended for a male patient during a voiding cystourethrogram?

   _____

8. What kVp range is recommended for an IVU? _____

9. True/False: There is a change in source–image receptor distance recommendations when placing a patient erect versus supine for an IVU anteroposterior (AP) projection.

10. True/False: The CR for an IVU anteroposterior (AP) projection is at the level of ASIS.

11. How is rotation determined on an IVU anteroposterior (AP) projection? _____

12. True/False: There is a smaller recommended collimation field size for a nephrogram compared to an AP scout.

    _____

13. At what stage of an IVU is the renal parenchyma best seen?

    A. 5 minutes after injection

    B. 10 minutes after injection

    C. After the postvoid projection

    D. Within 1 minute after injection

14. Where is the CR centered for a nephrogram?

    A. At the xiphoid process

    B. Midway between the xiphoid process and the iliac crest

    C. At the iliac crest

    D. At the axillary costal margin

15. Which specific position, taken during an IVU, places the left kidney parallel to the IR?

    _____

16. How much obliquity is required for the left/right posterior oblique (LPO/PRO) projections taken during an IVU?

    _____

17. Which position best demonstrates possible nephroptosis? _____

18. What CR angle is used for the AP projection taken during a cystogram?

    A. 20–25° caudad

    B. 5–10° cephalad

    C. 10–15° caudad

    D. 30–40° caudad

19. True/False: Contrast media should never be injected into the bladder under pressure but should be allowed to fill slowly by gravity in the presence of an attendant.

REVIEW EXERCISE F: Problem Solving for Technical and Positioning Errors

1. **Situation:** A radiograph of an AP scout projection of the abdomen, taken during an IVU, shows the symphysis pubis is cut off slightly. The abdomen is larger than the recommended collimation field size of 14 × 17 inches (35- × 43 cm). What should the technologist do in this situation?

    _____

    _____

2. **Situation:** A nephrogram is ordered as part of an IVU study. When the nephrogram image is processed, there is a minimal amount of contrast media within the renal parenchyma and the calyces are beginning to fill with contrast media. What specific problem led to this radiographic outcome?

    _____

    _____

3. **Situation:** A 45° RPO radiograph taken during an IVU shows that the left kidney is foreshortened. What modification is needed to improve this image during the repeat exposure?

    _____

    _____

4. **Situation:** An AP projection taken during the compression phase of an IVU shows the majority of the contrast media has left the collecting system of the kidneys. The technologist placed the pneumatic paddles near the umbilicus and ensured that they were inflated. What can the technologist do to ensure better retention of contrast media in the collecting system during the compression phase of future IVUs?

    _____

    _____

5. **Situation:** An AP axial projection radiograph taken during a cystogram shows the floor of the bladder is superimposed over the symphysis pubis. What can the technologist do to correct this problem during the repeat exposure?

_____

_____

6. **Situation:** A patient comes to the radiology department for an IVU. While taking the clinical history, the technologist learns the patient has renal hypertension. How must the technologist modify the IVU imaging sequence to accommodate this patient's condition?

_____

_____

7. **Situation:** A patient comes to the radiology department for an IVU. The AP scout shows an abnormal opacification near the lumbar spine that the radiologist suspects to be an abdominal aortic aneurysm. What should the technologist do about the ureteric compression phase of the study that is part of the procedure protocol?

_____

_____

8. **Situation:** A patient comes to the radiology department for an IVU. The patient history indicates he may have an enlarged prostate gland. Which projection will best demonstrate this condition?

_____

_____

9. **Situation:** A patient with a history of bladder calculi comes to the radiology department. A retrograde cystogram has been ordered. During the interview, the patient reports he had a severe reaction to contrast media in the past. What other imaging modality(-ies) can be performed to best diagnose this condition?

_____

_____

10. **Situation:** The same patient described in Question 9 may also have calculi in the kidney. What is the preferred imaging modality for this situation when iodinated contrast media cannot be used?

_____

_____

11. **Situation:** A patient comes to the radiology department for an IVU. As the patient's clinical history is being reviewed, it is discovered that he is diabetic. What additional question(s) should the patient be asked during the interview before the procedure?

_____

_____

12. **Situation:** During an IVU, the patient complains of a metallic taste and has a sudden urge to urinate. What action should the technologist take?

_____

_____

13. **Situation:** While reviewing the chart of a patient scheduled for an IVU, the technologist discovers that the BUN of the patient is 15 mg/100 mL with a creatinine level of 1.3 mg/dL and an eGFR of 90. Can this patient safely undergo an IVU?

_____

_____

PART III: LABORATORY EXERCISES

Although it is impossible to duplicate many aspects of urinary studies on a phantom in the lab, evaluation of actual radiographs and physical positioning is possible. You can gain experience in positioning and radiographic evaluation of these projections by performing exercises using radiographic phantoms and by practicing on other students (although you will not be taking actual exposures). Technologists must learn the positioning routine, room setup, and fluoroscopy procedure for their particular facility.

Laboratory Exercise A: Radiographic Evaluation

1. Using actual radiographs of IVU, cystogram, and retrograde urogram procedures provided by your instructor, evaluate each position for the following points (check off when completed).

_____ Evaluate the completeness of the study. (Are all pertinent anatomic structures included on the radiograph?)

_____ Evaluate for positioning or centering errors (e.g., rotation, off-centering).

_____ Evaluate for correct exposure factors and possible motion. (Is the contrast medium properly penetrated?)

_____ Determine whether patient rotation is correct for specific positions.

_____ Determine whether anatomic side markers and an acceptable degree of collimation is visible on the images.

Laboratory Exercise B: Physical Positioning

On another person, simulate performing all routine and special projections of the IVU as follows. Include the six steps listed below and described in the textbook. (Check off each when completed satisfactorily.)

Step 1. Appropriate collimation field size with correct side markers

Step 2. Correct CR placement and centering of part to CR and/or IR

Step 3. Accurate collimation

Step 4. Area shielding of patient (when required)

Step 5. Use of proper immobilizing devices when needed

Step 6. Approximate correct exposure factors, breathing instructions where applicable, and initiating exposure

Projections	Step 1	Step 2	Step 3	Step 4	Step 5	Step 6
• AP (recumbent and erect)	_____	_____	_____	_____	_____	_____
• LPO and RPO	_____	_____	_____	_____	_____	_____
• AP cystogram	_____	_____	_____	_____	_____	_____
• Lateral cystogram	_____	_____	_____	_____	_____	_____

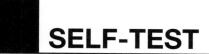

SELF-TEST

MY SCORE = _____ %

This self-test should be taken only after completing all of the readings, review exercises, and laboratory activities for a particular section. The purpose of this test is not only to provide a good learning exercise but also to serve as a strong indicator of what your final evaluation exam for this chapter will cover. It is strongly suggested that if you do not get at least a 90%–95% grade on each self-test, you should review those areas in which you missed questions before going to your instructor for the final evaluation exam.

1. The kidneys are _____ structures.
   A. Retroperitoneal
   B. Intraperitoneal
   C. Infraperitoneal
   D. Extraperitoneal

2. The ureters enter the _____ aspect of the bladder.
   A. Lateral
   B. Anterolateral
   C. Posterolateral
   D. Superolateral

3. The ureters lie on the _____ (anterior or posterior) surface of each psoas major muscle.

4. The kidneys lie at a _____ angle in relation to the coronal plane.

5. An abnormal drop of more than _____ inches, or _____ cm, in the position of the kidneys when the patient is erect indicates a condition termed *nephroptosis*.

6. The buildup of nitrogenous waste in the blood creates a condition called _____.

7. In 24 hours, how much urine do the kidneys normally produce?
   A. 2.5 L
   B. 180 L
   C. 0.5 L
   D. 1.5 L

8. The renal veins connect directly to the:
   A. Abdominal aorta
   B. Superior mesenteric vein
   C. Azygos vein
   D. Inferior vena cava

9. The 8 to 18 conical masses found within the renal medulla are called the _____.

10. The major calyces of the kidney unite to form the _____.

11. The microscopic unit of the kidney (of which there are more than 1 million in each kidney) is called the _____.

12. True/False: About 50% of the glomerular filtrate processed by the nephron is reabsorbed into the kidney's venous system.

13. True/False: The loop of Henle and collecting tubules are located primarily in the medulla of the kidney.

Chapter **14** Urinary System and Venipuncture: Self-Test

Copyright © 2025 by Elsevier Inc.
All rights reserved, including for text and data mining, AI training, and similar technologies.

14. The three constricted points along the length of the ureters where a kidney stone is most likely to lodge are:

    A. _____   B. _____   C. _____

15. The inner, posterior triangular aspect of the bladder that is attached to the floor of the pelvis is called the

    _____.

16. True/False: The retrograde ureterogram demonstrates the ureters, renal pelvis, and major and minor calyces.

17. Identify the structures labeled on this radiograph (Fig. 14.4).

    A. _____
    B. _____
    C. _____
    D. _____
    E. _____
    F. _____

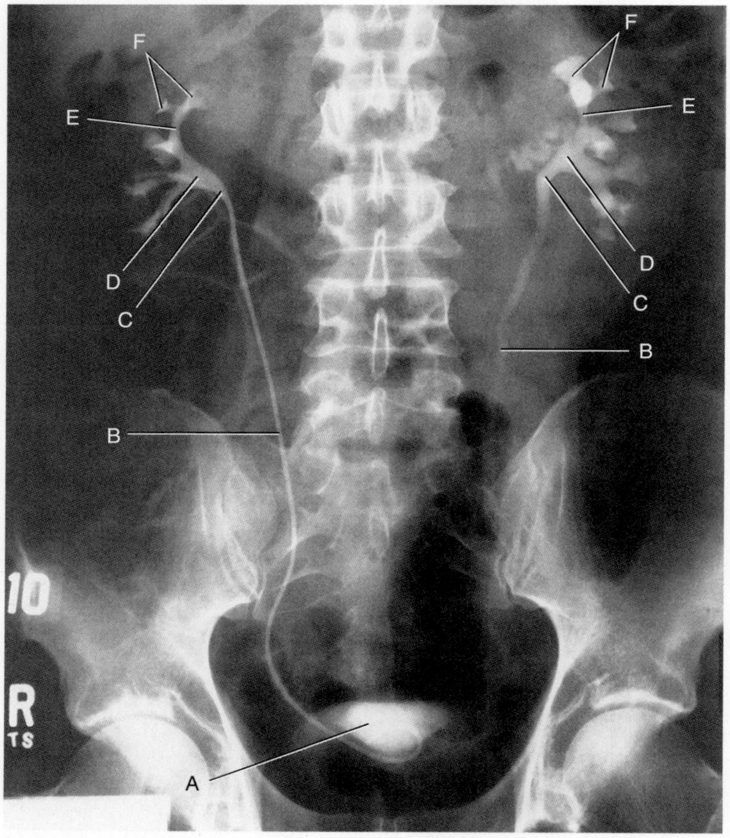

Fig. 14.4 Radiograph of the urinary system.

18. The term describing the radiographic procedure demonstrated on the radiograph in Fig. 14.4 is

    _____.

19. Under what circumstances should a pregnant patient have an IVU performed? _____

20. List the two classes of iodinated contrast media used for urinary studies. _____ and

    _____.

21. Match the following characteristics to the correct type of iodinated contrast media.

_____ A. Dissociates into two separate ions after injection   I. Ionic

_____ B. Possesses low osmolality   N. Nonionic

_____ C. Uses a salt as its cation

_____ D. Parent compound is an anion

_____ E. Is a high osmolar contrast media (HOCM)

_____ F. Produces a less severe contrast media reaction

_____ G. Diatrizoate is a common anion

_____ H. Does not contain a cation

_____ I. Creates a hypertonic condition in blood plasma

_____ J. Creates a near isotonic solution

22. The normal range of creatinine in an adult is:
    A. 2.0–3.4 mg/dL
    B. 0.6–1.5 mg/dL
    C. 8–25 mg/100 mL
    D. 0.1–1.25 mg/dL

23. How long must a patient with acute renal injury or an estimated glomerular filtration rate (eGFR) of ≤30 mL/min withhold from taking metformin after an iodinated contrast media procedure?
    A. 48 hours
    B. 2 hours
    C. 24 hours
    D. 72 hours

24. Hot flashes are classified as a:
    A. Side effect
    B. Local reaction
    C. Moderate systemic reaction
    D. Severe systemic reaction

25. Which of the following veins is not normally selected for venipuncture during an IVU?
    A. Basilic
    B. Cephalic
    C. Axillary
    D. Median cubital

26. At what angle is the needle advanced into the vein during venipuncture? _____

27. How long should the venipuncture site be cleaned with an alcohol wipe before needle insertion?
    A. 10 seconds
    B. 15 seconds
    C. 20 seconds
    D. 30 seconds

28. How high should the tourniquet be placed above the puncture site?
    A. 1–2 inches (2.5–5 cm)
    B. 3–4 inches (8–10 cm)
    C. 4–6 inches (10–15 cm)
    D. ½ inch (1.25 cm)

29. Which of the following conditions is considered high risk for an iodinated contrast media procedure?

A. Hematuria

C. Diabetes mellitus

B. Pheochromocytoma

D. Hypertension

30. What is the normal range for a patient's BUN?

A. 0.1–3.0 mg/100 mL

C. 5.0–7.5 mg/100 mL

B. 3.5–5.0 mg/100 mL

D. 8–25 mg/100 mL

31. What is the best course of action for a patient experiencing a mild systemic contrast media reaction?

A. Observe and reassure patient

C. Inform your supervisor

B. Call for immediate medical attention

D. Inform the referring physician

32. Which of the following is a symptom of a vasovagal reaction?

A. Itching

C. Cardiac arrhythmias

B. Angioedema

D. Urticaria

33. A true allergic reaction to iodinated contrast agents is classified as a(n):

A. Mild

C. Anaphylactic reaction

B. Vasovagal reaction

D. Local reaction

34. Tachycardia (>100 beats/min) is a symptom of a _____ type of reaction.

A. Side effect

C. Moderate systemic

B. Severe systemic

D. Local

35. Bradycardia (<60 beats/min) is a symptom of a(n) _____ type of systemic reaction.

A. Mild

C. Severe

B. Moderate

D. Organ-specific

36. Which of the following drugs may be given to minimize the risk for acute renal failure following a contrast media procedure?

A. Prednisone

C. Benadryl

B. Corticosteroid

D. Lasix

37. Metformin is a drug administered to patients with:

A. Sensitivity to iodine

C. Acute renal failure

B. Diabetes

D. Chronic renal failure

38. Which of the following drugs can be administered as part of the premedication protocol before an iodinated contrast media procedure?

A. Prednisone

C. Cipro

B. Zantac

D. Pentobarbital

39. Excretion of a diminished amount of urine in relation to the fluid intake is the general definition for:

A. Polyuria

C. Oliguria

B. Proteinuria

D. Nephroptosis

40. Constant or frequent involuntary passage of urine is termed:

A. Micturition

B. Urinary reflux

C. Retention

D. Urinary incontinence

41. The absence of a functioning kidney is called:

A. Renal agenesis

B. Renal failure

C. Nephroptosis

D. Oliguria

42. Complete cessation of urinary secretion by the kidneys is termed:

A. Micturition

B. Anuria

C. Urinary incontinence

D. Chronic renal failure

43. True/False: Adult forms of polycystic disease are inherent.

44. Hypernephroma is another term for:

A. Renal cell carcinoma

B. Wilms tumor

C. Hydronephrosis

D. Renal hypertension

45. Extravasation is classified as a _____ reaction.

A. Local

B. Mild

C. Moderate

D. Severe

46. Laryngeal swelling is classified as a:

A. Side effect

B. Mild level reaction

C. Moderate level reaction

D. Severe level reaction

47. True/False: Bladder carcinoma is three times more common in males than females.

48. Which of the following conditions may produce hydronephrosis?

A. Renal obstruction

B. Glomerulonephritis

C. Renal hypertension

D. BPH

49. Which of the following disorders is an example of a congenital anomaly of the urinary system?

A. Ectopic kidney

B. Pyelonephritis

C. Urinary tract infection

D. BPH

50. True/False: The patient should void before the IVU to prevent dilution of the contrast media in the bladder.

51. Which of the following conditions would contraindicate the use of ureteric compression?

A. Hematuria

B. Ureteric calculi

C. Urinary tract infection

D. Multiple myeloma

52. Typically, at what timing sequence during an IVU are the oblique projections taken? _____

53. Which projection(s) best demonstrate(s) the renal parenchyma? When should it (they) be taken?

54. Which procedure may require a Brodney clamp? _____

55. Which specific body position places the right kidney parallel to the IR? _____.

56. **Situation:** An AP projection taken during a retrograde cystogram shows that the symphysis pubis is superimposed over the floor of the bladder. What can be done during the repeat exposure to correct this problem?

_____

_____

57. **Situation:** Before the beginning of an IVU, the radiologist requests a nephrogram be taken as part of the study. At what point in the study should this projection be taken?

_____

_____

58. **Situation:** A patient comes to the radiology department for an IVU after abdominal surgery the day before. The IVU protocol requires that ureteric compression be used. What else can be done to achieve the same goal without using compression?

_____

_____

59. **Situation:** A radiograph of an RPO position taken during an IVU shows the left kidney is foreshortened and superimposed over the spine. What is the positioning error that led to this radiographic outcome?

_____

_____

14 Urinary System and Venipuncture

WORKBOOK SELF-TEST ANSWER KEY

1. A. Retroperitoneal
2. C. Posterolateral
3. Anterior
4. 30°
5. 2 inches; 5 cm
6. Uremia
7. D. 1.5 L
8. D. Inferior vena cava
9. Renal pyramids
10. Renal pelvis
11. Nephron
12. False (99% is reabsorbed.)
13. True
14. A. Ureteropelvic junction (UPJ)
    B. Near the brim of pelvis
    C. Ureterovesical junction (UVJ)
15. Trigone
16. False (primarily the ureter)
17. A. Urinary bladder
    B. Midureter
    C. Ureteropelvic junction (UPJ)
    D. Renal pelvis
    E. Major calyces
    F. Minor calyces
18. Retrograde pyelogram (note catheter in right ureter)
19. When the benefit of the procedure outweighs the risks of the radiation exposure
20. Ionic and nonionic
21. A. I
    B. N
    C. I
    D. I
    E. I
    F. N
    G. I
    H. N
    I. I
    J. N
22. B. 0.6–1.5 mg/dL
23. A. 48 hours
24. A. Side effect
25. C. Axillary
26. 20–45°
27. D. 30 seconds
28. B. 3–4 inches (8–10 cm)
29. B. Pheochromocytoma
30. D. 8–25 mg/100 mL
31. A. Observe and reassure patient
32. C. Cardiac arrhythmias
33. C. Anaphylactic reaction
34. C. Moderate systemic
35. C. Severe
36. D. Lasix (Furosemide)
37. B. Diabetes
38. A. Prednisone
39. C. Oliguria
40. D. Urinary incontinence
41. A. Renal agenesis
42. B. Anuria
43. True
44. A. Renal cell carcinoma
45. A. Local
46. D. Severe level reaction
47. True
48. A. Renal obstruction
49. A. Ectopic kidney
50. True
51. B. Ureteric calculi
52. 20 minutes following injection
53. Nephrogram; immediately after completion of injection
54. Retrograde urethrogram on a male patient
55. 30° left posterior oblique (LPO)
56. Angle the CR more caudally to project the symphysis pubis inferior to the bladder.
57. Between 30 seconds to 1 minute following the start of the bolus injection
58. Place the patient in a 15° Trendelenburg position during first aspect of procedure.
59. Overrotation of the body foreshortens the kidney and superimposes it over the spine.

15 Trauma, Mobile, and Surgical Radiography

This chapter has been divided into the following four sections:

1. Mobile X-Ray Equipment and Radiation Protection. Understanding the various types of mobile x-ray and fluoroscopy equipment used in trauma radiography (including use in surgery) is essential for technologists. Knowing and following safe radiation protection practices for workers around mobile equipment are especially important because of the unshielded environments in which mobile equipment is generally used (such as in the emergency room, in surgery, or in patients' rooms).

2. Trauma Positioning Principles and Fracture Terminology. Technologists should know the more common fracture terms included in this chapter to better understand patient histories and to ensure that the most appropriate projections are taken for demonstrating these fracture sites.

3. Trauma and Mobile Positioning and Procedures. This section describes specific positioning for each body part in which the patient cannot be moved from the recumbent position. Adaptation of central ray (CR) and image receptor (IR) placement as required is demonstrated and described for each body part.

4. Surgical Radiography. This section describes the role and responsibilities of the radiologic technologist in performing imaging in the surgical suite. Included are the following: essential surgical terminology, surgical radiographic equipment, various orthopedic fixation devices, and common surgical procedures that require radiographic support.

CHAPTER OBJECTIVES

After you have successfully completed the activities of this chapter, you will be able to:

_____ 1. Describe the two primary types of mobile radiographic units and their operating principles.

_____ 2. Explain the features, operating principles, and uses of mobile fluoroscopy units.

_____ 3. Describe the difference in exposure field levels with different orientations of the x-ray tube and intensifiers with the C-arm of a mobile fluoroscopy unit.

_____ 4. Explain why the anteroposterior (AP) projection orientation of the C-arm is not recommended.

_____ 5. Explain the three positioning principles that must be observed during trauma radiography.

_____ 6. Define and apply terms for specific types of fractures and soft tissue injuries.

_____ 7. List the projections taken for a postreduction study of the limbs, including open and closed reductions.

_____ 8. List projections for trauma and mobile procedures of the chest, bony thorax, and abdomen.

_____ 9. List projections for trauma and mobile procedures for various parts of the upper and lower limbs.

_____ 10. List projections for trauma and mobile procedures of the cervical, thoracic, and lumbar spine.

_____ 11. List trauma and mobile procedures for the skull and facial bones.

_____ 12. List the essential attributes of an effective surgical technologist.

_____ 13. Describe the role of the various members of the surgical team.

_____ 14. Differentiate between sterile and nonsterile environments in the surgical suite.

_____ 15. Define asepsis and describe methods and procedures to protect the integrity of the sterile environment.

_____ 16. Describe surgical attire that must be worn by the technologist before entering the operating suite, presurgical area, and recovery area.

_____ 17. Explain the preparation, cleaning, and safe use of radiographic equipment in surgery.

_____ 18. Describe common radiographic procedures performed in surgery, including required equipment, the role of the technologist, and surgical equipment and devices used during the procedure.

_____ 19. Match common surgical terms, orthopedic devices, and procedures to their correct definitions.

LEARNING EXERCISES

The following review exercises should be completed only after careful study of the associated pages in the textbook as indicated by each exercise. Answers to each review exercise are given at the end of this workbook.

REVIEW EXERCISE A: Mobile X-Ray Equipment and Radiation Protection (see textbook pp. 580–581 and pp. 610–612)

1. List the two primary types of mobile x-ray units.

   A. _____   B. _____

2. True/False: A fully charged battery-powered mobile unit has a driving range of up to 10 miles on level ground.

3. With battery-powered mobile unit types, how long does recharging take if the batteries are fully discharged?

   _____

4. Which type of mobile unit is lighter in weight? _____

5. What is the common term for a mobile fluoroscopy unit? _____

6. What are the two primary components of a mobile fluoroscopy unit (located on each end of the structure from which it derives its name)?

   A. _____   B. _____

7. Why should the mobile fluoroscopy unit not be placed in the AP projection ("tube-on-top" position)?

   _____

8. A. With the tube and intensifier in a horizontal position, at which side of the patient should the surgeon stand if he or she must remain near the patient—the x-ray tube side or the intensifier side?

   _____

   B. Why? _____

9. Of the two monitors found on most mobile fluoroscopy units, which is generally considered the "active" monitor—the right or the left? _____

10. True/False: The operator must determine image orientation on the mobile fluoroscopy monitors before the patient is brought into the room.

11. True/False: All mobile digital fluoroscopy units include the ability to magnify the image on the monitor during fluoroscopy.

12. A 30° C-arm tilt from the vertical perspective increases exposure to the head and neck regions of the operator by a factor of _____.

13. True/False: Automatic exposure control systems are not feasible with mobile fluoroscopy.

14. Name the feature that allows an image to be held on the monitor while also providing continuous fluoroscopy imaging and removing stationary structures from the viewing screen. _____

For Questions 15–19, review exposure field information in Figs. 15.1 and 15.2. (Also see the same exposure field drawings and charts in this chapter.)

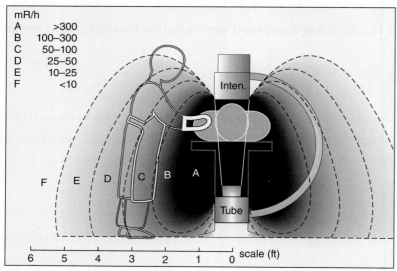

Fig. 15.1 Occupational exposure during mobile fluoroscopy, posteroanterior projection.

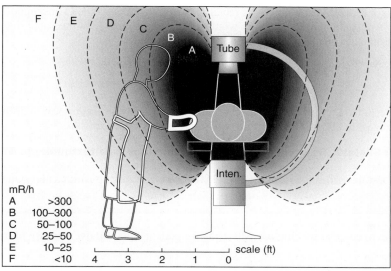

mR/h
A	>300
B	100–300
C	50–100
D	25–50
E	10–25
F	<10

scale (ft) 4 3 2 1 0

Fig. 15.2 Occupational exposure during mobile fluoroscopy, anteroposterior projection.

15. **Situation:** The C-arm is in position for a posteroanterior (PA) projection. What exposure field range would the operator receive at waist level standing 3 feet from the patient?

A. 20–25 mR/h

C. 50–100 mR/h

B. 25–50 mR/h

D. 100–300 mR/h

16. Approximately how much exposure at waist level would the operator receive with 5 minutes of fluoroscopy exposure standing 3 feet from the patient? (Hint: First convert mR/h to mR/min by dividing by 60; then multiply by minutes of fluoroscopy time.)

A. 5 mR

C. 25 mR

B. 60 mR

D. 2 mR

17. If a technologist receives 50 mR/h standing 3 feet from the mobile fluoroscopy unit, what would be the exposure rate if he or she moved back to a distance of 4 feet?

A. 10 mR/h

C. 100 mR/h

B. 25 mR/h

D. No significant difference

18. A technologist standing 1 foot from a mobile fluoroscopy unit is receiving approximately 400 mR/h. What is the total exposure to the technologist if the procedure takes 10 minutes of fluoroscopy time to complete?

_____

19. **Situation:** An operator receives 25 mR/h to the facial and neck region with the C-arm in position for a PA projection (intensifier on top). Approximately how much would the operator receive at the same distance if the C-arm were reversed to an AP projection position (tube on top)?

    A. 25–50 mR/h   C. 100–300 mR/h

    B. 50–100 mR/h   D. 300–500 mR/h

20. True/False: The intermittent mode used during mobile fluoroscopy procedures is helpful during procedures to produce brighter images, but it results in significantly increased patient exposure.

REVIEW EXERCISE B: Skeletal Trauma and Fracture Terminology (see textbook pp. 576–580)

1. Which single term best describes the primary difference between trauma positions and standard positioning?

   _____

2. What should be done to achieve specific projections if the patient cannot move because of trauma?

   _____

3. What is the minimum number of projections generally required for any trauma study?

   _____

4. How many joints must be included for an initial study of a long bone? _____

5. True/False: A follow-up postreduction radiograph of the middle portion of long bones should be collimated closely to the fracture region.

6. True/False: Digital radiography is well suited for emergency department (ED) and mobile procedures.

7. True/False: Nuclear medicine is effective in diagnosing certain emergency conditions such as pulmonary emboli.

8. True/False: For trauma patients who cannot be moved for conventional diagnostic imaging, other modalities, such as Diagnostic medical sonography (DMS) or nuclear medicine, may be used rather than trying to move the patient into specific positions.

9. What is defined as the displacement of a bone that is no longer within its normal articulation?

   _____

10. List the four regions of the body most commonly dislocated during trauma.

    A. _____   C. _____

    B. _____   D. _____

11. What is the correct term for a partial dislocation? _____

12. A forced wrenching or twisting of a joint that results in a tearing of supporting ligaments is a

    _____.

13. An injury in which there is no fracture or breaking of the skin is called a _____.

14. What is the term that describes the associative relationship between the long axes of fracture fragments?

    _____

15. Which term describes a type of fracture in which the fracture fragment ends are overlapped and not in contact?

    _____

16. A.   Which term describes the angulation of a distal fracture fragment toward the midline?

    _____

    B. Would this fracture angulation be described as a medial or a lateral apex? _____

17. What is the primary difference between a simple and a compound fracture? _____

18. List two types of incomplete fractures.

    A. _____   B. _____

19. Which type of comminuted fracture produces several separate wedge-shaped fragments?

    _____

20. What is the name of the fracture in which one fragment is driven into the other? _____

21. List the secondary name for the following fractures.

    A. Hutchinson fracture: _____

    B. Baseball fracture: _____

    C. Compound fracture: _____

    D. Depressed fracture: _____

    E. Simple fracture: _____

22. True/False: An avulsion fracture is the same as a chip fracture.

23. What type of reduction fracture does not require surgery? _____

24. Match each of the following types of fractures to its correct definition. (Use each choice only once.)

_____ 1. Greenstick   A. Fracture of proximal half of ulna with dislocation of radial head

_____ 2. Comminuted   B. Fracture of the base of the first metacarpal

_____ 3. Monteggia   C. Fracture of the pedicles of C2

_____ 4. Boxer   D. Fracture of distal radius with anterior displacement

_____ 5. Smith   E. Complete fracture of distal fibula, frequently with fracture of medial malleolus

_____ 6. Hutchinson   F. Fracture of lateral malleolus, medial malleolus, and distal posterior tip of tibia

_____ 7. Bennett   G. Incomplete fracture with broken cortex on one side of bone only

_____ 8. Avulsion   H. Fracture resulting in multiple (two or more) fragments

_____ 9. Depressed   I. Fracture of distal fifth metacarpal

_____ 10. Stellate   J. Intra-articular fracture of radial styloid process

_____ 11. Trimalleolar   K. Fracture of distal radius with posterior displacement

_____ 12. Compression   L. Indented fracture of the skull

_____ 13. Potts   M. Fracture resulting from a severe stress to a tendon

_____ 14. Colles   N. Fracture with fracture lines radiating from a center point

_____ 15. Hangman   O. Fracture producing a reduced height of the anterior vertebral body

25. A. Which specific named fracture does Fig. 15.3 illustrate? _____

    B. Which bone is most commonly fractured, and which displacement commonly occurs with this fracture?

    _____

    C. Describe the type of injury or fall that commonly results in this type of fracture.

    _____

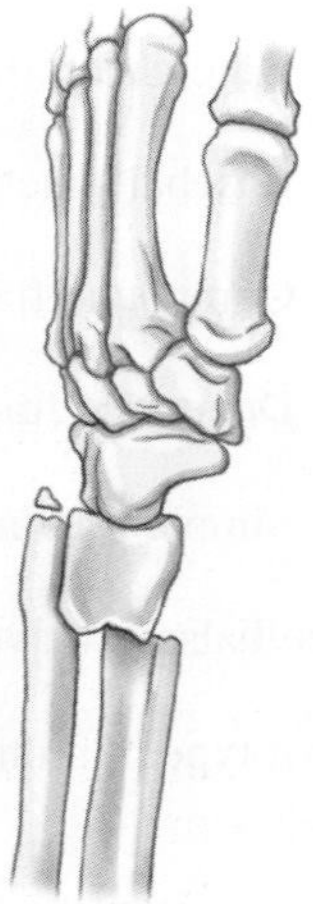

Fig. 15.3 Lateral wrist.

26. A. Which specific named fracture does Fig. 15.4 illustrate?

_____

B. Which bone(s) is (are) commonly fractured with this type of fracture?

_____

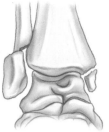

Fig. 15.4 Anteroposterior mortise ankle.

REVIEW EXERCISE C: Trauma and Mobile Positioning and Procedures (see textbook pp. 585–605)

1. How is the CR centered and aligned in relation to the sternum for an AP portable projection of the chest?

_____

2. A. A recommended collimation field size of 14 × 17 inches (35 × 43 cm) should be placed _____
   (landscape or portrait) for an AP portable chest on a sthenic or hypersthenic patient.

   B. Why? _____

3. True/False: Focused grids are recommended for mobile chest projections.

4. Which position can be used to replace the right anterior oblique of the sternum for the patient who cannot lie prone

   on the table but can be rotated into a semisupine position? _____

5. How must the grid be aligned to prevent grid cutoff when angling the CR mediolaterally for an oblique projection of
   the sternum when the patient cannot be rotated or moved at all from the supine position?

   _____

6. Other than the straight AP, what other projection of the ribs can be taken for the supine immobile patient who cannot

   be rotated into an oblique position? _____

7. Which of the following positions or projections best demonstrates free intra-abdominal air for the patient who cannot
   stand or sit erect?

   A. Left lateral decubitus   C. Right lateral decubitus

   B. AP kidneys, ureter, bladder (KUB)   D. Dorsal decubitus

8. Which of the following projections of the abdomen most effectively demonstrates a possible abdominal aortic
   aneurysm?

   A. Left lateral decubitus   C. Right lateral decubitus

   B. AP KUB   D. Dorsal decubitus

9. What is the disadvantage of performing a PA rather than an AP projection of the thumb?

_____

10. Which projections are taken for a postreduction study (casted) of the wrist? _____

11. True/False: A PA horizontal beam projection of the elbow can be taken for a patient with multiple injuries.

12. True/False: For a trauma lateral projection of the elbow, the CR must be kept parallel to the interepicondylar plane.

13. **Situation:** A patient with a possible fracture of the proximal humerus enters the emergency room. Because of multiple injuries, the patient is unable to stand or sit erect. What positioning routine should be performed to diagnose the extent of the injury?

_____

14. **Situation:** A patient with a possible dislocation of the proximal humerus enters the emergency room. Because of multiple injuries, the patient is unable to stand or sit erect. In addition to a routine AP projection, what second projection demonstrates whether the condition is an anterior or posterior dislocation?

_____

15. An AP oblique (scapular Y) projection taken AP supine for a trauma patient usually requires a _____-° rotation of the body away from the image receptor.

   A. 25–30   C. 50–60

   B. 45   D. 70

16. How much CR cephalic angulation should be used for an AP axial projection of the clavicle on a hypersthenic patient?

   A. 10°   C. 20°

   B. 15°   D. 25°

17. To ensure that the joints are opened up for an AP projection of the foot, how is the CR aligned?

   A. Perpendicular to the long axis of the tibia

   B. Perpendicular to the plantar surface

   C. 10° posteriorly from perpendicular to the plantar surface

   D. 10° posteriorly from perpendicular to the dorsal surface

18. **Situation:** An orthopedic surgeon orders a mortise projection of the ankle, but the patient has a severely fractured ankle and cannot rotate the ankle medially for the mortise projection. What can the technologist do to provide this projection without rotating the ankle?

_____

19. **Situation:** A patient with a possible dislocation of the patella enters the emergency room. What type of positioning routine should be performed on this patient that would safely demonstrate the patella?

_____

20. **Situation:** A patient with a possible fracture of the proximal tibia and fibula enters the emergency room. The routine AP and lateral projections are inconclusive. Because of severe pain, the patient is unable to rotate the leg from the AP position. What position or projection could be performed that would provide an unobstructed view of the fibular head and neck?

_____

377

21. To provide a lateral view of the proximal femur, which of the following projections would be performed on a trauma patient?

    A. Danelius-Miller method
    B. Fuchs method
    C. Waters method
    D. Ottonello method

22. How must the IR and grid be positioned for the inferosuperior (axiolateral) projection for the hip?

    _____

23. Which of the following projections demonstrates the odontoid process for the trauma patient who is unable to open the mouth yet can extend the skull and neck? (Subluxation and fracture have been ruled out.)

    A. Vertebral arch projection
    B. AP axial
    C. Judd method
    D. Fuchs method

24. **Situation:** A patient with injuries suffered in a motor vehicle accident enters the ED. The emergency room physician orders a lateral C-spine projection to rule out a fracture or dislocation. Because of the thickness of the shoulders, C6–C7 is not visualized. What additional projection can be taken safely to demonstrate this region of the spine?

    _____

25. **Situation:** A patient with a possible C2 fracture enters the emergency room on a backboard. The AP projection does not demonstrate C2. In addition, the patient cannot open his mouth because of a mandible fracture. Which projection can be performed safely to demonstrate this region of the spine?

    A. Swimmer method
    B. Judd method
    C. Vertebral arch projection
    D. 35–40° cephalad axial projection

26. Which projection will best demonstrate (with only minimal distortion) the pedicles of the cervical spine on a severely injured patient? _____

27. Identify the two CR angles for the AP axial trauma oblique projections of the cervical spine.

    A. _____ lateromedial
    B. _____ cephalad

28. True/False: A grid must be used with the AP axial trauma oblique projection for the cervical spine to reduce scatter radiation reaching the IR.

29. **Situation:** A patient with a possible basilar skull fracture enters the ED. The emergency room physician wants a projection that best demonstrates a sphenoid effusion. The patient cannot stand or sit erect. Which of the following projections would achieve this goal?

    A. AP skull
    B. Lateral recumbent skull
    C. Horizontal beam lateral skull
    D. Modified Waters projection

30. Which of the following projections of the skull would project the petrous ridges in the lower one-third of the orbits on a supine trauma patient?

    A. AP skull, CR 0° to orbitomeatal line (OML)
    B. AP axial, CR 15° caudad to OML
    C. AP axial, CR 15° cephalad to OML
    D. AP axial, CR 30° caudad to OML

31. True/False: The CR should not exceed a 30° caudad angle for the AP axial projection of the cranium to avoid excessive distortion of the cranial bones.

32. True/False: AP projections of the skull and facial bones will increase exposure to the thyroid gland as compared to PA projections.

33. How is the CR angled and where is it centered for the AP acanthioparietal (reverse Waters) projection of the facial bones?

_____

34. What type of CR angulation is required for the trauma version of an axiolateral projection of the mandible?

_____

35. **Situation:** A patient with a Monteggia fracture enters the emergency room. Which of the following positioning routines should be performed on this patient?

   A. AP and lateral thumb

   B. PA and horizontal beam lateral wrist

   C. AP and horizontal beam lateral lower leg

   D. PA or AP and horizontal beam lateral forearm

36. **Situation:** A patient with a possible greenstick fracture enters the emergency room. What age group does this type of fracture usually affect?

   A. Pediatric

   B. Young adult

   C. Middle age

   D. Elderly

37. **Situation:** A patient with a possible Potts fracture enters the emergency room. Which of the following positioning routines should be performed for this patient?

   A. AP and horizontal beam lateral lower leg

   B. PA and horizontal beam lateral wrist

   C. AP and lateral thumb

   D. Three projections of the hand

38. **Situation:** A patient is struck directly on the patella with a heavy object, and the patella is shattered. The resultant fracture most likely would be described as a:

   A. Burst fracture

   B. Compression fracture

   C. Stellate fracture

   D. Smith fracture

REVIEW EXERCISE D: Surgical Radiography (see textbook pp. 606–625)

1. List the four essential attributes of the successful surgical technologist.

   A. _____

   B. _____

   C. _____

   D. _____

2. Match the following roles to the correct member of the surgical team.

_____ 1. Scrub

_____ 2. Surgical assistant

_____ 3. Certified surgical technologist

_____ 4. Surgeon

_____ 5. Circulator

_____ 6. Anesthesiologist

A. Individual who assists the surgeon

B. Health professional who prepares the operating room (OR) by supplying it with the appropriate supplies and instruments

C. Individual who has the responsibility of ensuring the safety of the patient and monitoring physiologic functions and fluid levels of the patient during surgery

D. Individual who has primary responsibility for the surgical procedure and the well-being of the patient before, during, and immediately after surgery

E. Individual who prepares the sterile field, scrubs, and gowns for the members of the surgical team, and prepares and sterilizes the instruments before the surgical procedure

F. Individual who assists in the OR with the needs of the scrubbed members within the sterile field before, during, and after the surgical procedure

3. True/False: The technologist may violate the sterile environment in surgery if he/she is wearing sterile gloves, mask, and surgical scrubs.

4. True/False: The surgeon is responsible to maintain a safe radiation environment for all personnel in the OR.

5. True/False: The technologist has a moral and ethical responsibility to report any violations of the sterile field during surgery even if it was not noticed by another member of the surgical team.

6. True/False: Nonsterile items may be placed on the outer edges of a sterile field.

7. _____ consist(s) of the practice and procedures to minimize the level of infectious agents present in the surgical environment.

A. Asepsis

B. OSHA standards

C. Sterile practice

D. Surgical asepsis

8. Which parts of a sterile gown are considered sterile?

A. From the top of the shoulders to the knee

B. The sleeves and the waist region

C. The shoulders to the level of the sterile field, as well as the sleeve from the cuff to just above the elbow

D. The entire surgical gown

9. True/False: The entire OR table is considered sterile.

10. List the three measures that can be taken to maintain the sterile field when operating a mobile fluoroscopy unit in a surgical suite.

A. _____

B. _____

C. _____

11. True/False: Soft (canvas) shoes should be worn in surgery.

12. True/False: The pliable nose stripe on the surgical mask helps prevent the fogging of eyeglasses.

13. True/False: During most surgical procedures, the technologist is not required to wear protective eyewear.

14. True/False: Sterile gloves must be worn when handling a contaminated IR in surgery.

15. What type of equipment cleaner should not be used in surgery? _____

16. What is the primary disadvantage of using the "boost" feature during a mobile fluoroscopic procedure?

    _____

17. What is the primary advantage of using the "boost" feature during a mobile fluoroscopic procedure?

    _____

18. Which cardinal rule is most effective in reducing occupational exposure? _____

19. List the three terms describing the cardinal rules of radiation protection.

    A. _____   B. _____   C. _____

20. Which of the following measures is most effective (and practical) in limiting exposure with mobile fluoroscopy?
    A. Limit C-arm procedures to surgery cases only.
    B. Prevent nonradiologists from using the C-arm.
    C. Use intermittent or "foot-tapping" fluoroscopy.
    D. Limit all fluoroscopy procedures to no more than 10 minutes.

21. What anatomy is examined during an operative (immediate) cholangiogram? _____

22. What is the common name for the special tray device that holds the IR and grid during an operative

    cholangiogram? _____

23. How must the IR and grid be aligned if the OR table is tilted during an operative cholangiogram?

    _____

24. On average, how much contrast media is injected during an operative cholangiogram?

    _____

25. List the three advantages of laparoscopic cholecystectomy over traditional cholecystectomy.

    A. _____

    B. _____

    C. _____

26. Identify the anatomy of the biliary system labeled on this operative cholangiogram (Fig. 15.5).

A. _____

B. _____

C. _____

D. _____

E. _____

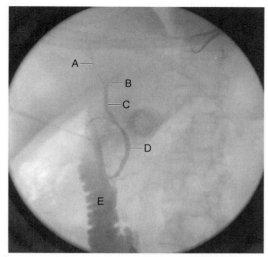

Fig. 15.5 Radiograph of an operative cholangiogram procedure.

27. A radiographic examination of the pelvicalyceal system only during surgery is termed:

A. Retrograde ureterogram

B. Antegrade pyelogram

C. Nephrostomy

D. Retrograde pyelogram

28. In what position is the patient placed during retrograde urography?

A. Left lateral recumbent position

B. Modified lithotomy position

C. Trendelenburg position

D. Reverse Trendelenburg position

29. Which of the following orthopedic procedures is considered nonsurgical?

A. Open reduction

B. External fixation

C. Closed reduction

D. Internal fixation

30. Which of the following orthopedic devices is classified as an external fixator?

    A. Intramedullary nail

    B. Cerclage wire

    C. Semitubular plate

    D. Ilizarov device

31. Which of the following orthopedic devices is often used during a hip pinning?

    A. Cannulated screw assembly

    B. Ilizarov device

    C. Kirschner wire

    D. Semitubular plate

32. Which of the following devices is often used to reduce femoral, tibial, and humeral shaft fractures?

    A. Intramedullary nail

    B. Cerclage wire

    C. Ilizarov device

    D. Compression screw

33. What is the name of the newer type of prosthetic device to replace a defective hip joint?

_____

34. A surgical procedure, performed to alleviate pain caused by bony neural impingement involving the spine, is termed

_____.

35. What is the name of the device used to stabilize the vertebral body in lieu of traditional spinal fusion?

_____

36. In what position is the patient placed during most cervical laminectomies? _____

37. List the two internal fixators commonly used during scoliosis surgery.

    A. _____   B. _____

38. Match each of the following surgical terms and devices to its correct definition.

_____ A. Orthopedic wire that tightens around the fracture site to reduce shortening of limb

_____ B. Narrow orthopedic screw designed to enter and fix cortical bone

_____ C. Large screw used in internal fixation of nondisplaced fractures of proximal femur

_____ D. Fabricated (artificial) substitute for a diseased or missing anatomic part

_____ E. Isolation drape that separates the sterile field from the nonsterile environment

_____ F. Soaking of moisture through a sterile or nonsterile drape, cover, or protective barrier

_____ G. Unthreaded (smooth) or threaded metallic wire used to reduce fractures of wrist (carpals) and individual bones of the hands and feet

_____ H. Orthopedic screw designed to enter and fix porous and spongy bone

_____ I. Creation of an artificial joint to correct ankyloses

_____ J. Electrohydraulic shock waves used to break apart calcifications in the urinary system

1. Arthroplasty

2. Cancellous screw

3. Cannulated screw

4. Cerclage wire

5. Cortical screw

6. ESWL

7. Kirschner wire

8. Prosthesis

9. Shower curtain

10. Strike through

39. Which type of pathology is addressed through a vertebroplasty?

A. Compression fracture of the vertebral body

B. Herniated intervertebral disk

C. Scoliosis

D. Spondylolysis

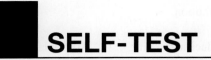
Directions: This self-test should be taken only after completing all of the readings, review exercises, and laboratory activities for a particular section. The purpose of this test is not only to provide a good learning exercise but also to serve as a strong indicator of what your final evaluation exam will be. It is strongly suggested that if you do not receive at least a 90%–95% grade on this self-test, you should review those areas in which you missed questions before going to your instructor for the final evaluation exam for this chapter.

1. From the list of possible fracture types listed here, indicate which fracture is represented on each drawing or radiograph by writing in the correct term where indicated (A–I):

   - Single (closed) fracture
   - Compound (open) fracture
   - Torus fracture
   - Greenstick fracture
   - Plastic fracture
   - Transverse fracture
   - Oblique fracture
   - Spiral fracture
   - Comminuted fracture
   - Impacted fracture
   - Baseball (mallet) fracture
   - Barton fracture
   - Bennett fracture
   - Colles fracture
   - Monteggia fracture
   - Nursemaid elbow fracture
   - Potts fracture
   - Avulsion fracture
   - Chip fracture
   - Compression fracture
   - Stellate fracture
   - Tuft fracture

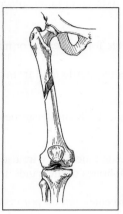

A. _____

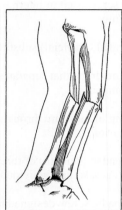

B. _____

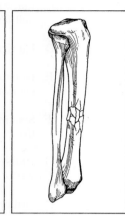

C. _____

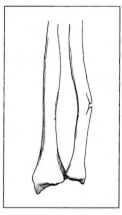

D. _____

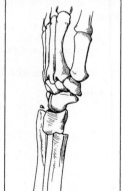

E. _____

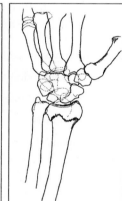

F. _____

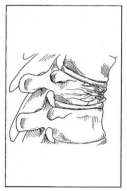

G. _____

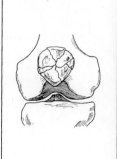

H. _____

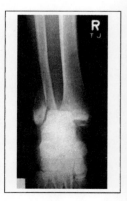

I. _____

385

2. A battery-powered, battery-operated mobile x-ray unit can climb a maximum incline of:

    A. 7°   C. 12°

    B. 10°   D. 15°

3. Which type of mobile radiography x-ray unit is self-propelled? _____

4. Which type of mobile x-ray unit is lighter weight? _____

5. True/False: C-arms are most generally stationary fluoroscopy units used in surgery.

6. True/False: The C-arm fluoroscopy unit can be rotated a maximum of 180°.

7. True/False: The AP projection with the x-ray tube placed directly above the anatomy during a C-arm procedure is recommended to minimize OID.

8. True/False: Digital C-arm units can store images on videotape or computer hard disk memory.

9. What is the term for the process of holding one image on the C-arm monitor while also providing continuous

    fluoroscopy? _____

10. Match each of the following fracture types to its correct definition (using each answer only once):

    _____ A. Fracture through the pedicles of C2   1. Nursemaid elbow

    _____ B. Fracture of proximal half of ulna with dislocation of radial head   2. Bennett

    _____ C. Fracture resulting from a disease process   3. Baseball

    _____ D. Fracture resulting in an isolated bone fragment   4. Pathologic

    _____ E. Subluxation of the radial head on a child   5. Hangman

    _____ F. Fracture along base of first metacarpal   6. Hutchinson

    _____ G. Fracture of distal phalanx with finger extended   7. Stress or fatigue

    _____ H. Also called a March fracture   8. Chip

    _____ I. Also called a chauffeur fracture   9. Monteggia

11. True/False: Any trauma study requires at least two projections as close as possible to 90° opposite from each other.

12. True/False: On an initial study of a long bone, both joints should be included for each projection.

13. True/False: Collimation on trauma cases can lead to cutoff of key anatomy and pathology, therefore it should be limited to the size of the IR.

14. The technologist must be at least _____ from the x-ray tube during a mobile radiographic procedure.

    A. 2 feet (0.6 m)   C. 6 feet (1.8 m)

    B. 4 feet (1.3 m)   D. 8 feet (2.4 m)

15. True/False: Wearing a protective lead apron is optional if the technologist is at least 8 feet (2.4 m) from both the x-ray tube and the patient during a mobile radiographic procedure.

16. True/False: The exposure dose is greater on the image intensifier side than on the x-ray tube side with the C-arm in the horizontal configuration.

17. True/False: A 30° tilt of the C-arm from the vertical perspective increases the dose by a factor of three to the head and neck region.

18. What final step should the technologist take before returning a trauma patient to the emergency room following a radiographic procedure?

    A. Review patient history

    B. Review examination requisition

    C. Check patient armband/identification

    D. Ensure side rails are up on the patient cart

19. True/False: The number of angiographies of the aortic arch for the trauma patient has declined because of the increased use of CT angiography.

20. A. What is the correct term for the displacement of a bone from a joint? _____

    B. What is the correct term for a partial displacement? _____

21. Which of the following fracture terms describes a situation in which the ends of fragments are aligned but are pulled apart and are not in contact with each other?

    A. Dislocation

    B. Lack of apposition

    C. Apex angulation

    D. Anatomic apposition

22. Which of the following fracture terms describes an angulation of a distal fracture end away from the midline?

    A. Valgus deformity

    B. Varus deformity

    C. Apex angulation

    D. Bayonet apposition

23. What is the primary source of radiation exposure to the technologist while using a C-arm? _____

24. **Situation:** A technologist receives 30 mR/h during a C-arm fluoroscopic procedure. What is the total exposure dose if the procedure takes 8 minutes of fluoroscopy time? _____

25. Radiologists often use the Salter-Harris system to classify _____ fractures.

    A. Pathologic

    B. Trimalleolar

    C. Stellate

    D. Epiphyseal

26. **Situation:** A patient with a possible pleural effusion in the right lung enters the emergency room. The patient is unable to stand or sit erect. What position would best demonstrate this condition?

    A. Right lateral decubitus

    B. AP supine

    C. Dorsal decubitus

    D. Semierect AP

27. Where is the CR centered for an AP semierect projection of the chest? _____

28. **Situation:** A patient with a crushing injury to the thorax enters the emergency room. The patient is on a backboard and cannot be moved. Which projections can be performed to determine whether the sternum is fractured?

29. **Situation:** A patient with possible ascites enters the emergency room. The patient is unable to stand or sit erect. Which of the following positions would best demonstrate this condition?

   A. AP supine KUB

   B. Dorsal decubitus

   C. Left lateral decubitus

   D. Prone KUB

30. What is the minimum number of projections required for a postreduction study of the wrist? _____

31. How is the CR aligned for a trauma lateral projection of the elbow? _____

32. Which lateral projection would best demonstrate the mid-to-distal humerus without rotating the limb?

   _____

33. How much rotation of the body, from a supine position, is generally required for a lateromedial scapula projection

   with a trauma patient who can be turned partially on her side? _____

34. To ensure that the CR is aligned properly for an AP trauma projection of the foot, the CR is angled

   _____.

35. **Situation:** A patient with a possible fracture of the ankle enters the emergency room. The patient cannot rotate the lower limb. What can be done to provide the orthopedic surgeon with a mortise projection of the ankle?

   _____

36. **Situation:** Following a postreduction of a fractured tibia/fibula, a postreduction study is ordered. A fiberglass cast was placed on the fractured leg. The original technique was 70 kVp at 4 mAs (analog system). Would the technologist be required to change their factors from the original technique?

   _____

37. Which of the following projections demonstrates the C1–C2 vertebra if the patient cannot open his mouth?

   A. 35–40° cephalad, AP axial projection

   B. Swimmer's lateral

   C. 15–20° cephalad, AP axial projection

   D. Articular pillar projection

38. **Situation:** A patient with a possible fracture of the cervical spine pedicles enters the emergency room. Which of the following projections will best demonstrate this region of the spine without moving the patient?

   A. Perform a swimmer's lateral

   B. Perform an articular pillar projection

   C. Perform a Fuchs method

   D. Perform AP axial trauma oblique projections

39. What is the name of the device that is designed for 2D fluoroscopic and 3D imaging?

   A. C-arm

   B. O-arm

   C. Portable x-ray unit

   D. PACS

40. Which of the following facial bone projections will best demonstrate air-fluid levels in the maxillary sinuses for a patient unable to stand or sit erect?

    A. AP acanthioparietal

    B. Trauma, horizontal beam lateral

    C. AP modified acanthioparietal

    D. AP axial

41. A. On a horizontal beam lateral trauma skull projection, should the IR be placed portrait or landscape to the patient?

    _____

    B. Where should the CR be centered for this lateral skull projection? _____

42. **Situation:** A patient with a possible compression fracture of the lumbar spine enters the emergency room. Which specific projection of the lumbar spine series would best demonstrate this fracture?

    A. AP

    B. Left posterior oblique (LPO) and right posterior oblique (RPO)

    C. Lateral

    D. AP L5–S1 projection

43. **Situation:** A patient with a possible Barton fracture comes to the radiology department. Which of the following positioning routines would best demonstrate this?

    A. AP or PA and lateral wrist

    B. AP, mortise, and lateral ankle

    C. AP and lateral foot

    D. AP and lateral lower leg

44. **Situation:** A patient enters the emergency room with a possible radial head dislocation. The arm is immobilized with the elbow flexed at 90°. Which of the following projections best demonstrates the radial head free of superimposition of the ulna without having to extend the elbow?

    A. AP partial flexion

    B. Trauma axiolateral projection

    C. Jones method

    D. Lateromedial projection

45. For successful surgical radiographic exposures, clear communication must be established among the surgeon, technologist, and:

    A. Scrub

    B. CST

    C. Circulator

    D. Anesthesiologist

46. CST is the acronym for _____.

47. Suctioning, tying, and clamping blood vessels, as well as assisting in cutting and suturing tissues, are the general duties of the:

    A. CST

    B. Circulator

    C. Surgical assistant

    D. Scrub

48. The absence of infectious organisms is the definition for:

    A. Surgical cleanliness

    B. Sepsis

    C. Asepsis

    D. Surgical sterility

49. What portion(s) of the OR table is (are) considered sterile?

    A. Only the level of the tabletop

    B. Entire table

    C. Tabletop and half of the base

    D. None of the table

50. True/False: Scrubs worn in radiology may be also worn in surgery.

51. True/False: Scrub covers must be removed before entering the surgical suite.

52. True/False: The technologist can wear nonsterile gloves when handling the IR and surgical cover following a procedure.

53. Imaging equipment permanently stored in surgery must be cleaned at least:

    A. Daily   C. Monthly

    B. Bimonthly   D. Weekly

54. Which of the following techniques best reduces the dose to the surgical team during a C-arm procedure?

    A. Use boost function whenever possible   C. Use intermittent fluoroscopy

    B. Place tube in vertical position above patient   D. Lower kVp as much as possible

55. What is the primary benefit of the "pulse mode" on a digital C-arm unit? _____

56. **Situation:** An image taken during an operative cholangiogram shows that the biliary ducts are superimposed over the spine. The surgeon wants the ducts projected away from the spine. Which of the following positions may eliminate this problem during the repeat exposure?

    A. Shallow RPO   C. AP

    B. Shallow LPO   D. Horizontal beam lateral

57. True/False: Laparoscopic cholecystectomy is not suited for every patient and condition.

58. Retrograde urography is a _____ (nonfunctional or functional) examination of the urinary system.

59. A retrograde pyelogram is a specific radiographic examination of the _____ system.

60. ORIF is the abbreviation for _____.

61. Which of the following devices helps maintain the sterile environment in surgery during a C-arm–guided hip pinning?

    A. Shower curtain   C. Cassette cover

    B. Mylar shield   D. Good cleaning of equipment before procedure

62. Which of the following orthopedic devices is used to stabilize a midfemoral shaft fracture?

    A. Austin Moore prosthesis   C. Interbody fusion cages

    B. Intramedullary rod   D. Cannulated screw

63. Which of the following devices is an example of an external fixator?

    A. Interbody fusion cage   C. Modular bipolar prosthesis

    B. Thompson prosthesis   D. Ilizarov device

64. Which of the following procedures does not require the use of mobile fluoroscopy?

    A. Hip pinning

    B. Intramedullary rod insertion

    C. Open reduction of tibia

    D. All of the above require fluoroscopic guidance

65. Which of the following devices can be used for spinal fusion surgery rather than the use of a pedicle screw?

    A. Austin Moore prosthesis

    B. Cannulated screw

    C. Dynamic compression plate

    D. Interbody fusion cage

66. Which spinal procedure may require the use of Harrington or Luque rods?

    A. Scoliosis corrective surgery

    B. Microdiscectomy

    C. Spinal fusion

    D. All of the above

67. An unthreaded (smooth) or threaded metallic wire, used to reduce fractures of the wrist (carpals), is called

_____.

68. A special OR table used for hip pinnings and other orthopedic procedures to provide traction to the involved limb is termed _____.

69. DHS is an abbreviation for _____.

15 Trauma, Mobile, and Surgical Radiography

WORKBOOK SELF-TEST ANSWER KEY

1. A. Spiral fracture
   B. Compound fracture
   C. Comminuted fracture
   D. Greenstick fracture
   E. Colles fracture
   F. Impacted fracture
   G. Compression fracture
   H. Stellate fracture
   I. Potts fracture
2. A. 7°
3. Battery-operated, battery-driven
4. Standard power source
5. False (mobile fluoroscopy units)
6. True
7. False (PA [x-ray tube placed under the anatomy] is recommended because of less exposure to the operator and less OID.)
8. True
9. Road mapping
10. A. 5
    B. 9
    C. 4
    D. 8
    E. 1
    F. 2
    G. 3
    H. 7
    I. 6
11. True
12. True
13. False
14. C. 6 feet (1.8 m)
15. False
16. False (greater on the tube side)
17. False (by a factor of four)
18. D. Ensure side rails are up on the patient cart.
19. True
20. A. Dislocation
    B. Subluxation
21. B. Lack of apposition (distraction)
22. A. Valgus deformity
23. Scatter radiation from the patient
24. 4 mR ($30 \div 60 \times 8 = 4$)
25. D. Epiphyseal
26. A. Right lateral decubitus
27. 3–4 inches (8–10 cm) below the jugular notch
28. 15–20° lateromedial angle and horizontal beam lateral projections
29. C. Left lateral decubitus
30. Two
31. Parallel to the interepicondylar plane
32. A horizontal beam lateromedial projection
33. 25–30°, or until the CR can be projected parallel to the scapular blade (wing)
34. 10° posteriorly from perpendicular to the plantar surface of the foot
35. Perform a cross-angle CR projection of the ankle, with CR 15–20° lateromedial from the long axis of the foot.
36. Yes, the technique should be increased 3–4 kVp to account for the additional thickness of the part.
37. A. 35–40° cephalad, AP axial projection
38. D. Perform AP axial trauma oblique projections
39. B. O-arm
40. B. Trauma, horizontal beam lateral
41. A. Horizontal
    B. 2 inches (5 cm) superior to EAM
42. C. Lateral
43. A. AP or PA and lateral wrist
44. B. Trauma axiolateral projection
45. D. Anesthesiologist
46. Certified surgical technologist
47. C. Surgical assistant
48. C. Asepsis
49. A. Only the level of the tabletop
50. False
51. True
52. True
53. D. Weekly
54. C. Use intermittent fluoroscopy
55. Reducing patient dose
56. A. Shallow RPO
57. True
58. Nonfunctional
59. Pelvicalyceal
60. Open reduction with internal fixation
61. A. Shower curtain
62. B. Intramedullary rod
63. D. Ilizarov device
64. D. All of the above require fluoroscopic guidance.
65. D. Interbody fusion cage
66. A. Scoliosis corrective surgery
67. A Kirschner wire
68. Fracture or orthopedic table
69. Dynamic hip screw

16 Pediatric Radiography

Positioning considerations are unique to pediatric radiography and present a definite challenge for all technologists. Children cannot be handled and positioned like miniature adults. They have special needs and require patience and understanding. Their anatomic makeup is vastly different from that of adults, especially the skeletal system. The bony development (ossification) of children goes through specific growth stages from infancy to adolescence. These need to be understood by technologists so that the appearance of the normal growth stages can be recognized. Examples of normal bone development patterns at various ages are included in this chapter and in the textbook.

The routine and optional projections and positions are much different for children than for adults. You need to know and understand these differences to be able to visualize the essential anatomy of children of various ages.

The most obvious differences for children when compared with adults are the methods of positioning and immobility. Small children cannot simply be instructed to remain stationary in certain positions or to hold their breath during the exposure. You will need to learn how to relate to children and to communicate with them to gain their cooperation without forceful immobilization.

Special immobilization techniques need to be learned along with the use of various types of commonly available immobilization equipment. Specialized restraining devices available in many departments will be explained and demonstrated in this chapter.

Radiation protection for these small patients must also be a major concern because the younger the child, the more sensitive the tissues are to radiation. Thus accurate collimation is essential. High-speed image receptor (IR) should also be used if applicable, and repeats must be minimized. Keeping all child doses as low as possible is even more important than in adult radiography. Therefore careful study of this chapter and related clinical experience are essential before you attempt a radiographic examination on a small child or infant. As a student, you may have limited opportunities to observe and assist with pediatric patients during your training. This makes learning and mastering the information provided in this chapter of the textbook and this workbook-laboratory manual even more important.

CHAPTER OBJECTIVES

After you have successfully completed the activities of this chapter, you will be able to:

_____ 1. List the steps and process of the technologist's introduction to the child and parent and the potential role of the parent during the child's examination.

_____ 2. Define the term nonaccidental trauma (NAT) and describe the role of technologists based on individual state guidelines if they suspect child abuse.

_____ 3. Identify the more common commercial immobilization devices and explain their function.

_____ 4. List the most common types of ancillary devices used for immobilization.

_____ 5. List the four steps of "mummifying" an infant. Perform this procedure on a simulated patient.

_____ 6. Define terms relating to bone development or ossification and identify the radiographic appearance and the normal stages of development of secondary growth centers.

_____ 7. Identify methods for reducing patient and guardian doses and repeat exposures during pediatric procedures.

_____ 8. Identify alternative imaging modalities and procedures performed on pediatric patients.

_____ 9. List the common clinical indications for radiographic examinations of the pediatric chest, upper and lower limbs, pelvis and hips, skull, and abdomen.

_____ 10. For select forms of pathology of the pediatric skeletal system, determine whether manual exposure factors would increase, decrease, or remain the same.

_____ 11. Describe positioning, technical factors, any potential shielding requirements, and immobilization techniques for procedures of the chest, skeletal system, and abdomen.

_____ 12. List general patient preparation requirements for procedures of the pediatric abdomen, including specific minimum patient preparation requirements for the upper gastrointestinal (GI), lower GI, and genitourinary procedures.

_____ 13. List the types and quantities of contrast media based on age as recommended for upper GI, lower GI, and genitourinary procedures.

_____ 14. Using an articulated pediatric mannequin, correctly immobilize and position a patient.

_____ 15. Perform examinations of the chest, abdomen, upper limb, lower limb, pelvis and hips, and skull.

_____ 16. According to established evaluation criteria, critique and evaluate radiographs provided by your instructor for each of the previously mentioned examinations.

_____ 17. Discriminate between acceptable and unacceptable radiographs and describe how positioning or technical errors can be corrected.

LEARNING EXERCISES

The following review exercises should be completed only after careful study of the associated pages in the textbook as indicated by each exercise. Answers to each review exercise are given at the end of this workbook.

PART I: INTRODUCTION TO PEDIATRIC RADIOGRAPHY

REVIEW EXERCISE A: Immobilization, Ossification, Radiation Protection, Pre-Exam Preparation, and Clinical Indications (see textbook pp. 628–638)

1. List the two important general factors that produce a successful pediatric radiographic procedure.

   A. _____

   B. _____

2. List the three possible roles for the parent during a pediatric procedure.

   A. _____

   B. _____

   C. _____

3. True/False: Parents should never be in the radiographic room with their child.

4. True/False: The technologist should always use the shortest exposure time possible during pediatric procedures.

5. True/False: The parent has the right to refuse the use of immobilization devices.

393

6. A device with an adjustable type of bicycle seat and two clear plastic body clamps is called

   _____.

7. For what is the immobilization device described in Question 6 most commonly used?

   _____

8. Why is tape is not recommended for immobilization purposes placed directly on children?

   _____

9. When adhesive tape is used to immobilize a child (if not placed directly over the parts to be radiographed), what two methods are used to prevent the adhesive tape from injuring the skin?

   A. _____

   B. _____

10. Briefly describe the four steps for "mummifying" a child.

    1. _____

    2. _____

    3. _____

    4. _____

11. Primary centers of bone formation (ossification) involving the midshafts of long bones are called

    _____.

12. Secondary centers of ossification of the long bones are called _____.

13. The area in which bone growth in length occurs is termed the _____.

14. What are three reasons for a Bone Age Study?

    1. _____

    2. _____

    3. _____

15. The most common image evaluated for a Bone Age Study is a _____ of the _____.

16. Around what age will the capitate and hamate begin to ossify and be seen radiographically?

    A. At birth   C. 14 months–3 years

    B. 3–14 months   D. 3–9 years

17. What are the names of the two, more specific, measurements for bone age?

    1. _____   2. _____

18. What are five of the six specific classifications of child abuse?

1. _____

2. _____

3. _____

4. _____

5. _____

19. How can rib fractures be a radiographic indication of child abuse?

_____

20. List three safeguards to help reduce repeat exposures during pediatric procedures.

A. _____   B. _____   C. _____

21. What three safeguards can be used to reduce the patient dose during pediatric procedures?

A. _____   B. _____   C. _____

22. Sometimes a primary technologist and assisting technologist work together. Match each of the following duties with the correct technologist.

_____ 1. Initiates exposures   A. Primary technologist

_____ 2. Positions the patient   B. Assisting technologist

_____ 3. Processes the images

_____ 4. Positions the tube and collimates

_____ 5. Sets exposure factors

_____ 6. Instructs the parents

23. True/False: Clothing, bandages, and diapers generally do not need to be removed from the regions being radiographed on pediatric patients because they do not cause artifacts on the radiographs (as long as metallic fasteners are not present).

24. True/False: A "babygram" is an acceptable alternative to the skeletal survey.

25. Grids (or virtual grids) should only be used, on pediatric patients, with a body part more than _____.

26. True/False: CT is a valuable imaging modality when slight differences in soft tissue densities must be demonstrated.

27. Beyond radiography, what other imaging modality is used to diagnose congenital hip dislocations in the newborn?

    A. Diagnostic medical sonography (DMS)   C. Nuclear medicine (NM)

    B. CT   D. Magnetic resonance imaging (MR)

28. Which of the following imaging modalities is most effective in diagnosing pyloric stenosis in children?

    A. Diagnostic medical sonography (DMS)   C. Functional MRI (fMRI)

    B. Helical CT   D. Nuclear medicine (NM)

29. Functional MRI (fMRI) has been used to detect disorders in all the following conditions except:

    A. Autism   C. Hydrocephalus

    B. Tourette syndrome   D. Attention deficient hyperactivity disorder

30. Match each of the following pathologic disorders of the pediatric chest with the best definition or description. (Use each choice only once.)

    _____ A. Meconium aspiration   1. Bacterial infection can lead to closure of the upper airway

    _____ B. Hyaline membrane disease   2. Also known as respiratory distress syndrome

    _____ C. Asthma   3. Inherited disease leading to clogging of bronchi

    _____ D. Epiglottitis   4. May develop during stressful births

    _____ E. Cystic fibrosis   5. Viral infection leading to labored breathing and dry cough

    _____ F. Croup   6. Foreign object breathed into the air passages

    _____ G. Aspiration   7. Airways narrowed by stimuli

31. Match each of the following pathologic disorders of the pediatric skeletal system to the best definition or description.

    _____ A. Meningocele   1. Decreased bone formation at growth plates

    _____ B. Kohler bone disease   2. Abnormally soft bones

    _____ C. Craniostenosis   3. Spinal cord protrudes through an opening

    _____ D. Talipes   4. Prematurely closed cranial sutures

    _____ E. Osteogenesis imperfecta   5. Disease of epiphyseal and growth plate

    _____ F. Achondroplasia   6. Protrusion of meninges through opening

    _____ G. Myelomeningocele   7. Inflammation of navicular in the foot

    _____ H. Osteochondrosis   8. Congenital deformity of the foot

32. Match each of the following clinical indications of the pediatric abdomen to the best definition or description.

_____ A. Ileus

_____ B. Pyloric stenosis

_____ C. Necrotizing enterocolitis (NEC)

_____ D. Atresias

_____ E. Polycystic kidney disease

_____ F. Hirschsprung disease

_____ G. Wilms tumor

1. May result in repeated, forceful vomiting

2. Characterized by the absence of rhythmic contractions of the large intestine

3. Condition characterized by the absence of an opening in an organ

4. Cancer of the kidney of embryonal origin

5. Obstruction caused by the lack of contractile movement of the intestinal wall

6. Inflammation of the inner lining of the intestine

7. Many cysts form on the kidneys

33. Indicate whether the following pathologic conditions require that manual exposure factors be increased (+), decreased (−), or remain the same (0).

_____ A. Idiopathic juvenile osteoporosis

_____ B. Osteogenesis imperfecta

_____ C. Osteomalacia

34. What is meconium?

A. Pancreatic enzymes

B. Blood and lymph

C. Dark green secretion of the liver and intestinal glands mixed with amniotic fluid

D. Pus and dead blood cells

35. True/False: Malignant bone tumors are rare in young children.

PART II: RADIOGRAPHIC POSITIONING

REVIEW EXERCISE B: Pediatric Positioning of the Chest, Skeletal System, and Skull (see textbook pp. 639–650)

1. True/False: If available, the Pigg-O-Stat should be used rather than relying on parental assistance during a pediatric chest examination.

2. Complete the following technical factors for an anteroposterior (AP) or posteroanterior (PA) pediatric chest.

A. Grid or nongrid? _____

B. kVp range: _____

C. Recommended collimation field size and/or IR—portrait or landscape? _____

D. Source–image receptor distance (SID), AP supine chest: _____

E. SID, PA erect chest: _____

3. What kVp range is generally used for a lateral chest? _____

4. Should a grid be used for a 2-year-old child's lateral chest? _____

397

5. The Pigg-O-Stat can be used effectively for an erect PA and lateral chest from infancy to approximately

   _____ years of age.

6. When should a chest exposure be initiated for a crying child? _____

7. Which radiographic structures are evaluated to determine rotation on a PA projection of the chest?

   _____

8. How is the x-ray tube aligned for a lateral projection of the chest if the patient is on a Tam-em board?

   _____

9. True/False: A well-inspired, erect chest radiograph taken on a young pediatric patient visualizes only six to seven ribs above the diaphragm.

10. True/False: The entire upper limb is commonly included on an infant rather than individual exposures of specific parts of the upper limb.

11. True/False: Except for survey exams, individual projections of the elbow, wrist, and shoulder should generally be taken on older children rather than including these regions on a single projection.

12. Match the following pathologic indicators with the correct radiographic procedure.

    _____ A. Atelectasis   1. Chest

    _____ B. Kohler disease   2. Upper or lower limb

    _____ C. Cystic fibrosis

    _____ D. Talipes

    _____ E. Respiratory distress syndrome (RDS)

13. Which single radiographic position provides a lateral projection of bilateral lower limbs for the nontraumatic

    pediatric patient? _____

14. Which radiographic projections (and method) are performed for the infant with congenital clubfeet?

    _____

15. True/False: It is important to place the foot into true AP and lateral positions when performing a clubfoot study.

16. True/False: Post-exposure cropping of an image due to poor collimation complies with ALARA principles.

17. What is the recommended collimation field size for a skull routine on a 6-year-old patient?

    _____

18. Which of the following CR angulations places the petrous ridges in the lower one-third of the orbits with an AP reverse Caldwell projection of the skull?

    A. 15 degrees cephalad to orbitomeatal line (OML)   C. CR perpendicular to OML

    B. 15 degrees caudad to OML   D. 30 degrees cephalad to OML

19. Which of the following clinical indicators applies to a pediatric skull series?

    A. Osteomyelitis

    B. CHD

    C. Craniosynostosis

    D. Hyaline membrane disease

20. Which skull positioning line is placed perpendicular to the film for an AP Towne 30 degrees caudal projection of the skull?

    A. Infraorbitomeatal line

    B. OML

    C. Mentomeatal line

    D. Acanthiomeatal line

21. True/False: Parental assistance for skull radiography is preferred rather than using head clamps and a mummy wrap on a pediatric patient.

22. True/False: Children older than 5 years of age can usually hold their breath after a practice session.

23. Correct centering for the following can be achieved by placing the CR at the level of which structure or landmark?

    A. AP, PA, or lateral chest: _____

    B. AP abdomen (infants and small children): _____

    C. AP supine abdomen (older children): _____

    D. AP skull: _____

REVIEW EXERCISE C: Positioning of the Pediatric Abdomen and Contrast Media Procedures (see textbook pp. 651–660)

1. A backward flow of urine from the bladder into the ureters and kidneys is called

    _____.

2. True/False: Small retention enema tips can be used on infants during a barium enema to help barium retention.

3. What type of contrast media is recommended for reducing an intussusception? _____

4. What is the maximum height of the barium enema bag above the tabletop before the beginning of the procedure?

    _____

5. True/False: The chest and abdomen are generally almost equal in circumference in the newborn.

6. True/False: Bony landmarks in infants are easy to palpate and locate.

7. True/False: It is difficult to distinguish the small bowel from the large bowel on a plain abdomen on an infant.

8. True/False: The radiographic contrast on a pediatric abdominal radiograph is high compared with that of an adult abdominal radiograph.

9. Complete the recommended NPO fasting before the following pediatric contrast media procedures.

    A. 1-year-old upper GI: _____

    B. 2-month-old upper GI: _____

    C. Infant lower GI: _____

    D. Pediatric intravenous urogram (IVU): _____

10. List five conditions that contraindicate the use of laxatives or enemas in preparation for a lower GI study.

   A. _____

   B. _____

   C. _____

   D. _____

   E. _____

11. Place an X next to the clinical indicators that apply for an AP abdomen (KUB).

   _____ A. Croup   _____ E. Mastoiditis

   _____ B. NEC   _____ F. Hepatomegaly

   _____ C. Intussusception   _____ G. Appendicitis

   _____ D. Foreign body localization   _____ H. Hydrocephalus

12. Where is the CR centered for an erect abdomen on a small child? _____

13. A. What is the minimum kVp for an AP abdomen projection of a newborn without a grid?

   _____

   B. A grid is required for a pediatric AP abdomen if the abdomen measures more than _____ cm.

14. Which of the following projections of the abdomen best demonstrates the prevertebral region?

   A. AP supine KUB   C. Dorsal decubitus abdomen

   B. PA prone KUB   D. AP erect abdomen

15. A malignant tumor of the kidney common in children under the age of 5 years is:

   A. Wilms tumor   C. Ewing sarcoma

   B. Adenocarcinoma   D. Teratoma

16. What is the most common clinical indication for a voiding cystourethrogram?

   _____

17. Which of the following conditions is caused by inflammation of the inner lining of the large or small bowel, resulting in tissue death?

   A. NEC   C. CHD

   B. Intussusception   D. Meconium ileus

18. Which of the following procedures or projections should be performed for a possible meconium ileus?

   A. IVU procedure   C. Upper GI series

   B. AP supine abdomen   D. Acute abdomen series

19. True/False: A piece of lead vinyl can be placed beneath the child's lower pelvis during conventional fluoroscopy to reduce the gonadal/mean bone marrow dose.

20. How much barium should be administered to each of the following patients for an upper GI series?

    A. Infants: _____

    B. Adolescents: _____

21. What might the only recourse be if a pediatric patient refuses to drink barium for an upper GI series?

    _____

22. True/False: The transit time of the contrast media for reaching the cecum during a small bowel series on a 3-year-old child is approximately 2 hours.

23. True/False: Latex enema tips should be used for barium enemas for children younger than 1 year of age.

24. Which projections are frequently performed during a voiding cystourethrogram (VUG) on a pediatric patient?

    _____

25. True/False: A radionuclide study for vesicourethral reflux provides a smaller patient dose compared with a fluoroscopic voiding cystourethrogram.

REVIEW EXERCISE D: Problem Solving and Analysis

1. **Situation:** A young child is sent to the radiology department for a skull series. The guardian states she is willing to hold her child during the exposures; however, the guardian is 8 months pregnant. What should the technologist do next?

   A. Place a 0.5-mm lead apron on the guardian and allow her to hold her child.

   B. The technologist should hold the child during each exposure and have the guardian wait outside.

   C. Have another (nonradiology) health professional hold the child and have the guardian wait outside the room.

   D. Have a radiography student hold the child and have the guardian wait outside the room.

2. **Situation:** A 3-year-old child comes to the radiology department for an erect abdomen examination. He is unable to remain still for the exposures. Which immobilization device should be used for this patient?

   A. Tam-em board   C. Plexiglas hold-down paddle

   B. Pigg-O-Stat   D. Have another technologist hold child

3. **Situation:** A child comes to the radiology department with possible croup. Which of the following procedures best demonstrates this condition?

   A. AP and lateral upper airway   C. PA and lateral chest

   B. Erect abdomen   D. Sinus series

4. **Situation:** A newborn is diagnosed with RDS. Which of the following procedures is commonly performed for this condition?

   A. Abdomen   C. CT of head

   B. Functional MRI (fMRI)   D. Chest

5. **Situation:** A child comes to the radiology department with a clinical history of Legg–Calvé–Perthes disease. Which of the following projections best demonstrates this condition?

   A. PA and lateral chest   C. AP and lateral hip

   B. Supine and erect abdomen   D. AP and lateral bilateral lower limbs

6. **Situation:** A child comes to the radiology department with a clinical history of Kohler bone disease. Which of the following radiographic routines demonstrates this condition?

   A. Foot

   B. Shoulder

   C. Lumbar spine

   D. Cervical spine

7. **Situation:** A child comes to radiology with a clinical history of talipes equinovarus. Which of the following positioning routines and/or methods is often performed for this condition?

   A. Coyle method

   B. Erect AP knee projections

   C. AP and lateral foot—Kite method

   D. AP and lateral hip

8. **Situation:** Which radiographic procedure is often performed for Hirschsprung disease?

   A. Upper GI

   B. MR

   C. Cystourethrography

   D. Barium enema

9. **Situation:** Which radiographic procedure is often performed for pyloric stenosis?

   A. Barium enema

   B. Evacuative proctography

   C. Enteroclysis

   D. Upper GI

10. Which of the following modalities is most effective in detecting signs of autism?

    A. Functional MRI (fMRI)

    B. Ultrasound

    C. Spiral CT

    D. Nuclear medicine

PART III: LABORATORY EXERCISES

Exercises A and B must be performed in a radiographic laboratory or a general diagnostic room in the radiology department. General immobilization paraphernalia must be available (i.e., tape, sheets or large towels, sandbags, various sizes and shapes of positioning sponge blocks, retention bands, head clamps, stockinettes, and Ace bandages). More common commercial immobilization devices, such as the Tam-em board or the Pigg-O-Stat (or similar devices), are optional if available. At least one of these devices should be made available for student use.

Exercise C can be performed if optimal and less than optimal pediatric radiographs are available.

Laboratory Exercise A: Immobilization

For this section you will need some type of large articulated doll or mannequin to use as your patient. The doll should have arms and legs that are flexible (similar to those of a child). This does not need to be a phantomlike doll because radiographs will not be taken, but it will be used to simulate immobilization techniques and positioning for various body parts.

Check off each of the following activities as you complete them.

_____ 1. Complete the four steps of "mummifying."

_____ 2. Immobilize your patient correctly with the Velcro straps to restrain the upper and lower limbs and also to secure immobilization across the pelvic region.

_____ 3. Pigg-O-Stat (if available)

Laboratory Exercise B: Physical Positioning

This section again requires the use of a large articulated pediatric mannequin. Practice the following projections or positions until you can perform them accurately and without hesitation. Place a check mark by each activity when you have achieved it.

Include the details listed in the following as you simulate the routine projections for each exam that follows. Assume that the patient will not cooperate and that forceful immobilization is required. Use suggested immobilization techniques.

_____Correct collimation field size (appropriate for size of "patient")

_____Correct centering of part to IR

_____Correct SID and location and angle of central ray

_____Selection of appropriate restraining devices and application of the same

_____Correct placement of markers

_____Correct use of contact shielding, when applicable.

_____Accurate collimation to body part of interest

_____Approximate correct exposure factors

Examination	*Immobilization*
_____ 1. AP chest, supine	Tam-em board or sandbags and/or stockinette and "Ace" bandages
_____ 2. Lateral chest, patient	Sandbags and tape, or retention band recumbent in lateral position

If Tam-em board is available:

_____ 3. Lateral chest, patient supine, horizontal beam CR	Tam-em board

If Pigg-O-Stat is available:

_____ 4. PA chest erect, 72-inch (180-cm) SID	Pigg-O-Stat
_____ 5. Lateral chest erect, 72-inch (180-cm) SID	Pigg-O-Stat
_____ 6. AP abdomen, erect	Pigg-O-Stat
_____ 7. AP abdomen, supine	Tam-em board, or tape, sandbags, and retention band
_____ 8. AP and lateral upper limb	Tape, sandbags, and/or retention band (from shoulder to hand)
_____ 9. AP and lateral lower limb	Tape, sandbags, and/or retention band (from hips to feet). Sitting on pad using tape
_____ 10. AP and lateral feet (such as follow-up exams for clubfeet)	Tape and sandbags and/or retention band
_____ 11. AP pelvis and hips	Tape and sandbags and/or retention band
_____ 12. Lateral hips	Head clamps or tape for head. Mummification and sandbags or retention band for limbs and body
_____ 13. AP skull, 15 degrees AP, and 30 degrees Towne	Head clamps or tape for head. Mummification and sandbags or retention band for limbs and body
_____ 14. Lateral skull, turned into lateral position	
_____ 15. Lateral skull, horizontal beam in supine position	Tam-em board and tape for head position

Laboratory Exercise C: Anatomy Review and Critique Radiographs of the Abdomen

Use the radiographs provided by your instructor. These should include optimal-quality and less-than-optimal quality radiographs of each of the following: chest, supine and erect abdomen, AP and lateral upper limb, AP and lateral pelvis and hips, AP and lateral lower limb, and AP and lateral skull.

Radiographs of the pelvis and upper and lower limbs of patients of various ages should be included to demonstrate the normal ossification or growth stages from infancy to adolescence.

Place a check mark by each of the following steps when completed.

_____ 1. Examine normal stages of growth by the appearance of the epiphyses in the pelvis and the long bones of the upper and lower limbs. Estimate the approximate age of the patient by the appearance of such epiphyses.

_____ 2. Critique each radiograph based on evaluation criteria provided for each projection in the textbook. Pediatric radiographs require a wider range of acceptable positioning criteria than for adults. Part centering and specific central ray locations are not as critical for pediatric radiographs because multiple anatomic parts or bones are included on one IR. This is possible because detailed views of joint areas are not as important because these secondary growth areas are not yet fully developed. Thus, complete limbs can be included on one film.

The following criteria guidelines can be used and checked as each radiograph is evaluated. Determine the corrections or adjustments in positioning or exposure factors that are necessary to bring those less-than-optimal radiographs up to a more desirable standard.

Radiographs

1	2	3	4	5	6

Criteria Guidelines

a. Correct field size as appropriate for age and size of patient?

b. Correct orientation of part to IR?

c. Acceptable alignment and/or centering of part to IR?

d. Correct CR angle where appropriate (such as for an AP skull)?

e. Evidence of collimation?

f. Pertinent anatomy well visualized?

g. Evidence of motion?

h. Optimal exposure (density and/or contrast)?

i. Patient ID with date and side markers visible without superimposing essential anatomy?

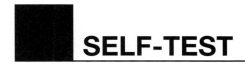

SELF-TEST

MY SCORE = _____ %

Directions: This self-test should be taken only after completing all of the readings, review exercises, and laboratory activities for a particular section. The purpose of this test is not only to provide a good learning exercise but also to serve as a strong indicator of what your final evaluation exam will be. It is strongly suggested that if you do not receive at least a 90%–95% grade on this self-test, you should review those areas in which you missed questions before going to your instructor for the final evaluation exam for this chapter.

1. At what age can most children be talked through a radiographic examination without purposeful immobilization?

   A. 1 year   C. 3 years

   B. 18 months   D. 5 years

2. At the first meeting between the technologist and the patient (accompanied by an adult), which of the following generally should not be discussed?

   A. Introduce yourself.

   B. Take the necessary time to explain what you will be doing.

   C. Discuss the possible forceful immobilization that will be needed if the child will not cooperate.

   D. Describe the total amount of radiation the patient will receive with the specific exam if it has to be repeated because of a lack of cooperation.

   E. All of these steps must be taken.

3. Which of the following is not the name of a known commercially available immobilization device?

   A. Posi-Tot   C. Pigg-O-Stat

   B. Tam-em board   D. Hold-em Tiger

4. The most suitable immobilization device for erect chests and/or the abdomen is the:

   A. Posi-Tot   C. Pigg-O-Stat

   B. Tam-em board   D. Hold-em Tiger

5. List the three factors that reduce the number of repeat exposures with pediatric patients.

   A. _____   B. _____   C. _____

6. Which immobilization device or method should be used for an erect 1-year-old chest procedure? Assume these devices are available.

   A. Tam-em board   C. Pigg-O-Stat

   B. Hold-down paddle   D. Parent holding child

7. Two common terms for the classic metaphyseal lesion, which may indicate child abuse, are _____ and _____.

8. If the technologist suspects child abuse, he or she should:

   A. Ask the parent when the abuse occurred

   B. Report the abuse immediately to the necessary state officials as required by the state

   C. Refuse to do the examination or touch the child until a physician has examined the patient

   D. Do none of the above

9. Complete the following as related to ossification by matching the correct term with the description. (More than one choice per blank may be used.)

   E = Epiphysis; D = Diaphysis; EP = Epiphyseal plate

   _____ 1. Primary centers

   _____ 2. Secondary centers

   _____ 3. Space between primary and secondary centers

   _____ 4. Occurs before birth

   _____ 5. Continues to change from birth to maturity

10. At birth, which of the following is not radiographically demonstrated?

    A. Metacarpals

    B. Radius

    C. Ulna

    D. Lunate

11. Which of the following procedures can be performed to evaluate children for attention deficient hyperactivity disorder?

    A. Helical CT

    B. Functional MRI (fMRI)

    C. 3D ultrasound

    D. Nuclear medicine

12. Match each of the following conditions to its correct definition or statement. (Use each choice only once.)

_____ A. Croup

_____ B. Cystic fibrosis

_____ C. Epiglottitis

_____ D. Osteochondrosis

_____ E. Osteogenesis imperfect

_____ F. Salter-Harris fracture

_____ G. Osteomalacia

_____ H. Hirschsprung disease

_____ I. Wilms tumor

_____ J. Neuroblastoma

_____ K. Pyelonephritis

_____ L. Atresia

_____ M. Craniosynostosis

1. Tumor that usually occurs in children younger than 5 years of age

2. Group of diseases affecting the epiphyseal growth plates

3. Fracture involving the epiphyseal plate

4. A common condition in children between the ages of 1 and 3, caused by a viral infection

5. Premature closure of the skull sutures

6. Second-most common form of cancer in children younger than 5 years of age

7. Bacterial infection of the upper airway that may be fatal if untreated

8. Congenital defect in which an opening into an organ is missing

9. Inherited disease leading to clogging of bronchi

10. Bacterial infection of the kidney

11. Also known as congenital megacolon

12. Also known as rickets

13. Inherited condition that produces very fragile bones

13. Indicate whether the following pathologic conditions require that manual exposure factors be increased (+), decreased (-), or remain the same (0):

_____ A. Idiopathic juvenile osteoporosis

_____ B. Osteomalacia

_____ C. Osteogenesis imperfecta

14. Which of the following imaging modalities is effective in detecting signs of autism?

A. CT

B. Diagnostic medical sonography (DMS)

C. Nuclear medicine

D. Functional MRI (fMRI)

15. True or False: Performing an erect chest x-ray for air/fluid levels is not important for pediatric patients.

16. What is the kVp range for a pediatric study of the upper limb? _____

17. True/False: A hand routine for a 7-year-old child would be the same as for an adult patient.

18. True/False: For a bone survey of a young child, both limbs are commonly radiographed for comparison.

19. Which radiographic technique or method is performed to study congenital clubfoot radiographically?

_____

20. What is the name of the study that includes multiple images for suspected child abuse?

_____

21. Match the following examinations with the clinical indicators with which they are most likely associated. (Answers may be used more than once.)

_____ A. Intussusception   1. Chest

_____ B. NEC   2. Abdomen

_____ C. Atelectasis   3. Upper and lower limbs

_____ D. Premature closure of fontanelles   4. Pelvis and hips

_____ E. CHD   5. Skull

_____ F. Cystic fibrosis

_____ G. Meconium ileus

_____ H. Legg–Calvé–Perthes disease

_____ I. Asthma

_____ J. Bronchiectasis

_____ K. Hyaline membrane disease

22. How much is the CR angled to the OML for an AP axial (Towne) projection of the skull?

   A. 15 degrees   C. 25 degrees

   B. None   D. 30 degrees

23. Where is the CR centered for a lateral projection of the pediatric skull?

   A. At the EAM   C. 1 inch (2.5 cm) above the EAM

   B. Midway between the glabella and inion   D. ¼ inch (2 cm) anterior and superior to the EAM

24. The NPO fasting period for a 6-month-old infant before an upper GI is:

   A. 4 hours   C. 1 hour

   B. 3 hours   D. 6 hours

25. Other than preventing artifacts in the bowel, what is the other reason that solid food is withheld for 4 hours before a pediatric IVU?

_____

26. Which of the following conditions contraindicates the use of laxatives before a contrast media procedure?

   A. Gastritis   C. Appendicitis

   B. Blood in stool   D. Diverticulosis

27. Where is the CR centered for a KUB on:

A. An 8-year-old child? _____

B. A 3-month-old infant? _____

28. Where is the CR centered for a PA and lateral pediatric chest projection? _____

29. What is the recommended amount of barium administered to an infant who is having an upper GI?

_____

30. How is barium instilled into the large bowel for a barium enema study on an infant?

_____

31. What is the bowel prep for a pediatric VCUG? _____

32. When is urinary reflux most likely to occur during a VCUG? _____

33. For a young pediatric small bowel study, the barium normally reaches the ileocecal region in

_____ hour(s).

34. A VCUG on a child is most commonly performed to evaluate for (A) _____ and is generally scheduled to be completed (B) _____ (before or after) an IVU or ultrasound study of the kidneys.

35. True/False: Using immobilization devices is one method to help reduce the chance of repeat exposures.

36. True/False: There should be no attempt to straighten out the abnormal alignment of the foot during a clubfoot study.

37. **Situation:** Which radiographic procedure is commonly performed for epiglottitis?

A. Sinus series

B. AP and lateral upper airway

C. CT of the chest

D. Functional MRI (fMRI)

38. **Situation:** Which of the following radiographic routines and/or procedures best demonstrates Osgood–Schlatter disease?

A. Barium enema

B. AP and lateral hip

C. Upper GI

D. AP and lateral knee

39. **Situation:** A 2-year-old child comes to the radiology department for a routine chest examination. While removing the child's shirt, you notice a human bite mark on the upper arm. What should you do next?

A. Call hospital security.

B. Inform the supervisor or physician.

C. Interview the parents about the injury.

D. Interview the child about the injury.

40. Which of the following conditions can be diagnosed prenatally with diagnostic medical sonography?

A. Tourette syndrome

B. Vesicoureteral reflux

C. Spina bifida

D. Autism

16 Pediatric Radiography

1. C. 3 years
2. D. Describe the total amount of radiation the patient will receive with the specific examination if it has to be repeated because of a lack of cooperation.
3. D. Hold-em Tiger
4. C. Pigg-O-Stat
5. A. Proper immobilization
   B. Short exposure times
   C. Accurate manual technique charts
6. C. Pigg-O-Stat
7. Corner fracture and bucket-handle fracture
8. D. Do none of the above
9. 1. D
   2. E
   3. EP
   4. D
   5. E and EP
10. D. Lunate
11. B. Functional MRI (fMRI)
12. A. 4
    B. 9
    C. 7
    D. 2
    E. 13
    F. 3
    G. 12
    H. 11
    I. 1
    J. 6
    K. 10
    L. 8
    M. 5
13. A. (–)
    B. (–)
    C. (–)
14. D. Functional MRI (fMRI)
15. False
16. 50–60 kVp
17. True
18. True
19. Kite method
20. Skeletal Survey
21. A. 2
    B. 2
    C. 1
    D. 5
    E. 4
    F. 1
    G. 2
    H. 4
    I. 1
    J. 1
    K. 1
22. D. 30 degrees
23. B. Midway between glabella and inion
24. A. 4 hours
25. To diminish the risk of aspiration from vomiting
26. C. Appendicitis
27. A. Level of iliac crest
    B. 1 inch (2.5 cm) above umbilicus
28. Mammillary (nipple) level
29. 6–12 ounces
30. Manually, very slowly, using a 60-mL syringe and a No. 10 French flexible silicone catheter
31. No bowel preparation is required.
32. When the bladder is full and when voiding
33. 1 hour
34. A. Vesicoureteral reflux
    B. Before
35. True
36. True
37. B. AP and lateral upper airway
38. D. AP and lateral knee
39. B. Inform the supervisor or physician.
40. C. Spina bifida

A1

17 Angiography and Interventional Procedures

This chapter, which includes extensive detailed and somewhat complex anatomy and procedural information, is an excellent introduction to angiography and interventional procedures. It provides effective preparation and a good overview for the additional clinical training and experience that a cardiovascular technologist will need.

CHAPTER OBJECTIVES

After you have successfully completed the activities of this chapter, you will be able to:

_____ 1. List the divisions and components of the circulatory system.

_____ 2. List the three functions of the cardiovascular system.

_____ 3. On drawings, identify the components of the pulmonary and general systemic circulation.

_____ 4. Identify the four chambers of the heart, associated valves, and coronary circulation.

_____ 5. List and identify the four arteries supplying blood to the brain and the three branches arising from the aortic arch.

_____ 6. List the major branches of the external and internal carotid arteries and the primary divisions of the brain supplied by each.

_____ 7. On drawings, identify the major veins of the neck draining blood from the head and neck region.

_____ 8. List the major venous sinuses found in the cranium.

_____ 9. List the four segments of the thoracic aorta and describe the three common variations of the aortic arch.

_____ 10. List and identify the five major branches of the abdominal aorta.

_____ 11. List and identify the major abdominal veins.

_____ 12. List and identify the major arteries and veins of the upper and lower limbs.

_____ 13. Identify the six steps for the Seldinger technique.

_____ 14. Identify the equipment and personnel generally found in an angiographic room.

_____ 15. Identify the clinical indications, contraindications, and general procedure for cerebral angiography.

_____ 16. Identify the indications, catheterization technique, and general procedure for thoracic and abdominal angiography.

_____ 17. Identify the clinical indications, contraindications, and general procedure for peripheral angiography.

_____ 18. Identify specific examples of vascular and nonvascular interventional procedures.

LEARNING EXERCISES

Complete the following review exercises after reading the associated pages in the textbook as indicated by each exercise. Answers to each review exercise are provided at the end of this workbook.

REVIEW EXERCISE A: Anatomy of Vascular System, Pulmonary and Systemic Circulation, and Cerebral Arteries and Veins (see textbook pp. 662–668)

1. List the two major divisions or components of the circulatory system.

   A. _____   B. _____

2. List the body system or part supplied by the following four divisions of the circulatory system.

   A. Cardio _____   C. Pulmonary _____

   B. Vascular _____   D. Systemic _____

3. List the three functions of the cardiovascular system.

   A. _____

   B. _____

   C. _____

4. Identify the major components of the general cardiovascular circulation as labeled in Fig. 17.1.

   A. _____

   B. _____

   C. _____

   D. _____

   E. _____

   F. _____

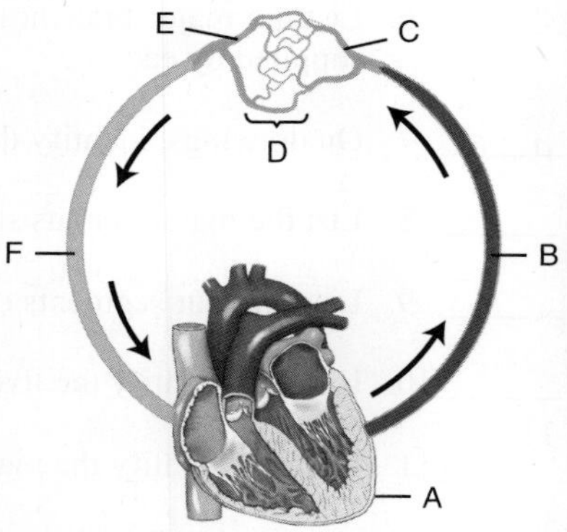

Fig. 17.1 Components of cardio-vascular circulation.

5. Which of the six general components of the circulatory system identified in

   Question 4 carry oxygenated blood to body tissue? _____

6. Which of the six general components of the circulatory system carry deoxygenated blood?

   _____

7. For each of the following three blood components, list the function and the common term (unless no other term exists).

	Common Term	*Function*
1. Erythrocytes	A. _____	B. _____
2. Leukocytes	A. _____	B. _____
3. Platelets	A. (No other term given)	B. _____

411

8. Plasma, the liquid portion of blood, consists of (A) _____ % water and

   (B) _____ % plasma protein and salts, nutrients, and oxygen.

9. Identify the chambers of the heart and the associated blood vessels (arteries and veins) as labeled in Fig. 17.2.

   A. _____ (chamber)

   B. _____ (chamber)

   C. _____ (chamber)

   D. _____

   E. _____

   F. _____

   G. _____

   H. _____

   I. _____

   J. _____ (chamber)

   K. _____

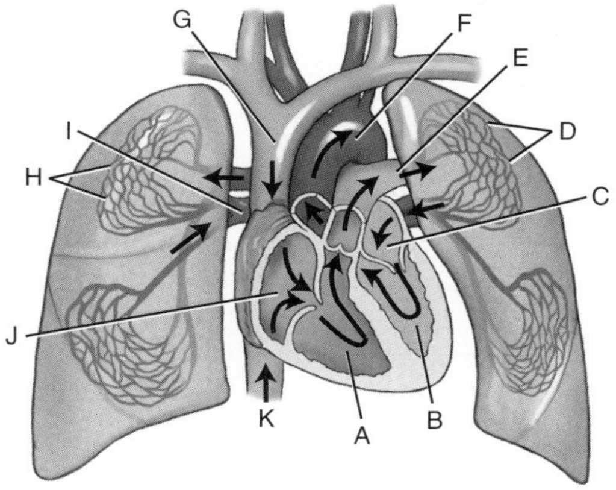

Fig. 17.2 Heart and pulmonary circulation (frontal view).

   Questions 10 and 11 also relate to Fig. 17.2.

10. In general, arteries carry oxygenated blood, and veins carry deoxygenated blood. The exceptions to these rules are as follows:

    A. The _____ that carry(-ies) deoxygenated blood to the lungs.

    B. The _____ that carry(-ies) oxygenated blood back to the left atrium of the heart.

11. A. Blood from the upper body returns to the heart through the _____.

    B. Blood from the abdomen and the lower limbs returns through the _____.

    C. Both of these major veins enter the _____ of the heart.

12. Identify the four major valves between the following heart chambers and associated vessels.

    A. Between right atrium and right ventricle: _____

    B. Between right ventricle and pulmonary arteries: _____

    C. Between left atrium and left ventricle: _____

    D. Between left ventricle and aorta: _____

13. A. The arteries that deliver blood to the heart muscle are the _____.

    B. These arteries originate at the _____.

14. List the three major branches of the coronary sinus.

   A. _____   B. _____   C. _____

15. Identify the labeled arteries in Fig. 17.3.

   A. _____

   B. _____

   C. _____

   D. _____

   E. _____

   F. _____

   G. _____

   H. _____

   I. _____

   J. _____

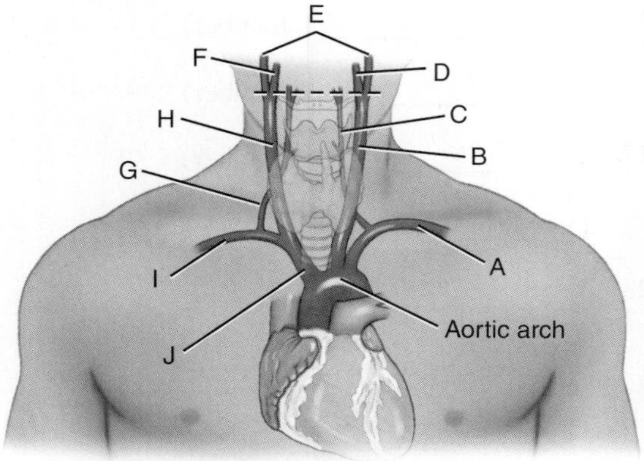

Fig. 17.3 Arterial branches of the aortic arch.

16. List the four major arteries supplying blood to the brain (important radiographically on a four-vessel angiogram).

   A. _____   C. _____

   B. _____   D. _____

17. List the three major branches of arteries arising from the arch of the aorta that supply the brain with blood.

   A. _____   B. _____   C. _____

18. True/False: The brachiocephalic artery bifurcates to form the right common and right vertebral arteries.

19. True/False: The level for bifurcation of the common carotid artery into the internal and external carotid arteries is at the level of C3–C4.

20. Any injection of the common carotid inferior to the bifurcation would result in filling both the

   _____ and _____ arteries.

21. What is the name of the S-shaped portion of the internal carotid artery near the petrous portion of the temporal bone?

   A. Carotid sinus   C. Carotid body

   B. Carotid canal   D. Carotid siphon

22. List the two end branches of the internal carotid artery.

   A. _____   B. _____

23. The _____ artery supplies much of the forebrain with blood.

24. The _____ supply(-ies) the posterior circulation of the brain.

25. The two vertebral arteries unite to form the single _____ artery.

26. Which of the two major branches of each internal carotid artery (anterior cerebral or middle cerebral arteries) supplies the lateral aspects of the cerebral hemispheres? _____

27. The anterior and middle cerebral arteries superimpose one another to a greater extent on the _____ (lateral or frontal) view.

28. Identify the labeled arteries in Fig. 17.4.

   A. _____

   B. _____

   C. _____

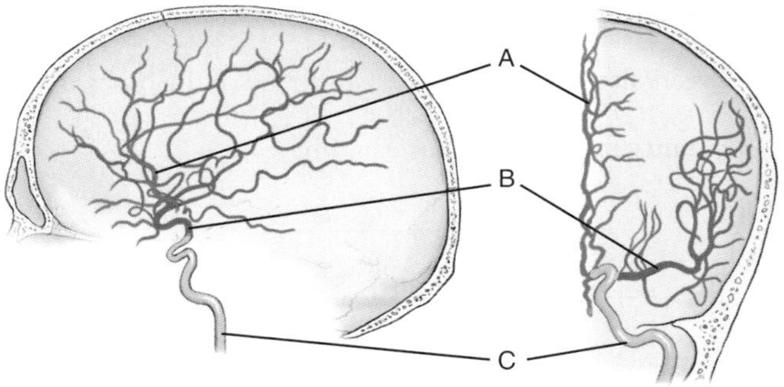

Fig. 17.4 Major cerebral arterial systems.

29. The posterior brain circulation communicates with the anterior circulation at the base of the brain in an arterial circle configuration called the arterial circle (Fig. 17.5). Identify the five arteries, or branches, that make up the arterial circle (circle of Willis) (labeled 1–5 on this drawing).

   1. _____

   2. _____

   3. _____

   4. _____

   5. _____

   6. A. Name the gland (labeled A) located in the center of the arterial circle (circle of Willis). _____

      B. The right and left _____ enter the cranium through the foramen magnum.

      C. They then unite to form this single _____ artery.

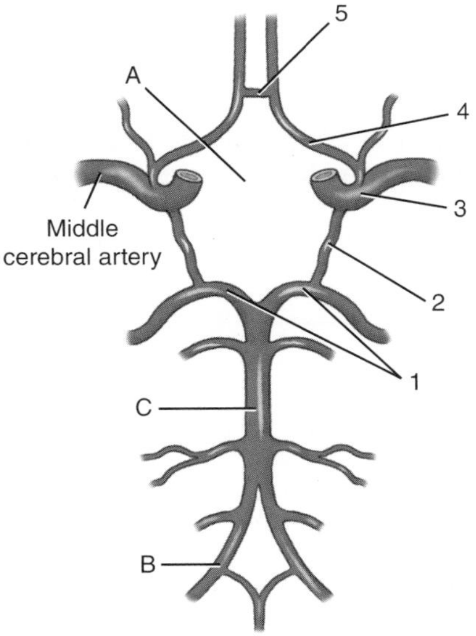

Fig. 17.5 Structure identification of the arterial circle (circle of Willis).

30. List the three pairs of major veins draining the head, face, and neck region.

   A. _____

   B. _____

   C. _____

31. A. The three pairs of major veins described in Question 30 join the subclavian vein to form the

   _____ vein.

   B. This vein joins the equivalent vein on the other side to form the _____, which

   returns blood to the _____ of the heart.

32. True/False: The venous sinuses found in the brain are situated between layers of the dura mater.

33. Identify the venous sinuses in Fig. 17.6.

   A. _____

   B. _____

   C. _____

   D. _____

   E. _____

   F. _____

   G. _____

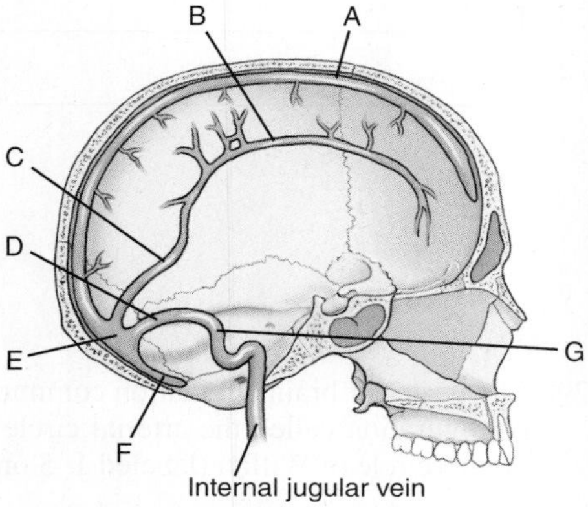

Fig. 17.6 Venous sinuses in the brain.

REVIEW EXERCISE B: Anatomy of Thoracic and Abdominal Arteries and Veins, Portal System, and Upper and Lower Limb Arteries and Veins (see textbook pp. 669–672)

1. List the four segments of the thoracic section of the aorta as labeled in Fig. 17.7.

   A. _____

   B. _____

   C. _____

   D. _____

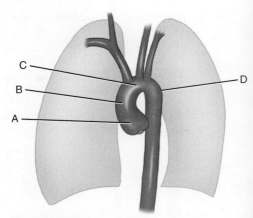

Fig. 17.7 Four segments of the aorta.

2. List the three common variations of the aortic arch that may be visualized during thoracic angiography and are demonstrated in Fig. 17.8.

A. _____

B. _____

C. _____

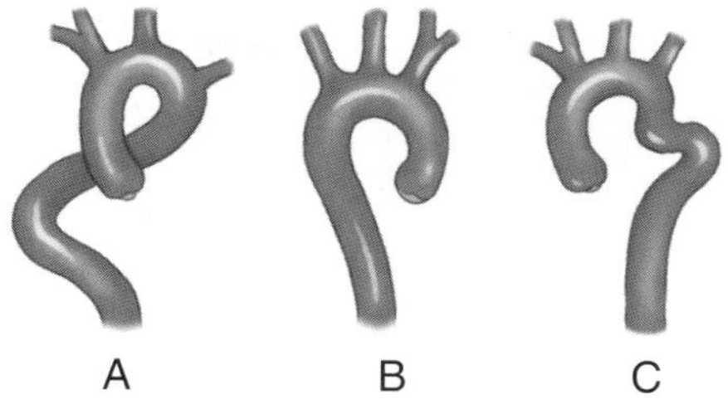

Fig. 17.8 Variations of the aortic arch.

3. Which of the following veins receives blood from the intercostal, bronchial, esophageal, and phrenic veins?

   A. Pulmonary veins

   B. Azygos vein

   C. Inferior vena cava

   D. Superior vena cava

4. List the five major branches of the abdominal aorta, labeled 1–5 in Fig. 17.9 (listed in order from most superior to most inferior).

   1. _____

   2. _____

   3. _____

   4. _____

   5. _____

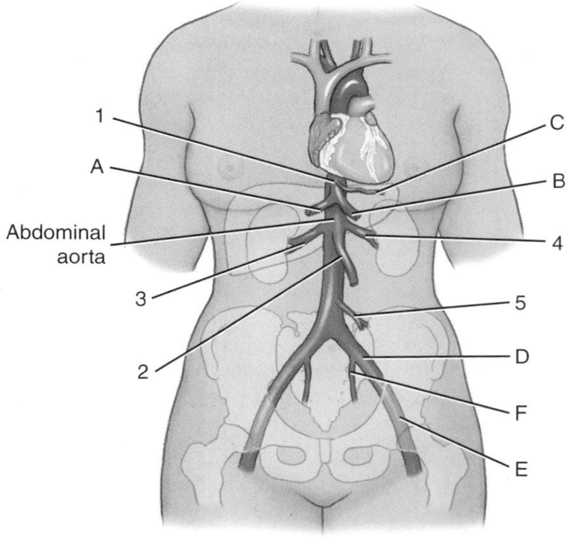

Fig. 17.9 Branches and divisions of the abdominal aorta.

5. At what approximate level does the descending aorta pass through the diaphragm to become the abdominal aorta?

   A. T9

   B. T12

   C. L2

   D. L3

6. List the three organs supplied with blood from the celiac artery, labeled A–C (Fig. 17.9).

A. _____

B. _____

C. _____

List the divisions of the abdominal aorta as it enters the pelvic region, labeled D–F (Fig. 17.9).

    D. _____

    E. _____

    F. _____

7. The distal abdominal aorta bifurcates at the approximate level of the _____ vertebra.

8. Venous blood is returned to the heart from structures below the diaphragm through the inferior vena cava. Identify the major venous tributaries to the inferior vena cava, as labeled on Fig. 17.10.

    A. _____

    B. _____

    C. _____

    D. _____

    E. Inferior vena cava

    F. _____

    G. _____

    H. _____

    I. _____

    J. _____

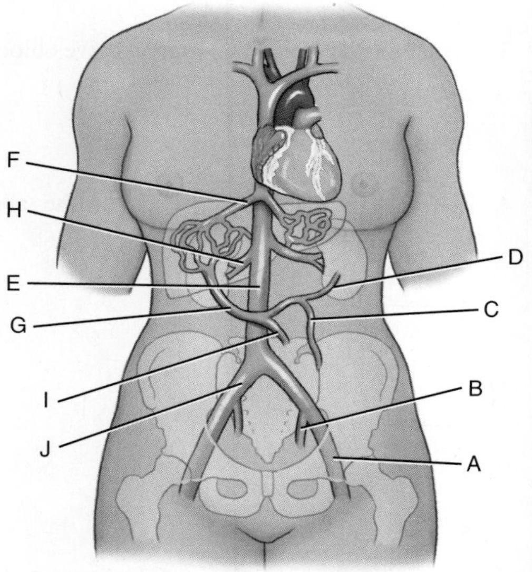

Fig. 17.10 Tributaries to the inferior vena cava.

9. Identify the following veins (A, B, D, and E) that make up the hepatic portal system, as labeled in Fig. 17.11. (Hint: A and B are the two major veins that unite to form the hepatic portal vein [C].)

    A. _____

    B. _____

    C. _____

    D. _____ drain "filtered" blood from the liver and return it to the

    E. _____

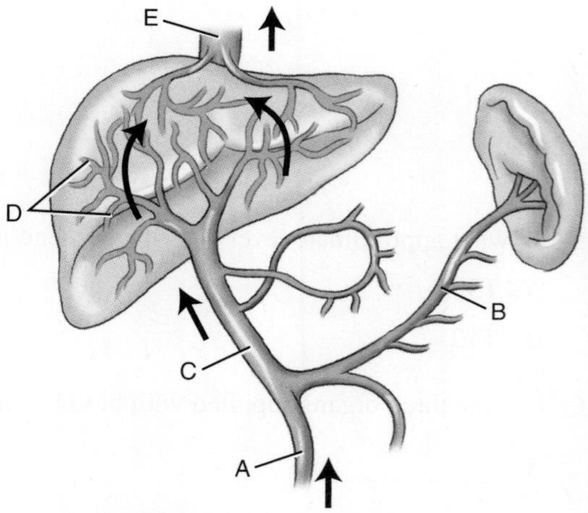

Fig. 17.11 Hepatic portal system.

10. Identify the following upper limb arteries (Fig. 17.12).

On the right side of the body, the (A) _____ artery gives rise to the (B) _____ artery.

Identify the following primary arteries of the upper limb, labeled C–F.

C. _____

D. _____

E. _____

F. _____

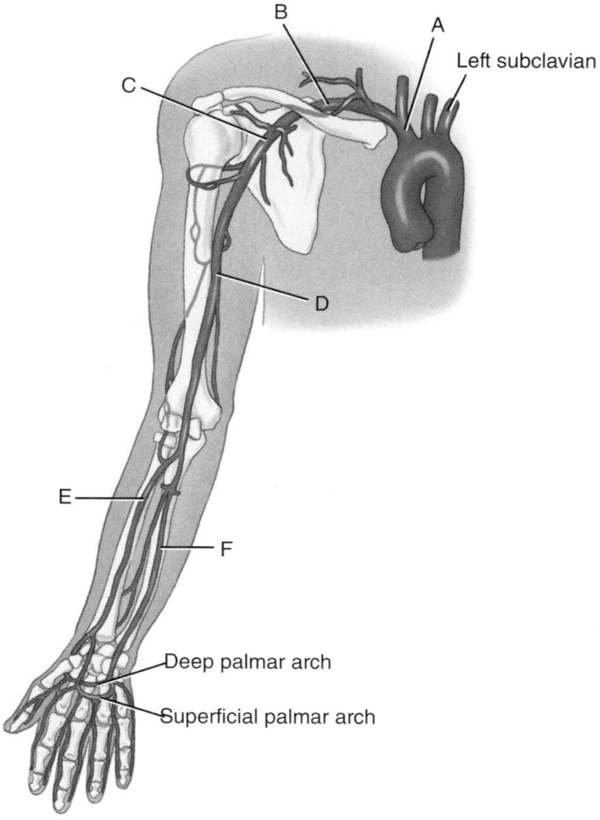

Fig. 17.12 Upper limb arteries.

11. Identify the upper limb veins labeled on Fig. 17.13. The venous system of the upper and lower limbs may be divided into two sets. For the upper limb these begin with:

A. _____ and

B. _____, which form two parallel drainage channels.

Identify the veins returning blood to the heart, labeled C–G in Fig. 17.13.

C. _____

D. _____

E. _____

F. _____

G. _____

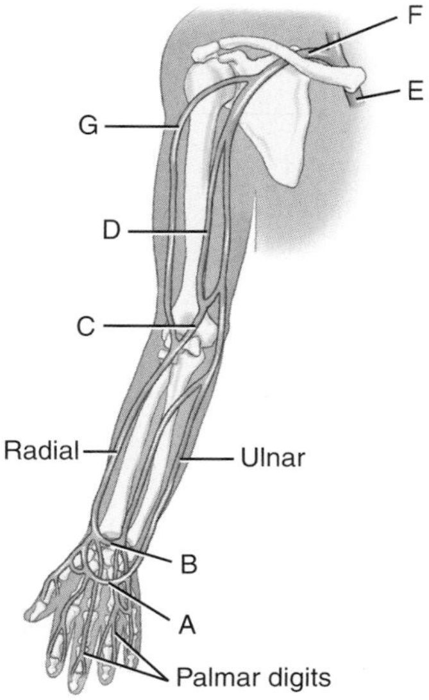

Fig. 17.13 Upper limb veins.

12. The vein most commonly used to draw blood at the elbow is the _____. (Hint: This is one of the veins [A–G] identified in Fig. 17.13.)

Lower Limb Arteries (Fig. 17.14)

13. The lower limb arterial system begins at the

   A. _____ artery and continues as the

   B. _____ artery and it divides into the

   C. _____ and

   D. _____ arteries in the area of the proximal and midfemur. At the knee, the femoral artery becomes the

   E. _____ artery, which continues into the foot as the

   F. _____ artery.

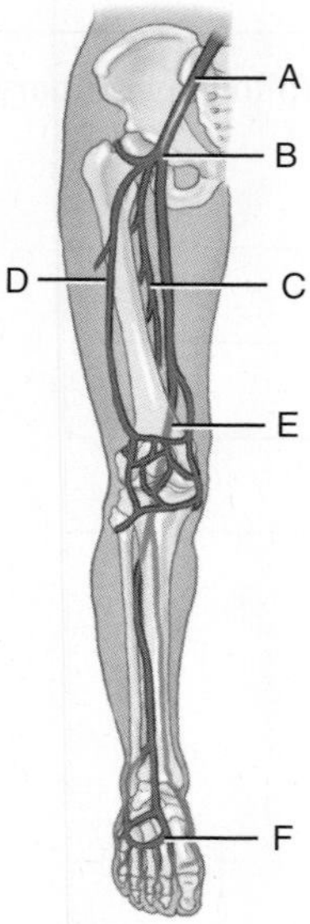

Fig. 17.14 Lower limb arteries.

Lower Limb Veins (Fig. 17.15)

14. Identify the following labeled veins of the lower limb.

   A. _____

   B. _____

   C. _____

   D. _____

   E. _____

   F. _____

   G. _____

   H. _____

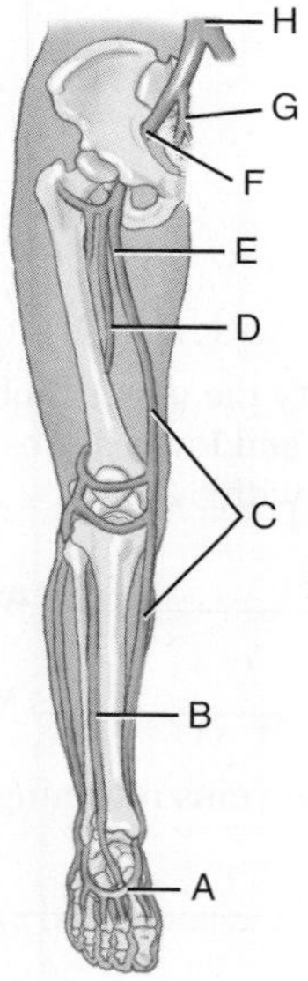

Anterior view
Fig. 17.15 Lower limb veins.

15. The longest vein in the body is the _____ of the lower limb. (Hint: This is one of the labeled veins in Fig. 17.15.)

REVIEW EXERCISE C: Angiographic Procedures, Equipment, and Supplies (see textbook pp. 673–687)

1. Which of the following individuals is (are) not normally part of the angiographic team?

   A. Scrub nurse/technologist

   B. Respiratory therapist

   C. Technologist

   D. Radiologist

2. What are the two specialties, according to the ARRT, interventional technologists are divided into?

   A. _____

   B. _____

3. True/False: An interventional technologist must have a thorough understanding of sterile technique and may be asked to "Scrub In" to assist the interventional physician.

4. A common method or technique for introducing a needle and/or catheter into the blood vessel for angiographic procedures is called the _____.

5. In the correct order, list the six steps of the technique identified in Question 4.

   A. _____

   B. _____

   C. _____

   D. _____

   E. _____

   F. _____

6. Which of the following vessels is preferred for arterial vessel access for the majority of angiographic procedures?

   A. Femoral artery

   B. Brachial artery

   C. Axillary artery

   D. Common carotid artery

7. What is the primary purpose of premedicating the patient before an angiographic procedure?

   A. Reduce the risk for bleeding

   B. Reduce the risk for infection

   C. Help the patient relax

   D. All of the above

8. What type of contrast media is used for most angiographic procedures? _____

9. List the six most common complications associated with angiography.

   1. _____

   2. _____

   3. _____

   4. _____

   5. _____

   6. _____

10. Generally, where is the femoral artery punctured during an arterial catheterization procedure?

   A. Just superior to the inguinal ligament
   B. Just inferior to the inguinal ligament
   C. At the midpoint of the inguinal ligament
   D. 2 inches superior to the popliteal artery

11. What is the minimum amount of time a patient should remain on bed rest following an invasive angiographic procedure?

   A. 1 hour
   B. 3 hours
   C. 4 hours
   D. 6 hours

12. At what angle should the head of the bed or stretcher be elevated following an invasive angiographic procedure?

   A. 10 degrees
   B. 15 degrees
   C. 20 degrees
   D. 30 degrees

13. True/False: Most pediatric angiographic procedures require heavy sedation.

14. What are the three radiation protection devices required for the angiography team?

   1. _____
   2. _____
   3. _____

15. Outlets for _____ and _____ should be located on the walls of the room near the work area.

16. The two types of C-arm configurations include:

   A. _____

   B. _____

17. True/False: The table does not need to provide access to the patient from all sides.

18. Digital subtraction angiography (DSA) provides the opportunity to remove _____ to show only the vessel(s) of interest containing contrast media.

19. List three postprocessing options with digital imaging to improve or modify the image.

   A. _____

   B. _____

   C. _____

20. Flow rate for an automatic electromechanical injector is affected by viscosity of contrast media, injector pressure,

   and _____ and _____ of the catheter.

21. The two purposes of the heating device on an electromechanical injector are as follows:

   A. _____

   B. _____

22. True/False: Multislice computed tomography can produce thinner slices and increase resolution of computed tomography angiography (CTA) images.

23. True/False: CTA does not require the use of iodinated contrast media to demonstrate vascular structures.

24. True/False: Nuclear medicine complements other angiographic modalities even though it provides little anatomic detail.

25. True/False: Color duplex Diagnostic medical sonography (DMS) is effective in demonstrating thrombus formation in the circle of Willis in the adult.

26. True/False: Magnetic resonance imaging (MR) may use carbon dioxide when iodinated contrast media is contraindicated.

27. True/False: Magnetic resonance angiography requires the use of special contrast media to demonstrate vasculature.

28. True/False: Rotational angiography units move around the anatomy up to 360 degrees during the procedure.

29. True/False: Carbon dioxide is recommended instead of iodinated contrast media for carotid angiography.

30. True/False: Gadolinium is recommended for renal angiography for patients with known renal disease.

REVIEW EXERCISE D: Interventional Imaging Procedures (see textbook pp. 688–696)

1. List the five common clinical indicators for cerebral angiography.

   A. _____

   B. _____

   C. _____

   D. _____

   E. _____

2. The point of bifurcation is of special interest to the radiologist; at this point, the internal carotid artery is more

   _____ (medial or lateral) when compared with the external carotid on an anteroposterior

   (AP) projection.

3. List four vessels commonly demonstrated during cerebral angiography.

   A. _____

   B. _____

   C. _____

   D. _____

4. List the three phases of cerebral circulation that can be visualized during cerebral angiography.

   A. _____

   B. _____

   C. _____

5. List five specific pathologies that are common indications for thoracic and pulmonary angiography.

   A. _____

   B. _____

   C. _____

   D. _____

   E. _____

6. True/False: Pulmonary arteriography is commonly performed for pulmonary emboli.

7. Which vessel is most often catheterized for a pulmonary angiogram?
   - A. Femoral vein
   - B. Femoral artery
   - C. Subclavian vein
   - D. Axillary artery

8. The preferred puncture site for a thoracic aortogram is the:
   - A. Femoral vein
   - B. Pulmonary vein
   - C. Pulmonary artery
   - D. Femoral artery

9. The preferred puncture site for a pulmonary arteriogram is:
   - A. Femoral vein
   - B. Pulmonary vein
   - C. Pulmonary artery
   - D. Femoral artery

10. What is the average amount of contrast media injected during a thoracic angiogram?
    - A. 5–8 mL
    - B. 10–15 mL
    - C. 20–25 mL
    - D. 30–50 mL

11. To prevent superimposition of the aortic arch with surrounding structures during a thoracic aortogram, a

    _____ left anterior oblique is often performed.
    - A. 5–10 degrees
    - B. 15–20 degrees
    - C. 45 degrees
    - D. 60 degrees

12. Coronary angiography is typically a study of the:
    - A. Coronary arteries
    - B. Aortic arch
    - C. Coronary veins
    - D. Chambers of the heart

13. Which vessel is commonly catheterized for access to the right side of the heart? _____

14. The average imaging rate during angiocardiography is:
    - A. 2–3 frames per second
    - B. 8–10 frames per second
    - C. 15–30 frames per second
    - D. 45–60 frames per second

15. Which of the following terms describes the pumping efficiency of the left ventricle?

    A. Ejection fraction

    B. Systolic contraction ratio

    C. Ejection coefficient

    D. Myocardial perfusion ratio

16. The term for an angiographic study of the superior and inferior vena cava is _____.

17. List five common clinical indicators for abdominal angiography.

    A. _____

    B. _____

    C. _____

    D. _____

    E. _____

18. The common puncture site for selective abdominal angiography is the _____ using the Seldinger technique.

19. Superselective abdominal angiography can be performed to visualize specific branches (and associated organs) of the abdominal aorta. Which three branches are most commonly catheterized for this purpose?

    A. _____

    B. _____

    C. _____

20. True/False: Venograms are rarely performed today because of increased use of color duplex ultrasound.

21. To study the left upper limb arteries, the catheter is passed from the aortic arch into the:

    A. Left common carotid

    B. Left brachiocephalic vein

    C. Left vertebral artery

    D. Left subclavian artery

22. True/False: Respiration is suspended for the angiographic imaging of the lower limb.

23. Define interventional imaging procedures.

    _____

24. Interventional procedures are considered a benefit to patients because of:

    A. Increased cost of the procedures

    B. Shorter hospital stays

    C. Longer recovery times

    D. A poor second choice to surgery

25. True/False: Interventional angiographic procedures are performed primarily for providing diagnostic information and secondarily for treatment of disease.

424

26. True/False: Interventional imaging procedures are most commonly performed in surgery.

27. How can uterine fibroid embolization help prevent the need for a patient to undergo a hysterectomy?

28. Indicate whether the following interventional procedures are vascular or nonvascular.

_____ 1. Percutaneous transluminal angioplasty (PTA)   A. Vascular procedure

_____ 2. Infusion therapy   B. Nonvascular procedure

_____ 3. Percutaneous biliary drainage (PBD)

_____ 4. Percutaneous gastrostomy

_____ 5. Stent placement

_____ 6. Embolization

_____ 7. Percutaneous abdominal drainage

_____ 8. Nephrostomy

_____ 9. Thrombolysis

_____ 10. Percutaneous needle biopsy

_____ 11. Kyphoplasty

_____ 12. Transjugular intrahepatic portosystemic shunt (TIPS)

29. How is the hepatic portal system accessed during a TIPS procedure? _____

30. What type of medication can be used during infusion therapy to control bleeding?

_____

31. What type of devices are often used to retrieve urethral stones? _____

32. What is the name of the procedure performed to restore the collapsed portion of a vertebral body?

_____

33. What specific device is placed within the collapsed vertebrae to restore their height and structure for the TIPS procedure identified in Question 32? _____

34. What type of catheter is used for transluminal angioplasty? _____

35. What is the correct term describing the interventional procedure for dissolving a blood clot?

    _____

36. Which of the following pathologic indications is most common for performing a PBD?

    A. Biliary obstruction
    B. Suppurative cholangitis

    C. Posttraumatic biliary leakage
    D. Unresectable malignant disease

37. True/False: Percutaneous abdominal drainage procedures have a success rate of only 50%.

38. True/False: Percutaneous gastrostomy is performed primarily for patients who are unable to eat orally.

39. Which of the following processes "ablate" tumor tissue during radiofrequency ablation (RFA)?

    A. Freezing
    B. Chemical dissolving tissue

    C. Low-intensity gamma radiation
    D. Frictional heating

Directions: This self-test should be taken only after completing all of the readings, review exercises, and laboratory activities for a particular section. The purpose of this test is not only to provide a good learning exercise but also to serve as a strong indicator of what your final evaluation exam will be. It is strongly suggested that if you do not receive at least a 90%–95% grade on this self-test, you should review those areas in which you missed questions before going to your instructor for the final evaluation exam for this chapter.

1. The two arteries that deliver blood to the heart muscle are:

   A. Right and left pulmonary veins

   B. Right and left brachiocephalic arteries

   C. Right and left pulmonary arteries

   D. Right and left coronary arteries

2. Which of the following arteries does not originate directly from the arch of the aorta?

   A. Brachiocephalic

   B. Left subclavian

   C. Left common carotid

   D. Right common carotid

3. Each common carotid artery bifurcates into the internal and external arteries at the level of the:

   A. C3–C4 vertebra

   B. C5–C6 vertebra

   C. C1–C2 vertebra

   D. Foramen magnum

4. Which of the following arteries arises from the brachiocephalic artery rather than the aortic arch?

   A. Right vertebral

   B. Left vertebral

   C. Right common carotid

   D. Left common carotid

5. The external carotid does not supply blood to the:

   A. Anterior portion of the brain

   B. Facial area

   C. Anterior neck

   D. Greater part of the scalp and meninges

6. Two branches of each internal carotid artery, which are well visualized with an internal carotid arteriogram, are the:

   A. Posterior and middle cerebral arteries

   B. Anterior and middle cerebral arteries

   C. Right and left vertebral arteries

   D. Facial and maxillary arteries

7. The two vertebral arteries enter the cranium through the foramen magnum and unite to form the:

   A. Brachiocephalic artery

   B. Vertebrobasilar artery

   C. Arterial circle

   D. Basilar artery

8. The basilar artery rests on the clivus of the _____ bone.

   A. Ethmoid

   B. Parietal

   C. Temporal

   D. Sphenoid

9. Which of the following veins do not drain blood from the head, face, and neck regions?

A. Right and left internal jugular veins

B. Right and left vertebral veins

C. Internal and external cerebral veins

D. Right and left external jugular veins

10. The superior and inferior sagittal sinuses join certain other venous sinuses, such as the transverse sinus, at the base of the brain to become the:

A. External jugular vein

B. Internal jugular vein

C. Subclavian vein

D. Vertebral vein

11. Which vein receives blood from the intercostal, esophageal, and phrenic veins?

A. Superior vena cava

B. Inferior vena cava

C. Azygos vein

D. Brachiocephalic vein

12. Which vessels carry oxygenated blood from the lungs back to the heart?

A. Pulmonary veins

B. Pulmonary arteries

C. Coronary arteries

D. Aorta

13. Match the following abdominal arteries with the labeled parts shown in Fig. 17.16.

_____ 1. Inferior mesenteric

_____ 2. Superior mesenteric

_____ 3. Left renal

_____ 4. Right renal

_____ 5. Common hepatic

_____ 6. Celiac (trunk) artery

_____ 7. Left common iliac

_____ 8. Left internal iliac

_____ 9. Left external iliac

_____ 10. Left gastric

_____ 11. Abdominal aorta

_____ 12. Splenic

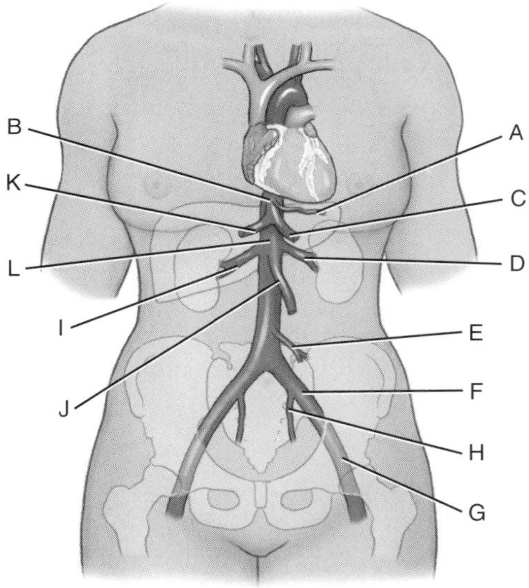

Fig. 17.16 Abdominal arteries.

14. True/False: The right subclavian artery arises directly from the aortic arch.

15. What is another term for the aortic bulb?

A. Aortic stem

B. Aortic confluence

C. Aortic root

D. Aortic sphincter

16. How many segments make up the thoracic aorta?

A. Three

B. Four

C. Five

D. Two

17. A condition in which the aortic arch is located in the right side of the thorax is a variation termed:

    A. Left circumflex aorta

    B. Inverse aorta

    C. Pseudocoarctation

    D. Situs inversus

18. Which of the following vessels carries blood from the intestine to the liver for filtration?

    A. Portal vein

    B. Hepatic veins

    C. Superior mesenteric vein

    D. Inferior vena cava

19. True/False: The cephalic vein is most commonly used for venipuncture.

20. True/False: The great (long) saphenous vein is the longest vein in the body.

21. True/False: The thoracic duct is the largest lymph vessel in the body.

22. Solid food should be withheld for approximately _____ hours before an angiographic procedure.

    A. 1

    B. 4

    C. 8

    D. 24

23. Which of the following vessels is most often punctured for the Seldinger technique?

    A. Abdominal aorta

    B. Femoral vein

    C. Femoral artery

    D. Axillary artery

429

24. Match each of the following terms with its definition or description.

_____ 1. Also known as red blood cells

_____ 2. Component of blood that helps repair tears in blood vessel walls and promotes blood clotting

_____ 3. Carries deoxygenated blood from the right ventricle of the heart to the lungs

_____ 4. Heart valve found between the left atrium and left ventricle

_____ 5. Heart valve found between the right atrium and right ventricle

_____ 6. The vessels that provide blood to the heart muscle

_____ 7. The artery that bifurcates to form the right common carotid and right subclavian arteries

_____ 8. The artery that primarily supplies blood to the anterior neck, scalp, and meninges

_____ 9. The artery that bifurcates into the anterior and middle cerebral arteries

_____ 10. The aspect of the sphenoid bone on which the basilar artery rests

_____ 11. The membranous portion of the dura mater containing the superior sagittal sinus

_____ 12. The artery that forms the left gastric, hepatic, and splenic arteries

_____ 13. The vein created by the splenic and superior mesenteric veins

_____ 14. The vessel that carries oxygenated blood from the lungs to the left atrium of the heart

A. Brachiocephalic artery

B. Pulmonary veins

C. Celiac artery

D. Coronary arteries

E. Superior vena cava

F. Portal vein

G. Falx cerebri

H. Inferior mesenteric artery

I. Coronary sinus

J. External carotid artery

K. Tricuspid (right atrioventricular) valve

L. Clivus

M. Mitral (left atrioventricular or bicuspid) valve

N. Erythrocytes

O. Pulmonary artery

P. Platelets

Q. Internal carotid artery

25. Injection flow rate in angiography is *not* affected by:

A. Viscosity of contrast media

B. Length and diameter of catheter

C. Body temperature

D. Injection pressure

26. Which of the following imaging modalities will best demonstrate velocity of blood flow within a vessel?

A. CTA

B. Color duplex Diagnostic medical sonography (DMS)

C. MR

D. CO_2 angiography

27. What is the minimum amount of time a patient should remain on bed rest following an angiographic procedure?

A. 1 hour

B. 4 hours

C. 8 hours

D. 24 hours

28. Which of the following is generally not found in the angiography unit?

    A. Island-type table
    B. Digital fluoroscopy
    C. Portable x-ray unit
    D. Electromechanical injector

29. True/False: Digital subtraction demonstrates only the bony anatomy during an angiographic study.

30. True/False: Multislice CT scanning does not require arterial puncture and catheter insertion to demonstrate vascular structures.

31. True/False: Contrast media must be used during magnetic resonance angiography.

32. True/False: CO_2 angiography requires the use of a special injector.

33. Which of the following is *not* a clinical indicator for cerebral angiography?

    A. Vascular lesions
    B. Aneurysm
    C. Coarctation
    D. Arteriovenous malformation

34. True/False: The three vascular phases visualized during cerebral angiography should be arterial, capillary, and venous.

35. Pulmonary arteriography is most often performed to diagnose:

    A. Heart valve disease
    B. Pulmonary emboli
    C. Arteriovenous malformation
    D. Coarctation of the aorta

36. The most common vascular approach during pulmonary arteriography is the.

    A. Femoral vein
    B. Femoral artery
    C. Superior vena cava
    D. Axillary artery

37. Which of the following positions prevents superimposition of the proximal aorta and aortic arch during a thoracic aortogram?

    A. 45 degrees right posterior oblique
    B. 45 degrees left posterior oblique
    C. 45 degrees left anterior oblique
    D. Lateral

38. During angiocardiography, the catheter is advanced from the aorta into the:

    A. Superior vena cava
    B. Right ventricle
    C. Left ventricle
    D. Brachiocephalic artery

39. The imaging rate during angiocardiography is:

    A. 1–3 frames per second
    B. 4–8 frames per second
    C. 10–12 frames per second
    D. 15–30 frames per second

40. Which of the following would not be a common pathologic indicator for abdominal angiography?

    A. Aneurysm
    B. Stenosis or occlusions of the aorta
    C. Trauma
    D. Bowel obstruction

41. A peripherally inserted central catheter (PICC) line can remain in the patient up to:

    A. 7 days
    B. 30 days
    C. 180 days
    D. 6 months

42. The tip of a central line is placed near the:

    A. Left ventricle

    B. Right atrium

    C. Brachiocephalic vein

    D. Inferior vena cava

43. For upper limb angiograms, the catheter is advanced along the:

    A. Right carotid artery

    B. Inferior vena cava

    C. Iliac vein of the affected side

    D. Abdominal and thoracic aorta

44. True/False: Angiographic lower limb imaging can only be conducted unilaterally.

45. True/False: A clinical indication for a transcatheter embolization includes stopping active bleeding at a specific site.

46. The most common pathologic indication for chemoembolization is to treat:

    A. Brain aneurysm

    B. Stenosed vessels

    C. Arteriovenous malformation

    D. Hepatic malignancies

47. Match the following descriptions to the correct term or interventional procedure. (Use each choice only once.)

    _____ A. Intravascular administration of drugs

    _____ B. Device to extract urethral stones

    _____ C. Procedure to dissolve blood clots

    _____ D. Technique to restrict uncontrolled hemorrhage

    _____ E. Technique to decompress obstructed bile duct

    _____ F. Direct puncture and catheterization of the renal pelvis

    _____ G. Placement of an extended feeding tube into the stomach

    1. Embolization

    2. Nephrostomy

    3. Infusion therapy

    4. Snare wire loop

    5. Percutaneous gastrostomy

    6. Thrombolysis

    7. Percutaneous biliary drainage

48. True/False: A vena cava filter is placed superior to the renal veins to prevent renal vein thrombosis.

49. True/False: RFA is ideal for treating tumors in the liver and lung.

17 Angiography and Interventional Procedures

1. D. Right and left coronary arteries
2. D. Right common carotid
3. A. C3–C4 vertebra
4. C. Right common carotid
5. A. Anterior portion of the brain
6. B. Anterior and middle cerebral arteries
7. D. Basilar artery
8. D. Sphenoid
9. C. Internal and external cerebral veins
10. B. Internal jugular vein
11. C. Azygos vein
12. A. Pulmonary veins
13. 1. E
    2. J
    3. D
    4. I
    5. K
    6. B
    7. F
    8. H
    9. G
    10. A
    11. L
    12. C
14. False (from the brachiocephalic artery)

15. C. Aortic root
16. B. Four
17. B. Inverse aorta
18. A. Portal vein
19. False (median cubital vein)
20. True
21. True
22. C. 8
23. C. Femoral artery
24. 1. N
    2. P
    3. O
    4. M
    5. K
    6. D
    7. A
    8. J
    9. Q
    10. L
    11. G
    12. C
    13. F
    14. B
25. C. Body temperature
26. B. Color duplex Diagnostic medical sonography (DMS)
27. B. 4 hours
28. C. Portable x-ray unit
29. False. (It demonstrates only the vessels of interest that contain contrast media.)

30. True
31. False (does not have to be used)
32. True
33. C. Coarctation
34. True
35. B. Pulmonary emboli
36. A. Femoral vein
37. C. 45 degrees LAO
38. C. Left ventricle
39. D. 15–30 frames per second
40. D. Bowel obstruction
41. D. 6 months
42. B. Right atrium
43. D. Abdominal and thoracic aorta
44. False. (It can be performed bilaterally or unilaterally.)
45. True
46. D. Hepatic malignancies
47. A. 3
    B. 4
    C. 6
    D. 1
    E. 7
    F. 2
    G. 5
48. False (placed inferior to the renal veins)
49. True

A1

18 Computed Tomography

This chapter presents the general principles of computed tomography (CT) and the various equipment systems in use today. A study of soft tissue anatomy of the central nervous system (CNS) as viewed in axial sections is included. An introduction to the purpose; pathologic indications; and procedure of cranial, thoracic, abdominal, and pelvic CT is also covered in this chapter. Selected sectional images of these three regions are presented.

CHAPTER OBJECTIVES

After you have successfully completed the activities of this chapter, you will be able to:

_____ 1. Identify the evolution and advances in CT systems.

_____ 2. List the major components of a CT system.

_____ 3. Explain the basic operating principles of CT imaging, including x-ray transmission, data acquisition, image reconstruction, window width, window level, and slice thickness.

_____ 4. Define and calculate the pitch ratio for a volume CT scan using different variables.

_____ 5. List the two general divisions of the CNS.

_____ 6. Identify the specialized cells (neurons) of the nervous system and describe their specific parts and functions.

_____ 7. List the specific membranes or coverings of the CNS and identify the meningeal spaces or potential spaces associated with them.

_____ 8. List the three primary divisions of the brain.

_____ 9. List the four major cavities of the ventricular system and identify specific structures and passageways of the ventricular system.

_____ 10. Identify select gray and white matter structures in the brain.

_____ 11. Describe the concept of the blood–brain barrier.

_____ 12. List the 12 cranial nerves.

_____ 13. List three advantages of CT over conventional radiography.

_____ 14. Identify the scan parameters for cranial CT studies.

_____ 15. Identify specific structures of the brain, seen on axial drawings, photographs, and CT sectional images.

_____ 16. Describe various specialized CT procedures to include purpose, procedure, and scan parameters.

LEARNING EXERCISES

Complete the following review exercises after reading the associated pages in the textbook as indicated by each exercise. Answers to each review exercise are provided at the end of this workbook.

REVIEW EXERCISE A: Basic Principles of Computed Tomography (see textbook pp. 698–703)

1. True/False: CAT scan is still an accurate name for computed tomography.

2. The primary changes between generations of CT relates to the _____ and

   _____.

3. Which technology replaced high-tension cables and allowed for continuous rotation of the x-ray tube?

   A. Slip rings
   B. Microswitches
   C. Detectors
   D. Gantry

4. True/False: Noninvasive studies of the heart are possible with multislice CT.

5. True/False: Volume CT scanners are limited to one 360-degree rotation per slice in the same direction.

6. True/False: Terms such as "helical" and "spiral" are vendor-specific terms for volume CT scanners.

7. Which of the following is not an advantage of multislice CT scanners?

   A. Reduced scan time
   B. Improved spatial and temporal resolution
   C. Decreased necessary dose of contrast medium
   D. Low-cost system to operate

8. Reconstruction of patient data into alternative planes (coronal, sagittal, three-dimensional) is termed:

   A. Algorithmic reconstruction
   B. 3D reconstruction
   C. Multiplanar reconstruction
   D. Modulated reconstruction

9. Which of the following uses two different x-ray tubes, separated by 90 degrees, each imaging at a specific kVp level?

   A. Dual-energy CT
   B. Dual-source CT
   C. Mobile CT
   D. PACS

10. List the three primary components of a computed tomographic system.

    A. _____   B. _____   C. _____

11. Which part of the CT system houses the x-ray tube, detector array, and collimators? _____

12. The central opening in the CT support structure at which the patient is scanned is called the _____.

13. List the scintillation materials that make up the solid-state detector array. _____

14. With multidetector CT systems, actual thickness of a tomographic slice is determined by:

    A. Size of detector row
    B. Prepatient collimator
    C. Effective focal spot
    D. Postpatient collimator

15. With a 512- × 512-image matrix, the CT processor must perform _____ mathematical calculations per slice.

   A. 128
   B. 1280
   C. 187,818
   D. 262,144

16. Permanent image archiving for most modern CT systems is performed through a(n):

   A. Picture archiving and communication system
   B. Magnetic disk or tape
   C. Optical disk
   D. Laser printer

17. What do the detectors measure in a CT system? _____

18. What is the basic definition of the term *voxel?* _____

19. A voxel is _____-dimensional image of the tissue, whereas a pixel is a

   _____-dimensional representation of the reconstructed image.

20. The depth of the voxels is determined by:

   A. Slice thickness
   B. Speed of computer
   C. Actual scan time
   D. Size of the pixel

21. Data sets from image voxels are referred to as:

   A. Bytes
   B. Isotropic
   C. Dimensions
   D. Spatial differences

22. Air would have a _____ (higher or lower) differential absorption as compared with soft tissue.

23. CT numbers are a numerical scale that represents tissue _____.

24. List the general CT number or range for the following tissue types.

   A. Cortical bone _____

   B. White brain matter _____

   C. Blood _____

   D. Fat _____

   E. Lung tissue _____

   F. Air _____

   G. Water _____

25. Which medium serves as the baseline for CT numbers? _____

26. Match the most common appearance (level of brightness) of the following tissue types as displayed on a CT image.

_____ A. Bone   1. White

_____ B. Gray brain matter 2. Gray

_____ C. CSF   3. Black

_____ D. Iodinated contrast media

27. Window width (WW) controls:
   A. Displayed image density   C. Slice thickness
   B. Displayed image contrast   D. Total number of slices

28. Window level (WL) controls:
   A. Image brightness   C. Slice thickness
   B. Image contrast   D. Total number of slices

29. Pitch is defined as _____.

30. Pitch is a relationship between _____ and _____.

31. Calculate the pitch ratio using the following parameters: couch movement at a rate of 20 mm per second with a slice collimation of 10 mm. _____

32. The pitch ratio calculated in Question 31 is an example of:
   A. Undersampling   C. Perfect pitch
   B. Oversampling   D. Intermittent pitch

33. Which of the following parameters would produce a 0.5: 1.0 pitch ratio?
   A. 10-mm couch movement and 10-mm slice thickness
   B. 15-mm couch movement and 10-mm slice thickness
   C. 10-mm couch movement and 20-mm slice thickness
   D. 30-mm couch movement and 10-mm slice thickness

34. CT can detect tissue density differences as low as:
   A. $\leq 1\%$ C. 15%
   B. 10%   D. 20%

35. True/False: Both oral and intravenous contrast media can be given during a CT procedure.

36. How must the intravenous contrast media be administered during a multislice CT scan?
   A. Hand, bolus injection   C. Slow drip infusion
   B. Power injector   D. Fast drip infusion

37. True/False: A lower pitch results in lower patient dose.

436

Chapter **18 Computed Tomography**

REVIEW EXERCISE B: Clinical Applications of Computed Tomography (see textbook pp. 704–706)

1. List the four advantages of CT over conventional radiography.

   A. _____

   B. _____

   C. _____

   D. _____

2. A scanogram or topogram is another term for:

   A. CT scan of the head

   B. Scout view

   C. Warm-up procedure for scanner

   D. Calibration procedure for scanner

3. Approximately _____ % to _____ % of all cranial CTs require contrast media.

4. True/False: Oxygen deprivation of *2 minutes* will lead to permanent brain cell injury.

5. True/False: Iodinated contrast media are able to pass through the blood–brain barrier in the normal individual.

6. True/False: Iodinated contrast media are often required to visualize neoplasms during a head CT scan.

7. Which of the following substances will not pass through the blood–brain barrier?

   A. Proteins

   B. Glucose

   C. Oxygen

   D. Select ions found in the blood

8. True/False: Patient dose is higher for a CT scan of the head as compared with a routine skull series.

9. True/False: The higher the pitch ratio during a volume CT scan, the greater the patient dose.

10. What is the name of the technology that uses the optimal mAs per slice to minimize the patient dose during a CT scan?

    A. Modulation transfer function

    B. Scan-dose calibration

    C. Detector calibration

    D. Dose modulation

11. What is the primary goal of the Image Gently

    campaign?_____

12. True/False: If a technologist must remain in the CT imaging room during a procedure, they must wear protective lead apparel.

REVIEW EXERCISE C: Cranial Anatomy and Head CT Procedures (see textbook pp. 707–718)

1. The CNS can be divided into the following two main divisions:

   A. _____

   B. _____

2. A. The solid spinal cord terminates at the lower border of which vertebra? _____

   B. This tapered terminal area of the spinal cord is called the _____.

3. Why is the level of L3 and L4 a common site for a lumbar puncture?

   _____

4. Three membranes or layers of coverings called meninges enclose both the brain and the spinal cord. Certain important spaces or potential spaces are associated with these meninges. List these three meninges and three associated spaces as described below.

   Meninges

   Skull or cranium

   A. _____
      (Outer "hard" or "tough" layer)

   B. _____
      (Spiderlike avascular membrane)

   C. _____
      (Inner "tender" layer)

   Spaces

   D. _____
      (Space or potential space)

   E. _____
      (Narrow space containing thin layer of fluid)

   F. _____
      (Wider space filled with cerebrospinal fluid)

5. The outer "hard" or "tough" membrane has an inner and outer layer that are tightly fused except for certain larger spaces between folds or creases of the brain and skull, which provide for large venous blood channels called

   _____.

6. List the three primary structures of the brainstem.

   A. _____   C. _____

   B. _____

7. The CNS can be divided by appearance into white matter and gray matter, which can be differentiated by CT. The difference in appearance between these two is a result of their makeup. Describe this difference by indicating what each consists of:

   A. White matter: _____   B. Gray matter: _____

8. In general, the thin, outer cerebral cortex is (A) _____ matter, whereas the more centrally located brain tissue is (B) _____ matter.

9. The large cerebrum is divided into right and left hemispheres. Each hemisphere of the cerebrum is further divided into five lobes, with four of the lobes lying under the cranial bone of the same name. List these five lobes.

A. _____   D. _____

B. _____   E. _____

C. _____

10. The brain (encephalon) can be divided into three general divisions: the (1) forebrain, (2) midbrain, and (3) hindbrain. The forebrain and hindbrain are both divided into three divisions. List the three divisions of the forebrain and the hindbrain as labeled in Fig. 18.1. (Note: Secondary terms for these divisions as found in the textbook are included in parentheses.)

1. Forebrain   A. _____
   (Prosencephalon)   (Telencephalon)—largest division
   (Diencephalon)   B. _____
                      C. _____
2. Midbrain   (Mesencephalon)
3. Hindbrain   D. _____
   (Rhombencephalon) E. _____
                      F. _____

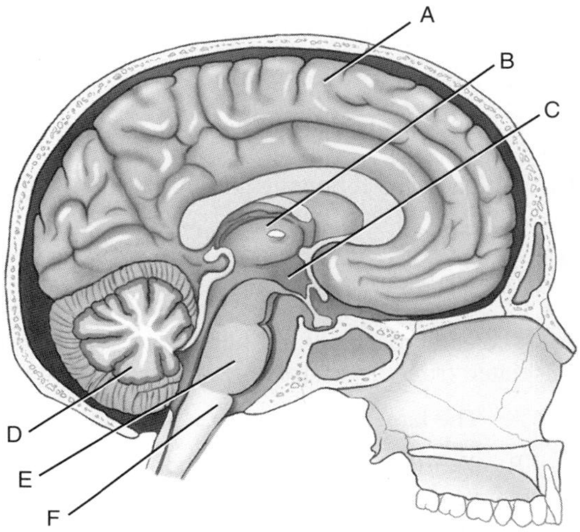

Fig. 18.1 Divisions of the forebrain and hindbrain, midsagittal view.

11. Identify the three lobes of the right cerebral hemisphere, as labeled A through C in Fig. 18.2. The deep fissure separating the two cerebral hemispheres is labeled D. (Note: There is a fold of dura mater, called the falx cerebri, which extends deep within this fissure and separates the two hemispheres that is visualized on CT scans.)

A. _____ lobe

B. _____ lobe

C. _____ lobe

D. _____ fissure

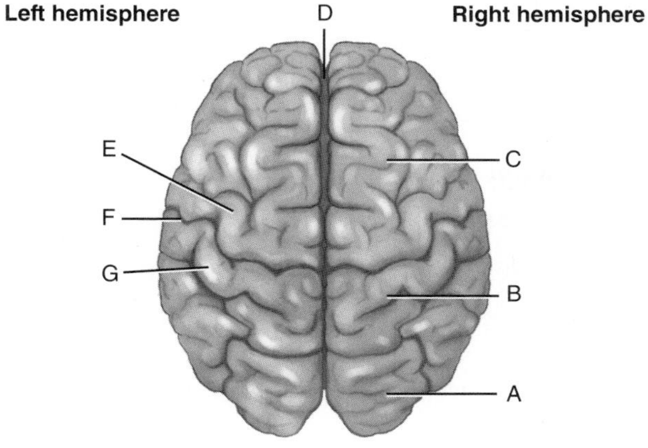

Fig. 18.2 Structures of the cerebral hemispheres.

12. The surface of each cerebral hemisphere contains numerous grooves and convolutions or raised areas. Identify labeled parts E through G in Fig. 18.2. Two of these raised areas, E and G, have specific names and are frequently demonstrated and identified on cranial CT scans. Part F is a shallow groove with a specific name.

    E. _____

    F. _____

    G. _____

13. What is the name of the arched mass of transverse fibers (white matter) that connects the two cerebral hemispheres?

    A. Falx cerebri

    B. Anterior central gyrus

    C. Central sulcus

    D. Corpus callosum

14. What is the name of the large groove that separates the cerebral hemispheres?

    A. Anterior central gyrus

    B. Longitudinal fissure

    C. Central sulcus

    D. Posterior central gyrus

15. Which of the following produces cerebrospinal fluid (CSF)?

    A. Pons

    B. Thalamus

    C. Choroid plexus

    D. Cerebellum

16. The cerebrospinal fluid-filled space and ventricular system are important in CT because these areas can be differentiated from tissue structures by their density differences.

    A. The larger spaces or areas within the CSF-filled space are called _____.

    B. The largest of these is the _____, located just posterior and inferior to the fourth ventricle.

17. The central midline portion of the brain connecting the midbrain, pons, and medulla to the spinal cord is called the

_____.

18. Which aspect of the brain serves as an interpretation center for certain sensory impulses?

    A. Midbrain

    B. Pituitary gland

    C. Thalamus

    D. Hypothalamus

19. The optic chiasma, the site at which some of the optic nerves cross to the opposite side, is located in the

_____, a division of the forebrain.

20. Which of the following is often referred to as the "master" gland?

    A. Pineal

    B. Pons

    C. Pituitary

    D. Corpus callosum

21. The pituitary gland is attached to the hypothalamus by the_____

22. Which aspect of the brain coordinates important motor functions such as coordination, posture, and balance?

    A. Pons

    B. Cerebellum

    C. Midbrain

    D. Cerebrum

23. Which aspect of the brain controls important body activities related to homeostasis?

    A. Pons   C. Thalamus

    B. Cerebellum   D. Hypothalamus

24. Which structure of the brain controls a wide range of body functions, including growth and reproductive functions?

    A. Pineal gland   C. Thalamus

    B. Pituitary gland   D. Hypothalamus

25. List the four groupings of cerebral nuclei (basal ganglia).

    A. _____   C. _____

    B. _____   D. _____

26. Ventricles: There are four major cavities in the ventricular system. These are labeled in Fig. 18.3 and demonstrate the four ventricles in relationship to other brain structures. Two of the ventricles are located within the right and left cerebral hemispheres (*A*); the remaining two are midline structures (*B* and *C*).

    The larger two ventricles (*A*) have four significant parts labeled *1, 2, 3,* and *6* in Fig. 18.4. The small ductlike structure (*4*) provides communication between ventricles, and number *5* indicates a connection between the third and fourth ventricles. An important gland (*8*) is also shown. Number *7* represents an important communication with the subarachnoid space on each side of the fourth ventricle.

    Identify the ventricles and their parts as labeled on these two drawings.

Fig. 18.3

    A. Right and left _____ ventricles

    B. _____ ventricle

    C. _____ ventricle

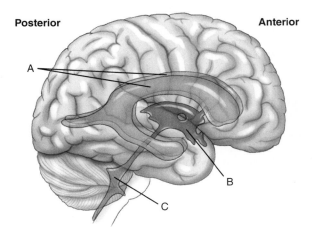

Fig. 18.3 Cavities in the ventricular system.

Fig. 18.4

1 _____ (occipital)

2 _____

3 _____ (frontal)

4 _____ (foramen)

5 _____

6 _____ (temporal)

7 _____

8 _____ (gland)

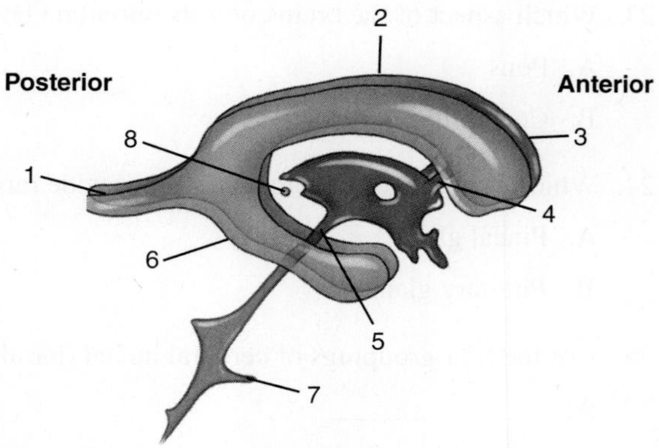

Fig. 18.4 Anatomy of the ventricles.

27. There are 12 pairs of cranial nerves, most of which originate from the brainstem and travel to various parts of the brain, controlling both sensory and motor functions. List these 12 pairs of cranial nerves.

A. _____   E. _____   I. _____

B. _____   F. _____   J. _____

C. _____   G. _____   K. _____

D. _____   H. _____   L. _____

28. Head CT images are viewed in what two window settings?

A. _____   B. _____

29. The most important aspect of positioning the head for cranial CT is to ensure there is no _____

and no _____ of the head.

30. Trauma to the skull may lead to a collection of blood accumulating under the dura mater called

_____.

31. Identify the labeled parts on this axial section through the region of the midventricular level (Fig. 18.5).

A. _____

B. _____

C. _____

D. _____

E. _____

F. _____

G. _____

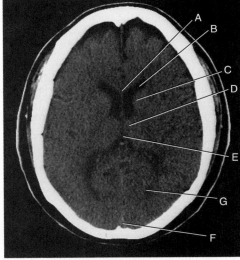

Fig. 18.5 Structure identification on an axial CT scan at midventricular level.

32. Identify the labeled parts on this axial section through the level of the middle third ventricle (Fig. 18.6).

A. _____

B. _____

C. _____

D. _____

E. _____

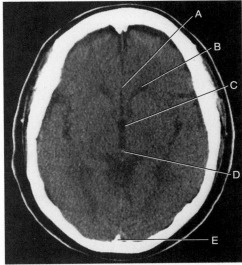

Fig. 18.6 Structure identification on an axial CT scan at mid-third-ventricle level.

REVIEW EXERCISE D: Additional and Specialized Computed Tomography Procedures and Computed Tomography Terminology (see textbook pp. 719–725)

1. CT scanning of the neck for a possible tumor of the nasopharynx requires slice thicknesses of no greater than:

   A. 2–3 mm
   B. 5 mm
   C. 7–10 mm
   D. 1 cm

2. True/False: Air may be injected into the joint for a CT scan of synovial joints.

3. Common pathologic indications for a CT study of the spine include the following *except:*

   A. Infection
   B. Spinal stenosis
   C. Spinal cord deformity
   D. Fracture of the vertebrae

4. When performing musculoskeletal CT examinations, which window setting(s) are used?

   A. Bone
   B. Soft Tissue
   C. Both A&B
   D. None of the above

5. True/False: Oral and IV contrast are used for abdominopelvic CT images of kidney stones.

6. True or False: 3D imaging requires a data set created during a volume acquisition.

7. What is the contrast medium of choice for most CT virtual endoscopic procedures? _____

8. Other than air, what other contrast media are often used for a CT colonography? _____

9. True/False: CT angiography (CTA) does not require the use of iodinated contrast media.

10. How much oral contrast media is instilled for a CT enterography?

    A. Up to 100 mL
    B. Up to 500 mL
    C. Up to 1000 mL
    D. Up to 2000 mL

11. What is the purpose of electrocardiogram gating during a cardiac CT scan? _____

12. True/False: Traditional coronary angiography remains the gold standard for the evaluation of the coronary arteries rather than cardiac CT.

13. True/False: The patient/table is stationary during CT fluoroscopy.

14. During CT fluoroscopy, partially reconstructed images are obtained and displayed at a rate of:

    A. 1–3 images per second
    B. 6–8 images per second
    C. 8–12 images per second
    D. 20–25 images per second

15. One of the most common applications for CT fluoroscopy is:

    A. CT myelography
    B. Gastrointestinal motility studies
    C. Virtual colonoscopy
    D. Biopsies

16. What is used to minimize exposure to the hands of the radiologist during a CT fluoroscopic biopsy?

    A. Lead gloves
    B. Low kVp
    C. Special filters
    D. Special needle holders

17. True/False: CT percutaneous biopsies have an equal accuracy rate as compared with surgical biopsies.

18. The success rate for CT percutaneous abscess drainage is approximately:

    A. 10%–15%   C. 50%–60%

    B. 20%–25%   D. 85%

19. Identify the name of the device that houses the CT x-ray tube, detectors, and collimators.

    _____

20. What is the term for a series of rows and columns of pixels that give form to the digital image?

    _____

21. What are the terms (more than one answer) for a preliminary image taken before a CT procedure?

    _____

22. A device that transmits electrical energy and allows continuous rotation of the CT x-ray tube for volumetric acquisition is called _____.

23. _____ controls the brightness of a CT-reconstructed image within a certain range.

24. _____ controls the gray level or contrast of a CT image.

25. _____ is a technique used to view vessels demonstrated during a CTA.

LABORATORY EXERCISES

This learning activity needs to be performed in a special procedures room equipped for CT. A supervising technologist or instructor should be present for this activity.

Laboratory Exercise: Positioning

Complete the following steps and place a check mark by each when completed.

_____ 1. Review the equipment in the room, noting the location of patient support equipment, such as oxygen, suction, the IV pole, and the emergency cart.

_____ 2. Role-play using another student as the patient. Prepare the "patient" by explaining the procedure, the breathing instructions that will be given, the sounds that will be experienced, and what he or she will see and experience as the patient is placed into the gantry aperture for the examination.

_____ 3. Place your patient on the table (couch) in a supine position with the arms above the head. Raise the patient and table to the correct height and slowly move into the gantry aperture until the x-ray beam trajectory coincides with the starting scan position for the part being examined. Using the intercom device, talk to the patient from the control console. Finally, remove your patient when the procedure is completed.

_____ 4. Review the controls and monitors at the operator console. Have someone demonstrate the image parameters and the other variables controlled by the technologist and explain how whole-body scanning is different from head CT scanning.

Directions: This self-test should be taken only after completing all of the readings, review exercises, and laboratory activities for a particular section. The purpose of this test is not only to provide a good learning exercise but also to serve as a strong indicator of what your final evaluation exam will be. It is strongly suggested that if you do not receive at least a 90%–95% grade on this self-test, you should review those areas in which you missed questions before going to your instructor for the final evaluation exam for this chapter.

1. X-ray tube movement was restricted in early CT scanners by:

    A. Gantry size

    B. Rotational speed

    C. Voltage levels

    D. High-tension cables

2. The general term used to describe the acquisition of a volume of data is:

    A. Volume scanning

    B. Whole-body scanning

    C. Single-slice acquisition

    D. Dual-energy scanning

3. Which devices in the volume CT scanners allow continual tube rotation in the same direction? _____

4. CT can detect tissue density differences as low as:

    A. 1%

    B. 5%

    C. 10%

    D. 20%

5. Which device shapes and limits the x-ray beam in the CT tube? _____

6. What must be done to the numeric data (CT numbers) to create the displayed CT image?

    _____

7. The three major components of the scan unit are:

    A. _____

    B. _____

    C. _____

8. Each tiny picture element in the display matrix is called a(n) _____.

9. Which of the following parameters *cannot* be varied by appropriate manipulation at the operator console?

    A. kVp

    B. Scan time

    C. Pitch ratio

    D. Vertical adjustment of table height

    E. Thickness of slice

10. What is the name of the 3D element that provides height, width, and depth to the display matrix of the digital image?

    A. Pixel

    B. Voxel

    C. Image volume

    D. Isotropic data set

11. True/False: Submillimeter slice thicknesses are possible with multislice CT scanners.

12. A 64-slice CT scanner can acquire up to _____ images per second.

    A. 64   C. 525

    B. 160   D. 1048

13. What does the detector actually measure in a CT system? _____

14. What substance serves as the baseline for CT numbers? _____

15. What is the CT number for the substance described in Question 31? _____

16. What is the CT number for fat?

    A. −100   C. +100

    B. −200   D. +250

17. Pitch is defined as a ratio between table speed and:

    A. Number of tube rotations   C. Slice thickness

    B. Size of total tissue acquisition   D. Tissue attenuation

18. Which one of the following pitch ratios represents "undersampling"?

    A. 1: 1   C. 0.5: 1

    B. 2: 1   D. 0.7: 1

19. True/False: CT exceeds the contrast resolution seen on a conventional radiograph.

20. Contrast media do not ordinarily cross the _____ barrier.

21. A. The parts of the neuron that conduct impulses toward the cell body are called _____.

    B. The part that conducts impulses away from the cell body is the _____.

22. Three protective membranes that cover or enclose the entire CNS are collectively called: _____

23. The three specific membranes from Question 2 are called (starting externally)

    A. _____

    B. _____

    C. _____

24. The various layers of the membranes just discussed have specific spaces of various sizes between these layers. Each has a specific name. Identify these various membrane layers and their associated spaces on Fig. 18.7.

A. _____

B. _____

C. _____

D. _____

E. _____

F. _____

G. _____

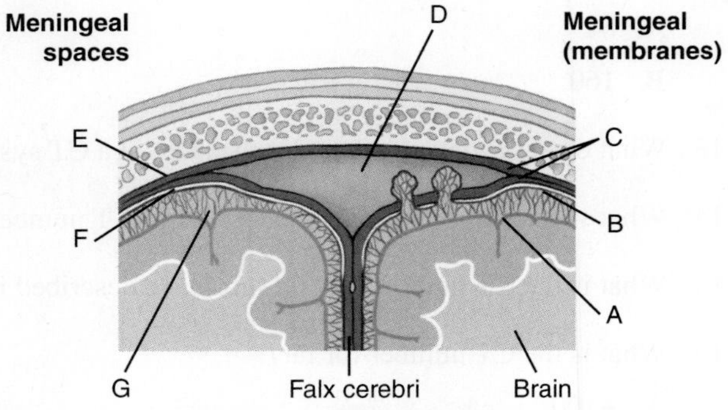

Fig. 18.7 Meninges and meningeal spaces.

25. Which of the spaces in question is normally filled with cerebrospinal fluid? _____

26. Match the following structures to the correct division of the brain.

_____ A. Pons   1. Forebrain

_____ B. Cerebellum   2. Midbrain

_____ C. Cerebrum   3. Hindbrain

_____ D. Thalamus

_____ E. Cerebral aqueduct

27. The largest division of the brain is the _____.

28. A deep fissure called the _____ separates the right and left cerebral hemispheres.

29. The fibrous band of white tissue deep within this fissure connecting the right and left cerebral hemispheres is called the _____.

30. The inner layers of dura mater within the longitudinal fissure join to form the _____.

31. Which of the following ventricle(s) is (are) located in the upper aspect of the cerebral hemispheres?

A. Lateral ventricles   C. Third ventricle

B. Fourth ventricle   D. Cisterna magna

32. The diamond-shaped fourth ventricle connects inferiorly with a wide portion of the subarachnoid space called the:

A. Interventricular foramen   C. Cisterna cerebellomedullaris

B. Lateral recesses   D. Cisterna pontis

33. Identify the ventricles, their parts, and their associated structures as labeled on both the lateral and top-view drawings (Figs. 18.8 and 18.9).

Ventricles

A. _____

B. _____

C. _____

Connecting passageways for CSF

a. _____

b. _____

c. _____

Parts of lateral ventricles

1. _____

2. _____

3. _____

4. _____

Small gland (only in Fig. 18.8)

5. _____

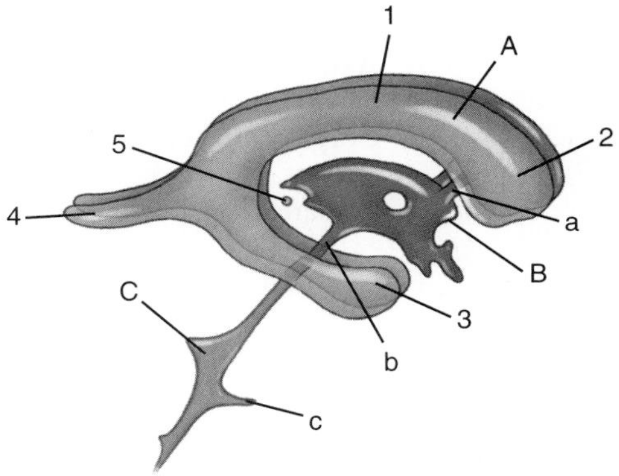

Fig. 18.8 Ventricles, lateral view.

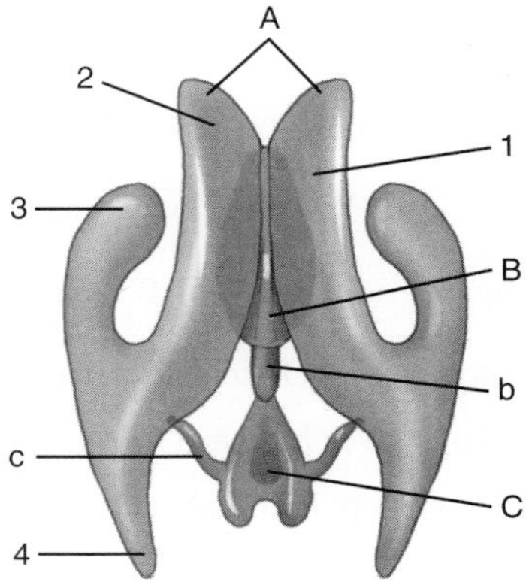

Fig. 18.9 Ventricles, superior view.

34. The condition known as _____ results from an abnormal accumulation of cerebrospinal fluid within the _____.

35. Enlarged regions of the subarachnoid space are called _____.

36. Identify the four lobes of the cerebrum as labeled in Fig. 18.10.

A. _____

B. _____

C. _____

D. _____

E. The fifth lobe, which is more centrally located and not shown in this drawing, is called the _____.

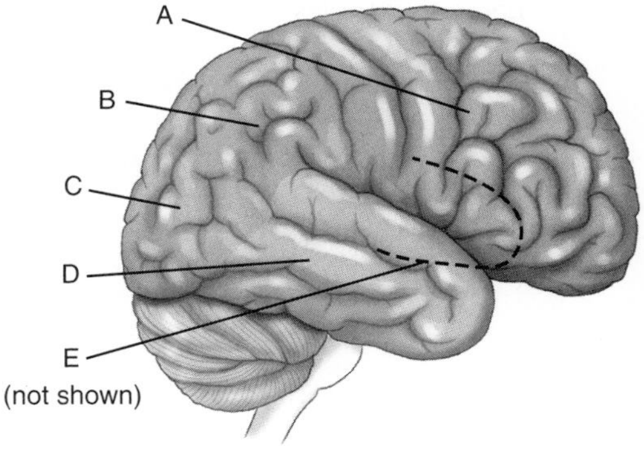

Fig. 18.10 Four lobes of the cerebrum.

449

37. Identify each of the following terms as either gray matter or white matter brain structures.

_____ A. Cerebral cortex

_____ B. Axons (fibrous parts of neuron)

_____ C. Corpus callosum

_____ D. Thalamus

_____ E. Centrum semiovale

_____ F. Cerebral nuclei

1. Gray matter

2. White matter

38. Which of the following pathologic indications does *not* apply to head CT?

A. Brain neoplasm

B. Brain atrophy

C. Multiple sclerosis

D. Trauma

E. All of the above apply

39. True/False: An intravenous injection of iodinated contrast media is often given during a CT enterography study.

40. Images produced during CTA are viewed with a technique termed _____.

41. What type of technical factors are used with CT fluoroscopy?

A. High kVp; high mA

B. Low kVp; high mA

C. High kVp; low mA

D. Low kVp; low mA

42. The typical slice thickness for a spine CT is:

A. 3 mm

B. 7 mm

C. 10 mm

D. 15 mm

43. A CT colonography requires the use of _____ as a contrast medium.

A. Barium sulfate

B. Iodinated rectal contrast

C. Air

D. All of the above

44. What is the chief disadvantage of CT colonography over conventional endoscopy?

A. Cost

B. Cannot biopsy or remove polyps

C. Bowel prep required

D. Time-consuming procedure

45. True/False: Special filters can be used during CT fluoroscopy to reduce patient skin dose during biopsies.

46. How long is the catheter left in place following a percutaneous abscess drainage procedure?

    A. 1 hour   C. 12 hours

    B. 6 hours   D. 24–48 hours

47. _____ is a method by which images acquired in the axial plane may be reconstructed in the coronal or sagittal plane.

48. _____ controls the gray level of an image (the contrast).

49. _____ is a computer that serves as a digital postprocessing station and/or an image review station.

18 Computed Tomography

WORKBOOK SELF-TEST ANSWER KEY

1. D. High-tension cables
2. A. Volume scanning
3. Slip rings
4. A. 1%
5. Prepatient collimator
6. Assign various shades of gray to the CT numbers based on tissue attenuation.
7. A. Gantry
   B. Computer
   C. Operator console
8. Pixel
9. D. Vertical adjustment of table height
10. B. Voxel
11. True
12. B. 160
13. Tissue attenuation
14. Water
15. Zero (0)
16. A. −100
17. C. Slice thickness
18. B. 2:1
19. True
20. Blood–brain
21. A. Dendrites
    B. Axon
22. Meninges

23. A. Dura mater
    B. Arachnoid mater
    C. Pia mater
24. A. Pia mater
    B. Arachnoid mater
    C. Dura mater
    D. Venous sinus
    E. Epidural space
    F. Subdural space
    G. Subarachnoid spaces
25. Subarachnoid space
26. A. 3
    B. 3
    C. 1
    D. 1
    E. 2
27. Cerebrum
28. Longitudinal fissure
29. Corpus callosum
30. Falx cerebri
31. A. Lateral ventricles
32. C. Cisterna cerebellomedullaris
33. A. Lateral
    B. Third
    C. Fourth
       a. Interventricular foramen
       b. Cerebral aqueduct
       c. Lateral recess
          1. Body
          2. Anterior horn
          3. Inferior (temporal) horn

       4. Posterior horn
       5. Pineal gland
34. Hydrocephalus; ventricles
35. Cisterns
36. A. Frontal
    B. Parietal
    C. Occipital
    D. Temporal
    E. Insula or central lobe
37. A. 1
    B. 2
    C. 2
    D. 1
    E. 2
    F. 1
38. C. Multiple sclerosis
39. True
40. Maximum intensity projection
41. C. High kVp; low mA
42. A. 3 mm
43. C. Air
44. B. Cannot biopsy or remove polyps
45. True
46. D. 24–48 hours
47. Multiplanar reconstruction (MPR)
48. Window width
49. Workstation

A1

19 Special Radiographic Procedures

This chapter discusses those additional diagnostic imaging procedures that are less common in most radiology departments. Arthrograms, biliary duct procedures, myelograms, long bone measurements, skeletal surveys, and digital tomosynthesis are largely being replaced with other imaging modalities such as computed tomography (CT) or magnetic resonance imaging (MR). However, in some departments, these procedures are still being performed in sufficient numbers that technologists must be familiar with them so that they can perform them when requested.

The anatomy for these procedures has been studied in previous chapters; therefore this chapter covers only the procedures themselves and the related positioning. The exception to this is the anatomy of the female reproductive organs as described in the section on hysterosalpingography.

CHAPTER OBJECTIVES

After you have successfully completed the activities of this chapter, you will be able to:

ARTHROGRAPHY

_____ 1. Identify the purpose, clinical indications, patient preparation, equipment, general procedure, and positioning routines related to knee arthrography.

_____ 2. Identify the purpose, clinical indications, patient preparation, equipment, general procedure, and positioning and imaging sequence related to shoulder arthrography.

BILIARY DUCT PROCEDURES

_____ 1. Describe the purpose, clinical indications, patient preparation, equipment, general procedure, and positioning and imaging sequence for the postoperative (T-tube or delayed) cholangiography.

_____ 2. Describe the purpose, clinical indications, patient preparation, equipment, general procedure, and the positioning and imaging sequence for an endoscopic retrograde cholangiopancreatography (ERCP).

HYSTEROSALPINGOGRAPHY

_____ 1. Identify specific aspects of the female reproductive system.

_____ 2. Identify the purpose, clinical indications, patient preparation, equipment, general procedure, and the positioning routines related to hysterosalpingography.

MYELOGRAPHY

_____ 1. Identify the purpose, clinical indications, contraindications, equipment, and general procedures related to myelography.

_____ 2. Identify positioning routines performed for lumbar, thoracic, and cervical myelography.

LONG BONE MEASUREMENT (HIP-TO-ANKLE)

_____ 1. Define long bone measurement and the purpose of this procedure.

_____ 2. Identify the specific positioning and procedure for lower limb long bone measurements.

SKELETAL SURVEY (BONE SURVEY)

_____ 1. Define skeletal survey and the purpose of this procedure.

_____ 2. Identify the specific positioning and procedure for a skeletal survey.

DIGITAL TOMOSYNTHESIS

_____ 1. Define digital tomosynthesis and the purpose of this imaging technique.

_____ 2. Describe the benefits of digital tomosynthesis.

_____ 3. Compare digital tomosynthesis to CT and conventional tomography.

LEARNING EXERCISES

The following review exercises should be completed only after careful study of the associated pages in the textbook as indicated by each exercise. Answers to each review exercise are provided at the end of this workbook.

REVIEW EXERCISE A: Arthrography (see textbook pp. 728–731)

1. Which classification of joints are studied with arthrography? _____

2. Other than conventional radiography of synovial joints (e.g., arthrography), which imaging procedure is preferred by

   physicians for studying synovial joints? _____

3. List the three common forms of knee injury that may require arthrography.

   A. _____

   B. _____

   C. _____

4. Give an example of nontraumatic pathology of the knee joint indicating arthrography.

   _____

5. What are the two primary contraindications for arthrography of any joint? _____

6. True/False: An arthrogram must be approached as a sterile procedure. Proper skin prep and sterility must be maintained.

7. True/False: After the contrast medium is introduced into the knee joint, the knee must *not* be flexed or exercised.

8. What is the normal appearance of synovial fluid?

9. List the two types of contrast media used for a knee arthrogram.

A. _____ B. _____

10. List the two routine projections for conventional radiographic projections used for knee arthrography.

A. _____ B. _____

11. A. On average, how many exposures are taken of each meniscus during fluoroscopy of the knee?

_____

B. How many degrees of rotation of the leg are used between exposures? _____

12. What four aspects of shoulder anatomy are demonstrated with shoulder arthrography?

A. _____ C. _____

B. _____ D. _____

13. What is the general name for the conjoined tendons of the four major shoulder muscles?

_____

14. What type of needle is commonly used for shoulder arthrograms? _____

15. List three clinical indications for a shoulder arthrogram.

A. _____

B. _____

C. _____

16. List the six projections frequently taken during a shoulder arthrogram.

A. _____ D. _____

B. _____ E. _____

C. _____ F. _____

REVIEW EXERCISE B: Biliary Duct Procedures (see textbook pp. 732–733)

1. Postoperative (T-tube) cholangiograms are usually performed to detect

A. Pancreatitis C. Liver cyst

B. Biliary stones D. Infected gallbladder

2. True/False: A surgeon usually performs T-tube cholangiography during a colectomy.

3. Which two blood chemistry values must be checked prior to a postoperative (T-tube) cholangiogram?

A. _____ B. _____

4. Why are the contrast media for a T-tube cholangiogram occasionally diluted before injection?

_____

5. True/False: Bile is sterile, and standard precautions do not apply when handling it.

6. **Situation:** A T-tube cholangiogram image demonstrates the biliary ducts superimposed over the spine. The patient is in an anteroposterior (AP) position. Which position would remove the ducts from the spine?

_____

7. Postoperative (T-tube) cholangiograms are generally performed _____.

8. Which of the following procedures might be performed during a postoperative (T-tube) cholangiogram?

   A. Removal of the gallbladder

   B. Removal of a liver cyst

   C. Removal of a biliary stone

   D. Catheterization of the hepatic portal vein

9. A. A radiographic procedure of examining the biliary and main pancreatic ducts is called a(n)

   _____. (Write out the full term.)

   B. What initials are commonly used as an abbreviation for this procedure? _____

   C. What type of special endoscope is commonly used for this procedure? _____

   D. Which member of the health care team usually performs this procedure? _____

   E. Why should a patient remain NPO at least 1 hour after this procedure? _____

10. Which condition of the pancreas may contraindicate an ERCP? _____

REVIEW EXERCISE C: Hysterosalpingography (see textbook pp. 734–736)

1. The hysterosalpingogram (HSG) is a radiographic study of the _____ and

   _____.

2. The uterus is situated between the _____ posteriorly and the

   _____ anteriorly.

3. List the four divisions of the uterus.

   A. _____

   B. _____

   C. _____

   D. _____

4. The largest division of the uterus is the _____.

5. The distal aspect of the uterus extending to the vagina is the _____.

6. List the three layers of tissue that form the uterus (from the innermost to the outermost layer).

   A. _____

   B. _____

   C. _____

7. Which of the following terms is not an aspect of the uterine tube?
   A. Cornu
   B. Ampulla
   C. Isthmus
   D. Infundibulum

8. True/False: Fertilization of the ovum occurs in the uterine tube.

9. True/False: The distal portion of the uterine tube opens into the peritoneal cavity.

10. Which of the following terms is used to describe the "degree of openness" of the uterine tube?
    A. Stenosis
    B. Patency
    C. Atresia
    D. Gauge

11. The most common pathologic indication for the HSG is _____.

12. In addition to the answer for Question 11, what are two other clinical indications for HSG?

    A. _____

    B. _____

13. List the three common types of lesions that can be demonstrated during an HSG.

    A. _____

    B. _____

    C. _____

14. The contrast medium preferred by most radiologists for an HSG is
    A. Water-soluble, iodinated
    B. Oil-based, iodinated
    C. Oxygen
    D. Nitrogen

15. What device might be needed to aid the insertion and fixation of the cannula or catheter during the HSG?

    _____

16. To help facilitate the flow of contrast media into the uterine cavity, in which position is the patient placed following

    the injection of contrast media? _____

17. In addition to the supine position, what two other positions may be imaged to adequately visualize the pertinent anatomy for an HSG?

    A. _____

    B. _____

18. Where is the central ray (CR) centered for radiographic projections taken during an HSG using a recommended collimation field size of 10- × 12-inch (25- × 30-cm)?

    A. At level of anterior superior iliac spine   C. Iliac crest

    B. Symphysis pubis   D. 2 inches (5 cm) superior to the symphysis pubis

REVIEW EXERCISE D: Myelography (see textbook pp. 737–740)

1. Myelography is a radiographic study of the:

    A. _____

    B. _____

2. List the four common lesions or clinical indications demonstrated during myelography.

    A. _____   C. _____

    B. _____   D. _____

3. Of the four clinical indications just mentioned, which is the most common for myelography?

    _____

4. True/False: Myelography of the cervical and thoracic spinal regions is most common.

5. List the four common contraindications for myelography.

    A. _____   C. _____

    B. _____   D. _____

6. To reduce patient anxiety, a sedative is usually administered _____ hour(s) before the procedure.

7. What type of radiographic table must be used for myelography? _____

8. Into which spinal space is the contrast medium introduced during myelography?

    _____

9. List the two common puncture sites for contrast media injection during myelography.

    A. _____

    B. _____

10. Which of the puncture sites from Question 9 is preferred? _____

11. What is the patient's general body position for each of the following punctures? (Note: There may be more than one acceptable answer for each.)

    A. Lumbar _____

    B. Cervical _____

12. Why is a large positioning block placed under the abdomen for a lumbar puncture in the prone position?

    _____

13. Which type of contrast medium is most commonly used for myelography? _____

14. The contrast medium in Question 13 provides good radiopacity up to _____ after injection.
    A. 20 minutes
    B. 30 minutes
    C. 1 hour
    D. 8 hours

15. What dosage range of contrast medium is usually injected for myelography?
    A. 8–10 mL
    B. 20–30 mL
    C. 9–15 mL
    D. Approximately 1 mL

16. Indicate the correct sequence of events for a myelogram by numbering the following steps in order (from 1 to 8).

    _____ A. Introduce needle into subarachnoid space

    _____ B. Collect cerebrospinal fluid and send to laboratory

    _____ C. Take overhead radiographic images

    _____ D. Explain procedure to the patient

    _____ E. Introduce contrast medium

    _____ F. Have patient sign informed consent form

    _____ G. Take fluoroscopic images

    _____ H. Prepare patient's skin for puncture

17. Which position is performed to demonstrate the region of C7 during a cervical myelogram?

    _____

18. Why should the patient's head and neck remain hyperextended during cervical myelography?

    _____

19. True/False: Generally, AP supine, posteroanterior prone, or horizontal beam lateral projections are not taken during thoracic spine myelography.

20. Complete the following for suggested routine projections (following fluoroscopy and spot filming) for the different levels of the spine.

Projection/Position	Level of CR
1. Cervical region	_____
2. Thoracic region	_____
3. Lumbar region	_____

21. True/False: Myelography has been largely replaced by MR and CT.

22. How is the contrast medium removed from the body after myelography?

_____

REVIEW EXERCISE E: Hip-to-Ankle Long Bone Measurement (see textbook p. 741)

1. What is the major reason hip-to-ankle long bone measurement studies are conducted?

_____

2. If surgery is indicated, how might long bone measurement imaging help with planning?

_____

3. What is the recommended source–image receptor (IR) distance for long bone measurement studies of hip-to-ankle?

_____

4. What radiographic tools may be used to promote even x-ray absorption from hip to ankle with long bone

measurements? _____

5. How far apart should the lateral malleoli be with the patient standing for long bone measurement images?

_____

6. What is the angle and placement of the central ray for hip-to-ankle long bone measurement images?

_____

REVIEW EXERCISE F: Radiographic Skeletal Survey (Bone Survey) (see textbook p. 742)

1. What is a skeletal survey? _____

2. What are some indications for a skeletal survey? _____

3. Which of the following is not considered part of the appendicular skeleton?

A. Humeri   C. Hands

B. Thorax   D. Lower Legs

459

4. Which of the following is considered part of the axial skeleton?

   A. Forearms

   B. Femurs

   C. Feet

   D. Lumbosacral spine

5. True/False: Radiographic skeletal surveys may be performed as the initial imaging procedure.

6. True/False: Radiographic skeletal surveys may be performed following a positive finding on radionuclide bone scan.

REVIEW EXERCISE G: Digital Tomosynthesis (see textbook p. 743)

1. Which of the following has digital tomosynthesis not been applied to?

   A. Angiographic

   B. Gastric

   C. Orthopedic

   D. Breast

2. True or False. Digital tomosynthesis (DTS) often delivers a higher dose than CT and is more expensive.

3. How does digital tomosynthesis (DTS) work?

   _____

   _____

4. What is the main advantage of DTS over conventional tomography?

   _____

   _____

5. True/False: The data acquired during DTS may acquire as many as 60 images in a single linear sweep.

6. What is the name of the fundamental principle behind DTS whereby the position or direction of an object appears to differ when viewed from different positions? _____

7. What is the limitation of standard x-ray that DTS addresses? _____

LABORATORY EXERCISES

The following exercises involve two procedures for which supplies and equipment are most commonly available to students.

Exercise: Hip-to-Ankle Long Bone Measurement

1. Using a lower limb radiographic phantom (if available), produce long bone measurement radiographs of the following:

   _____ Unilateral lower limb (AP projection of hip, knee, and ankle on one IR with a correctly placed Bell-Thompson ruler)

   _____ Bilateral lower limbs (AP projections of hips, knees, and ankles on one IR with correctly placed Bell-Thompson ruler (if available)

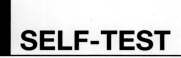

Directions: This self-test should be taken only after completing all of the readings, review exercises, and laboratory activities for a particular section. The purpose of this test is not only to provide a good learning exercise but also to serve as a strong indicator of what your final evaluation exam will be. It is strongly suggested that if you do not receive at least a 90%–95% grade on this self-test that you review those areas in which you missed questions before going to your instructor for the final evaluation exam for this chapter.

1. List the two synovial types of joints most commonly examined with an arthrogram.

   A. _____   B. _____

2. List the two contraindications for an arthrogram.

   A. _____   B. _____

3. An indication of a possible Baker cyst suggests the need for an arthrogram procedure for the

   _____.

4. List the two types of contrast media commonly used for a knee arthrogram.

   A. _____   B. _____

5. What is the purpose of flexing the knee gently after the contrast medium has been injected for an arthrogram

   procedure? _____

6. How many exposures are made, and how much is the leg rotated, between each exposure for horizontal beam knee arthrograms?

   A. Number of exposures per meniscus: _____

   B. Degrees of rotation between exposures: _____

7. The term *rotator cuff* refers to what structures of the shoulder? _____

8. What type of needle is most often used to introduce contrast media during a shoulder arthrogram?

   _____

9. List the overhead projections that may be requested for a shoulder arthrogram.

   Scout

   A. _____

   Post-injection

   B. _____

   C. _____

   D. _____

   E. _____

   F. _____

10. How is the contrast medium instilled into the biliary ducts during an ERCP? _____

11. Other than a radiologist, what type of physician often performs ERCP? _____

12. What is the most common clinical reason for performing a T-tube cholangiogram?

   _____

13. Which of the following conditions may contraindicate an ERCP?
   A. Biliary obstruction   C. Jaundice
   B. Stone in main pancreatic duct   D. Pseudocyst

14. List the four divisions of the uterus.

   A. _____   C. _____

   B. _____   D. _____

15. Which of the following is *not* a tissue layer of the uterus?
   A. Osseometrium   C. Endometrium
   B. Myometrium   D. Serosa

16. True/False: The uterine tubes are connected directly to the ovaries.

17. List the three contraindications for Hysterosalpingography (HSG).

   A. _____

   B. _____

   C. _____

18. True/False: An oil-based contrast medium is preferred for the majority of HSG.

19. True/False: Hysterosalpingography can be a therapeutic procedure in correcting certain obstructions within the uterine tube.

20. List the four common lesions or conditions diagnosed through a myelogram.

   A. _____   C. _____

   B. _____   D. _____

21. List the four contraindications for a myelogram.

   A. _____   C. _____

   B. _____   D. _____

22. The most common clinical indication for a myelogram is

   A. Benign tumors   C. Herniated nucleus pulposus (HNP)

   B. Spinal cysts   D. Bony injury to the spine

23. In which space is the contrast medium injected during a myelogram? _____

24. Which position will move the contrast media column from the lumbar to the cervical region during a myelogram?

   A. Fowler   C. Trendelenburg

   B. Left lateral decubitus   D. Prone

25. What is the most common spinal puncture site for a lumbar myelogram?

   A. L3–L4   C. L4–L5

   B. L1–L2   D. L5–S1

26. A cervical puncture is indicated for an upper spinal region myelogram if:

   A. The patient has severe lordosis

   B. The patient has mild scoliosis

   C. The patient has HNP of the L4–L5 level

   D. The patient has complete blockage at the T-spine level

27. The absorption of the water-soluble contrast media into the vascular system of the body begins approximately

   _____ minutes after injection and is totally undetectable radiographically after

   _____ hours.

28. Which position is performed during a cervical myelogram to demonstrate the C7–T1 region?

   _____

29. The formal term for a radiographic study to compare the bilateral lower limbs is _____.

30. True/False: To measure the length of a long bone properly, the entire lower limb should be included on a single projection.

31. True/False: Movement of the body part between exposures compromises the long bone study.

32. True/False: If a long bone study of both lower limbs is ordered, the use of two metal rulers is recommended with both limbs exposed at the same time on the same IR.

33. What is the proper name for the filter used to promote consistent x-ray absorption with long bone measurement images? _____

34. List several indications for a radiographic skeletal survey.

_____

35. Define digital tomosynthesis. _____

36. True/False. Digital tomosynthesis delivers a continuous exposure.

37. In DTS, how many images can be acquired in a single linear sweep?
    A. 10
    B. 20
    C. 40
    D. 60

38. True/False. DTS removes overlapping structures.

19 Special Radiographic Procedures

WORKBOOK SELF-TEST ANSWER KEY

1. A. Knee
   B. Shoulder
2. A. Sensitivity to iodine
   B. Sensitivity to local anesthetics
3. Knee
4. A. Iodinated water soluble
   B. Carbon dioxide, oxygen, or room air
5. To provide a thin, even coating of positive contrast media over the soft tissues of the knee joint
6. A. 9
   B. 20 degrees
7. The conjoined tendons of the four major shoulder muscles
8. 2¾- to 3½-inch spinal needle
9. A. AP internal and external rotation shoulder scout
   B. AP internal rotation
   C. AP external rotation
   D. Glenoid fossa AP oblique (Grashey method) projection
   E. Transaxillary (inferosuperior axial) projection
   F. Intertubercular (bicipital) groove projection (Fisk method)
10. Through a special catheter introduced through the duodenoscope
11. Gastroenterologist
12. To detect postoperatively any residual stones in the biliary ducts that may have gone undetected during the cholecystectomy
13. D. Pseudocyst
14. A. Fundus
    B. Corpus or body
    C. Isthmus
    D. Cervix (neck)
15. A. Osseometrium
16. False (connected to the uterus at the cornu)
17. A. Acute pelvic inflammatory disease
    B. Active uterine bleeding
    C. Pregnancy
18. False (Water-soluble iodinated contrast is preferred.)
19. True
20. A. Herniated nucleus pulposus (HNP)
    B. Cancerous or benign tumors
    C. Cysts
    D. Possible bone fragments (trauma)
21. A. Blood in the cerebrospinal fluid
    B. Arachnoiditis
    C. Increased intracranial pressure
    D. Recent lumbar puncture (within the past 2 weeks)
22. C. Herniated nucleus pulposus (HNP)
23. Subarachnoid space
24. C. Trendelenburg
25. A. L3–L4
26. D. The patient has complete blockage at the T-spine level
27. 30 minutes; 24 hours
28. Horizontal beam swimmer's lateral (cervicothoracic projection)
29. Hip-to-ankle long bone measurement
30. True. (Iliac crest to inferior calcaneus.)
31. False
32. False
33. Wedge filter
34. To accurately identify the focal and diffuse abnormalities of the skeleton such as evaluation of fractures, bone lesions, metabolic bone disease, skeletal dysplasia, developmental changes, or anatomic variants
35. Multiple very low-dose x-ray projection images acquired from different angles during a single linear sweep of the x-ray tube across a stationary detector
36. False. DTS pulses x-ray exposures at different tube angles.
37. D. 60
38. True

20 Diagnostic and Therapeutic Modalities

This chapter introduces select alternative diagnostic and therapeutic imaging modalities, including nuclear medicine (NM), positron emission tomography (PET), radiation oncology (therapy), diagnostic medical sonography (DMS), mammography, bone densitometry, and magnetic resonance imaging (MR). The information and review exercises contained in this chapter are intended to introduce students to basic concepts related to each of these modalities. Basic definitions, physical principles, clinical applications, and technologist responsibilities will be covered.

A more extensive presentation is provided in the MR section, which introduces MR terminology and the basics of MR physics and instrumentation. The important clinical aspects related to personnel and patient safety are discussed. An introduction to the imaging parameters that affect the quality of the images and clinical applications of MR is included.

CHAPTER OBJECTIVES

Nuclear Medicine (NM)

_____ 1. Identify basic operating principles related to NM imaging.

_____ 2. List the purpose, radionuclide used, and pathologic indications demonstrated with select NM procedures.

_____ 3. List specific responsibilities for members of the NM team.

Positron Emission Tomography (PET)

_____ 1. Describe the PET imaging process.

_____ 2. Identify the different types of radionuclides used in PET imaging.

_____ 3. Describe the basic operating principles of PET imaging.

_____ 4. Identify the pathologic conditions best demonstrated with PET imaging.

_____ 5. Define terms and concepts specific to nuclear medicine technology.

Radiation Oncology (Therapy)

_____ 1. Distinguish between internal and external types of radiation therapy.

_____ 2. Identify the energy level, characteristics, and advantages of the major types of radiation therapy units.

_____ 3. List the specific responsibilities of radiation oncology team members.

Diagnostic Medical Sonography (DMS)

_____ 1. Identify basic operating principles related to ultrasound.

_____ 2. List the characteristics, advantages, and disadvantages of specific types of ultrasound systems.

_____ 3. List the purpose, transducer used, and pathologic indications demonstrated with select ultrasound procedures.

Mammography

_____ 1. List statistics for breast cancer in the United States and worldwide.

_____ 2. Describe the recommendations from the American Cancer Society and American College of Radiology (ACR) in regard to mammography.

_____ 3. Describe the impact of the Mammography Quality Standards Act (MQSA) on mammography facilities and mammographers.

_____ 4. On drawings and radiographs, identify the specific anatomy of the female breast.

_____ 5. Identify specific regions of the breast using the quadrant and the clock systems.

_____ 6. List the three general categories of breast tissue according to their tissue composition, age of the patient, and radiographic density (brightness).

_____ 7. Identify the three classifications of the breast.

_____ 8. Describe the general patient preparation concerns before a mammogram.

_____ 9. Identify key questions that should be asked as part of the taking of the clinical history before a mammogram.

_____ 10. List the technical considerations and equipment essential for quality images of the breast.

_____ 11. Identify the diagnostic benefits of breast compression and the precautions when applying compression.

_____ 12. Identify the principal means by which patient dose can be decreased or controlled during mammography.

_____ 13. Compare and contrast the advantages and disadvantages of film-screen and digital mammography.

_____ 14. List the benefits of using computer-aided detection (CAD) in mammographic interpretation.

_____ 15. Identify alternative imaging modalities available to study the breast, including advantages and disadvantages of each system.

_____ 16. Describe the basic and special projections most commonly performed in mammography and include patient positioning, central ray (CR) placement, and anatomy demonstrated.

_____ 17. Describe the Eklund method for imaging breasts with implants.

_____ 18. List the average skin dose and mean glandular dose (MGD) range for each projection of the breast as described in the textbook.

_____ 19. Define specific types of breast pathology.

_____ 20. List the American College of Radiology nomenclature of terms and abbreviations for mammographic positioning.

_____ 21. Given mammographic images, identify specific positioning and exposure factor errors.

Mammography Positioning and Image Critique

_____ 1. Using a peer in a simulated setting, position for basic and special mammographic projections.

_____ 2. Using appropriate radiographic phantoms, produce satisfactory radiographs of specific positions (if equipment is available).

466

_____ 3. Critique and evaluate mammographic images based on the five divisions of radiographic criteria: (1) anatomy demonstrated, (2) position, (3) collimation field size and CR, (4) exposure, and (5) anatomic image markers.

_____ 4. Distinguish between acceptable and unacceptable mammographic images based on exposure factors, motion, collimation, positioning, or other errors.

Bone Densitometry (BD)

_____ 1. List the major components of bone and their function.

_____ 2. List common clinical and pathologic indicators for osteoporosis.

_____ 3. Define and list the risk factors for fracture risk and osteoporosis.

_____ 4. List the World Health Organization (WHO) criteria for the diagnosis of osteoporosis.

_____ 5. List and describe the general types of agents approved by the US Food and Drug Administration (FDA) for the treatment and prevention of osteoporosis and also the specific drugs approved under each type.

_____ 6. Identify the most common types of equipment, methods, and techniques for determining bone mineral density (BMD).

_____ 7. Define and describe the meaning of the two terms DXA precision and DXA accuracy as used in the performance of bone densitometry procedures.

Magnetic Resonance Imaging (MR)

_____ 1. Explain how MR produces an image.

_____ 2. Compare the process of MR image production with that of other imaging modalities.

_____ 3. Explain how a tissue signal is generated and received from body tissues.

_____ 4. Explain how image contrast is produced in the MR image.

_____ 5. Identify basic MR safety considerations.

_____ 6. Identify information to include when preparing a patient for an MR exam.

_____ 7. Identify the type of contrast agent used in MR.

_____ 8. State the appearance of specific tissue types on both T1- and T2-weighted images.

_____ 9. Define the terms and pathologic indications related to MR.

_____ 10. Explain the purpose and applications of functional MRI (fMRI).

LEARNING EXERCISES

The following review exercises should be completed only after careful study of the associated pages in the textbook as indicated by each exercise. Answers to each review exercise are provided at the end of this workbook. Imaging modality separates the review exercises.

REVIEW EXERCISE A: Nuclear Medicine and PET (see textbook pp. 746–752)

1. A group of radioactive drugs used in the diagnosis and treatment of disease is termed

_____.

2. True/False: NM examines physiologic functions of an organ on the molecular level.

467

3. How are the materials that are identified in Question 1 introduced into the body?

 A. Inhaled

 B. Ingested

 C. Instilled

 D. All of the above

4. The most common nuclide used in NM procedures is:

 A. Sulfur colloid

 B. Iodine 123 (^{123}I)

 C. Technetium 99 m

 D. Thallium

5. Technetium 99 m allows target tissue to return to background radiation levels within:

 A. 6 hours

 B. 12 hours

 C. 24 hours

 D. 48 hours

6. Nuclear medicine (NM) can produce _____ imaging which are a single "snapshot", and _____ imaging which provides a series of images in sequence like frames of a movie.

7. SPECT is an abbreviation for _____.

8. The typical patient dose for most diagnostic nuclear medicine procedures ranges between _____ and _____.

9. A bone scan can detect a postinjury fracture up to _____.

10. A common genitourinary nuclear medicine study is performed for:

 A. Kidney transplants

 B. Renal cyst

 C. Pyelonephritis

 D. All of the above

11. An NM procedure to evaluate the motility of both solids and liquids through the GI tract is termed a(n) _____ study.

 A. Hepatobiliary iminodiacetic acid

 B. Gastric emptying

 C. Gastroesophageal reflux

 D. GI flow

12. Which of the following NM procedure assesses blood flow to the myocardium under stress and resting conditions?

 A. Cardiac diffusion imaging

 B. Myocardial perfusion imaging

 C. SPECT

 D. Electrocardiogram

13. Which of the following radiopharmaceuticals is administered for a nuclear thyroid uptake scan?

 A. Technetium 99 m

 B. Thallium

 C. Sodium iodide 123 (^{123}I)

 D. NeoTect

14. Match the following responsibilities with the correct NM team member.

_____ A. Properly disposes of contaminated materials

_____ B. Calibrates nuclear medicine imaging equipment

_____ C. Performs statistical analysis of study data

_____ D. Administers radionuclide to patient

_____ E. Interprets procedure

_____ F. Often serves as department radiation safety officer

_____ G. Licensed to acquire and use radioactive materials

_____ H. Reviews all dosimetry records

_____ I. Performs audits on the recordkeeping

_____ J. Digitally processes the images

1. Nuclear medicine technologist

2. Nuclear medicine physician

3. Health physicist

4. Radiation safety officer

15. Match each of the following NM terms to its correct definition (use each choice only once).

_____ A. Synonym for a product of decay

_____ B. Time required for the disintegration of half of the original activity of a nuclide

_____ C. Type of atom whose nucleus disintegrates spontaneously

_____ D. External indication of a device designed to enumerate ionizing events

_____ E. SI unit of radioactivity

_____ F. Stage in a reaction in which the concentration of the reactive species is no longer changing

_____ G. Traditional or standard unit of radioactivity

_____ H. Spontaneous nuclear transmutation characterized by the emission of energy and/or mass from the nucleus

1. Becquerel

2. Radionuclide

3. Daughter

4. Curie

5. Equilibrium

6. Half-life

7. Disintegration

8. Count

16. PET is an acronym for _____.

17. PET is a process that demonstrates:

A. Anatomic appearance of tissues and organs

B. Molecular makeup of tissues

C. Metabolic and biochemical changes in tissue

D. Pathologic processes of brain tissue only

18. True/False: The PET scanner produces radiation with an intensity of 5.11 MeV.

19. PET uses radioactive compounds that emit _____ during the radioactive decay process.

A. Electrons

B. Positrons

C. Two gamma rays

D. Neutrinos

20. The disappearance of the electron–positron pair and, in their place, two 511-keV photons that travel out in opposite directions, is termed _____.

21. The PET scanner detector array measures:

    A. Emitted photons

    B. Electrons

    C. Positrons

    D. Neutrons

22. PET combined with CT allowing imaging of biochemical functions is termed _____.

23. PET uses radioactive compounds, which include oxygen and nitrogen, as well as:

    A. Selenium and iron

    B. Hydrogen and iodine

    C. Carbon and argon

    D. Carbon and fluorine

24. PET radioactive compounds measure all of the following vital cellular biochemical processes except:

    A. Oxygen use

    B. Tissue perfusion

    C. Cellular reproduction

    D. Glucose metabolism

25. Match each of the following PET tracer compounds to the cellular function that it measures (different compounds may measure the same biologic process).

    _____ A. Glucose metabolism

    _____ B. Blood flow/perfusion

    _____ C. Amino acid metabolism

    _____ D. Blood flow, blood volume, and oxygen consumption

    1. ^{13}N-ammonia

    2. ^{18}F-fluorodeoxyglucose (FDG)

    3. ^{15}O-water

    4. ^{11}C-methionine

26. What is the name of the device required to produce the PET radioactive compounds?

    _____

27. Most PET tracers have a half-life of:

    A. 120 seconds–110 minutes

    B. 10–60 seconds

    C. 15 minutes–8 hours

    D. 8–12 hours

28. True/False: PET is superior to MR in demonstrating anatomic structures of the brain.

29. True/False: PET can be used to investigate the location of seizure sites in patients with epilepsy who are not responding to drug therapy.

30. PET plays an important role in the initial diagnosis and _____ of malignancy.

    A. Destruction

    B. Prevention

    C. Staging

    D. Cure

31. True/False: In PET imaging, active tumor growth leads to a decreased uptake of ^{18}F-FDG.

32. True/False: Decreased uptake of an ammonia tracer in the heart tissue may indicate that coronary artery disease is present.

33. Two common radionuclides used for PET perfusion coronary artery disease studies include ¹³N-ammonia and

    _____.

    A. ⁸²Rbn chloride

    B. ¹⁵O-water

    C. ¹⁸F-FDG

    D. ¹¹C-methionine

34. True/False: PET/CT scanners can determine the location of an atherosclerotic lesion and its impact on cardiac perfusion.

35. True/False: Generally, malignant cells have an accelerated glucose metabolism.

36. PET brain mapping is performed to:

    A. Identify possible tumors in the brain

    B. Distinguish between the gray and white matter of the brain

    C. Identify the transmission or impulse patterns of the brain

    D. Identify the location of key motor and sensory regions of the brain

37. In patients with Alzheimer disease, glucose metabolism is dramatically _____ (increased or decreased) in several key areas of the brain.

38. Coregistration is another term for:

    A. PET image manipulation

    B. Increased tracer uptake in the brain

    C. Artifact seen on certain PET images

    D. Fusion technology

39. PET may be combined with a(n) _____ study to determine if any epileptic activity is present.

40. True/False: It is possible to acquire functional PET and anatomic CT images in the same scanning session when the correct technology is used.

REVIEW EXERCISE B: Radiation Oncology (Therapy) (see textbook pp. 753–754)

1. True/False: The goal of radiation oncology is to deliver a tumoricidal dose while sparing normal tissue.

2. Candidates for radiation therapy are scheduled for _____, which is a procedure performed by the radiation therapist to prepare the patient for treatment.

3. Identify the dimensional imaging techniques relied upon for the development of modern treatment plans:

    A. _____

    B. _____

4. Which type of radiation therapy provides high doses of radiation to a prescribed treatment area without significant dose to surrounding tissues? _____

5. Modern linear accelerators are capable of producing images from these two modalities to confirm localization of treatment area.

    A. _____

    B. _____

6. _____ is the radiation treatment for brain tumors.

7. What is the term for the maximum dose delivered to a tumor with proton therapy?

   A. Cobalt-60 peak

   B. Megavoltage radiation peak

   C. Uranium 235 peak

   D. Bragg Peak

8. 4D imaging takes into account movement of the tumor caused by _____ functions.

9. SBRT is the abbreviation for _____.

10. _____ is a technique to administer radiation directly to the region of interest using a multileaf collimator to direct an individual radiation beam.

11. What is the new radiation therapy technique that allows for prescription of narrowly defined margins around the tumor? _____

12. Another term for brachytherapy is _____.

REVIEW EXERCISE C: Diagnostic Medical Sonography (DMS) (see textbook pp. 755–760)

1. List four additional terms for diagnostic medical sonography.

   A. _____

   B. _____

   C. _____

   D. _____

2. Diagnostic medical sonography (DMS) uses high-frequency sound waves in the range between _____ and _____ MHz or higher.

3. What is the fundamental purpose or function of the transducer?

   _____.

4. True/False: A diagnostic medical transducer serves as both a transmitter and a receiver of sound waves.

5. True/False: Lower frequency transducers permit greater penetration for imaging organs within the abdominal cavity.

6. List the three major imaging specialty areas that are within Diagnostic medical sonography.

   A. _____

   B. _____

   C. _____

7. True/False: DMS is not the preferred modality for the male and female reproductive system.

8. What is the chief advantage in using DMS for obstetric and pediatric patients?

   _____

9. True/False: The origins of diagnostic medical sonography can be traced back to World War I with the development of SONAR.

10. After which war did the medical use of ultrasound become more prevalent? _____

11. What is SONAR often referred to as? _____

12. Improvements in which technology is closely aligned with the evolution of diagnostic medical sonography?

   A. SONAR
   B. Transducers
   C. Computers
   D. X-ray

13. Which generation of sonographic equipment introduced grayscale imaging?

   A. A-mode
   B. B-mode
   C. Real-time dynamic
   D. Doppler

14. Which type of ultrasound system is used to examine the structure and behavior of flowing blood?

   A. A-mode
   B. B-mode
   C. Real-time dynamic
   D. Doppler

15. Elastography is performed for the assessment of:

   A. Muscular injuries
   B. Arterial wall calcification
   C. Meniscal tears in the knee joint
   D. The stiffness of normal versus abnormal tissues

16. True/False: DMS can use microbubbles of gas encased in lipids as a contrast agent.

17. True/False: DMS has limitations to where it can be used due to the immobility.

18. True/False: Thermal index, or TI, refers to the heating of the face of a transducer.

19. True/False: Mechanical index, or MI, refers to changes in cell structure.

20. The safety goal for each sonographic procedure performed is to use the least amount of scan time with the

   _____.

21. True/False: ALARA principles apply to diagnostic medical sonography.

22. True/False: Air is an efficient medium for sound waves to travel.

23. True/False: The weight of a patient may be a factor that relates to image quality.

24. Diagnostic medical sonography is highly diagnostic for studies of all of the following structures except the:

   A. Liver
   B. Stomach
   C. Gallbladder
   D. Uterus

25. True/False: DMS of the breast is effective in distinguishing a cystic structure from a solid mass.

   _____

26. DMS is very effective in evaluating the Achilles tendon for tears.

27. What is placed between the transducer and the anatomy to prevent air distortion of the ultrasound signal?

   A. Water bath

   B. Nitrogen gas

   C. Gel

   D. Saline disk

28. True/False: DMS can visualize the pediatric brain.

29. Match each of the following sonographic terms to its correct definition (use each choice only once).

   _____ A. Uses heat to destroy tissues

   _____ B. Alteration in sound frequency or wavelength

   _____ C. Acoustic energy that travels through a medium

   _____ D. An anatomic object that does not produce any echoes

   _____ E. Ultrasound images that demonstrate dynamic motion

   _____ F. Highly reflective (echogenic) structures as compared with the surrounding structures

   _____ G. Acoustic energy that is reflected from a structure back toward the transducer

   _____ H. An anatomic structure or region of the body that highly reflects sound energy

   _____ I. An aspect of acoustic energy reflected back toward the source or origin

   _____ J. An anatomic object that produces fewer echoes than normal

   1. Anechoic
   2. Backscatter reflected by moving structures
   3. Doppler effect
   4. Echogenic
   5. Hyperechoic
   6. Hypoechoic
   7. Real-time imaging
   8. High-intensity focused ultrasound
   9. Wave
   10. Reflection

30. What is the term used to describe an irregular structure containing a spectrum of grays?

   A. Homogeneous

   B. Heterogeneous

   C. Hypoechoic

   D. Hyperechoic

MAMMOGRAPHY

REVIEW EXERCISE A: Breast Cancer, Mammography Quality Standards Act, Anatomy of the Breast, and Breast Classifications (see textbook pp. 761–765)

1. Radiographic examination of the mammary gland or breast is called _____.

2. The American Cancer Society recommends that women older than the age of _____ should have a screening mammogram performed.

    A. 35

    B. 40

    C. 45

    D. 50

3. The MQSA, which went into effect on October 1, _____, was passed to ensure a high-quality mammography service that requires certification by the secretary of the Department of Health and Human Services.

    A. 1992

    B. 1993

    C. 1994

    D. 1995

4. There were _____ new cases of breast cancer documented worldwide in 2020.

5. Men have a _____% chance of developing breast cancer as compared with a woman's risk.

6. Research indicates that after a breast cancer tumor has reached a size of _____ cm, it has often metastasized.

7. Breast cancer accounts for _____ of all new cancers detected in women.

    A. 12%

    B. 15%

    C. 30%

    D. 50%

8. In Canada, mammography guidelines are set by the _____.

9. Which of the following mammography facilities are exempt from MQSA standards?

    A. Medicare facilities

    B. VA facilities

    C. Not-for-profit facilities

    D. No facilities are exempt

10. The junction of the inferior part of the breast with the anterior chest wall is called the

    _____.

11. The pigmented area surrounding the nipple is the _____.

12. Breast tissue extending into the axilla is called the tail of the breast or the _____.

13. In the average female breast, the _____ (craniocaudal or mediolateral) diameter is usually greater.

14. Using the clock localization system, five o'clock on the right breast would be in what quadrant?

    _____

15. Based on the clock system method, a suspicious mass at two o'clock on the right breast would be at

    _____ o'clock if it were in a similar position on the left breast.

16. What is the large muscle commonly seen on a mammogram that is located between the bony thorax and the mammary gland? _____

17. Two fibrous sheets of tissue join together just posterior to the breast to form the _____ space.

18. What is the function of the mammary gland? _____

19. List the three tissue types found in the female breast.

    A. _____   B. _____   C. _____

20. Various small blood vessels, fibrous connective tissues, ducts, and other small structures seen on finished mammograms are collectively called _____.

21. Bands of fibrous tissue passing through the breast tissue are known as _____.

22. Classify the following types of breasts into one of the three general categories: fibroglandular (FG), fibrofatty (FF), or fatty (F).

    _____ 1. 20 years, no children   _____ 5. 50 years, two children

    _____ 2. 35 years, no children   _____ 6. Male

    _____ 3. 35 years, three children   _____ 7. 35 years, lactating

    _____ 4. 25 years, pregnant   _____ 8. 10 years

23. Which is the least dense of the following tissues: fibrous, glandular, or adipose? _____

24. Identify the labeled parts within this sagittal section drawing (Fig. 20.1).

    A. _____

    B. _____

    C. _____

    D. _____

    E. _____

    F. _____

    G. _____

    H. _____

    I. _____

    J. _____

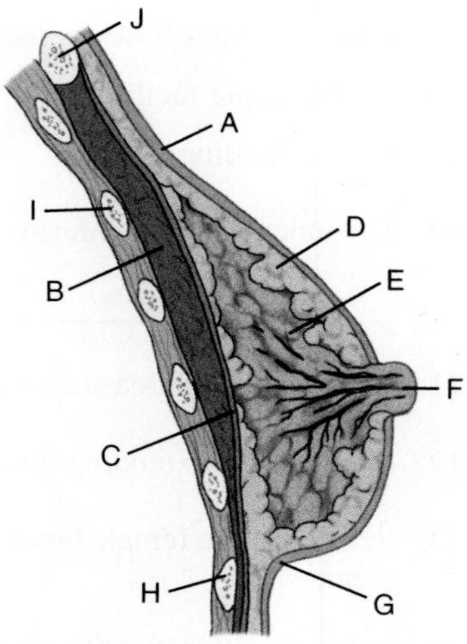

Fig. 20.1 Sagittal section of the breast.

25. Identify the labeled parts in Fig. 20.2.

A. _____

B. _____

C. _____

D. _____

E. _____

F. _____

G. _____

H. _____

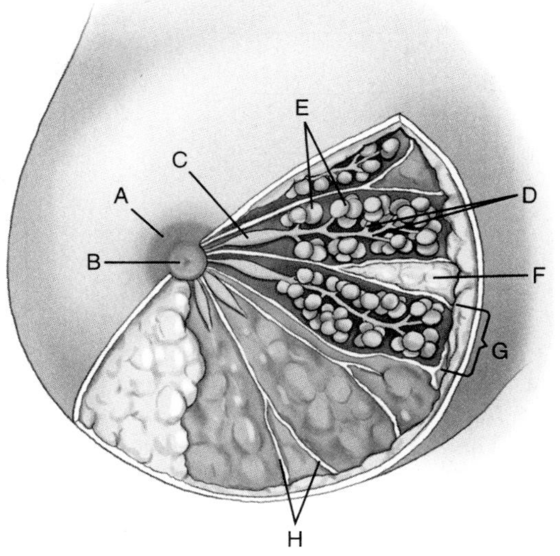

Fig. 20.2 Cutaway anterior view of the breast.

26. The glandular tissue of the breast is divided into _____ lobes.

27. Which portion of the breast is nearest to the chest wall (apex or base)? _____

28. Which portion of the breast is nearest to the nipple (apex or base)? _____

29. What are the two determinants that contribute to the exposure factors in mammography?

A. _____

B. _____

30. What is one of the strongest risk factors associated with breast cancer and makes cancer diagnosis most challenging?
_____

REVIEW EXERCISE B: Mammography: Patient Preparation, Technical Considerations, Alternative Modalities, and Radiographic Positioning (see textbook pp. 766–780)

1. Other than jewelry and clothing, what substances must be removed from the patient's body before mammography to prevent artifacts? _____

2. True/False: Certain lotions with glitter may produce artifacts on the mammographic image.

3. List the six questions that should be included in taking the patient's history before a mammogram.

   A. _____

   B. _____

   C. _____

   D. _____

   E. _____

   F. _____

4. True/False: The apex of the breast is much thicker and contains denser tissues than at the base.

5. The central ray is usually directed through the _____ of the breast.

6. The focal spot size on a dedicated mammography unit is usually between _____ and

   _____ mm.

7. Typically, compression applied to the breast is _____ to _____
   pounds of pressure.

8. List the six benefits of applying breast compression during mammography.

   A. _____

   B. _____

   C. _____

   D. _____

   E. _____

   F. _____

9. How does breast compression improve image quality or resolution?

   A. _____

   B. _____

10. Magnification is performed during mammography primarily to:

    A. Increase signal-to-noise ratio   C. Reduce dose per projection

    B. Magnify specific regions of interest   D. Demonstrate the deep chest wall

11. What are the three factors used to determine dose to the breast?

    A. _____

    B. _____

    C. _____

12. True/False: Digital mammography has superior spatial resolution as compared to analog (film-screen) systems.

478

13. To minimize patient dose, the ACR recommends a repeat rate of less than:

    A. 2%   C. 10%

    B. 5%   D. 15%

14. True/False: Mean Glandular Dose (MGD) is often referenced in mammography because glandular tissue is most sensitive to radiation.

15. What is the three-part hallmark of good analog (film-screen) mammography (i.e., what are the three image qualities that need to be present on a diagnostic mammogram)?

    A. _____   B. _____   C. _____

16. Which of the following is not an advantage of digital mammography over film-screen?

    A. Information is quickly available on the screen for making a diagnosis.

    B. Image storage is easier and less bulky, and access is much quicker.

    C. Overall spatial resolution is higher.

    D. Ability to localize small lesions and guide the radiologist during biopsy.

17. Which of the following, used in digital mammography, allows the technologist to use higher kVp without compromising image contrast?

    A. Algorithms   C. Compression

    B. Contrast   D. Anode heel

18. The type of contrast media used during contrast-enhanced mammography is:

    A. Microbubbles   C. Saline

    B. Gadolinium   D. Iodinated

19. What is the name of the device that captures the image with direct digital mammography?

    _____

20. True/False: Contrast in mammography is not useful for the detection of tumors.

21. Studies have shown that using computer-aided detection (CAD) as a second reader to interpret screening mammograms improves the cancer detection rate by as much as:

    A. 10%   C. 20%

    B. 15%   D. 30%

22. The major benefit of DMS (sonomammography) of the breast is _____.

23. True/False: Functional imaging uses a radiopharmaceutical.

24. True/False: Scintimammography is considered unreliable for any lesion smaller than 1 cm.

25. Scintimammography uses which radionuclide?

    A. Cardiolyte   C. Thallium

    B. Iodine 131   D. Technetium-99m-sestamibi

26. A second type of nuclear medicine procedure called sentinel node studies is performed to:

    A. Determine whether a malignant lesion is present in the breast

    B. Detect metastasis to a lymph node surrounding the breast

    C. Distinguish between a benign and a malignant tumor of the breast

    D. Diagnose a lymphoma

27. What type of radionuclide is often used with sentinel node studies?

    A. Sulfur colloid   C. Sestamibi

    B. Technetium   D. FDG

28. PET studies of the breast can detect early cancerous cells by measuring the rate of:

    A. Oxygen metabolism   C. Glucose (sugar) metabolism

    B. Phosphorus metabolism   D. Osmosis through the cell membrane

29. The primary difference between breast-specific gamma imaging (BSGI) and scintimammography is

    _____.

30. List the two major disadvantages of using positron emission tomography (PET) mammography as a breast-screening tool.

    A. _____

    B. _____

31. True/False: Patients with the BRCA1 and BRCA2 genes have reduced risk of developing breast cancer.

32. List the three disadvantages in using MR to study the breast.

    A. _____

    B. _____

    C. _____

33. Which of the following technologies produces a 3D image of the breast tissue?

    A. Direct digital radiography   C. Sentinel node study

    B. Digital breast tomosynthesis   D. Sonomammography

34. The most common form of benign tumor of the breast is

    A. Fibroadenoma   C. Fibrocystic lesion

    B. Adenocarcinoma   D. Adenosarcoma

35. The most common form of breast cancer is

    A. Fibroadenoma   C. Infiltrating (invasive) ductal carcinoma

    B. Intraductal papilloma   D. Lobular carcinoma

36. Which of the following breast lesions has well-defined margins?

    A. Gynecomastia   C. Fibroadenoma

    B. Lobular carcinoma   D. Infiltrating ductal carcinoma

37. True/False: Gynecomastia primarily involves the male breast.

38. What are the two routine projections performed for screening mammograms?

   A. _____   B. _____

39. What surface landmark determines the correct height for the placement of the image receptor (IR) for the CC

   projection? _____

40. Anatomic side markers and patient identification information need to be placed near the

   _____ side of the breast.

41. In the CC projection, what structure must be in profile? _____

42. In the CC projection, the head should be turned _____ (toward or away from) the side
   being radiographed.

43. Which routine projection taken during a screening mammogram demonstrates more of the pectoral muscle?

   _____

44. For an average-sized breast, how much CR/IR angulation is used for the mediolateral oblique (MLO) projection?

   _____

45. True/False: The desired patient position for the MLO projection is seated.

46. For the MLO projection, the arm of the side being examined should be placed:
   A. On the hip   C. Resting on top of the head
   B. Forward, toward the front of the body   D. Behind the back, palm out

47. Which special projection is usually requested when a lesion is seen on the MLO but not on the CC projection?

   _____

48. In both the CC and the mediolateral projections, the central ray is generally directed to the

   _____ of the breast.

49. What is the most frequently requested special projection of the breast? _____

50. Which projection most effectively shows the axillary aspect of the breast? _____

51. How much is the CR/IR angled from vertical for the mediolateral, true lateral projection?

   _____

52. True/False: Mark each of the following statements either T for true or F for false.

_____ A. It is important that all skinfolds be smoothed out and all wrinkles and pockets of air removed on each projection for the breast.

_____ B. Because the base of the breast is shown clearly on the CC projection, this area does not need to be shown on the MLO projection.

_____ C. The axillary aspect of the breast is usually well visualized on the CC projection.

_____ D. Mammography is usually performed in the standing position.

_____ E. Because of a short exposure time, the patient does not need to be completely motionless during the exposure.

_____ F. With breast implants, the use of AEC often results in an underexposed image.

_____ G. In the CC projection, the chest wall must be pushed firmly against the IR.

_____ H. Standard CC and MLO projections should be performed on patients who have breast implants.

_____ I. Compression should not be used on patients with breast implants.

_____ J. The mediolateral projection is recommended to demonstrate air/fluid structures in the breast.

53. Which technique (method) is commonly used for the breast with an implant? _____

54. During the procedure identified in Question 53, what must be done to allow the anterior aspect of the breast to be compressed and properly visualized? _____

55. If a lesion is too deep toward the chest wall and cannot be visualized with a laterally exaggerated craniocaudal projection, a(n) _____ projection should be performed.

A. MLO

B. CC

C. Mediolateral

D. Axillary tail

56. Identify the correct positioning term or description for each of the following ACR abbreviations.

A. MLO _____

B. SIO _____

C. AT _____

D. CC _____

E. RL _____

F. LM _____

G. XCCL _____

H. LMO _____

I. ID _____

REVIEW EXERCISE C: Critique Radiographs of the Breast

These questions relate to the radiographs found in this exercise. Evaluate these radiographs for the radiographic criteria categories (1–5) that follow. Describe the corrections needed to improve the overall image. The major, or "repeatable," errors are specific errors that indicate the need for a repeat exposure, regardless of the nature of the other errors.

A. **CC projection** (Fig. 20.3)

Description of possible error:

1. Anatomy demonstrated:

_____

2. Part positioning:

_____

3. Collimation field size and central ray:

_____

4. Exposure:

_____

5. Anatomical side markers:

_____

Repeatable error(s):

_____

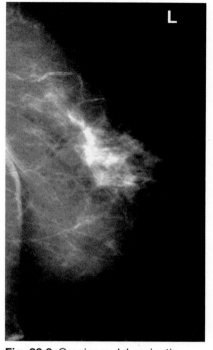

Fig. 20.3 Craniocaudal projection.

B. **MLO projection** (Fig. 20.4)

Description of possible error:

1. Anatomy demonstrated:

_____

2. Part positioning:

_____

3. Collimation field size and central ray:

_____

4. Exposure:

_____

5. Anatomical side markers:

_____

Repeatable error(s):

_____

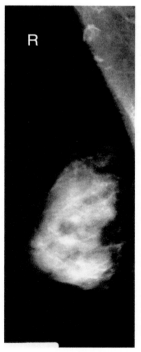

Fig. 20.4 Mediolateral oblique projection.

C. **CC projection** (Fig. 20.5)

Description of possible error:

   1. Anatomy demonstrated:

   _____

   2. Part positioning:

   _____

   3. Collimation field size and central ray:

   _____

   4. Exposure:

   _____

   5. Anatomical side markers:

   _____

Repeatable error(s):

_____

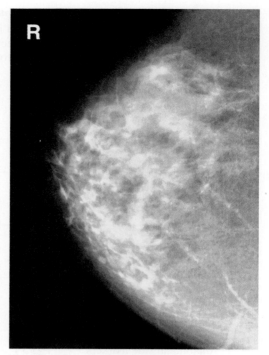

Fig. 20.5 Craniocaudal projection.

D. **MLO projection** (Fig. 20.6)

Description of possible error:

   1. Anatomy demonstrated:

   _____

   2. Part positioning:

   _____

   3. Collimation field size and central ray:

   _____

   4. Exposure:

   _____

   5. Anatomical side markers:

   _____

Repeatable error(s):

_____

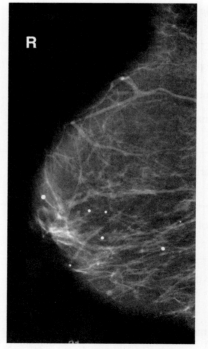

Fig. 20.6 Mediolateral oblique projection.

E. **CC projection** (Fig. 20.7)

Description of possible error:

1. Anatomy demonstrated:

_____

2. Part positioning:

_____

3. Collimation field size and central ray:

_____

4. Exposure:

_____

5. Anatomical side markers:

_____

Repeatable error(s):

_____

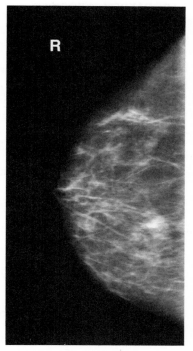

Fig. 20.7 Craniocaudadl projection.

F. **CC projection** (Fig. 20.8)

Description of possible error:

1. Anatomy demonstrated:

_____

2. Part positioning:

_____

3. Collimation field size and central ray:

_____

4. Exposure:

_____

5. Anatomical side markers:

_____

Repeatable error(s):

_____

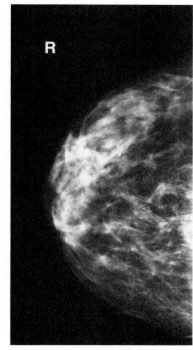

Fig. 20.8 Craniocaudal projection.

LABORATORY EXERCISES

Exercise A that follows needs to be performed in the radiology department where the mammography machine is located. Part B can be performed in a classroom or in any room where illuminators are available.

Laboratory Exercise A: Positioning

For this section you need another person to act as your "patient." Male and female students should be separated for this exercise, and students can be fully clothed for the simulated positioning. A clinical instructor must be present. Include each of the following during this exercise (check off when completed).

_____ Manipulate the x-ray imaging system into all the positions and become familiar with the locks and devices.

_____ Place or exchange the compression cone on the x-ray machine.

_____ Place an IR into the cassette holder.

_____ Place a fist on the IR tray and compress it by using the compression device. (This should be performed so that the student can sense the pressure of the device.)

_____ Place another student in position and simulate the CC, MLO, laterally exaggerated craniocaudal, and mediolateral positions.

_____ Optional: If the department or school has a breast phantom, perform the basic and special mammogram positions.

Laboratory Exercise B: Image Critique and Evaluation

Your instructor will provide various breast radiographs for these exercises. Some will be optimal-quality radiographs that meet all or most of the evaluation criteria described for each projection in the textbook. Others will be of less than optimal quality, and others will be unacceptable, requiring a repeat exam. Evaluate each radiograph as specified in the following.

Radiographs

1	2	3	4	5	6	*Criteria Guidelines*
_____	_____	_____	_____	_____	_____	a. Correct alignment and centering of part
_____	_____	_____	_____	_____	_____	b. Pectoral muscle included
_____	_____	_____	_____	_____	_____	c. Tissue thickness distributed evenly
_____	_____	_____	_____	_____	_____	d. Optimal compression noted
_____	_____	_____	_____	_____	_____	e. Dense areas adequately penetrated
_____	_____	_____	_____	_____	_____	f. High tissue contrast and optimal resolution noted
_____	_____	_____	_____	_____	_____	g. Absence of artifacts
_____	_____	_____	_____	_____	_____	h. Markers in proper position; accurate patient identification, including date and left or right anatomical side marker
_____	_____	_____	_____	_____	_____	i. Based on acceptable variances to criteria factors, determine which of these radiographs are acceptable and which are unacceptable and should have been repeated. (Place a check mark if the radiograph needs to be repeated.)

BONE DENSITOMETRY

REVIEW EXERCISE: Bone Densitometry (see textbook pp. 781–787)

1. According to the National Osteoporosis Foundation, the number of adults over 50 years old expected to be affected by osteoporosis by year 2030 is _____.

2. Bone strength is determined by which two factors?

   A. _____

   B. _____

3. For osteoporosis to be visible on conventional radiographs, a loss of _____% to _____% of the trabecular bone must occur.

4. Cells responsible for new bone formation are called _____, and cells that help to break down and remove old bone are _____.

5. By the age of approximately _____ years, more bone is being removed than is being replaced by new bone formation.

6. Bone matrix is _____% collagen and _____% other proteins.

7. The quantity or mass of bone measured in grams is the definition for _____.

8. The purpose of bone densitometry is to:

   A. Establish the diagnosis of osteoporosis

   B. Assess the response to osteoporosis therapy

   C. Measure BMD

   D. All of the above

9. Clinical indications for bone densitometry include all of the following except:

   A. Estrogen deficiency in women

   B. Hyperparathyroidism

   C. Vertebral abnormalities

   D. Polycystic kidney disease

10. True/False: A sedentary lifestyle can lead to osteoporosis.

11. Place a check mark next to each of the following that are *not* risk factors for low bone mass as identified in the textbook

    _____ A. Family history of osteoporosis

    _____ B. Excessive physical activity

    _____ C. Low sodium and niacin intake

    _____ D. Smoking

    _____ E. Low body weight

    _____ F. Alcohol consumption

    _____ G. High-fat diet

    _____ H. Low calcium intake

    _____ I. Height greater than 6 feet (180 cm)

    _____ J. Previous fractures

12. True/False: Women on estrogen replacement therapy (ERT) are at greater risk for acquiring osteoporotic fractures.

13. True/False: Bone strength and bone density are directly proportional.

14. True/False: Patients who have undergone intestinal bypass surgery are at greater risk for acquiring an osteoporotic fracture.

15. Osteoporosis in postmenopausal, Caucasian women is defined by the WHO as a BMP value of:

    A. 1.0 standard deviation below the average for the young normal population

    B. 1.5 standard deviations below the average for the same age and sex population

    C. 2.0 standard deviations below the average for the same age and sex population

    D. 2.5 standard deviations below the average for the young normal population

16. A T-score is defined as _____.

17. A T-score no lower than −1.0 indicates

    A. Normal bone

    B. Osteoporosis

    C. Osteopenia

    D. Severe osteoporosis

18. BMD reporting for premenopausal females or males younger than 50 should be reported in

    _____ rather than T-scores.

19. Which of the following drugs is administered as a stimulator for new bone growth and reduces the risk for vertebral fracture?

    A. Estrogen

    B. Parathyroid hormone analog (PTH 1-34)

    C. Calcitonin

    D. Alendronate

20. True/False: ERT is classified as an antiresorptive agent.

21. List the three most common diagnostic systems used for bone densitometry.

    A. _____

    B. _____

    C. _____

22. Which of the following is considered the gold standard for measuring bone density?

    A. Quantitative computed tomography (QCT)

    B. Dual-energy x-ray absorptiometry (DXA)

    C. Quantitative ultrasound (QUS)

    D. Dual-energy photon absorptiometry

23. True/False: Current DXA systems use a pencil x-ray beam to reduce dose to the patient.

24. In what units of measurement is patient dose delivered during bone densitometry procedures using an x-ray

    source? _____

25. Effective dose delivered during a bone density exam of both the spine and the hip is

_____ μSv.

26. A Z-score produced during a DXA scan compares the patient's bone density with that of:
    A. An average, young, healthy individual with peak bone mass
    B. An average individual of the same sex and age
    C. A person with a slight degree of osteoporosis
    D. A person with a severe degree of osteoporosis

27. QCT involves a scan taken between the vertebral levels of:
    A. C4–T5
    B. T7–T12
    C. T12–L5
    D. L5–S1

28. True/False: QCT permits 3D analysis of the scanned region of the spine.

29. True/False: QCT produces less patient dose as compared to DXA.

30. QCT provides BMD measurements of _____ and _____ bone.

31. An average patient dose with QCT is approximately _____.

32. The most common anatomic site selected for QUS is the
    A. Spine
    B. Femur
    C. Calcaneus (Os calcis)
    D. Pelvis

33. Which of the following bone densitometry methods results in no radiation to the patient?
    A. DXA
    B. QCT
    C. QUS
    D. None of the above

34. Central or axial analysis using DXA or QCT includes bone density measurements of the:

    A. _____

    B. _____

35. True/False: Severe scoliosis or kyphosis might result in less accurate results for bone densitometry procedures.

36. True/False: New DXA technology allows for bilateral hips to be scanned concurrently; therefore, a hip prosthesis should not compromise the quality of the study.

37. True/False: If a patient has severe scoliosis, DXA can be performed on the forearm to gain a true measurement of BMD.

38. True/False: DXA of the hip requires the lower limb to be rotated 45° internally.

39. True/False: A patient history of hyperparathyroidism is considered a contraindication for a DXA scan.

40. Another term for *precision* in regard to the ability of a DXA system to obtain repeated measurements on the same patient is

   A. Reliability
   B. Reproducibility
   C. Validity
   D. Duplicity

41. Which of the following factors has the greatest impact of precision during a DXA scan?

   A. Patient positioning
   B. Exposure factors
   C. Postprocessing algorithm
   D. Quality of x-ray beam

42. Typically, the accuracy of a DXA system is better than _____%.

43. Vertebral fractures are most common in patients older than the age of _____.

44. Which region of the body is scanned during a vertebral fracture assessment study?

   A. Thoracolumbar spine
   B. Pelvis
   C. Bilateral hips
   D. Ribs and sternum

45. Which of the following anatomical regions is examined during an FRAX assessment?

   A. T12 or L1
   B. Femoral neck or total hip
   C. L3 or L5
   D. Femoral neck or humerus

46. True/False: A patient must be on pharmacologic treat for osteoporosis for an FRAX assessment.

MAGNETIC RESONANCE IMAGING

REVIEW EXERCISE A: Physical Principles of MR and MR Magnets (see textbook pp. 788–793)

1. MR uses _____, _____, and a _____to generate cross-sectional slices.

2. True/False: MR and CT are similar in that they produce cross-sectional imaging and use ionizing radiation.

3. Which of the following sequences will generate an image showing a fatty lesion as an area with bright signal?

   A. T1
   B. T2
   C. T3
   D. T4

4. What is the mathematical process used reconstruct the raw-data matrix?_____

5. A. Which nucleus is most suitable for MR? _____

   B. Why? _____

6. Which component of the nucleus is affected by radio waves and static magnetic fields?

   _____

7. Define *precession* by comparing it to another, more well-known phenomenon. _____

8. The rate of precession of a proton in a magnetic field _____ (increases or decreases) as the strength of the magnetic field increases.

9. What two terms can precessional frequency also be known as?

A. _____

B. _____

10. The sum of all magnetic moments is known as_____

11. True/False: Image quality improves as net magnetization increases.

12. Matching the radiowave frequency to the rate of the precessing nuclei is an example of the concept of

_____.

13. True/False: All protons will resonate in clinical MR scanners.

14. What are the two actions an RF excitation pulse accomplishes?

A. _____

B. _____

15. Relaxation of the nuclei as soon as the radiofrequency pulse is turned off can be divided into two categories:

_____ and _____.

16. T1 relaxation is known as _____ (transverse or longitudinal), or spin-lattice, relaxation.

17. T2 relaxation is known as _____ (transverse or longitudinal), or spin-spin, relaxation.

18. The quantity of hydrogen nuclei per given volume of tissue is referred to as the _____.

19. What are the three types of magnets used for MR?

A. _____

B. _____

C. _____

Which is the most common for MR? _____

20. Which of the following is the unit of measurement for a magnetic field?

A. Watt   C. Tesla

B. Edison   D. Ohm

21. At the 5 G (Gauss) line, what is the T (Tesla)?

A. .05   C. .005

B. .005   D. .0005

22. Which MR magnet type uses cryogens?

A. Permanent   C. Superconducting

B. Resistive   D. Open bore

REVIEW EXERCISE B: Patient Aspects: Contraindications, Preparation, Anxiety, Monitoring, MR Safety, and Pulse Sequences (see textbook pp. 793–800)

1. An MR examination is contraindicated for patients having which of the following?

   A. Electronic and electronic conductive metals

   B. External medication pumps

   C. Implanted medication pumps

   D. Any of the above

2. True/False: An MR examination is impossible for any patient with a contraindicated device such as a pacemaker.

3. What must be obtained before an MR examination is performed? _____

4. Who reviews the patient screening form to determine if any contraindications are present?

   A. Schedular   C. MR technologist

   B. Tech aide   D. Referring physician

5. Which of the following must the patient remove before entering the MR suite?

   A. Metallic jewelry   C. Credit card

   B. Cell phone   D. All of the above

6. Which of the following is not helpful in reducing patient anxiety?

   A. Explain the examination   C. Use restraints

   B. Move the patient slowly into the magnet   D. Provide an alarm (squeeze) ball

7. Which of the following sedatives is an example of an oral benzodiazepine?

   A. Versed   C. Xanax

   B. Fentanyl   D. Benadryl

8. Match the MR safety zones to their descriptions

   A. Public area where safety screening is performed (i.e., Changing rooms)_____   1. Zone I

   B. Inside the MR magnet room_____   2. Zone II

   C. Accessible public areas _____   3. Zone III

   D. Near the magnet room (MR control area)_____   4. Zone IV

9. Which MR personnel must have training on RF and contrast agent safety?

   A. Level 0   C. Level 2

   B. Level 1   D. Non-MR

10. Who is responsible for establishing the necessary training and identifies who qualifies for Level 1 and Level 2 personnel?

    A. Radiologist   C. Radiation Safety Officer

    B. Technologist   D. MR Medical Director

11. What is the term used to describe a ferrous object being pulled at a high speed into the MR magnet due to strong magnetic attraction? _____.

12. True/False: In the event of a code, it is recommended to leave the patient in Zone IV.

13. What are the two actions a magnetic object placed in the MR field subject to?

    A. _____

    B. _____

14. In the event of an unknown metallic object in the eye, which modality is used for a screening image?
    A. X-ray
    B. CT
    C. DMS
    D. A or B

15. What is defined as the RF power absorbed per unit mass on an object?_____

16. Which of the following is SAR measured in?
    A. Tesla
    B. Gauss
    C. Watts per kilogram
    D. Ohms

17. Which operating mode is considered safe for all patients?
    A. Normal
    B. First Level Controlled
    C. Second Level Controlled
    D. Third Level Controlled

18. Which of the following is the total accumulated amount of energy that is deposited into the body?
    A. SAR
    B. SED
    C. kVp
    D. Gd-DTPA

19. True/False: Direct skin contact with the side of the bore can cause a burn.

20. True/False: Pregnancy is not an absolute contraindication for an MR procedure.

21. Which of the following are used for MR contrast?
    A. Iodine
    B. Air
    C. Gadolinium
    D. Lead

22. How long after injection of MR contrast should the imaging procedure be completed?
    A. Within 15 minutes
    B. Within 30 minutes
    C. Within 1 hour
    D. Within 3 hours

23. Which of the following tests measure how well the kidneys filter blood by removing waste and extra water?
    A. CBC
    B. Lipid panel
    C. eGFR
    D. TSH

24. What are the three parameters that determine tissue contrast in MR images?

   A. _____

   B. _____

   C. _____

25. What are the three primary pulse sequences?

   A. _____

   B. _____

   C. _____

REVIEW EXERCISE C: MR Examinations (see textbook: pp. 800–809)

1. What are the three fundamental sequences of the brain?

   A. _____

   B. _____

   C. _____

2. Which of the following is not anatomy seen on an MR of the brain?

   A. Basal ganglia
   B. Pons

   C. Internal auditory canal
   D. Intervertebral discs

3. Which of the following suppresses CSF to better visualize conditions such as multiple sclerosis?

   A. T1
   B. T2

   C. FLAIR
   D. PD

4. Which of the following is acquired pre- and post- contrast for comparison?

   A. T1
   B. T2

   C. FLAIR
   D. PD

5. Which of the following is not anatomy seen on an MR of the spine?

   A. Nerve roots
   B. Pons

   C. CSF
   D. Vertebral foramina

6. What MR examination enables the radiologist to evaluate major arteries? _____

7. What MR examination enables the radiologist to evaluate veins? _____

8. Which of the following is visualized on an MRA of the brain?

   A. Aorta
   B. SVC

   C. Circle of Willis
   D. Loop of Henle

9. Complete the list of five structures best demonstrated in MR for musculoskeletal imaging.

  A. Soft tissue

  B. _____

  C. _____

  D. _____

  E. _____

10. Which of the following clinical indications would MR be used for?

  A. Osteonecrosis

  B. Tears in the meniscus

  C. Avascular necrosis

  D. Any of the above

11. True/False: When using respiratory triggering, erratic breathing has no impact on imaging time.

12. Which of the following is not a clinical indication for an MR of the body (abdomen/pelvis)?

  A. Rotator cuff tear

  B. Cirrhosis

  C. Adenomyosis

  D. Adrenal lesions

13. True/False: Breast MR is a supplemental exam performed in conjunction with routine screening.

14. What is the optimal timeframe for performing a breast MR on a premenopausal woman?

  A. During menstruation

  B. 1–6 days from the start of menstruation

  C. 7–14 days from the start of menstruation

  D. 15–20 days from menstruation

15. MR cardiac imaging is used to evaluate cardiac _____ and _____.

16. Diffusion-weighted imaging (DWI) is based on measuring random motion of _____ in a voxel of tissue.

17. True/False: Diffusion-weighted imaging (DWI) cannot differentiate between acute and chronic stroke.

18. Diffuse tensor imaging (DTI) can be used to trace the 3D path of _____

19. What are the two terms typically associated with functional imaging?

  A. _____

  B. _____

20. Match the following MR terms with the correct definition.

_____ A. Frequency at which the nuclear spins precess around the direction of the outer magnetic field

_____ B. Physiologically controlled imaging; synchronization of imaging with a time window so that a particular even or signal will be selected and others eliminated.

_____ C. Defines the angle of the excitation for a pulse sequence.

_____ D. Antennas used to send RF pulses or receive MR signals.

_____ E. Magnetic field outside the magnet that does not contribute to imaging.

_____ F. An item that has been demonstrated to pose no known hazards in a specified MR environment with specific conditions of use.

_____ G. Static main magnetic field of an MR system.

_____ H. Mathematical procedure for reconstructing images from raw data.

_____ I. The time between the excitation pulse of a sequence and the resulting echo.

_____ J. Coils used to generate magnetic gradient fields.

1. B0

2. Coil

3. Echo time (TE)

4. Flip angle

5. Fourier transform (FT)

6. Fringe field

7. Gating

8. Gradient coils

9. Larmor frequency

10. MR conditional

21. Match the following MR terms with the correct definition.

_____ A. Time between two excitation pulses.

_____ B. SI unit for magnetic field strength.

_____ C. Tissue-specific time constant that describes the return of the longitudinal magnetization to equilibrium.

_____ D. Wobbling motion that occurs when a spinning object is the subject of an external force.

_____ E. The RF energy absorbed per time unit and per kilogram.

_____ F. Chronological order of RF pulses and gradient pulses used to excite the volume to be measured, generate the signal, and provide spatial encoding.

_____ G. Ability to differentiate neighboring tissue structures.

_____ H. Tissue-specific time constant that describes the decay of transverse magnetization in an ideal homogeneous magnetic field.

_____ I. A vector quantity given by the vector project of the force and the position vector where the force is applied.

_____ J. Exchange of energy between two systems at a specific frequency.

1. Precession

2. Pulse sequence

3. Relaxation time (TR)

4. Resonance

5. Spatial resolution

6. Specific absorption rate

7. T1 relaxation

8. T2 relaxation

9. Tesla

10. Torque

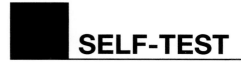

SELF-TEST

Directions: This self-test should be taken only after completing all of the readings, review exercises, and laboratory activities for a particular section. Please note: The self-test is divided into sections specific to each imaging modality described in the chapter. The purpose of this test is not only to provide a good learning exercise but also to serve as a good indicator of what your final evaluation exam will be. It is strongly suggested that if you do not achieve at least a 90%–95% grade on this self-test, you should review those areas in which you missed questions before going to your instructor for the final evaluation exam for this chapter.

NUCLEAR MEDICINE AND PET

1. One of the most common radionuclides used in NM is

   A. Thallium

   B. Technetium 99 m

   C. Cardiolite

   D. Sulfur colloid

2. What type of imaging device, used in NM, provides a 3D image of anatomic structures?

   A. Single-photon emission computed tomography (SPECT) camera

   B. B-mode unit

   C. Linear accelerator

   D. Real-time scanner

3. An abnormal region detected during a NM bone scan is often described as a(n)

   A. Signal void

   B. Hot spot

   C. Acoustic shadow

   D. Region of high attenuation

4. Which of the following is a common clinical indicator for a nuclear medicine gastrointestinal study?

   A. Duodenal ulcer

   B. Bezoar

   C. Hepatobiliary disease

   D. Ileus

5. How is the heart typically stressed during a nuclear cardiac perfusion study?

   A. Giving the patient a radiopharmaceutical

   B. Giving the patient Valium

   C. Giving the patient Lasix

   D. Having the patient run on a treadmill

6. Which radiopharmaceutical is administered during a thyroid uptake study?

   A. Technetium 99 m

   B. Sodium iodide (^{123}I)

   C. Sulfur colloid

   D. Thallium

7. Which of the following duties is *not* a typical responsibility of the nuclear medicine technologist?

   A. Calibrating imaging equipment

   B. Processing images

   C. Administering radionuclides

   D. Decontaminating area after spills

8. A device for accelerating charged particles in a circular orbit to high energies by means of an alternating electric field is a:

A. Cyclotron

C. Linear accelerator

B. Particle accelerator

D. Pulsed accelerator

9. A helium nucleus, consisting of two protons and two neutrons, is a(n):

A. Alpha particle

C. Beta particle

B. Neutrino

D. Radionuclide

10. A type of atom whose nucleus disintegrates spontaneously is a(n):

A. Alpha particle

C. Radiopharmaceutical

B. Beta particle

D. Radionuclide

11. PET demonstrates the _____ of the body's organs and tissues.

A. Anatomy

C. Physiology

B. Biochemical function

D. Chemical structure

12. What is produced when a positron and an electron join and then undergo annihilation?

A. X-ray

C. Radionuclide

B. Alpha particle

D. Two 511-keV photons

13. Which of the following elements is *not* used in the PET imaging process?

A. Hydrogen

C. Fluorine

B. Carbon

D. Oxygen

14. Which of the following biochemical compounds is used to gauge glucose metabolism in tissues during a PET scan?

A. ^{15}O-water

C. ^{18}F-FDG

B. ^{13}N-ammonia

D. ^{11}C-methionine

15. Most PET tracers have a half-life of:

A. 1–13 seconds

C. 150–320 seconds

B. 120 seconds–110 minutes

D. 8–12 hours

16. True/False: Malignant cells have a high rate of glucose metabolism.

17. True/False: During an epileptic seizure, there is a decrease in sugar (glucose) use at the seizure site in the brain.

18. Brain mapping is a PET procedure used to identify:

A. Primary tumors

C. Critical motor or sensory regions

B. Metastatic spread

D. Regions of brain responsible for dementia

19. True/False: Central nervous system tumors examined with PET demonstrate decreased glucose metabolism.

20. True/False: Dementia, when studied with PET, is demonstrated by decreased glucose metabolism in aspects of the brain.

21. The most common form of coregistration, or fusion technology, is the use of:

    A. PET/MR
    B. CT/MR
    C. PET/x-ray
    D. PET/CT

Radiation Oncology

22. Which of the following treats tumors in slices?

    A. Linear accelerator
    B. Tomotherapy
    C. Intraoperative radiation therapy (IORT)
    D. Cobalt-60 unit

23. Stereotactic radiation therapy is intended to:

    A. Treat only deep tumors
    B. Treat only superficial tumors
    C. Treat tumors only during surgery
    D. Deliver doses in minimal treatment fractions

24. True/False: Brachytherapy uses radioisotopes that may be placed in tissues.

25. Which of the following radiation therapy type deposits its energy to a maximum dose as it passes through the patient?

    A. Proton therapy
    B. Bradytherapy
    C. Megavoltage radiation therapy
    D. Tomotherapy

Diagnostic Medical Sonography

26. Which of the following is *not* an alternative term for medical ultrasound?

    A. Echosonography
    B. Sonography
    C. Piezosonography
    D. Ultrasonography

27. Diagnostic medical sonography operates at a frequency range from:

    A. 1–5 kHz
    B. 25–50 kHz
    C. 1–17 kHz
    D. 2–20 MHz

28. Which generation of ultrasound equipment first introduced grayscale imaging?

    A. A-mode
    B. B-mode (patient-mode)
    C. Real-time dynamic
    D. Doppler

29. An ultrasound transducer converts _____ energy to ultrasonic energy.

    A. Electrical
    B. Heat
    C. Light
    D. Magnetic

30. Which sonographic technique allows for organs and vascular structures to be accurately mapped, measured, and imaged?

    A. Doppler
    B. Transesophageal echocardiography (TEE)
    C. Extended focused assessment with sonography for trauma (EFAST)
    D. Sound navigation and ranging (SONAR)

31. True/False: A higher-frequency transducer increases penetration through the anatomy but produces lower image resolution.

32. True/False: A simple cyst is an example of a *hyperechoic* structure.

499

33. True/False: Breast sonography is used primarily to distinguish between solid and cystic masses.

34. What is the term used to describe a smooth structure with similar grays throughout?

    A. Heterogeneous

    B. Homogeneous

    C. Hyperechoic

    D. Hypoechoic

Mammography

35. What does the acronym MQSA represent, and what year did it go into effect? _____

36. Which health facilities (if any) are exempt from the MQSA requirements? _____

37. In 1992 the American Cancer Society recommended that all women older than the age of

    _____ undergo an annual screening mammography.

38. Currently, one in _____ American women will develop breast cancer sometime during her life.

39. The junction between the inferior aspect of the breast and the chest wall is called the

    _____.

40. In which quadrant of the breast is the tail, or axillary prolongation, found? _____

41. Using the clock system, one o'clock in the left breast would correspond to _____ in the right breast.

42. Which large muscle is located directly posterior to the breast? _____

43. What is the function of the mammary gland? _____

44. Name the bands of connective tissue passing through the breast tissue to provide support.

    _____

45. Which of the three breast tissue types (described in textbook) is the least dense radiographically?

    _____

46. What is the term used by radiologists for various small structures (blood vessels, etc.) seen on the mammogram?

    _____

47. Which term describes the thickest portion of the breast near the chest wall? _____

48. Which of the following tissue types would be found in the breasts of a 25-year-old pregnant female?

    A. Fibroglandular

    B. Fibrofatty

    C. Fatty

    D. Cystic

49. Which of the following tissue types would be found in the breasts of a 35-year-old female who has borne two children?

    A. Fibroglandular

    B. Fibrofatty

    C. Fatty

    D. Cystic

50. The male breast would be classified as:

    A. Fibroglandular   C. Fatty

    B. Fibrofatty   D. Cystic

51. Which of the following tissue types requires more compression during mammography as compared with the others?

    A. Fibrofatty   C. Fatty

    B. Fibroglandular   D. Cystic

52. Identify the anatomy and tissues labeled in Fig. 20.9.

    A. _____

    B. _____

    C. _____

    D. _____

    E. Which basic mammogram projection is demonstrated in

       Fig. 20.9? _____

    F. The right-side marker on this mammogram is correctly

       placed on the _____ side of the breast.

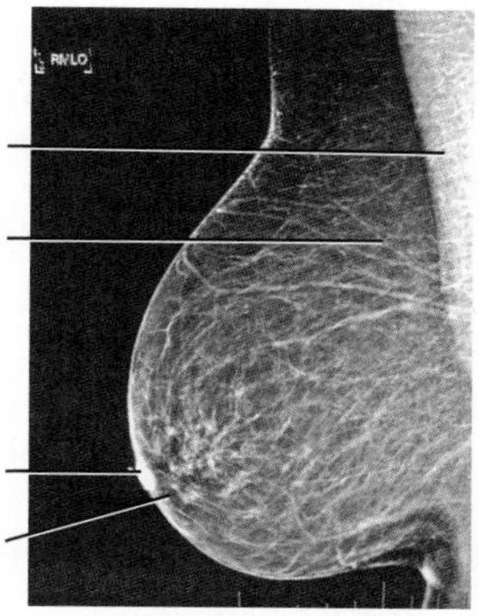

Fig. 20.9 Breast anatomy on a mammogram.

53. The target material commonly used in most mammographic x-ray tubes is _____.

54. To take maximum advantage of the anode-heel effect, the anode side of the x-ray tube should be over the

    _____ (base or apex) of the breast.

55. True/False: AEC can be used for most mammographic projections.

56. True/False: Compression of the breast improves image quality by reducing scatter radiation.

57. True/False: A grid (or virtual grid) is generally not used for mammography.

58. What size of focal spot should be used for magnification of small breast nodules or tissue samples?
    _____

59. What is the magnification factor for an exposure with a source–object distance (SOD) of 20 inches (50 cm) and a

    source–image receptor distance (SID) of 40 inches (100 cm)? _____

60. What is the dose unit most referenced in mammography consisting of the average dose to the patient's glandular tissue?

    A. REM   C. SAR

    B. MGD   D. Columbs

61. Which imaging modality is best suited to distinguish a cyst from a solid mass within the breast?

    _____

62. Which imaging modality is best suited to diagnose an extracapsular rupture of a breast implant?

    _____

63. True/False: Breast imaging using diagnostic medical sonography has been performed since the mid-1970s.

64. True/False: The primary means of reducing patient dose during mammography is to use higher mAs.

65. True/False: One reason that mammoscintigraphy is not ordered more frequently is the high number of false positives reported with this procedure.

66. Which of the following radionuclides is used during a BSGI study?
    A. Sulfur colloid   C. Technetium
    B. Sestamibi   D. Iodine 131

67. Carcinoma of the breast is divided into two categories: _____ and

    _____.

68. Which of the following refers to the exaggerated craniocaudal (lateral) projection?
    A. LECC   C. LCC
    B. LXCC   D. XCCL

69. What is the abbreviation for a mediolateral oblique projection?

70. List the two routine projections taken during a screening mammogram.

    A. _____   B. _____

71. Which of the routine projections taken during a mammogram best demonstrates the pectoral muscle?

    _____

72. True/False: Higher kVp can be used in digital imaging without affecting image quality.

73. Which projection best demonstrates the axillary aspect of the breast?

74. What is the abbreviation for the special projection, lateromedial oblique, often used with pacemaker

    patients? _____

75. The use of AEC when performing a projection with a breast implant in place can lead to

    _____ (overexposure or underexposure) of the breast.

76. A. The technique of "pinching" the breast to push an implant posteriorly to the chest wall is known as the

    _____ method.

    B. What is the correct term and abbreviation for this method? _____

502

77. What other special projection can be taken if a lesion is too deep into the axillary tail aspect of the chest wall to be seen with an exaggerated craniocaudal projection? (Include the correct ACR term and abbreviation.)

_____

78. Identification markers should always be placed near the _____.

79. How is the opposite breast prevented from superimposing the breast being examined on the MLO projection?

_____

80. With a large breast, which of the two routine projections is most likely to require two images to include all the breast tissue? _____

81. Which projection is usually requested when a lesion is seen on the MLO but not on the CC projection?

_____

82. What soft-tissue landmark determines the correct height for placement of the IR for the CC projection?

_____

83. Which of the following projections is recommended for demonstrating and evaluating air-fluid levels in structures of the breast?

A. CC
B. MLO

C. Mediolateral (true lateral)
D. XCCL

84. **Situation:** A mammogram is performed for a patient with breast implants. The resultant images are overexposed. The following factors were used: 28 kVp, AEC, grid, and gentle compression. Which of the following modifications would produce more diagnostic images during the repeat study?

A. Lower the kVp.
B. Do not use a grid.

C. Use manual exposure factors.
D. Do not use breast compression.

85. What device or system is part of direct digital mammography?

A. Imaging plate
B. Image intensifier

C. Bucky tray
D. Flat panel detector

86. True/False: The spatial resolution of digital mammography nearly equals that of film-screen imaging.

87. CAD is an acronym for _____.

88. It is reported that CAD can improve the breast cancer detection rate as much as _____%.

89. What type of radionuclide is used with mammoscintigraphy?

A. Technetium-99m-sestamibi
B. Iodine 131

C. Sulfur colloid
D. Gadolinium

90. Which imaging modality produces sectional images of the breast with a 3D appearance?

A. Mammoscintigraphy
B. Digital breast tomosynthesis

C. Sonomammography
D. BSGI

91. True/False: Patient dose from a PET scan of the breast is comparable to that of a film-screen mammogram.

92. Which of the following imaging modalities is most effective in studying the breast with implants?

    A. Diagnostic medical sonography

    B. PET mammography

    C. MR

    D. IR-screen mammography

93. One of the major disadvantages of using MR as a breast-screening tool is:

    A. Higher patient dose

    B. High false-positive rate

    C. Patient discomfort

    D. Length of the exam

94. The most common form of breast cancer is:

    A. Fibroadenoma

    B. Infiltrating sarcoma

    C. Lobular carcinoma

    D. Infiltrating ductal carcinoma

Bone Densitometry

95. Which of the following is not a risk factor for osteoporosis?

    A. Excessive physical activity

    B. Alcohol consumption

    C. Low body weight

    D. Low calcium intake

96. Newer DXA uses:

    A. Fan-beam x-ray source

    B. Positron-emission source

    C. Pencil-thin x-ray source

    D. Super-voltage x-ray source

97. A T-score obtained with the DXA system compares the patient with a(n):

    A. Average patient of the same age, sex, and ethnic background

    B. Young healthy individual with peak bone mass

    C. Young healthy individual of the same sex and ethnic background

    D. Patient with severe osteoporosis

98. True/False: The dose for QCT is lower than DXA.

99. The anatomic area most commonly scanned with QUS is the _____.

100. What specific cells are responsible for bone resorption? _____

101. Which of the following factors often leads to advanced bone loss?

    A. Being a female over the age of 21 years

    B. Undergoing hormone replacement therapy

    C. Undergoing glucocorticoid therapy

    D. Undergoing cardiac rehab

102. How much trabecular loss is needed before it becomes visible on a radiograph?

    A. 5%–10%

    B. 20%–30%

    C. 30%–50%

    D. >50%

103. A T-score acquired during a DXA scan of lower than −1.0 but higher than −2.5 indicates:

    A. Normal BMD

    B. Osteopenia

    C. Osteoporosis

    D. Severe osteoporosis

504

104. True/False: Estrogen often stimulates new bone formation.

105. What is the average effective dose delivered to a patient during a bone density scan of the spine and hip?

    A. 5 μSv
                          C. 1–30 Seiverts

    B. 10–30 μSv
                      D. 1–3 mSv

106. True/False: QUS is only recommended as a screening process.

107. Which vertebral region(s) is (are) analyzed during a DXA scan?

    A. T12
                          C. L1–L4

    B. Between T7 and L1
            D. L4–S1

108. The ability of a DXA system to obtain consistent BMD values of repeated measurements of the same patient is called _____.

109. True/False: If trabecular and cortical bone is being evaluated, QCT is the method of choice.

110. True/False: QCT of the hip is most valuable to predict future hip fracture.

111. The presence of _____ prevents the accurate measurement of the BMD of an extremity.

    A. Cancer
                          C. Metallic prosthesis

    B. Paget disease
                      D. Osteoporosis

112. True/False: Single-energy photon absorptiometry is no longer used in clinical practice.

113. Parathyroid hormone analog (PTH 1-34) (teriparatide, brand name Forteo) is provided to patients with osteoporosis to:

    A. Heal hip fractures
                      C. Relieve pain

    B. Stimulate bone formation
          D. Reduce bone loss

114. Boniva belongs to a group of drugs termed:

    A. Calcitonin
                          C. Teriparatide

    B. Selective estrogen receptor modulators
    D. Bisphosphonates

Magnetic Resonance Imaging

115. The MR image represents differences in the number of:

    A. X-rays attenuated
                   C. Frequencies of nuclei

    B. Nuclei and the rate of their recovery
    D. Radio waves

116. The MR process excites the nuclei in the body with:

    A. X-rays
                         C. Sound waves

    B. Radio frequencies waves
          D. Visible light

117. The most common nuclei in the body that are used to receive and re-emit radio waves are:

    A. Hydrogen
                        C. Oxygen

    B. Carbon
                          D. Phosphorus

118. The nuclei that receive and reemit radio waves are under the influence of:

    A. Gravitational force

    B. The sun and the planets

    C. X-ray energy

    D. A static magnetic field

119. Which of the following properties results in a nucleus behaving like a small magnet?

    A. An even number of neutrons and protons

    B. An odd number of neutrons or protons

    C. An even number of electrons

    D. The presence of a magnet

120. Precession of the magnetic nuclei occurs because of:

    A. Oscillation in the presence of other atoms

    B. Regression under the influence of a magnet

    C. The influence of a static magnetic field

    D. Ionization-exposed atoms

121. A precessing nucleus produces _____ in a nearby loop of wire.

    A. An alternating current

    B. A dipole

    C. A direct current

    D. Magnetic regression

122. Precession of magnetic nuclei can be altered by the application of:

    A. X-rays

    B. Radio frequencies

    C. Microwaves

    D. Visible light

123. Resonance occurs when radio waves are:

    A. Of the same frequency as the precessing nuclei

    B. At the same rate as T1 relaxation

    C. At the same rate as T2 relaxation

    D. Received by an antenna

124. The angle of precession of the nuclei is altered because the:

    A. Nuclei must be vertical

    B. Magnetic force dominates

    C. Electrostatic properties of the nuclei dominate

    D. MR signal is strongest when nuclei are in a horizontal or transverse plane

125. Emitted signals from the exposed nuclei are _____ and sent to the computer.

    A. Evaluated

    B. Received by an RF coil (antenna)

    C. In resonance

    D. Precessing

126. The _____ among T1, T2, and proton density signals of tissues produce(s) contrast in the MR image.

    A. Similarities

    B. Phase

    C. Differences

    D. Frequency

127. In T2 relaxation, the spins of the exposed nuclei:

    A. Are vertical in orientation

    B. Move to the north

    C. Are reduced in density

    D. Become out of phase with one another

128. In T1 relaxation, the spins of the exposed nuclei:

    A. Are relaxing back to a vertical orientation

    B. Stay in a horizontal position

    C. Are reduced in density

    D. Become out of phase with one another

506

129. Proton density refers to the _____ of hydrogen nuclei.
    A. Quality
    B. Quantity
    C. Phase
    D. Wavelength

130. The signal strength and thus the brightness of points in the image are primarily determined by:
    A. Differences in T1 and T2 relaxation rates of tissues
    B. Differences in spin density of tissues
    C. The longitudinal component of nuclei
    D. Exposure of the nuclei to the static magnetic field

131. Common strengths of magnets used in MR range from:
    A. 0.2 to 7 tesla
    B. 5 to 7 tesla
    C. 12 to 15 tesla
    D. 15 to 20 tesla

132. Which of the following types of MR magnets requires the use of cryogens?
    A. Permanent
    B. Superconducting magnets
    C. Resistive
    D. Open magnets

133. TR can be defined simply as:
    A. Time reversal
    B. Repetition time
    C. Timing range
    D. Time of resonance

134. TE can be defined simply as:
    A. Echo phase
    B. Time net
    C. Temporary echo
    D. Echo time

135. TR and TE have a profound influence on:
    A. Image noise deletion
    B. Image contrast
    C. Signal averaging
    D. Image density

136. One tesla equals:
    A. 10,000 times the Earth's magnetic field
    B. .00005 gauss
    C. 10 gauss
    D. 10,000 gauss

137. Which of the following is *not* a similarity between MR and CT?
    A. The outward appearance of the unit
    B. The use of a computer to analyze information
    C. The use of ionizing radiation
    D. Images viewed as a slice of tissue

138. What zone is the area near the magnet room and where the technologist's console is?
    A. Zone I
    B. Zone II
    C. Zone III
    D. Zone IV

139. What type of objects are a concern when placed within the fringe field?
    A. Ferromagnetic
    B. Titanium
    C. Molded plastic
    D. Those containing water or other fluids

140. What category would an implanted device (i.e., pacemaker) be allowed in the MR environment if certain precautions are met?

    A. MR-Safe

    B. MR-Conditional

    C. MR-Unsafe

    D. There are no conditions where a pacemaker is allowed in MR.

141. What zone is inside the room where the MR magnet is?

    A. Zone I   C. Zone III

    B. Zone II   D. Zone IV

142. The most important MR safety contraindication in regard to the torquing of metallic objects is:

    A. Intra-abdominal surgical staples   C. Ferromagnetic intracranial aneurysm clips

    B. Stainless steel femoral rods   D. Titanium hip prosthesis

143. Local heating of tissues (referred to as *SAR*) is measured in:

    A. W/kg   C. RF frequency

    B. Joules/kg   D. W/cm^2

144. A contrast agent commonly used for MR examinations is:

    A. Iodine 131   C. Gadolinium oxysulfide

    B. Lanthanum oxybromide   D. Gadolinium-diethylenetriaminepentaacetic acid

145. Contrast agents are generally used in conjunction with:

    A. T1-weighted pulse sequences   C. Spin density–weighted pulse sequences

    B. T2-weighted pulse sequences   D. All of the above

146. True/False: Contrast media used in MR carry a higher risk for allergic reaction as compared with iodinated contrast agents.

147. Which of these pathologic conditions would indicate the use of contrast media during an MR procedure?

    A. Cerebral bleed   C. Herniated nucleus pulposus

    B. C-spine fracture   D. Inflammatory conditions of spine

148. True/False: T1-weighted images demonstrate free air within the abdominal cavity.

149. An inversion recovery pulse sequence is used to null the signal from:

    A. Water   C. Muscle

    B. Bone   D. Cartilaginous

150. One type of Echoplanar Imaging (EPI) sequence is also known as a:

    A. FLAIR   C. HASTE

    B. Single shot   D. MRV

151. MR of the brain allows visualization of:

    A. White matter disease   C. Small calcifications

    B. Acute cerebral bleeds   D. Skull anomalies

508

152. MR of the brain includes the use of a standard head coil and:

    A. Prone position

    B. Cardiac gating

    C. Sedation

    D. T1-weighted and T2-weighted pulse sequences

153. MR of the spine is not best for evaluating which of the following?

    A. Bone marrow changes

    B. Cord abnormalities

    C. Disk herniation

    D. Degree of scoliosis present in spine

154. MR of the joints or limbs demonstrates all of the following except:

    A. Ligaments

    B. Tendons

    C. Muscle

    D. Cortical bone

155. The largest drawback to MR of the abdomen is:

    A. Motion artifacts

    B. Metallic implants

    C. Coil selection

    D. Sequence times

156. True/False: High-field strength MR magnets can produce up to 7 tesla.

157. True/False: An MR technologist is considered an MR Level 2 personnel.

158. A stray magnetic field that exists outside the MR gantry is the definition for:

    A. RF field

    B. Fringe field

    C. Magnetic field

    D. Field of influence

159. fMRI is performed to study:

    A. Anatomy of the brain

    B. Specific functions of the brain

    C. Processes such as language, vision, movement, hearing, and memory

    D. All of the above

160. True/False: fMRI of the brain exceeds the spatial resolution seen with PET and SPECT images.

20 Diagnostic and Therapeutic Modalities

NUCLEAR MEDICINE AND PET

1. B. Technetium-99m
2. A. Single-photon emission computed tomography (SPECT) camera
3. B. Hot spot
4. C. Hepatobiliary disease
5. D. Having the patient run on a treadmill
6. B. Sodium iodide (^{123}I)
7. A. Calibrating imaging equipment
8. A. Cyclotron
9. A. Alpha particle
10. D. Radionuclide
11. B. Biochemical function
12. D. Two 511-keV photons
13. A. Hydrogen
14. C. ^{18}F-FDG
15. B. 120 seconds–110 minutes
16. True
17. False
18. C. Critical motor or sensory regions
19. False
20. True
21. D. PET/CT

RADIATION ONCOLOGY

22. B. Tomotherapy
23. D. Deliver doses in minimal treatment fractions
24. True
25. C. Megavoltage radiation therapy

SONOGRAPHY

26. C. Piezosonography
27. D. 2 to 20 MHz
28. B. B-mode (patient-mode)
29. A. Electrical
30. A. Doppler
31. False (Decreased penetration but higher resolution)
32. False. (Simple cyst is anechoic.)
33. True
34. True

MAMMOGRAPHY

35. Mammography Quality Standards Act; 1994
36. Only Veterans Administration (VA) facilities are exempt.
37. 40
38. Eight
39. Inframammary fold
40. Upper outer quadrant (UOQ)
41. 11 o'clock
42. Pectoralis major muscle
43. Lactation or production of milk
44. Cooper (suspensory) ligaments
45. Adipose (fatty)
46. Trabeculae
47. Base
48. A. Fibroglandular
49. B. Fibrofatty
50. C. Fatty
51. A. Fibrofatty
52. A. Glandular tissue
    B. Nipple
    C. Adipose (fatty) tissue
    D. Pectoral muscle
    E. Mediolateral oblique (MLO)
    F. Axillary
53. Molybdenum
54. Apex
55. True
56. True
57. False. (A grid or virtual grid is used because of the large amount of scatter and secondary radiation.)
58. 0.1 mm
59. Two times the original size of the object
60. B. MGD
61. Diagnostic medical sonography (DMS)
62. Magnetic resonance imaging (MR)
63. True
64. False. (Patient dose is reduced primarily by minimizing repeats.)
65. True
66. B. Sestamibi
67. Noninvasive and invasive
68. D. XCCL
69. MLO
70. A. Craniocaudal (CC)
    B. Mediolateral oblique (MLO)
71. Mediolateral oblique projection
72. True
73. Exaggerated craniocaudal or lateral (XCCL) projection
74. LMO
75. Overexposure
76. A. Eklund
    B. Implant-displaced (ID)
77. Axillary tail (AT) view
78. Axillary side
79. Have patient hold the breast back with her opposite hand.
80. MLO (mediolateral oblique)
81. XCCL (exaggerated craniocaudal, or lateral)
82. Inframammary fold at its upper limits
83. C. Mediolateral (true lateral)
84. C. Use manual exposure factors.
85. D. Flat-panel detector
86. True
87. Computer-aided detection
88. 15%
89. A. Technetium-99m-sestamibi
90. B. Digital breast tomosynthesis
91. False
92. C. MR
93. B. High false-positive rate
94. D. Infiltrating ductal carcinoma

BONE DENSITOMETRY

95. A. Excessive physical activity
96. A. Fan-beam x-ray source

97. B. Young healthy individual with peak bone mass
98. False.
99. calcaneus or Os calcis
100. Osteoclasts
101. C. Undergoing glucocorticoid therapy
102. C. 30%–50%
103. B. Osteopenia
104. False (Estrogen inhibits resorption)
105. A. 5 μSv
106. True
107. C. L1–L4
108. Precision (or reproducibility)
109. True
110. False. (DXA of the hip is most valuable to predict future hip fracture.)
111. C. Metallic prosthesis
112. True
113. B. Stimulate bone formation
114. D. Bisphosphonates

MAGNETIC RESONANCE IMAGING

115. B. Nuclei and the rate of their recovery
116. B. Radio frequencies waves
117. A. Hydrogen
118. D. A static magnetic field
119. B. An odd number of neutrons or protons
120. C. The influence of a static magnetic field
121. A. An alternating current
122. B. Radio frequencies
123. A. Of the same frequency as the precessing nuclei
124. D. MR signal is strongest when nuclei are in a horizontal or transverse plane.
125. B. Received by an RF coil (antenna)
126. C. Differences
127. D. Become out of phase with one another
128. A. Are relaxing back to a vertical orientation (within the magnetic field)
129. B. Quantity
130. A. Differences in T1 and T2 relaxation rates of tissues
131. A. 0.2 to 7 tesla
132. B. Superconducting magnets
133. B. Repetition time
134. D. Echo time
135. B. Image contrast
136. D. 10,000 gauss
137. C. The use of ionizing radiation
138. D. Interaction of magnetic fields with ferrometallic objects and tissues
139. A. Ferromagnetic
140. B. MR-Conditional
141. D. Zone IV
142. C. Ferromagnetic intracranial aneurysm clips
143. A. W/kg
144. D. Gadolinium-diethylenetriamine pentaacetic acid
145. A. T1-weighted pulse sequences
146. False
147. D. Inflammatory conditions of spine
148. False
149. A. Water
150. B. Single shot
151. A. White matter disease
152. D. T1-weighted and T2-weighted pulse sequences
153. D. Degree of scoliosis present in spine
154. D. Cortical bone
155. A. Motion artifacts
156. True
157. True
158. B. Fringe field
159. D. All of the above
160. True

Answers to Review Questions

CHAPTER 1

Review Exercise A: General, Systemic, and Skeletal Anatomy and Arthrology

1. Chemical level
2. A. Epithelial
   B. Connective
   C. Muscular
   D. Nervous
3. A. Skeletal
   B. Circulatory
   C. Digestive
   D. Respiratory
   E. Urinary
   F. Reproductive
   G. Nervous
   H. Muscular
   I. Endocrine
   J. Integumentary
4. 1. C
   2. E
   3. H
   4. G
   5. I
   6. D
   7. J
   8. F
   9. B
   10. A
5. True
6. A. Integumentary
7. C. Integumentary
8. A. Axial skeleton
   B. Appendicular skeleton
9. False (206)
10. False (part of appendicular)
11. True
12. True
13. A. Long bones
    B. Short bones
    C. Flat bones
    D. Irregular bones
14. D. Periosteum
15. C. Medullary aspect
16. C. Periosteum
17. A. Diaphysis (body)
    B. Epiphyses
18. False (20–25 years)
19. C. Metaphysis

20. A. Synarthrosis
    B. Amphiarthrosis
    C. Diarthrosis
21. A. Fibrous
    B. Cartilaginous
    C. Synovial
22. 1. C
    2. A
    3. C
    4. A
    5. B
    6. C
    7. A
    8. B
    9. B
    10. C
23. A. Plane (gliding)
    B. Ginglymus (hinge)
    C. Pivot (trochoid)
    D. Ellipsoid (condylar)
    E. Saddle (sellar)
    F. Ball and socket (spheroidal)
    G. Bicondylar
24. 1. E
    2. B
    3. F
    4. A
    5. D
    6. G
    7. C
    8. B
    9. C
    10. E
    11. G
    12. D
25. Body habitus
26. B. Sthenic
27. D. Hyposthenic
28. True
29. Bariatrics
30. False

Review Exercise B: Positioning Terminology

1. Radiograph
2. Central ray (CR)
3. Anatomic
4. Median or midsagittal
5. Midcoronal
6. Transverse, axial, or horizontal

7. True
8. Posterior or dorsal; anterior or ventral
9. A. Projection
10. C. Position
11. True
12. True
13. Lateral position
14. Left posterior oblique (LPO)
15. Right anterior oblique (RAO)
16. Dorsal decubitus (left lateral)
17. Right lateral position
18. Left lateral decubitus (PA)
19. 1. H
    2. G
    3. F
    4. I
    5. B
    6. D
    7. J
    8. C
    9. E
    10. A
20. Anteroposterior (AP)
21. Axial
22. (Apical) lordotic position
23. Dorsiflexion
24. False (inward, toward midline)
25. 1. B
    2. A
    3. A
    4. A
    5. A
    6. B
    7. B
    8. A
    9. B
    10. A
26. A. Extension
    B. Radial deviation
    C. Plantar flexion
    D. Inversion
    E. Medial (internal) rotation
    F. Adduction
    G. Pronation
    H. Protraction
    I. Elevation
27. 1. F
    2. D
    3. G

510

Answers to Review Questions

Copyright © 2025 by Elsevier Inc.
All rights reserved, including those for text and data mining, AI training, and similar technologies.

4. E
5. C
6. J
7. I
8. H
9. A
10. B
28. A. Patient identification and date
    B. Anatomic side markers
29. False
30. D. Any of the above

Review Exercise C: Positioning Principles

1. Code of ethics
2. True
3. True
4. B. ARRT
5. A. **A**nnounce
   B. **C**ommunicate
   C. **E**xplain
6. A. A minimum of two projections 90 degrees from each other
   B. A minimum of three projections when joints are in the prime interest area
7. A. 3
   B. 2
   C. 3
   D. 2
   E. 2
   F. 3
   G. 2
   H. 2
   I. 3
   J. 1 (see text)
8. A. (d) Two
   B. (c) Rather than move the forearm for additional projections, place the image receptor and x-ray tube as needed for a second projection 90 degrees from the first projection.
9. Topographic landmarks
10. True
11. True
12. True
13. False
14. False
15. True

Review Exercise D: Imaging Principles

1. A. Technical factors
   B. Radiographic technique
2. Receptor exposure
3. A. mAs
4. Kilovoltage (kVp)

5. Milliseconds
6. False. The highest kVp and lowest mAs should be used.
7. Source to image distance (SID)
8. D. Intensity will decrease by a factor of 4
9. Grids
10. Doubling
11. C. 15%
12. 4 inches (10 cm), unless using virtual grid software
13. False
14. A. Reducing radiation dose to the patient
    B. Optimal image quality
15. A. Exposure indicator (EI)
16. 1. The recommended EI range for a given area of interest
    2. If the EI value of their imaging system has a direct or inverse relationship to radiation exposure
    3. How to adjust exposure factors based on the generated EI
17. Spatial resolution
18. Blur or unsharpness
19. A. Focal spot size
    B. Source–image receptor distance (SID)
    C. Object–image receptor distance (OID)
20. Penumbra
21. 1. Detail
    2. Recorded detail
    3. Image sharpness
    4. Definition
22. Motion (voluntary and involuntary)
23. B. Breathing
24. D. Any of the above
25. Focal spot
26. Motion
27. A. Decrease OID
28. D. 0.3-mm focal spot and 40-inch (100 cm) SID
29. Distortion
30. False (There is always some degree of penumbra caused by OID and divergence of the x-ray beam.)
31. A. SID
    B. OID
    C. Object IR alignment
    D. Central ray placement
32. False (increase distortion)
33. False (increase distortion)
34. True

35. A. 40 inches (100 cm)
36. B. 72 inches (180 cm)
37. True
38. False
39. True
40. True

Review Exercise E: Digital Imaging Characteristics

1. False
2. True
3. True
4. Pixel
5. Matrix
6. A. Increase
7. Contrast
8. False
9. True
10. False
11. D. Contrast resolution
12. C. Application of processing algorithms
13. B. Contrast resolution
14. Detective quantum efficiency (DQE)
15. D. 1
16. 1. Intensity of the x-ray beam
    2. Amount of tissue irradiated
    3. Type and thickness of the tissue
17. False. Digital receptors are more sensitive to low radiation; therefore controlling scatter is important.
18. True.
19. Exposure latitude
20. True
21. Noise
22. Signal-to-noise ratio
23. Low-SNR
24. C. Mottle
25. Electronic noise

Review Exercise F: Digital Imaging Components, Postprocessing Options, and Image Archiving

1. C. Computed radiography
2. True
3. B. Analog-to-digital converter (ADC)
4. C. Electrons
5. False
6. True
7. True
8. A. Bright light
9. Archiving
10. Digital radiography (DR)
11. 1. Amorphous selenium
    2. Amorphous silicon

12. B. Indirect
13. D. Both A and B
14. True
15. True
16. False
17. True
18. 1. D
    2. E
    3. A
    4. C
    5. F
    6. B
19. D. Algorithms
20. False
21. Width; Level
22. A. Annotation
    B. Edge enhancement
    C. Image reversal (invert image)
    D. Magnification
    E. Smoothing
    F. Subtraction
23. Picture archiving Communication system
24. A. Digital imaging Communications medicine
    B. Radiology information system
    C. Hospital information system
    D. Direct or digital radiography
25. A. Display matrix
    B. Exposure latitude
    C. Windowing
    D. Penumbra
    E. Exposure indicator
    F. Bit depth
    G. Distortion
    H. Kilovoltage
    I. Noise
    J. Spatial resolution (detail, sharpness, or definition)
    K. Postprocessing
26. A. Radiology information system
    B. Image receptor
    C. Object image distance
    D. Source image receptor distance (SID)
    E. Automatic exposure control
    F. Hospital information system
27. A. 5
    B. 7
    C. 3
    D. 2
    E. 1
    F. 4
    G. 6

Review Exercise G: Radiation Protection

1. A. TIME—Minimize radiation beam on time
   B. DISTANCE—Maximize distance from the radiation source of both patients and staff
   C. SHIELDING—Use shielding on staff and patients
2. Roentgen or Coulombs per kilogram (C/kg)
3. Air kerma (replaced exposure as preferred quantity)
4. Gray (rad)
5. Effective dose
6. 1 (one)
7. 50 mSv (5 rem) per year
8. True.
9. A. Coulombs per kilogram (C/kg) of air
   B. Gray (Gy)
   C. Sievert (Sv)
10. A. 0.03 Gy
    B. 4.48 mGy
    C. 0.38 Sv
    D. 150 mSv
11. A. 0.5 mSv (50 mrem)
    B. 5 mSv (500 mrem)
12. 1 mSv (0.1 rem) per year
13. B. 10%
14. A. Thermoluminescent dosimeter
    B. Optically stimulated luminescence (dosimeter)
15. As low as reasonably achievable
16. A. Family member (if not pregnant)
17. True
18. True
19. True
20. False (considers dose risk to all organs)
21. C. AP abdomen
22. C. Retrograde pyelogram
23. C. Poor communication between technologist and patient
24. A. Carelessness in positioning
    B. Selection of incorrect exposure factors
25. A. Inherent
    B. Added
26. Aluminum or copper (or combination of both)
27. C. 2.5 mm aluminum
28. False (2%, not 10%)

29. True
30. True
31. A. Volume of tissue directly irradiated is diminished
    B. Amount of accompanying scatter radiation is decreased
32. True
33. False. Consult with the radiologist before proceeding with the examination
34. A. Head CT
35. False
36. True
37. D. 95%–99%
38. D. All of the above are true.
39. D. 10 R/min (air kerma rate of 88 mGy/min)
40. Must not exceed 20 R/min (air kerma rate of 176 mGy/min)
41. C. 1–3 R/min (air kerma rate of 8.8–26 mGy/min)
42. 1. Dose area product (DAP)
    2. Cumulative total dose
43. Dose area product (DAP)
44. B. 3 Gy (300 rad)
45. True
46. C. Behind the radiologist (fluoroscopist)
47. Keep the receptor as close as possible to the patient. (Also, some experts recommend wearing a thyroid shield along with a protective apron.)
48. 0.5-mm lead (Pb) equivalent
49. True
50. False (Image Gently) is intended to reduce unnecessary dose to children.)

CHAPTER 2

Review Exercise A: Radiographic Anatomy of the Chest

1. A. Sternum
   B. Clavicles
   C. Scapulae
   D. Ribs
   E. Thoracic vertebrae
2. A. Vertebra prominens (spinous process on seventh cervical [C7] vertebra)
   B. Jugular notch (upper portion of sternum)
3. A. Pharynx
   B. Trachea
   C. Bronchi
   D. Lungs

4. A. Thyroid cartilage
   B. Larynx
   C. Sternum
   D. Scapula
   E. Clavicle
5. A. Nasopharynx
   B. Oropharynx
   C. Laryngopharynx
6. Epiglottis
7. Anteriorly
8. Hyoid
9. A. Right
   B. It is larger in diameter and more vertical.
10. A. Carina
    B. T4–5
11. Alveoli
12. A. Pleura
    B. Parietal pleura
    C. Pulmonary or visceral pleura
    D. Pleural cavity
    E. Pneumothorax
13. A. Base
    B. Hilum (hilus)
    C. Apex (apices)
    D. Costophrenic angle
14. Presence of liver on right
15. A. Thymus gland
    B. Heart and great vessels
    C. Trachea
    D. Esophagus
16. A. Thymus
    B. Arch of aorta
    C. Heart
    D. Inferior vena cava
    E. Superior vena cava
    F. Thyroid
    G. Trachea
    H. Esophagus
17. Pericardial sac or pericardium
18. Ascending, arch, and descending aorta
19. A. Apex of left lung
    B. Trachea
    C. Carina
    D. Heart
    E. Left costophrenic angle
    F. Right hemidiaphragm (or base)
    G. Hilum
    H. Apex of lungs
    I. Hilum
    J. Heart
    K. Right and left hemidiaphragm
    L. Right and left costophrenic angles (superimposed)

20. A. Left mainstem bronchus
    B. Descending aorta
    C. T5 (fifth thoracic vertebra)
    D. Esophagus
    E. Region of carina
    F. Right main stem bronchus
    G. Superior vena cava
    H. Ascending aorta
    I. Sternum

Review Exercise B: Technical Considerations

1. Hypersthenic
2. D. Hyposthenic and asthenic
3. 10 ribs
4. A. Necklace
   B. Bra
   C. Religious medallion around neck
   F. Hair fasteners
   G. Oxygen lines
5. True
6. True
7. 110–125 kVp
8. False
9. E. All of the above
10. Should be able to see faint outlines of at least middle and upper vertebrae and ribs through heart and other mediastinal structures
11. False (heart may be located in right thorax)
12. Situs inversus
13. C. Pigg-O-Stat
14. A. 70–85 kVp, short exposure time
15. True
16. False (Centering for bariatric patient is at the same location—T7)
17. Second
18. A. Small pneumothorax
    B. Fixation or lack of normal diaphragm movement
    C. Presence of a foreign body
    D. Distinguishing between opacity in rib or lung
19. A. To allow diaphragm to move down farther
    B. To show possible air and fluid levels in the chest
    C. To prevent engorgement and hyperemia of the pulmonary vessels
20. Erect position allows abdominal organs to drop, allowing the diaphragm to move farther down and the lungs to aerate more fully.
21. Reduces distortion and magnification of the heart and other chest structures
22. C. Symmetric appearance and location of sternoclavicular joints
23. Extend the neck upward
24. A. Left
    B. Right
    C. Left
25. Prevents upper arm soft tissues from being superimposed over upper chest fields
26. 1½ –2 inches (5 cm)
27. Vertebra prominens, 8 inches (20 cm) for male, 7 inches (18 cm) for female
28. A. Landscape
    B. Portrait
29. B. Jugular notch
30. True
31. False (should be equal)
32. False (greater width)
33. True
34. True
35. False
36. False
37. 1. F
    2. J
    3. E
    4. I
    5. G
    6. L
    7. K
    8. B
    9. D
    10. C
    11. A
    12. H
38. D. Air bronchogram sign
39. Left lung atelectasis +
    Lung neoplasm 0
    Severe pulmonary edema +
    RDS or ARDS (HMD in infants) +
    Reactivation (secondary) tuberculosis (slight increase) +
    Advanced emphysema –
    Large pneumothorax 0
    Pulmonary emboli 0
    Primary tuberculosis 0
    Advanced asbestosis 0
40. B. Emphysema
41. D. AP lordotic

513

Review Exercise C: Positioning of the Chest

1. Places the heart closer to the image receptor to reduce magnification of the heart
2. T7
3. Scapulae
4. A left lateral better demonstrates the heart region
5. Greater than 1 cm (½–¾ inch)
6. A. Caudad (±5 degrees)
   B. Sternum
7. Pleural effusion
8. Left lateral decubitus
9. Pneumothorax
10. Right lateral decubitus (affected side up)
11. Rule out calcifications or masses beneath the clavicles
12. AP axial projection, central ray 15–20 degrees cephalad
13. A. RAO
    B. LPO
14. Left, 60 degrees
15. False (A grid is recommended.)
16. Level of C6–C7, midway between thyroid cartilage and jugular notch
17. Scatter
18. Lift the breasts up and outward and then remove her hands as she leans against the chest board (image receptor) to keep them in the position.
19. False
20. Engorgement, hyperemia

Review Exercise D: Problem Solving for Technical and Positioning Errors

1. Right rotation. The patient is rotated into a slight RAO position.
2. The lungs are underinflated. Explain to the patient the need for a deep inspiration, and take the exposure on the second deep inspiration.
3. A. The 78 kVp is too low. The recommended kVp range is 110–125.
   B. Increase the kVp and reduce the mAs for the repeat exposure.
4. Center the central ray higher (to the level of T7, which will be found 7–8 inches below the vertebra prominens). Make sure the image receptor is centered to the central ray and the top collimation light border is at the vertebra prominens.
5. B. Decrease the kVp moderately (– –).
6. C. Increase the kVp slightly (+).
7. Ensure placement of the correct right or left anatomic side marker on the image receptor, because the heart and other thoracic structures may be transposed from right to left.
8. Determine which hemidiaphragm (right or left) is more posterior or more anterior. The left hemidiaphragm can frequently be identified by visualization of the gastric air bubble or the inferior heart shadow, both of which are associated with the left hemidiaphragm.
9. Right lateral decubitus; in a patient with hemothorax (fluid), the side of interest should be down.
10. AP and lateral upper airway projections
11. AP lordotic
12. Inspiration and expiration PA projections and/or a lateral decubitus AP chest with affected side up
13. C. Erect PA and lateral
14. AP semiaxial projection; CR is angled 15–20 degrees cephalad to project the clavicles above the apices and to clearly demonstrate the possible tumor.
15. Both the LPO and RAO oblique positions will best demonstrate or elongate the left lung.

Review Exercise E: Critique Radiographs of the Chest

A. PA chest (Fig. 2.5)
   Description of possible error:
   1. Anatomy demonstrated: Left costophrenic angle is missing.
   2. Part positioning: Landscape alignment of the IR is required to have the entire chest anatomy displayed.
   3. Collimation and CR: Centering is acceptable. No evidence of collimation.
   4. Exposure: Acceptable exposure factors. Could be increased for better penetration of mediastinum and surrounding soft tissues.
   5. Anatomic side markers: side marker evident
      Repeatable error(s): Criterion 1
B. Lateral chest (Fig. 2.6)
   Description of possible error:
   1. Anatomy demonstrated: Aspect of apical region is obscured by soft tissues of upper arm.
   2. Part positioning: Rotation of thorax is evident by poor superimposition of posterior ribs.
   3. Collimation and CR: Absence of collimation
   4. Exposure: There appears to be involuntary or voluntary motion.
   5. Anatomic side markers: Absent from image
      Repeatable error(s): Criteria 1, 2, 4, and 5

CHAPTER 3

Review Exercise A: Abdominopelvic Anatomy

1. Psoas muscles
2. Gastro-
3. A. Duodenum
   B. Jejunum
   C. Ileum
4. Ileum
5. Right lower, cecum
6. Descending colon, rectum
7. B. Spleen
8. A. Pancreas
   B. Liver
   C. Gallbladder
9. Posteriorly
10. B. Spleen
11. Presence of liver on right
12. Suprarenals (adrenal)
13. False (intravenous urogram [IVU]). IVP is a study of the collecting system of the kidneys specifically.
14. Peritoneum
15. Retroperitoneal
16. D. Mesentery
17. C. Greater omentum

18. 1. A
    2. C
    3. B
    4. A
    5. C
    6. B
    7. A
    8. C
    9. B
    10. A
    11. B
    12. B
19. A. RUQ
    B. LUQ
    C. LLQ
    D. LUQ
    E. LUQ
    F. RLQ
    G. LUQ
20. C. Umbilical
21. A. Pubic
22. A. Ischial tuberosity
    B. Greater trochanter
    C. Iliac crest or crest of ilium
    D. Anterior superior iliac spine (ASIS)
    E. Symphysis pubis
23. Superior border; 1½ (inches), 1–4 (cm), distal
24. Symphysis pubis
25. Inferior costal margin
26. Interspace between L4 and L5
27. A. Stomach
    B. Jejunum
    C. Ileum
    D. Region of ileocecal
    E. Duodenum
    F. Duodenal bulb
28. A. Liver
    B. Ascending colon
    C. Right kidney
    D. Right ureter
    E. Right psoas muscle
    F. L2-L3 vertebra
    G. Left kidney
    H. Left ureter
    I. Descending colon
    J. Small intestine (jejunum)

Review Exercise B: Shielding, Exposure Factors, and Positioning

1. A. Patient breathing
   B. Patient movement during exposure
2. Careful breathing instructions
3. Peristaltic action of the bowel
4. Use the shortest exposure time possible.

5. False
6. False
7. D. Any of the above
8. B. Females
9. ASIS; Symphysis pubis
10. C. 80–85 kVp, grid, 40-inch (100-cm) SID
11. D. All of the above
12. True
13. False
14. False
15. C. Computed tomography (CT)
16. A. Ultrasound
17. A. Ultrasound
18. 1. E
    2. D
    3. F
    4. C
    5. B
    6. A
    7. G
19. 1. F
    2. E
    3. A
    4. C
    5. D
    6. B
20. Iliac crest
21. Expiration
22. A. Iliac wings
    B. Obturator foramina (if visible)
    C. Ischial spines
    D. Outer rib margins
23. Hypersthenic body type
24. True
25. False. Patient may have situs inversus in which the liver is on the patient's left.
26. To increase the room for expansion of the abdominal organs within the abdominal cavity
27. C. Pancreas
28. Increased object image receptor distance (OID) of kidneys on PA
29. Left lateral decubitus (free air best visualized in upper right abdomen in area of liver)
30. To allow intra-abdominal air to rise or abnormal fluids to accumulate
31. Dorsal decubitus
32. Lateral position
33. A. AP supine
    B. AP erect or lateral decubitus abdomen
    C. PA erect chest
34. PA chest

35. Two-projection/way abdomen; AP supine abdomen, and left lateral decubitus
36. C. PA, erect chest for free air under diaphragm
37. 2 inches (5 cm) above iliac crest; axilla
38. 1–2 inches (3–5 cm)
39. B. Long scale
40. False. Short exposure time best controls peristalsis

Review Exercise C: Problem Solving for Technical and Positioning Errors

1. No. A KUB must include the symphysis pubis on the radiograph to ensure that the bladder is seen. The positioning error involves centering of the central ray to the iliac crest. The technologist should also palpate the symphysis pubis (if permitted by institutional policy) or greater trochanter to ensure that it is above the bottom of the cassette.
2. The technologist needs to lower the kilovoltage to 80 ± 5 kVp and reduce the milliamperage and exposure time (review digital imaging concepts in Chapter 1).
3. The blurriness may be caused by involuntary motion. To control this motion, the technologist needs to increase the milliamperage and decrease the exposure time (e.g., 400 mA at 1/10 second).
4. Patient was rotated into a slight right posterior oblique (RPO) position. (The downside ilium will appear wider.)
5. The three-projection/way acute abdominal series, including the anteroposterior (AP) supine and erect abdomen and posteroanterior (PA) erect chest projections.
6. The two-projection/way acute abdomen series: AP supine abdomen and left lateral decubitus.
7. A KUB would be performed with the correct exposure factors to visualize the possible stone.
8. A bedside portable left lateral decubitus projection could be performed to demonstrate any fluid levels in the abdomen.

515

9. A. The erect AP abdomen position best demonstrates air-fluid levels. Ascites produces free fluid in the intraperitoneal cavity.
10. B. Because the patient may have renal calculi in the distal ureters and urinary bladder, gonadal shielding cannot be used.
11. D. Repeat the exposure using two 14- × 17-inch (35 × 43 cm) image receptors placed in landscape orientation. The bariatric patient often requires this type of IR placement for abdomen studies.
12. B. Decrease the mAs. Because trapped air is easier to penetrate than soft tissue with x-rays, reducing the mAs will prevent overexposing the radiograph.
13. C. KUB and lateral abdomen. With any foreign body study, two projections 90 degrees opposite are recommended to pinpoint the location of the foreign body.

Review Exercise D: Critique Radiographs of the Abdomen

A. AP KUB (Fig. 3.4)
   Description of possible error: Poor centering and collimation
   1. Anatomy demonstrated: Floor of urinary bladder is not included on radiograph
   2. Part positioning: Slight tilt of the pelvis
   3. Collimation and CR: Poor collimation and centering is too high (not at iliac crest)
   4. Exposure: Slightly under exposed
   5. Anatomic side markers: Present
      Repeatable error(s): None. The benefit of the additional exposure would add dose to the pediatric patient.
B. AP erect abdomen (Fig. 3.5)
   Description of possible error: Critical anatomy not included due to poor centering. Possible motion on image

1. Anatomy demonstrated: The hemidiaphragm not demonstrated
2. Part positioning: Tilt of pelvis evident
3. Collimation and CR: CR is centered too low. Collimation is not evident
4. Exposure: Voluntary motion is present. A shorter exposure time and breathing instructions are indicated.
5. Anatomic side markers: The left or right side marker is absent.
   Repeatable error(s): Criteria 1, 3, 4, and 5

CHAPTER 4

Review Exercise A: Anatomy of Hand and Wrist

1. A. 14
   B. 5
   C. 8
   D. 27
2. A. Proximal phalanx
   B. Distal phalanx
3. A. Proximal phalanx
   B. Middle phalanx
   C. Distal phalanx
4. A. Head
   B. Body (shaft)
   C. Base
5. A. Base
   B. Body (shaft)
   C. Head
6. Interphalangeal joint
7. Metacarpophalangeal (MCP) joints
8. A. Fifth carpometacarpal (CMC) joint
   B. Body of third metacarpal
   C. Head of fifth metacarpal
   D. Fourth metacarpophalangeal (MCP) joint
   E. Head of proximal phalanx of fifth digit
   F. Base of middle phalanx of fourth digit
   G. Distal interphalangeal (DIP) joint of fourth digit
   H. Body of middle phalanx of second digit
   I. Proximal interphalangeal (PIP) joint of second digit
   J. Body of distal phalanx of first digit

   K. Interphalangeal (IP) joint of first digit
   L. Metacarpophalangeal (MCP) joint of first digit
   M. Head of first metacarpal
   N. Second carpometacarpal (CMC) joint
   O. First carpometacarpal (CMC) joint
9. A. 8
   B. 1
   C. 5
   D. 4
   E. 3
   F. 6
   G. 7
   H. 2
10. Capitate
11. Hamulus or hamular process
12. Scaphoid
13. Pisiform
14. A. 3
    B. 9
    C. 2
    D. 5
    E. 1
    F. 8
    G. 6
    H. 7
    I. 4
15. A. Body of first metacarpal (thumb)
    B. Carpometacarpal joint of first digit
    C. Trapezium
    D. Scaphoid
    E. Lunate
    F. Radiocarpal (wrist) joint (between radius and carpals)

Review Exercise B: Anatomy of the Forearm, Elbow, and Distal Humerus

1. A. Radius
   B. Ulna
2. A. U
   B. U
   C. H
   D. H
   E. U
   F. U
   G. U
   H. H
3. Proximal radioulnar joint
4. A. Trochlea
   B. Capitulum
5. Olecranon fossa
6. A. Trochlear sulcus (groove)

B. (a) Capitulum
    (b) Trochlea
C. Trochlear notch
7. A. 1
    B. 5
    C. 1
    D. 2
    E. 2
    F. 4
    G. 1
    H. 3
8. Diarthrodial, 4 (four)
9. True
10. Radial collateral ligament
11. A. Ulnar deviation
    B. Radial deviation
12. Ulnar deviation
13. The proximal radius crosses over the ulna.
14. A. Scaphoid fat stripe
    B. Pronator fat stripe
15. A. Elbow flexed 90 degrees
    B. Optimal exposure factors used
    C. In a true lateral position
16. False (A nonvisible fat pad suggests a negative exam.)
17. True
18. False
19. Posteroanterior (PA) and oblique wrist
20. Lateral wrist
21. A. Radial tuberosity
    B. Radial neck
    C. Capitulum
    D. Lateral epicondyle
    E. Olecranon fossa
    F. Medial epicondyle
    G. Trochlea
    H. Coronoid tubercle
    I. Olecranon process
    J. Superimposed humeral epicondyles
    K. Radial head
    L. Radial neck
    M. Radial tuberosity
    N. *Outer ridges of trochlea and capitulum
    O. *Trochlear sulcus (groove)
    P. *Trochlear notch
22. A. Radial tubercle (tuberosity)
    B. Radial neck
    C. Radial head
    D. Capitulum
    E. Lateral epicondyle
    F. Coronoid process
    G. Trochlea
    H. Olecranon process

Review Exercise C: Positioning of the Fingers, Thumb, Hand, and Wrist

1. A. Low to medium (60 to 80 kVp)
    B. Short exposure time
    C. Small focal spot
    D. 40 inches (100 cm)
    E. 4 inches (10 cm)
    F. 5–7 kVp
    G. 8–10 kVp
    H. 3–4 kVp
    I. Soft tissue, trabecular
2. Collimation borders should be visible on all four sides if the image receptor (IR) is large enough to allow this without cutting off essential anatomy.
3. B, D, E, F
4. True. Trauma patients can be radiographed on the table or stretcher.
5. True (Ensure that adults are given a lead apron to wear during exposures)
6. Arthrography
7. PA, PA oblique, and lateral
8. Distal aspect of metacarpals
9. A. Symmetric appearance of both sides of the shafts of phalanges and distal metacarpals
    B. Equal amounts of tissue on each side of the phalanges
10. A. Perform the medial oblique rather than lateral oblique to decrease OID.
    B. Perform a thumb-down lateral (mediolateral projection) to decrease OID.
11. Proximal interphalangeal (PIP) joint
12. D
13. The AP position produces a decrease in OID and increased resolution.
14. PA oblique
15. 8 × 10 inches (18 × 24 cm). (Collimation specific to thumb region)
16. Metacarpophalangeal
17. True
18. C. First metacarpophalangeal (MCP) joint
19. A. Base of first metacarpal
20. A. Modified Robert's method
    B. 15 degrees proximal
21. A. Third MCP joint

22. 1 inch (2.5 cm)
23. True
24. Fan lateral
25. Lateral in extension
26. 15 degrees proximal toward the ulna
27. D. Rheumatoid arthritis
28. PA stress (Clenched PA) of the wrist
29. 45 degrees
30. Anteroposterior (AP) projection (with the hand slightly arched)
31. Excessive lateral rotation from PA
32. B. Pott's
33. 10–15 degrees, proximally
34. C. 20 degrees
35. 25° to 30 degrees
36. PA projection with radial deviation
37. Tangential inferosuperior or Gaynor-Hart projection
38. 45 degrees
39. 90 degrees

Review Exercise D: Clinical Indications of the Fingers, Thumb, Hand, and Wrist

1. A. Barton fracture
    B. Multiple myeloma
    C. Osteoporosis
    D. Skier's thumb
    E. Achondroplasia
    F. Boxer's fracture
    G. Osteopetrosis
    H. Colles fracture
2. A. 4
    B. 2
    C. 3
    D. 1
    E. 5
3. Osteoporosis (−)
    Osteopetrosis (+)

Review Exercise E: Positioning of the Forearm, Elbow, and Humerus

1. AP and lateral
2. False
3. Parallel
4. Two AP projections (partially flexed), one with humerus parallel to IR and one with forearm parallel to IR
5. AP oblique with 45-degree lateral rotation
6. Palm Up (Supinated)
7. AP oblique with 45-degree medial rotation

8. Lateral, flexed 90 degrees
9. Two projections—central ray perpendicular to humerus and central ray perpendicular to forearm (acute flexion projections)
10. 45 degrees laterally
11. 45 degrees toward shoulder
12. 45 degrees away from shoulder
13. 80 degrees of flexion
14. The rotational position of the hand and wrist

Review Exercise F: Problem Solving for Technical and Positioning Errors

1. Use a small focal spot and minimum 40-inch (100-cm) SID to produce a higher quality study.
2. Rotation
3. Excessive lateral rotation
4. PA forearm projection was performed rather than AP.
5. The central ray needs to be angled 15 degrees proximally, toward the elbow.
6. The elbow is rotated medially.
7. Increase lateral rotation of the elbow to separate the radius from the ulna.
8. The forearm and humerus are not on the same horizontal plane.
9. Coyle method for radial head (lateral elbow, central ray 45 degrees toward shoulder)
10. PA and lateral-in-extension projection
11. AP and lateral forearm projections to include the wrist
12. Two AP projections with acute flexion and a lateral projection
13. Modified Robert method
14. Carpal canal position (Gaynor-Hart method)
15. AP axial projection (Brewerton method)
16. PA stress (Folio method) projection
17. Tangential projection—carpal bridge projection
18. Trauma axial lateral projection—Coyle method for coronoid process

Review Exercise G: Critique Radiographs of the Upper Limb

A. PA hand (Fig. 4.12)
  1. Because of rotation and flexion, the anatomy of hand is distorted and the joints are not open.

2. Fingers flexed preventing clear assessment of joint spaces. Medial rotation of hand distorts the proximal phalanges and metacarpals.
3. No collimation evident on this printed radiograph; centering satisfactory for hand
4. Exposure factors are acceptable.
5. No anatomic side marker
  Repeatable error(s): Criteria 1 (anatomy demonstrated) and 2 (part positioning)

B. Lateral wrist (Fig. 4.13)
  1. All pertinent anatomic structures included
  2. Upper limb rotated slightly; radius and ulna not directly superimposed; metacarpals not all superimposed
  3. No collimation evident on this printed radiograph; centering slightly off; central ray centered to the distal carpal region; includes too much forearm
  4. Acceptable selected exposure factors
  5. Anatomic side marker evident on this projection
  Repeatable error(s): 2 (rotation) and 3 (centering)

C. AP Elbow (Fig. 4.14)
  1. All essential anatomic structures included
  2. Elbow is rotated laterally, evident by slight separation of proximal radius and ulna
  3. No collimation borders evident; central ray centering excellent for elbow
  4. Optimal exposure factors
  5. No anatomic side marker evident on this projection
  Repeatable error(s): Criteria 2 (rotation) and 5 (unless markers are visible elsewhere on radiograph)

D. PA wrist with ulnar deviation (Fig. 4.15)
  Note: This demonstrates a radial deviation for the ulnar side carpals (the opposite of the ulnar deviation for scaphoid).
  1. Aspect of pisiform cut off laterally

2. Poor positioning due to radial rather than ulnar deviation
3. Central ray centering error—central ray centered over scaphoid and medial carpals; would have excellent collimation if central ray were centered correctly
4. Excellent exposure factors
5. Evidence of satisfactory anatomic marker
  Repeatable error(s): Criteria 1 (anatomy demonstrated) and 3 (centering)

E. PA forearm—pediatric (Fig. 4.16)
  1. All pertinent anatomic structures not included because of PA projection being performed over AP
  2. Poor part positioning because proximal radius crossing over ulna as a result of PA projection being performed
  3. No collimation evident on this printed radiograph; acceptable central ray centering.
  4. Exposure factors are satisfactory.
  5. Anatomic side marker evident
  Repeatable error(s): Criteria 1 (anatomy demonstrated) and 2 (Note: Individual who is immobilizing infant's hand should wear lead glove or use mechanical restraint.)

F. Lateral elbow (Fig. 4.17)
  1. All pertinent anatomic structures demonstrated
  2. Elbow hyperflexed (beyond 90 degrees) and not true lateral; too much distance between parts of concentric circles 1 and 2; trochlear notch space not open
  3. Satisfactory collimation (i.e., collimation that is evident); central ray centering slightly off center to the elbow joint
  4. Acceptable exposure factors
  5. Anatomic side marker partially off radiograph and unacceptable (unless it is demonstrated on the actual radiograph)
  Repeatable error(s): Criteria 2 (part positioning) and 5 (unless marker is more visible on actual radiograph)

518

CHAPTER 5

Review Exercise A: Radiographic Anatomy of the Humerus and Shoulder Girdle

1. A. Proximal humerus
   B. Scapula
   C. Clavicle
2. A. Intertubercular sulcus (bicipital groove)
   B. Greater tubercle (tuberosity)
   C. Head of humerus
   D. Anatomic neck
   E. Lesser tubercle (tuberosity)
   F. Surgical neck
   G. Neutral (Neither the greater nor lesser tubercle is in profile.)
3. A. Sternal extremity
   B. Body (shaft)
   C. Acromial extremity
4. Male
5. A. Lateral angle
   B. Superior angle
   C. Inferior angle
6. Costal
7. Axilla
8. A. Infraspinous fossa
   B. Supraspinous fossa
9. Synovial (diarthrodial)
10. A. Ball and socket (Spheroidal)
    B. Plane
    C. Plane
11. 1. C
    2. A
    3. A
    4. B
    5. B
    6. C
    7. A
    8. C
12. A. Lateral angle (head)
    B. Scapulohumeral joint (glenohumeral joint)
    C. Acromion
    D. Coracoid process
    E. Suprascapular notch
    F. Superior angle
    G. Medial (vertebral)
    H. Lateral (axillary)
    I. Ventral (costal)
    J. Dorsal (posterior)
    K. Spine of scapula
    L. Acromion
    M. Coracoid process
    N. Body (blade, wing, or ala)
    O. Inferior angle
13. A. Coracoid process
    B. Scapulohumeral
    C. Acromion
    D. Greater tubercle
    E. Lesser tubercle
    F. Lateral border
    G. Internal rotation (lesser tubercle is in profile medially)
    H. Lateral perspective
    I. Perpendicular
    J. Body of scapula
    K. Spine of scapula and acromion
    L. Coracoid process
    M. Body (shaft) of humerus
    N. Scapular Y lateral-posterior oblique projection
14. A. Coracoid process
    B. Glenoid cavity (fossa)
    C. Spine of scapula
    D. Acromion
    E. Inferosuperior axial projection (Lawrence method)
    F. 90 degrees

Review Exercise B: Positioning of the Humerus and Shoulder Girdle

1. 1. A
   2. C
   3. B
   4. A
   5. C
   6. A
   7. B
   8. B
   9. A
2. A. Neutral
   B. External
   C. Internal
3. A. True
   B. False
   C. False
   D. False
   E. True
   F. False
   G. True
4. C. 80–90 kVp
5. D. Boomerang compensating filter
6. A. Parent or guardian
7. True (to reduce OID and part distortion)
8. True (See Chapter 18)
9. True
10. True
11. False
12. True
13. 1. D
    2. B
    3. G
    4. A

5. C
6. F
7. E
14. 1. G
    2. E
    3. F
    4. H
    5. I
    6. B
    7. D
    8. A
    9. C
15. D. Osteoporosis
16. True
17. False
18. A. Supraspinatus
19. A. AP, external rotation
    B. AP, internal rotation
20. CR perpendicular to IR, directed to 1 inch (2.5 cm) inferior to coracoid process
21. Transthoracic lateral projection for humerus
22. B. Rotate affected arm externally approximately 45 degrees
23. A. 25–30 degrees medially
24. Anterior oblique; Grashey method
25. A. Fisk modification
26. Perpendicular to the glenoid cavity (fossa). This is between the AC joint and the superior angle of the scapula, approximately 5–15 degrees medially
27. D. Posterior oblique (Scapular Y) projection
28. Tangential projection— Supraspinatus Outlet; Neer method or Apical AP axial projection
29. B. 30 degrees caudad
30. C. Posterioanterior (PA) axial transaxillary projection (Bernageau method)
31. A. 5–15 degrees
32. D. 10–15 degrees cephalad
33. False (30 degrees caudad)
34. True
35. True
36. False
37. False (10–15 degrees cephalad)
38. False
39. Superior angle of the scapula and the AC joint articulation
40. AP apical oblique axial projection
41. Superior
42. More (CR angle)
43. Fracture of clavicle

44.
  1. C
  2. B
  3. D
  4. A
  5. C
  6. E
45. C. Suspected AC joint separation
46. D. No CR angle
47. CR perpendicular to midscapula, 2 inches (5 cm) inferior to coracoid process, or to level of axilla, and approximately 2 inches (5 cm) medial from lateral border of patient
48. D. None. CR perpendicular to the IR
49. True
50. False (arm location along with CR centering are different)

Review Exercise C: Problem Solving for Technical and Positioning Errors

1. Increase to 80 kVp and decrease mAs to 10. Ensure the humeral epicondyles are perpendicular to the IR.
2. Increase central ray cephalic angle. Based on body habitus, CR angle will range between 15 and 30 degrees cephalad.
3. Ensure that the affected arm is abducted 90 degrees and use a breathing technique.
4. Supinate the hand and ensure that the epicondyles are parallel to the IR for a true AP.
5. Increase rotation of body toward the IR. Palpate the superior angle of the scapula and AC joint articulation and ensure that the imaginary plane between these points is perpendicular to the IR.
6. Increase rotation of affected shoulder toward IR between 35 and 45 degrees.
7. Angle the central ray 10–15 degrees cephalad to separate the shoulders.
8. The routine includes an AP of the right shoulder and humerus, without rotation (neutral rotation), and a supine, horizontal beam, right transthoracic shoulder. Note: In those cases in which the opposite arm cannot be elevated or extended, a supine

posterior oblique scapular Y lateral projection could also be used as a second option for a lateral shoulder position (see Chapter 15).

9. Possible positioning options: Inferosuperior axial projection with exaggerated external rotation, inferosuperior axial projection (Clements modification), and AP apical oblique axial projection (Garth method)
10. A. AP apical oblique axial (Garth method)
    B. Posterior oblique (Scapular Y) lateral
    C. Anterior oblique (Grashey method)
11. B. MR
12. C. Diagnostic medical sonography (DMS)
13. The humeral epicondyles were not placed perpendicular to the plane of the IR.
14. Use orthostatic (breathing) exposure technique to create blurring of ribs and lung markings.
15. Transthoracic lateral projection for humerus
16. Anterior dislocation of the proximal humerus

Review Exercise D: Critique Radiographs of the Humerus and Shoulder Girdle

A. AP clavicle (Fig. 5.11)
   1. All of clavicle demonstrated
   2. Rotation of body toward the patient's right, superimposing sternal end over the spine and creating overall distortion of the clavicle and associated joints
   3. Collimation not evident. Central ray centered too low (inferiorly), which also adds to distorted appearance of clavicle. No sign of collimation.
   4. Acceptable but slightly underexposed exposure factors
   5. Missing (or not visible) anatomic side marker
      Repeatable error(s):
      2 (rotation), 3 (incorrect centering), and 5 (missing anatomic side marker)

B. AP shoulder—external rotation (Fig. 5.12)
   1. All pertinent anatomic structures demonstrated
   2. Greater tubercle is not in profile but note fracture of scapular neck. No rotation of the proximal humerus should be used. Transthoracic lateral projection should be performed to provide 90 degrees opposite perspective.
   3. No evidence of collimation
   4. Acceptable but slightly overexposed
   5. Anatomic side marker is present
      Repeatable error(s):
      None (considering the degree of trauma). Transthoracic lateral or Scapular Y lateral projection should be performed to provide another perspective.
C. AP scapula (Fig. 5.13)
   1. Inferior angle of scapula cut off at bottom edge of radiograph
   2. Arm must be abducted at 90-degree angle to body
   3. Collimation not evident; need to center central ray and cassette to include the entire scapula
   4. Underexposed scapula and slight blurring of ribs, not evident from orthostatic technique
   5. Missing (or not visible) anatomic side marker
      Repeatable error(s):
      1 (anatomy), 2 (positioning), 3 (centering), 4 (exposure), and 5 (anatomic side marker)
D. AP humerus (Fig. 5.14)
   1. Distal humerus is not included.
   2. Correct part positioning for AP projection, but centering is off
   3. Evidence of collimation on one side only, indicating incorrect centering; central ray and IR centering too lateral and proximal
   4. Acceptable

5. Acceptable; anatomic side marker partially seen on radiograph
   Repeatable error(s): 1 (anatomy) and 3 (centering)
   Position: AP projection, external rotation

CHAPTER 6

Review Exercise A: Radiographic Anatomy of the Foot and Ankle

1. A. 14
   B. 5
   C. 7
   D. 26
2. A. Phalanges of the foot are smaller.
   B. The joint movements of the foot are more limited than those of the hand.
3. Tuberosity of base of the fifth metatarsal
4. The plantar surface of the foot near the first metatarsophalangeal joint
5. Calcaneus
6. Subtalar or talocalcaneal
7. A. Posterior facet
   B. Anterior facet
   C. Middle facet
8. Sinus tarsi or tarsal sinus
9. 1. B
   2. F
   3. D
   4. G
   5. E
   6. B
   7. G
   8. A
   9. C
   10. B
10. A. Sinus tarsi (tarsal sinus)
    B. Talus
    C. Navicular
    D. Lateral cuneiform
    E. Base of first metatarsal
    F. Body (shaft) of first metatarsal
    G. Sesamoid bone
    H. Metatarsophalangeal (MTP) joint of first digit
    I. Distal phalanx of first digit
    J. Tuberosity at base of fifth metatarsal
    K. Cuboid
    L. Calcaneal tuberosity
    M. AP 45-degree medial oblique

N. Tuberosity of calcaneus
O. Lateral process of calcaneus
P. Peroneal trochlea (trochlear process)
Q. Lateral malleolus of fibula
R. Sustentaculum tali
S. Talocalcaneal joint
T. Plantodorsal (axial) projection of calcaneus
11. False (five)
12. B. Cuboid
13. A. Longitudinal arch
    B. Transverse arch
14. Achilles tendon
15. A. Talus
    B. Tibia
    C. Fibula
16. Ankle mortise
17. A. Tibial plafond
18. False
19. Saddle (sellar)
20. A. Tuberosity at base of fifth metatarsal (see fracture on radiograph in Fig. 6.3)
    B. Lateral malleolus of fibula
    C. Distal tibiofibular joint
    D. Medial malleolus of tibia
    E. Talus
    F. Calcaneus
    G. Sinus tarsi (tarsal sinus)
    H. Talus
    I. Tibial plafond
    J. Anterior tubercle
    K. Navicular
    L. Cuboid
    M. AP mortise, 15- to 20-degree medial rotation

Review Exercise B: Radiographic Anatomy of the Lower Leg, Knee, and Distal Femur

1. Tibia
2. Tibial tuberosity
3. Adductor tubercle
4. Fibular notch
5. Tibial plateau
6. D. 10–20
7. Apex or styloid process
8. Lateral malleolus
9. Patella
10. A. Intercondylar sulcus
    B. Trochlear groove
11. Intercondylar fossa or notch
12. Because the medial condyle extends lower or more distally than the lateral condyle of the femur
13. C. Adductor tubercle

14. A. Medial epicondyle
    B. Lateral epicondyle
15. Popliteal region
16. False
17. True
18. False
19. Quadriceps femoris muscle
20. A. Patellofemoral
    B. Femorotibial
21. A. Fibular (lateral) collateral
    B. Tibial (medial) collateral
    C. Anterior cruciate
    D. Posterior cruciate
22. Medial and lateral menisci
23. A. Suprapatellar bursa
    B. Infrapatellar bursa
24. 1. A
    2. A
    3. C
    4. C
    5. A
    6. A
    7. B
    8. D
    9. A
    10. B
25. 1. C
    2. C
    3. D
    4. D
    5. F
    6. E
26. A. Fibular notch of tibia (also may be identified as distal tibiofibular joint)
    B. Body (shaft) of fibula
    C. Articular facets (or tibial plateau)
    D. Lateral condyle of tibia
    E. Intercondyloid eminence (tibial spine)
    F. Medial condyle of tibia
    G. Tibial tuberosity
    H. Anterior crest of body (shaft of tibia)
    I. Medial malleolus
    J. Lateral malleolus
    K. Body (shaft) of fibula
    L. Neck of fibula
    M. Head of fibula
    N. Apex or styloid process of fibula
    O. 10–20 degrees
    P. Tibial tuberosity
    Q. Body (shaft) of tibia
    R. Medial malleolus
    S. Lateral condyle of femur
    T. Patellar surface of femur

521

U. Medial condyle of femur
V. Patellofemoral joint space
W. Patella
X. Tangential (patellofemoral joint)
27. A. Base of patella
   B. Apex of patella
   C. Tibial tuberosity
   D. Neck of fibula
   E. Head of fibula
   F. Apex or styloid process of fibula
   G. Superimposed medial and lateral condyles
   H. Patellar surface/intercondylar sulcus or trochlear groove
   I. Adductor tubercle
   J. Lateral femoral condyle
   K. Medial femoral condyle
28. A. 1
   B. 4
   C. 2
   D. 3

Review Exercise C: Positioning of the Foot and Ankle

1. True
2. False
3. True. However, if it is done, lead masking should be used.
4. True
5. False
6. False
7. False (may produce artifacts on images)
8. A. 9
   B. 8
   C. 10
   D. 7
   E. 1
   F. 5
   G. 6
   H. 3
   I. 2
   J. 4
9. Chondromalacia patellae
10. Rickets
11. A. 7
    B. 3
    C. 8
    D. 1
    E. 5
    F. 4
    G. 2
    H. 6
12. A. Foot
13. Opens up the interphalangeal and metatarsophalangeal joint spaces
14. Base of third metatarsal

15. Tangential projection
16. 15–20 degrees
17. Opens up metatarsophalangeal and certain intertarsal joints
18. True
19. Second to fifth
20. AP oblique with medial rotation
21. AP oblique with lateral rotation
22. Lateromedial
23. AP and lateral weight-bearing projections
24. 40 degrees cephalad
25. 45 degrees cephalad (anterior) to exit at the base of the fifth metatarsal
26. 1 inch (2.5 cm) inferior to medial malleolus
27. C. Lateral aspect of joint
28. To demonstrate a possible fracture of the fifth metatarsal tuberosity (a common fracture site)
29. 15–20 degrees (medially)
30. Intermalleolar line or plane
31. 45-degree AP oblique with medial rotation
32. B. Projected over the posterior aspect of the distal tibia
33. AP stress projections
34. False
35. True

Review Exercise D: Positioning of the Tibia, Fibula, Knee, and Distal Femur

1. AP and lateral projections
2. A fracture may also be present at the proximal tibia or fibula in addition to the distal portion.
3. C. Diagonal
4. B. 3–5 degrees cephalad
5. A. ½ inch (1.25 cm) distal to apex of patella
6. C. AP oblique, 45-degree medial rotation
7. Medial (internal)
8. B. 5 degrees cephalad
9. B. 20–30 degrees
10. Improper angle of the central ray or lack of support of the lower leg to keep entire lower limb in same plane.
11. Overrotation (toward the IR) or underrotation of the knee (away from IR)
12. Adductor tubercle on posterolateral aspect of the medial femoral condyle
13. AP or PA weight-bearing knee projections

14. C. MR
15. A. Holmblad
16. 40-degree flexion
17. Distortion caused by poor central ray-to-IR alignment and increased OID for AP axial projection
18. B. 10 degrees caudad
19. D. 45 degrees
20. C. 60–70 degrees
21. D. None. CR is perpendicular to IR
22. True
23. 5–10 degrees
24. 30° from horizontal
25. A. 55 degrees
    B. 90 degrees
26. D. None. CR is perpendicular to IR.
27. 1. F
    2. E
    3. D
    4. G
    5. C
    6. A
    7. B
28. A. Rosenberg method
29. True
30. D. None

Review Exercise E: Problem Solving for Technical and Positioning Errors

1. Central ray is not angled correctly; adjust central ray angle to keep it perpendicular to metatarsals (anterior arch of foot).
2. Overrotation of foot (toward the medial direction)
3. Increase cephalad angle of the central ray to correctly elongate the calcaneus.
4. Possibly a spread of the ankle mortise caused by ruptured ligaments
5. Underrotation of the ankle (toward the medial direction). The described appearance is that of a true AP ankle with little or no obliquity.
6. Angling the central ray correctly to keep it parallel to the articular facets (tibial plateau)
7. The wrong oblique position of the knee was obtained. This description is that of a laterally or externally oblique position of the knee.

522

8. Underrotation of knee (excessive rotation of patella away from the IR)
9. An AP lateral oblique projection with 30 degrees of external rotation will separate the bases of the first and second metatarsals and separate the first and second cuneiforms.
10. Repeat the AP projection to ensure the ankle joint is demonstrated.
11. Rotation of the affected limb or incorrect CR angle to match the degree of flexion of the lower limb
12. Decrease the amount of flexion of the knee to only 5–10 degrees.
13. An AP or PA weight-bearing bilateral knee projection will best evaluate the joint spaces.
14. AP and lateral weight-bearing foot projections
15. AP and lateral weight-bearing projections of the foot
16. Intercondylar fossa projections, including the PA axial projections (Holmblad, Rosenberg, and/or Camp Coventry methods) demonstrate the entire knee joint and intercondylar fossa region, which may be hiding "joint mice."
17. The lateral knee projection will best demonstrate any separation of the tibial tuberosity from the shaft of the tibia.
18. By angling the central ray 5–7 degrees cephalad, the medial femoral condyle will be superimposed with the lateral condyle. If CR angulation was used on the initial projection, increase the amount of angle with the repeat exposure. The technologist could also elevate the ankle and lower limb to same plane as the long axis of femur.
19. The superoinferior sitting tangential method is best suited for this patient. While remaining in the wheelchair, the patient's knees can be flexed, the IR can be positioned on a footstool, and the CR is placed vertically above the knees.

20. The most common error with the tangential (inferosuperior) projection is hyperflexion of the knee, which draws the patella into the intercondylar sulcus. Flexion of the lower limb should not exceed 45 degrees. Another possible error is that the CR is not parallel to the joint space.

Review Exercise F: Critique Radiographs of the Lower Limbs

A. Bilateral tangential patella (Fig. 6.10)
1. Portion of each patella superimposed over intercondylar sulcus of femur
2. Excessive flexion of knee is most likely cause of superimposition of patella with patellar surface of femur.
3. Evidence of collimation; correct central ray centering and IR placement; may be an error in central ray angle, which would have contributed to the superimposition. No evidence of collimation
4. Underexposed
5. Anatomic side marker present
Repeatable error(s):1 (anatomy demonstrated), 2 (part positioning), and 3 (CR angle) (possibly four-exposure)

B. Plantodorsal (axial) calcaneus (Fig. 6.11)
1. Possible fracture of calcaneus. All pertinent anatomy is seen.
2. Positioning is acceptable but foot is plantar flexed.
3. Off centering of part to IR is too anterior. Better centering would lead to more concise collimation.
4. Acceptable exposure factors
5. No anatomic side marker visible
Repeatable error(s): None (Note: Centering was incorrect but not repeatable.)

C. AP mortise ankle (Fig. 6.12)
1. Mortise of ankle is not demonstrated.
2. Excessive medial rotation superimposes lateral malleolus over lateral aspect of talus.

3. No collimation evident. Centering is correct.
4. Acceptable exposure factors
5. Anatomic side marker visible Repeatable error(s): 2 (part positioning). (The ankle must not be rotated and side markers must be used.)

D. AP lower limb (pediatric) (Fig. 6.13)
1. Note fracture of distal femur. All anatomy demonstrated.
2. Positioning is correct for AP projection.
3. No collimation is used. Centering is correct for entire lower limb. Unprotected hand used to immobilize the lower limb: Unacceptable practice
4. Acceptable exposure factors
5. Anatomic side marker visible Repeatable error(s): 3 (radiation protection issue) (not a repeatable error in this situation)

E. Lateral knee (Fig. 6.14)
1. All pertinent anatomic structures included, but patellofemoral joint not open (presence of superimposition of patella over lateral condyle because of rotation)
2. Rotation of anterior knee away from image receptor (underrotation); almost total superimposition of proximal fibula; visibility of adductor tubercle identifies medial condyle as being posterior; hyperflexed knee (should be flexed only 15–20 degrees rather than the almost 45 degrees used in this radiograph)
3. No evidence of collimation; correct central ray centering and IR placement
4. Acceptable exposure factors
5. Anatomic side marker present Repeatable error(s): 1 (anatomy demonstrated) and 2 (part positioning)

F. AP medial oblique knee (Fig. 6.15)
1. Anatomy of knee is demonstrated including proximal patellofemoral joint space.

2. Acceptable rotation of anterior knee toward image receptor (overrotation); separation of proximal fibula from tibia; outline of adductor tubercle on medial condyle also anterior to lateral condyle
3. No evidence of collimation; correct central ray centering and IR placement
4. Acceptable exposure factors
5. Anatomic side marker present
   Repeatable error(s): 1 (anatomy demonstrated) and 2 (rotation)

CHAPTER 7

Review Exercise A: Anatomy of Femur, Hips, and Pelvic Girdle

1. Femur
2. Fovea capitis
3. Medial; posteriorly
4. 15–20
5. True
   A. Right and left hip bones, sacrum, and coccyx
   B. Right and left hip bones
   C. (a) ossa coxae, (b) innominate bones
6. A. Ilium
   B. Ischium
   C. Pubis
7. Acetabulum, midteens
8. A. Crest of ilium (iliac crest)
   B. Anterior superior iliac spine (ASIS)
9. Ischial tuberosity
10. Symphysis pubis
11. Obturator foramen
12. A. 1 inch (2.5 cm)
    B. 1½–2 inches (4–5 cm)
13. Pelvic brim
14. A. False pelvis
    B. True pelvis
15. A. Supports the lower abdominal organs and fetus
    B. Forms the actual birth canal
16. A. Inlet (superior aperture)
    B. Cavity
    C. Outlet (inferior aperture)
17. 1. B
    2. B
    3. A
    4. A

5. C
6. A
7. C
8. A
18. Cephalopelvimetry
19. Diagnostic medical sonography (ultrasound)
20. 1. F
    2. F
    3. M
    4. M
    5. M
    6. F
21. A. Synovial, diarthrodial, ball and socket
    B. Synovial, amphiarthrodial, limited
    C. Cartilaginous, amphiarthrodial, limited
    D. Cartilaginous, synarthrodial, nonmovable
22. A. Crest, IL
    B. ASIS, IL
    C. Greater trochanter
    D. Body, IS
    E. Superior ramus, P
    F. Ischial tuberosity, IS
    G. Inferior ramus, P
    H. Obturator foramen
    I. Body, P
    J. Body, IL
    K. Wing (ala), IL
    L. Right sacroiliac (SI) joint
    M. Ischial spine, IS
    N. Sacrum
    O. Body, IL
    P. Posterior superior iliac spine (PSIS), IL
    Q. Posterior inferior iliac spine, IL
    R. Greater sciatic notch, IL
    S. Ischial spine, IS
    T. Lesser sciatic notch, IS
    U. Ischial tuberosity, IS
    V. Ramus, IS
    W. Inferior ramus, P
    X. Acetabulum, IS, IL, P
    Y. Anterior inferior iliac spine, IL
    Z. ASIS, IL

Review Exercise B: Positioning of Femur, Hips, Pelvis, and Sacroiliac Joints

1. A. ASIS
   B. Symphysis pubis (or greater trochanter if palpation of this landmark is not permitted by institution)
2. Approximately 2.5 inches (6–7 cm) below the midpoint of the line
3. ASIS; 1–2 inches (3–5 cm); symphysis pubis and/or greater trochanter; 3–4 inches (8–10 cm)
4. 15–20
5. Lesser trochanter should not be visible, or should only be slightly visible, on the radiograph.
6. The patient's foot is rotated externally.
7. AP pelvis
8. Use a shaped ovarian shield with top of shield at level of ASIS and bottom at symphysis pubis.
9. The top of the shield should be placed at the inferior margin of the symphysis pubis.
10. Pincer, Cam, Combined
11. It reduces patient dose.
12. It reduces radiographic contrast.
13. B. DDH (development dysplasia of hip)
14. True
15. False. (The size of the bony pelvis is not proportional to the girth and dimensions of the soft tissue that surrounds it.)
16. A. Diagnostic medical sonography (DMS)
17. D. Nuclear medicine (NM)
18. A. 7
    B. 5
    C. 4
    D. 2
    E. 6
    F. 1
    G. 3
19. C. Compensating filter
20. A. CT
21. True. If an AP and lateral femur study is ordered, both joints must be demonstrated on each projection.
22. Midway between ASIS and symphysis pubis
23. 2 inches (5 cm)
24. Rotation toward left side
25. Rotation toward right side
26. A. T
    B. NT
    C. NT

D. T

E. T

27. B. PA axial oblique
28. Internally 35 degrees
29. 45 degrees
30. 3 inches (7.5 cm) below level of ASIS (1 inch [2.5 cm] above symphysis pubis)
31. 14 × 17 inches (35 × 43 cm), landscape
32. Midfemoral neck (see positioning considerations for femoral neck localization in chapter)
33. B. 30–45 degrees cephalad
34. A. Acetabular fractures
35. D. 45 degrees
36. D. 12 degrees cephalad
37. C. PA 35–40 degrees toward affected side
38. True
39. Traumatic
40. It is flexed and elevated to prevent it from being superimposed over the affected hip.
41. C. Use of gonadal shielding
42. True
43. True
44. 15–20
45. A. Posterior oblique projections of acetabulum (Judet method)
    B. 0 degree (perpendicular)
46. AP axial outlet projection (Taylor method)
47. 1. D
    2. C
    3. F
    4. E
    5. B
    6. A
48. D. 20–30 degrees from vertical
49. True
50. 15 degrees from the vertical

Review Exercise C: Problem Solving for Technical and Positioning Errors

1. Rotate the lower limbs 15–20 degrees internally to place the proximal femurs in a true AP position. (With general chronic pain, the lower limbs usually can be rotated safely.)
2. The patient is rotated toward the left—left posterior oblique (LPO).
3. Repeat the exposure and only abduct the femur 20–30 degrees from vertical. (It will produce less distortion of the femoral neck.)
4. If possible, elevate the patient at least 2 inches (or 5 cm) by placing sheets or blankets beneath the pelvis.
5. A greater central ray angle is required. Female patients require a central ray angle of 30–45 degrees.
6. The PA axial oblique (Teufel method) or posterior oblique (Judet method) can be taken to demonstrate aspects of the acetabulum more completely.
7. When using automatic exposure control (AEC) for an AP pelvis projection, the left and right ionization chambers must be activated. The center chamber is over the less dense pelvic cavity, which may lead to an underexposed image.
8. Ensure that the central ray is centered to near the midline of the grid cassette and the face of the image receptor is perpendicular to the central ray.
9. Yes. Any orthopedic appliance or prosthesis must be seen in its entirety in both projections.
10. AP pelvis and axiolateral (inferosuperior) left hip. The AP pelvis radiograph should be taken initially without leg rotation; the radiograph must be reviewed by the physician and checked for fractures or dislocations before attempting an internal rotation of the left leg for the axiolateral (inferosuperior) projection.
11. AP pelvis and modified axiolateral—Clements-Nakayama method
12. Posterior oblique—Judet method. CT is often judged superior in detecting pelvic ring fractures.
13. AP axial for pelvic "outlet" (Taylor method) and AP axial for pelvic "inlet" projections and possibly the posterior oblique (Judet method) projections to provide another perspective of the inlet and outlet regions of the pelvis. (If unsure of the request routine, contact the physician for clarification.)
14. Palpate both ASIS and ensure they are equal distance from the tabletop. To verify no rotation is still present, ensure that the iliac wings are symmetric, as seen on the radiograph.
15. AP pelvis and bilateral modified Cleaves method

Review Exercise D: Critique Radiographs of the Femur and Pelvis

A. AP pelvis (Fig. 7.3)
   1. All anatomy of the pelvis is demonstrated.
   2. The lesser trochanters are visible, which indicates the lower limbs were not rotated 15–20 degrees medially.
   3. No collimation evident (acceptable) and CR centering was slightly off laterally (to the patient's right)
   4. Exposure factors are acceptable.
   5. Anatomic side marker evident. Repeatable error(s): 2 (Part/anatomy positioning)
   Note: Based on the lesser angle of the pubic arch, less flared iliac wings, and heart-shaped pelvic inlet, this is a **male pelvis**.

B. AP pelvis (Fig. 7.4)
   1. All anatomy of pelvis is demonstrated.
   2. No rotation of lower limbs evident by presence of lesser trochanters. But because of pelvic ring fracture involving pubis, inadvisable to rotate lower limbs. Fracture may have extended into acetabulum. Slight tilt of pelvis.
   3. No collimation evident (acceptable) and CR centering is acceptable.
   4. Exposure factors are acceptable.
   5. No anatomic side marker visible
   Repeatable error(s): 5 (anatomic side marker. Unsure side of fracture)
   Note: Based on a greater angle (80–85 degrees) of the pubic arch, flared iliac wings, and round pelvic inlet, this is a **female pelvis**.

525

C. Unilateral modified Cleaves method (performed cystography) (Fig. 7.5)
   1. All pertinent anatomy is demonstrated.
   2. Lower limb must not have been rotated into modified Cleaves method because of the severity of the fracture.
   3. No collimation evident, and it is needed to reduce exposure to abdomen. Note: Patient's right upper limb is in field. Centering is too low.
   4. Exposure factors are acceptable.
   5. Anatomic side marker is evident.
      Repeatable error(s): 2 (part positioning) and 3 (centering—if exposure is to be repeated for other reasons)
D. Bilateral abducted position (2-year-old) (Fig. 7.6)
   1. Left hip (assuming that this is the left side because the side marker is not visible) obscured by artifact (superimposition of patient's hand)
   2. Tilted pelvis (and note that the gonadal shield placement is useless for either males *or* females—a serious error for a small child)
   3. No visible collimation, which should be visible for this pediatric patient; central ray centering/image receptor placement too high for pelvis centering but acceptable for bilateral hip projection
   4. Very low contrast (may have been caused by not using a grid)
   5. No visible anatomic side marker
      Repeatable error(s): 1 (anatomy demonstrated)

CHAPTER 8

Review Exercise A: Radiographic Anatomy of the Cervical and Thoracic Spine

1. A. 7
   B. 12
   C. 5
   D. 1

   E. 1
   F. 26
2. A. Thoracic
   B. Sacral
3. A. Cervical
   B. Lumbar
4. 1. B and D
   2. A and C
   3. A and C
   4. B and D
   5. A
5. Lordosis
6. Scoliosis
7. Body; vertebral arch
8. Lamina
9. Intervertebral
10. Vertebral (spinal) canal
11. A. Medulla oblongata
    B. Lower border of L1
    C. Conus medullaris
12. Spinal nerves and blood vessels
13. A. Spinous process
    B. Lamina
    C. Transverse process
    D. Facet of superior articular process
    E. Pedicle
    F. Vertebral foramen
    G. Spinous process
    H. Facet of superior articular process
    I. Pedicle
    J. Body
    K. Inferior articular process
    L. Superior articular process
    M. Zygapophyseal joint
    N. Facet for head of rib (forms costovertebral joint)
    O. Intervertebral foramen
    P. Facet for rib articulation
    Q. Costovertebral joints
    R. Costotransverse joints
14. C. Zygapophyseal joints
15. False (T1 and T10–T12 have full facets)
16. False (between C1 and C2 visualized on a frontal or AP projection)
17. A. Annulus fibrosus
    B. Nucleus pulposus
18. Herniated nucleus pulposus (HNP)
19. A. C1: Atlas
    B. C2: Axis
    C. C7: Vertebra prominens
20. A. Transverse foramina
    B. Bifid spinous process
    C. Overlapping vertebral bodies
21. Articular pillar

22. Lateral mass
23. 90; 70–75
24. Atlanto-occipital articulation
25. Dens or odontoid process
26. Rotation of the skull
27. Presence of facets for articulation with ribs
28. T5–T8
29. A. Body, C4
    B. Dens (odontoid), C2
    C. Posterior arch and tubercle, C1
    D. Zygapophyseal joint, C5–C6
    E. Spinous process (vertebra prominens), C7
    F. Posterior arch and tubercle, C1
    G. Pedicle, C4
    H. Intervertebral foramen, C4–C5
30. 15 degrees cephalad

Review Exercise B: Positioning of the Cervical and Thoracic Spine

1. A. Manubrium
   B. Jugular (suprasternal) notch
   C. Body
   D. Sternal angle
   E. Xiphoid process
2. 1. H
   2. E
   3. F
   4. B
   5. D
   6. C
   7. A
   8. G
3. Thyroid, parathyroid glands, and breasts
4. A. Increase in exposure latitude (wider range of densities)
   B. Decrease in patient dose
5. True
6. False (Lead masking should be used even if close collimation is used.)
7. True
8. True
9. A. Keep vertebral column parallel to IR
10. B. Using a small focal spot
    C. Increasing SID
11. A. 9
    B. 10
    C. 4
    D. 8
    E. 2
    F. 6
    G. 1
    H. 7

I. 5

J. 3

12. A. Erect (AP/PA) and lateral spine including bending laterals
    B. Lateral cervical
    C. AP open mouth C1–C2
    D. Scoliosis series
    E. Lateral cervical spine
    F. AP and lateral of affected spine

13. Spondylitis is an inflammatory process of the vertebrae characterized by bony bridges between vertebrae (advanced stages). Spondylosis is a condition of the spine characterized by decreased vertebral joint space and arthritic changes of the zygapophyseal joints.

14. True

15. True

16. Myelography

17. Nuclear medicine

18. Lower margin of upper incisors and base of skull

19. False. The entire dens or odontoid process must be demonstrated. If trauma or injury is ruled out, the technologist could perform the AP or PA projection for the odontoid process to demonstrate the tip.

20. To open up the intervertebral disk spaces

21. C. Base of skull

22. True

23. A. Compensates for increased OID; reduces magnification
    B. Less divergence of x-ray beam to reduce shoulder superimposition of C7

24. 15 degrees cephalad

25. Right intervertebral foramina (upside)

26. Left intervertebral foramina (downside)

27. Rotate the skull into a near lateral position

28. 60–72 inches (150–180 cm)

29. Expiration; for maximum shoulder depression

30. Lateral, horizontal beam projection

31. Swimmer's method

32. To T1; 1 inch (2.5 cm) above the jugular notch anteriorly and level of vertebra prominens posteriorly

33. C5–T3

34. D. Hyperextension and hyperflexion lateral positions

35. If unable to demonstrate the upper portion of the odontoid process (dens) with the AP open mouth projection

36. AP "wagging jaw" projection (Ottonello method)

37. Correct use of anode-heel effect and use of compensating (wedge) filter

38. To blur out rib and lung markings that obscure detail of thoracic vertebrae

39. Right (downside)

40. C. Cervicothoracic position

41. True (anterior oblique (approx.) <5 mrad; posterior oblique <69 mrad)

42. B. Articular pillars (lateral masses of C-spine)

43. C. 20–30 degrees caudad

44. Lead mat or masking

45. Mentomeatal line (MML)

46. Right

47. 20 degrees from lateral position (70 degrees from plane of table or wall bucky)

Review Exercise C: Problem Solving for Technical and Positioning Errors

1. Excessive extension of the skull

2. Increase central ray angulation to 15 degrees cephalad.

3. When the lower intervertebral foramina are narrowed while the upper foramina are well demonstrated, the positioning error most often is underrotation of the upper body (shoulders). The upper body must be rotated 45 degrees.

4. Initiate exposure during suspended expiration and increase SID to 72 inches (180 cm).

5. Reduce mAs and increase exposure time to produce more blurring of the mandible.

6. Use of an orthostatic (breathing) technique to blur lung markings and ribs more effectively.

7. Use a compensating (wedge) filter with thicker part of filter placed over the upper thoracic spine to equalize the density along the thoracic spine.

8. Angle CR 3–5 degrees caudad.

9. Horizontal beam lateral projection

10. Hyperextension and hyperflexion lateral positions

11. Perform either the (AP) Fuchs or (PA) Judd method.

12. Cervicothoracic (swimmer's) lateral position

13. AP axial—vertebral arch (pillar) projection

14. AP open mouth projection. The patient's mouth must be carefully opened without any movement of the cervical spine.

15. Scoliosis series

Review Exercise D: Critique Radiographs of the Cervical and Thoracic Spine

A. AP open mouth (Fig. 8.5)
   1. Upper aspect of dens obscured by base of skull
   2. Overextension of skull, causing superimposition of base of skull over dens
   3. Collimation is poor, resulting in excessive exposure to face, eyes, and neck region; central ray and IR placement are too high
   4. Acceptable image receptor exposure and contrast
   5. Anatomic side marker
      Repeatable error(s): 1 (anatomy demonstrated), 2 (positioning), and 3 (CR and IR placement)

B. AP open mouth (Fig. 8.6)
   1. Upper aspect of dens and joint space obscured by front incisors
   2. Overflexion of skull causing superimposition of front incisors over top of dens
   3. Collimation too loose, resulting in excessive exposure to face, eyes, and neck region; slightly low central ray and IR
   4. Acceptable image receptor exposure and contrast
   5. No evidence of anatomic side marker
      Repeatable error(s): 1 (anatomy demonstrated) and 2 (positioning)

C. AP axial projection (Fig. 8.7)
   1. Distorted vertebral bodies and intervertebral joint spaces; base of skull superimposed over upper cervical spine

2. Overextension of skull and/or excessive central ray cephalic angle, which led to poor definition of vertebral bodies and joint spaces
   3. Evidence of collimation; slightly low central ray centering but correct IR placement
   4. Acceptable image receptor exposure and contrast
   5. Anatomical side marker is partially cut off
   Repeatable error(s): 1 (anatomy demonstrated), 2 (positioning), and 3 (Anatomical side marker not clearly demonstrated). Note: Unsure of the origin of the artifact seen on lower, left cervical spine region
D. Right posterior oblique (Fig. 8.8)
   1. Lower intervertebral joint spaces and foramina not clearly demonstrated
   2. Appears that body is underrotated from AP position (with appearance of upper rib cage suggesting underrotation rather than overrotation), an error that led to narrowing and obscuring of the lower intervertebral foramina.
   3. Collimation is evident. CR is centered too low.
   4. Acceptable image receptor exposure and contrast
   5. Anatomic side marker is evident
   Repeatable error(s): 1 (anatomy demonstrated), 2 (positioning), and 3 (CR centering)
E. Horizontal beam lateral (trauma) (Fig. 8.9)
   1. Aspect of C1 and dens cut off; C7–T1 not demonstrated
   2. Need to depress shoulders (because chin cannot be adjusted as a result of the trauma)
   3. No evidence of collimation except along anterior, upper margin; central ray centered too posterior, causing upper cervical spine to be cut off; IR placement centered too low

4. Acceptable image receptor exposure (poor contrast resulting from using a nongrid technique)
   5. No evidence of anatomic side marker
   Repeatable error(s): 1 (anatomy demonstrated), 2 (positioning), and 3 (CR centering)
F. AP for odontoid process—Fuchs method (Fig. 8.10)
   1. Upper part of odontoid process is not demonstrated.
   2. The skull and neck are overextended, which produces a poor image of the dens within the foramen magnum. There is slight tilt of the skull.
   3. The CR is centered too high and collimation is absent.
   4. Slightly underexposed
   5. No evidence of anatomic side marker
   Repeatable errors: 1 (anatomy demonstrated), 2 (positioning), 3 (CR centering), and 5 (no side marker)
G. AP thoracic spine (Fig. 8.11)
   1. Necklace is obscuring T1/2 region
   2. Positioning is acceptable
   3. CR is centered slightly high but acceptable
   4. Overexposed near the region of T1–T3
   5. Anatomic side marker is visible but placement may be obscuring costotransverse joint
   Repeatable errors: 1 (anatomy demonstrated), 4 (exposure), and 5 (anatomic side marker placement)

CHAPTER 9

Review Exercise A: Radiographic Anatomy of the Lumbar Spine, Sacrum, and Coccyx

1. Pars interarticularis
2. B. Intervertebral foramina
3. Lateral position
4. A. Pedicle
   B. Transverse process
   C. Superior articular process and facet

D. Lamina
   E. Spinous process
   F. Zygapophyseal joints
   G. Intervertebral foramina
5. 50 degrees for upper and 65 degrees for lower vertebrae to the midsagittal plane
6. Pelvic sacral foramina
7. Promontory
8. Cornua
9. 25–30 degrees
10. Coccyx
11. Base
12. A. Synovial, diarthrodial, plane, or gliding
    B. Cartilaginous, amphiarthrodial (slightly movable), none
13. A. Intervertebral disk space, L1–L2
    B. Spinous process, L2
    C. Transverse process, L3
    D. Region of lamina (body), L4
    E. Left ala of sacrum
    F. Left sacroiliac (joint)
    G. Body of L1
    H. Pedicles of L2
    I. Intervertebral foramina, L3–L4
    J. Intervertebral disk space, L5–S1
    K. Sacrum
    L. Inferior articular process, L3 (leg)
    M. Zygapophyseal joint, L4–L5
    N. Pars interarticularis, L3 (neck)
    O. Pedicle, L3 (eye)
    P. Transverse process, L3 (nose)
    Q. Superior articular process, L3 (ear)
14. A. Left zygapophyseal joints
    B. Left zygapophyseal joints
    C. Intervertebral foramina
    D. Right zygapophyseal joints
    E. Right zygapophyseal joints
15. 45 degrees, 65 degrees

Review Exercise B: Topographic Landmarks and Positioning of the Lumbar Spine, Sacrum, and Coccyx

1. 1. C
   2. E
   3. A
   4. B
   5. D
2. False
3. True

4. True
5. False (PA would open intervertebral joint spaces better.)
6. False (should be flexed)
7. True
8. False
9. True
10. A. 4
    B. 1
    C. 1 (and 3-myelography)
    D. 5
    E. 2
11. A. 8
    B. 3
    C. 1
    D. 2
    E. 4
    F. 7
    G. 6
    H. 5
12. Iliac crest
13. A. Sacroiliac (SI) joints are equidistant from the spine.
    B. Spinous process should be midline to the vertebral column (transverse processes are equal length)
14. 65-degrees
15. Right (upside)
16. Pedicle
17. Excessive rotation
18. Lateral
19. 5–8 degrees, caudad
20. With the sag or convexity of the spine closest to the IR
21. Reduces lumbar curvature, which opens the intervertebral disk space
22. True
23. 1½ inches (4 cm) inferior to iliac crest and 2 inches (5 cm) posterior to ASIS
24. 30 degrees cephalad
25. True
26. False [lower margin 1–2 inches (3–5 cm) below iliac crest]
27. True
28. D. Compensating filter
29. The convex side of the spine
30. 3–4 inches/8–10 cm
31. Pelvis
32. Hyperextension and hyperflexion lateral projections
33. B. 80–95
34. 15 degrees cephalad
35. 2 inches (5 cm) superior to pubic symphysis
36. A PA (prone) with 15 degrees caudad central ray angle

37. 2 inches (5 cm) superior to the symphysis pubis
38. 10 degrees caudad
39. False (need different central ray angles for AP projections; can combine lateral but not AP projections)
40. AP of sacrum and coccyx
41. Place lead blocker on tabletop behind patient.
42. Left
43. 25–30 degrees
44. D. 35 degrees cephalad
45. 1 inch (2.5 cm) medial from upside ASIS

Review Exercise C: Problem Solving for Technical and Positioning Errors

1. Rotation of the spine
2. Insufficient rotation of the spine (pedicle "eye" should be to midvertebral bodies)
3. If the patient has a wide pelvis, the central ray can be angled 5–8 degrees caudad.
4. Place additional support beneath the spine, or use a 5- to 8-degree caudad angle.
5. An increase in central ray angle is required to separate the coccyx from the symphysis pubis.
6. Decrease rotation of the body and spine.
7. AP or PA and collimated lateral projections would provide the best view of the L3 region. The central ray should be about 2 inches (5 cm) above the iliac crest.
8. A. Use high kVp technique.
   B. Perform a PA rather than an AP projection.
   C. Use breast shields.
9. Perform a PA rather than an AP projection and reverse the direction of the central ray from caudad to cephalad.
10. A lateral L5–S1 position would demonstrate the degree of forward displacement of L5 onto S1.
11. The CR should be angled 15–20 degrees cephalad.
12. Although AP and lateral projections of the lumbar spine are helpful, posterior or anterior oblique positions best

demonstrate advanced signs of spondylolysis.
13. B. MR
14. Hyperflexion and hyperextension lateral positions
15. Routine lumbar spine projections should be performed erect.

Review Exercise D: Critique Radiographs of the Lumbar Spine, Sacrum, and Coccyx

A. Lateral lumbar spine (Fig. 9.6)
   1. Posterior elements of upper lumbar spine cut off
   2. Patient positioned too far posterior
   3. Evident and acceptable collimation (could be collimated a little more tightly if centering were correct); central ray centering too anterior, causing posterior elements to become cut off
   4. Acceptable but slightly underexposed exposure factors
   5. Anatomic side marker cut off Repeatable errors: 1 (anatomy demonstrated), 2 (part positioning), 3 (CR centering), and 5 (missing anatomic side marker)

B. Lateral lumbar spine (Fig. 9.7)
   1. All structures demonstrated. Note: This patient has a transitional vertebra, which produces six lumbar vertebrae. Also, there is calcification of the abdominal aorta.
   2. Poor visibility of upper intervertebral joint spaces caused by poor positioning of upper thoracic. Often if the shoulders are not superimposed, there is closure of the upper joint spaces.
   3. Collimation not evident; acceptable central ray centering and IR placement
   4. Overexposed exposure factors
   5. No evidence of anatomic side marker (it may have been placed too low on IR) Repeatable errors: 2 (part positioning) and 5 (no anatomic side marker)

C. Lateral L5–S1 (Fig. 9.8)

529

1. All pertinent anatomic structures included
2. Excellent part and central ray centering
3. Additional collimation needed; L5–S1 joint space not open; may need waist support or central ray caudal angle
4. Poor contrast resolution of the L5–S1 joint space region
5. Evidence of anatomic side marker (better to place up and posterior to spine)
   Repeatable errors: 3 (collimation and part positioning) and 4 (exposure)

D. RPO lumbar spine (Fig. 9.9)
1. Posterior elements of upper lumbar spine cut off
2. Overrotated upper aspect of lumbar spine (eye of "Scottie dog" [pedicles] posterior and not centered to body)
3. Evidence of collimation; central ray centered too anterior; posterior elements of lumbar spine to become cut off
4. Acceptable exposure factors
5. No evidence of anatomic side marker
   Repeatable errors: 1 (anatomy demonstrated), 2 (part positioning), 3 (centering of CR and anatomy), and 5 (no anatomic side marker)

E. RPO lumbar spine (Fig. 9.10)
1. Entire lumbar spine demonstrated
2. Underrotated lumbar spine [eye of Scottie (pedicles) too anterior]
3. Collimation too loose and not evident (should be visible on sides); central ray centering and IR placement correct
4. Acceptable but slightly overexposed exposure factors
5. No evidence of anatomic side marker
   Repeatable error: 2 (part positioning)

F. LPO lumbar spine (Fig. 9.11)
1. Entire lumbar spine demonstrated but overrotation of spine obscures essential anatomy and joints

2. Excessive rotation
3. No evidence of collimation and incorrect centering of anatomy to IR
4. Acceptable
5. Right side marker is barely visible by distortion. May have been placed on sheet on table.
   Repeatable error(s): 2 (part positioning) and 3 (collimation and centering)

G. AP lumbar spine (Fig. 9.12)
1. All lumbosacral spine anatomy demonstrated
2. Slight tilt of hips
3. No collimation evident. CR centered slightly high.
4. Exposure factors acceptable
5. Anatomic side markers evident
   Repeatable error(s): None (although centering and positioning are not ideal)

H. PA erect lumbar spine-scoliosis study (Fig. 9.13)
1. All thoracolumbar spine is demonstrated.
2. Positioning for projection was correct.
3. Absence of any collimation and no breast shields in place. Collimation could have prevented needless exposure to cervical spine region and lower pelvis.
4. Exposure factors are acceptable.
5. Both left and right markers on image. May be confusing for interpretation
   Repeatable error(s): Absence of collimation and no breast shields in place. Because of added exposure to patient, it is not advisable to repeat exposure.

I. Lateral erect lumbar spine-scoliosis study (Fig. 9.14)
1. Thoracolumbar spine demonstrated
2. Arms were not raised away from thorax and are in field of view. This poor positioning may have increased the forward curvature of the thoracic spine region.
3. Absence of any collimation or use of breast shields. Collimation could have

prevented needless exposure to cervical spine region and lower pelvis.
4. Exposure factors are acceptable.
5. Left anatomic side is evident
   Repeatable error(s): Arms need to be raised and body placed as erect as possible. Absence of collimation and no breast shields in place.

CHAPTER 10

Review Exercise A: Radiographic Anatomy of the Bony Thorax, Sternum, and Ribs

1. A. Sternum
   B. Thoracic vertebra
   C. 12 pairs of ribs
2. A. Jugular (suprasternal or manubrial) notch
   B. Facet for sternoclavicular joint
   C. Facet for first rib
   D. Manubrium
   E. Sternal angle
   F. Xiphoid process
   G. Costal cartilage of seventh rib (last of "true" ribs)
   H. Tenth rib
   I. Costal cartilage of second rib
   J. Clavicle
3. Body
4. 40
5. 6 inches (15 cm)
6. A. T9–T10
   B. T4–T5
   C. Manubriosternal joint
7. Sternoclavicular joint
8. Costal cartilage
9. True ribs connect to the sternum by their own costal cartilage. False ribs are connected to the sternum via the costal cartilage of the seventh rib.
10. True
11. False (called the anterior or sternal end)
12. D. Tubercle
13. A. Artery
    B. Vein
    C. Nerve
14. A. Posterior or vertebral ends
    B. 3–5 inches (8–12 cm)
    C. First (anterior sternal end)
    D. Eighth or ninth
    E. 10

15. 1. B
    2. A
    3. B
    4. A
    5. A
    6. A
    7. C
16. Synovial
17. A. True ribs, 1–7
    B. False ribs, 8–12
    C. Floating ribs, 11–12
18. Each rib attaches to the sternum by its own costal cartilage
19. They do not connect to the sternum (thus the term "floating" ribs).
20. A. Vertebral end (posterior)
    B. Tubercles (for articulation with vertebrae)
    C. Axillary or angle portion of rib
    D. Costal groove
    E. Sternal end (anterior)
    F. Neck
    G. Head

Review Exercise B: Positioning of the Ribs and Sternum

1. True
2. False (less obliquity)
3. Approximately 15°
4. A. 70–85 kVp
   B. Low
   C. Long (3 to 4 seconds) with orthostatic (breathing) technique
5. It blurs lung markings and ribs, which improves the visibility of the sternum.
6. Increase in patient dose, especially skin dose
7. CT or nuclear medicine
8. A. Recumbent
   B. Expiration
   C. kVp range—75 to 85
9. Above
10. Away from
11. PA and anterior obliques (Placing the area of interest closest to the IR is one recommended routine.)
12. AP and RPO (to shift spine away from area of interest)
13. By taping a small, metallic "BB" or other opaque marker over the site of the injury
14. Erect PA and lateral chest
15. B. Pulmonary injury caused by blunt trauma to two or more ribs

16. B. Erect
17. A. Irregular bony margins
18. C. Depressed sternum resulting from congenital defect
19. A. Osteoblastic
20. False
21. True
22. A. Jugular notch (may also be known as the suprasternal or manubrial notch)
23. RAO; it places the sternum over the heart to provide a uniform background for added visibility of the sternum.
24. True. Rotation beyond 15–20 degrees will produce distortion of the sternum.
25. Midsternum (midway between jugular notch and xiphoid process)
26. LPO (oblique supine position)
27. 60–72 inches (150–180 cm); reduces magnification created by the long OID
28. B. The entire sternum should lie over the heart shadow adjacent to the spine.
29. B. Level of T2–T3 (3 inches (8 cm) distal to vertebra prominens)
30. D. Suspend respiration on expiration
31. 10–15 degrees from PA position
32. LAO
33. A. The nature of the trauma or patient complaint
    B. The location of the rib pain or injury
    C. Whether the injury was caused by trauma to the thoracic cavity
34. 3–4 inches (8–10 cm) below the jugular notch, level of T7
35. RAO or LPO elongates the left axillary ribs (and shifts the spine away from the injury site)
36. PA and LAO (to elongate the right axillary rib region)
37. 45 degrees
38. 72 inches (180 cm)
39. True
40. Left axially portion of the ribs
41. False. Perform the right lateral chest decubitus for a possible pneumothorax in the left thorax.
42. True (Affected side down to demonstrate any free fluid)

43. False. The right SC joint is projected closest to the spine with an RAO projection.
44. C. 15 inches (40 cm)
45. B. Hemothorax

Review Exercise C: Problem Solving for Technical and Positioning Errors

1. Underrotation of the patient
2. Lower the kVp to 70–85 to prevent overpenetration of the sternum.
3. Increase the exposure time (and lower the mA) to allow for greater blurring of the lung markings (perform orthostatic technique).
4. Have the patient bring the breasts to the side; hold them in this position with a wide bandage.
5. CT
6. 15- to 20-degree RAO sternum with orthostatic (breathing) technique; lateral sternum on inspiration; and 10- to 15-degree LAO of sternoclavicular joint with suspended inspiration
7. Suspend respiration during inspiration to move the diaphragm below the eighth ribs.
8. LPO and horizontal beam lateral projections (may use 15- to 20-degree mediolateral central angle if patient cannot be in oblique position)
9. Erect PA and LAO (or RPO) position with suspended inspiration
10. Recumbent PA (or AP if the patient cannot assume prone position) and RAO (or LPO) positions with suspended expiration
11. Because of patient condition, it is best to perform all positions erect and initiate exposure on full inspiration for upper ribs and full expiration for lower ribs. AP projections and both oblique positions (RPO and LPO) must be performed. It is recommended that kVp (manual technique used) for all projections be lowered because of the advanced osteoporosis.

531

12. A limited rib series will indicate the ribs that are fractured (and whether this has led to flail chest). Because the patient is restricted to a backboard, the oblique positions may not be possible. Note: With flail chest, the positions are best performed erect but patient's condition prevents it.

Review Exercise D: Critique Radiographs of the Bony Thorax

A. Bilateral ribs above diaphragm (Fig. 10.5)
    1. Ninth through eleventh ribs are cut off at left and right lateral margin.
    2. Tilt of body toward projected ribs numbers 9 and 10 below collimation field
    3. CR centering is acceptable.
    4. Acceptable exposure factors
    5. Anatomic side marker is evident.
       Repeatable errors: 1 (anatomy demonstrated) and 2 (positioning)
B. Oblique sternum (Fig. 10.6)
    1. All pertinent anatomic structures included
    2. Sternum is overrotated; sternum away from the spine and rotated beyond heart shadow and distorted (Note: Because of additional patient dose, some departments may choose not to repeat this projection given that the outline of the sternum is visible.)
    3. Collimation not completely evident; central ray centering and IR placement correct
    4. Acceptable exposure factors and processing
    5. No evidence of anatomic side marker
       Repeatable errors: 2 (positioning)
C. AP ribs below diaphragm (Fig. 10.7)
    1. Right lower ribs cut off; only lower three pair of ribs demonstrated, indicating diaphragm is too low from poor expiration

2. No elevation of diaphragm; need to take exposure during expiration with the patient in a recumbent position to raise the diaphragm to the highest level
3. No evidence of collimation; acceptable central ray centering, but IR should have been placed landscape to prevent lateral margins of ribs from being cut off.
4. Acceptable exposure factors and processing
5. Anatomic side marker evident but placed a little low and almost off the radiograph
   Repeatable errors: 1 (anatomy demonstrated) and 3 (IR placement)
D. Lateral sternum (Fig. 10.8)
    1. Lower aspect of sternum cut off
    2. Acceptable part positioning
    3. No evidence of collimation; central ray centering and IR placement too high, causing lower sternum to be cut off
    4. Acceptable exposure factors
    5. No evidence of markers
       Repeatable errors: 1 (anatomy demonstrated) and 3 (CR centering and IR placement)

CHAPTER 11

Review Exercise A: Radiographic Anatomy of the Cranium

1. A. 8
   B. 14
2. A. Frontal
   B. Right parietal
   C. Left parietal
   D. Occipital
3. A. Right temporal
   B. Left temporal
   C. Sphenoid
   D. Ethmoid
4. A. Frontal
   B. Right parietal
   C. Right temporal
   D. Sphenoid
   E. Ethmoid
   F. Left temporal
   G. Left parietal
   H. Occipital

5. A. Frontal
   B. Ethmoid
   C. Sphenoid
   D. Left temporal
   E. Left parietal
   F. Occipital
   G. Right parietal
   H. Right temporal
6. A. Crista galli
   B. Cribriform plate
   C. Perpendicular plate
   D. Lateral labyrinth (mass)
   E. Middle nasal conchae (turbinate)
7. Cribriform plate
8. Perpendicular plate
9. A. Anterior clinoid processes
   B. Lesser wing
   C. Greater wing
   D. Sella turcica
   E. Dorsum sellae
   F. Posterior clinoid process
   G. Clivis
   H. Foramen rotundum
   I. Foramen ovale
   J. Foramen spinosum
   K. Foramen magnum
   L. Optic foramen
   M. Lateral pterygoid process (plate)
   N. Pterygoid hamulus
   O. Medial pterygoid process (plate)
   P. Superior orbital fissure
   Q. Body of sphenoid (sinus)
10. Sella turcica
11. Dorsum sellae
12. Optic foramen
13. Medial and lateral pterygoid processes
14. Lateral projection
15. Orbital or horizontal portion
16. A. Coronal
    B. Squamosal
    C. Lambdoidal
    D. Sagittal
    E. Bregma
    F. Lambda
    G. Pterion
    H. Asterion
    I. Anterior
    J. Posterior
    K. Sphenoid
    L. Mastoid
17. Fibrous or synarthrodial
18. Sutural or wormian; lambdoidal
19. Supraorbital margin (SOM)
20. Ethmoidal notch

532

Answers to Review Questions

Copyright © 2025 by Elsevier Inc.
All rights are reserved, including those for text and data mining, AI training, and similar technologies.

21. Right and left parietals
22. Occipital
23. External occipital protuberance, or inion
24. Occipital condyles, or lateral condylar portions
25. A. Squamous
    B. Mastoid
    C. Petrous
26. False (petrous portion)
27. Top of the ear attachment (TEA)
28. Internal acoustic meatus
29. Cranial structures, PA axial (Caldwell) projection (Fig. 11.15)
    A. Supraorbital margins of right orbit
    B. Crista galli of ethmoid
    C. Sagittal suture—posterior skull
    D. Lambdoidal suture—posterior skull
    E. Petrous ridge
    F. Superior orbital fissure
    Cranial structures, lateral projection (Fig. 11.16)
    A. External acoustic meatus (EAM)
    B. Mastoid portion of temporal bone
    C. Occipital bone
    D. Lambdoidal suture
    E. Dorsum sellae
    F. Anterior clinoid processes
    G. Vertex of skull
    H. Coronal suture
    I. Frontal bone
    J. Orbital plates (frontal bone)
    K. Sella turcica
    L. Body of sphenoid bone: sphenoid sinus
    M. Petrous portion of temporal bone
    N. Greater wing of sphenoid bone

Review Exercise B: Specific Anatomy and Pathology of the Temporal Bone

1. A. Squamous
   B. Mastoid
   C. Petrous
2. Petrous portion
3. Auricle or pinna
4. 1 inch (or 2.5 cm)
5. Tympanic membrane (eardrum)
6. Auditory ossicles
7. Eustachian or auditory tube
8. To equalize the atmospheric pressure within the middle ear

9. Aditus
10. Tegmen tympani
11. Malleus (Hammer)
12. Stapes (Stirrup)
13. Incus (Anvil)
14. Oval or vestibular window
15. A. Hearing
    B. Equilibrium
16. Round or cochlear window
17. False
18. A. Malleus
    B. Incus
    C. Stapes
    D. Oval window
    E. Cochlea
    F. Round window
    G. Eustachian tube
    H. Tympanic cavity
    I. Tympanic membrane
    J. EAM or canal
19. A. 5
    B. 3
    C. 1
    D. 6
    E. 2
    F. 4
20. A. Expansion of the internal acoustic canal
21. B. Computed tomography (CT)

Review Exercise C: Radiographic Anatomy of the Facial Bones

1. A. Middle nasal conchae
2. Maxilla
3. A. Frontal process
   B. Zygomatic process
   C. Alveolar process
   D. Palatine process
4. Frontal process
5. Acanthion
6. Horizontal portion of the palatine bones
7. Frontal and ethmoid
8. Zygomatic or malar bones
9. B. Mandible
10. Lacrimal bones
11. Conchae, turbinates
12. False (Most of the nose is composed of cartilage.)
13. Septal cartilage, vomer (pushed laterally to one side)
14. A. 3
    B. 8
    C. 6
    D. 7
    E. 5
    F. 1
    G. 2

H. 4
Figs. 11.18 (Frontal view) and 11.19 (Side view).
    A. Nasal bones
    B. Lacrimal bones
    C. Zygomatic bones
    D. Maxillary bones
    E. Inferior nasal conchae
    F. Mandible
15. Vomer and the palatine bones
    Inferior surface view of the maxillae (Fig. 11.20)
    A. Pterygoid hamulus, sphenoid
    B. Right palatine process, right maxilla
    C. Left palatine process, left maxilla
    D. Horizontal portions, right and left palatine bones
16. Nasal septum (Fig. 11.21)
    A. Perpendicular plate of ethmoid
    B. Vomer
    C. Septal cartilage
17. Mandible (Fig. 11.22) and Lateral skull and mandible (Fig. 11.23)
    A. Condyle
    B. Neck
    C. Ramus
    D. Gonion or mandibular angle
    E. Body
    F. Mental foramen
    G. Mentum or mental protuberance
    H. Alveolar process
    I. Coronoid process
    J. Mandibular notch
    K. Temporal bone
    L. Temporomandibular joint (TMJ)
    M. External auditory meatus (EAM)
    N. Mastoid process
18. A. Lacrimal (facial)
    B. Ethmoid (cranial)
    C. Frontal (cranial)
    D. Sphenoid (cranial)
    E. Palatine (facial)
    F. Zygomatic (facial)
    G. Maxilla (facial)
19. H. Optic foramen
    I. Superior orbital fissure
    J. Inferior orbital fissure
    K. Sphenoid strut
20. 30 degrees, 37 degrees
21. Inferior orbital fissure
22. A. Superior orbital fissure
23. B. Optic nerve

Review Exercise D: Radiographic Anatomy of the Paranasal Sinuses

1. Antrum, antrum of Highmore
2. Maxillary
3. Between the inner and outer tables of the skull, posterior to the glabella
4. 6 years
5. Lateral masses or labyrinths
6. B. Osteomeatal complex
7. Sphenoid sinus
8. A. Nasal cavity (fossae)
   B. Maxillary sinuses
   C. Right temporal bone (squamous portion)
   D. Frontal sinuses
   E. Ethmoid sinuses
   F. Sphenoid sinuses
   G. Maxillary sinuses
   H. Ethmoid sinuses
   I. Frontal sinuses
   J. Squamous portion of left temporal bone
   K. Mastoid portion of left temporal bone
   L. Sphenoid sinus
   M. Roots of upper teeth (alveolar process)
9. A. Sphenoid sinus
   B. Maxillary sinuses
   C. Ethmoid sinuses
   D. Frontal sinus
   E. Frontal sinuses
   F. Sphenoid sinus
   G. Ethmoid sinuses
   H. Maxillary sinuses
10. Infundibulum
11. True
12. B. Prone

Review Exercise A: Skull Morphology, Topography, Pathology, and Positioning of the Cranium

1. A. Mesocephalic (c)
   B. Brachycephalic (b)
   C. Dolichocephalic (a)
2. Mesocephalic, 47 degrees
3. ±40 (<47 degrees)
4. False (CR angles and head rotations may be different)
5. 7–8 degrees; 7–8 degrees (same degrees of difference)
6. 1. G
   2. E
   3. J
   4. N

5. H
6. K
7. D
8. F
9. B
10. I
11. O
12. L
13. C
14. A
15. M
7. 75–90 kVp
8. A. Rotation
   B. Tilt
   C. Excessive neck flexion
   D. Excessive neck extension
   E. Incorrect central ray angulation
9. A. Rotation
   B. Tilt
10. A. Le Fort
11. A. CT
12. B. Diagnostic medical sonography (DMS)
13. D. Nuclear medicine (NM)
14. A. 3
    B. 5
    C. 6
    D. 1
    E. 2
    F. 4
    G. 7
15. A. Advanced Paget disease
16. Occipital
17. A. OML
18. C. Foramen magnum
19. D. Rotation
20. IOML; 37
21. Dorsum sellae and posterior clinoids should be projected into the foramen magnum.
22. 25 degrees cephalad
23. 2 inches (5 cm) above the EAM
24. B. Rotation
25. In the lower one-third of the orbits
26. Excessive flexion or insufficient central ray angle
27. 0 degree posteroanterior (PA)
28. Rule out any possible cervical fractures or subluxation.
29. Tilt of the skull
30. B. IOML
31. D. Lateral
32. C. 25- to 30-degree PA axial
33. C. Lateral
34. A. 1½ inches (4 cm) superior to the nasion
35. A. CT

Review Exercise B: Problem Solving for Technical and Positioning Errors of the Cranium

1. Rotation of skull present; rotation of patient's face toward left
2. Excessive extension or excessive caudad central ray angle—projects the petrous ridges lower than expected (should be in the lower third of the orbit)
3. Rotation of the patient's face (skull) to the left
4. Insufficient extension of the skull, or central ray was not perpendicular to IOML
5. Skull tilt
6. Skull rotation
7. Central ray angled <37 degrees to the IOML, or <30 degrees to the OML (would be caused by 30-degree angle to IOML). This error can be addressed with more flexion of the neck as well.
8. Collimated, lateral projection of the sella turcica
9. Right lateral projection of the skull
10. Should perform the PA axial projection (Haas method)
11. Horizontal beam (dorsal decubitus) lateral position—will demonstrate a possible air-fluid level in the sphenoid sinus
12. Diagnostic medical sonography (DMS)—a noninvasive means of evaluating the newborn's cranium
13. Either MR or CT can be performed.
14. Overangulation of the CR or excessive flexion of neck
15. No repeat exposure is required. Because of elongation of the facial mass with the AP axial projection for the skull, cutting off aspects of the mandible is acceptable.

PART III: RADIOGRAPHIC POSITIONING OF FACIAL BONES, MANDIBLE, AND PARANASAL SINUSES

Review Exercise A: Positioning of the Facial Bones

1. False (Best to perform erect)
2. True
3. False

4. True
5. False (It is used for this.)
6. False (Strong magnets in MR prohibit this.)
7. Blow-out fracture
8. Tripod
9. Dense petrous pyramids superimpose the orbits, obscuring facial bone structures.
10. C. Zygoma
11. Waters method
12. Orbits including infraorbital rims, bony nasal septum, maxillae, zygomatic bones, and arches
13. B. 30 degrees
14. Orbital rims and orbital floors
15. A. Reduces OID of facial bones
    B. Reduces exposure to anterior facial bones and neck structures such as thyroid glands
16. A. IR is placed in portrait orientation for facial bones but landscape for the cranium.
    B. CR is centered to the zygoma for facial bones and 2 inches (5 cm) above the EAM for the cranium.
17. Mentomeatal; 37 degrees
18. Acanthion
19. Nasion
20. Lips-meatal; 55 degrees
21. True
22. False (toward the affected side)
23. True
24. Maxillary sinuses; inferior orbital rims
25. Glabelloalveolar (GAL)
26. Zygomatic arches
27. 1 inch (2.5 cm) superior to nasion to pass through midarches (at level of gonion)
28. A. Rhese method
    B. Three-point landing
29. A. Cheek, nose, chin
    B. 53 degrees
    C. Acanthiomeatal
    D. Lower outer
30. 1. E
    2. C
    3. F
    4. A
    5. D
    6. B

Review Exercise B: Positioning of the Mandible and Temporomandibular Joints (TMJ)

1. True
2. Axiolateral oblique

3. Extend the chin
4. A. 30 degrees
   B. 45 degrees
   C. 0 degree, true lateral
   D. 10–15°
   E. 25° cephalad
5. Insufficient cephalic CR angle or skull tilt
6. Acanthion (at lips for PA projection)
7. Orbitomeatal line (OML)
8. True
9. False (cephalad)
10. Condyloid process
11. A. 35 degrees caudad
    B. 42 degrees caudad
12. 1 inch (2.5 cm) superior to glabella
13. SMV projection
14. Orthopantomography (panoramic tomography)
15. Narrow, vertical slit diaphragm
16. Infraorbitomeatal line (IOML)
17. Digital detector or photo-stimulable phosphor plate
18. True
19. True
20. B. Schuller
21. 25–30 degrees; caudad
22. A. Modified law
    B. 15 degrees
    C. 15 degrees
23. 40 degrees caudad
24. Midsagittal

Review Exercise C: Positioning of the Paranasal Sinuses

1. 75–85 kVp
2. A. Perform positions erect when possible
   B. Use horizontal x-ray beam
3. True
4. True
5. False
6. A. Lateral
   B. PA Caldwell
   C. Parietoacanthial (Waters method)
   D. SMV
7. Lateral
8. Horizontal x-ray beam
9. Frontal and anterior ethmoid
10. 15 degrees
11. A. Maxillary
    B. 37 degrees
12. Mentomeatal line (MML)
13. Just below the maxillary sinuses

14. Sphenoid, ethmoid, and maxillary sinuses
15. Level of the acanthion
16. The mouth (oral cavity) is open with the PA transoral projection.
17. Sphenoid sinuses
18. 1. C
    2. D
    3. E
    4. A
    5. B

Review Exercise D: Problem Solving for Technical and Positioning Errors for Facial Bones, Mandible, and Paranasal Sinuses

1. Rotation of the skull
2. No. The petrous ridges should be projected just below the maxillary sinuses. The patient's head needs to be extended more.
3. Rotation of the skull
4. Yes, this image meets the evaluation criteria for a 30-degree PA axial projection.
5. Excessive flexion of the head and neck or incorrect CR angle will project the glabella into the nasal bones. The CR must be parallel to the glabelloalveolar line.
6. The head was tilted. Ensure that the MSP is parallel to the image receptor.
7. No. Increase extension of the head and neck. The AML should be placed perpendicular to the IR to ensure that the optic foramen is open and is projected into the lower outer quadrant of the orbit (skull rotation is correct).
8. Insufficient rotation of the skull toward the IR. The skull should be rotated 30 degrees (from lateral position) toward the IR to prevent foreshortening of the body.
9. Parietoacanthial and R and L lateral projections. The parietoacanthial (Waters method) or the optional PA axial projections would demonstrate any possible septal deviation. The lateral projections would demonstrate any possible fracture of the nasal bones or anterior nasal spine. (The superoinferior tangential projection would provide an axial perspective but

535

is considered an optional projection in most departments and not part of the routine unless specifically requested.)

10. Modified parietoacanthial (modified Waters method) projection

11. Perform the oblique inferosuperior (tangential) projections. These projections are ideal to demonstrate a depressed fracture of the zygomatic arch. (Bilateral projections are generally taken for comparison.)

12. Angle CR to place it perpendicular to the IOML. Angle the image receptor to maintain a perpendicular relationship between the CR and the image receptor. This will prevent distortion of the anatomy.

13. The head and neck need to be extended more to project the petrous ridges below the ethmoid sinuses.

14. Rotation of the skull

15. Tilt of the skull

16. Increase extension of the head and neck to project the entire sphenoid sinus through the oral cavity.

17. None. The petrous ridges should be below the floors of the maxillary sinuses on a well-positioned parietoacanthial projection.

18. The most diagnostic projection is the horizontal beam lateral projection to demonstrate any air-fluid levels.

19. The PA transoral special projection in addition to the routine four sinuses projection series (the lateral, PA Caldwell, parietoacanthial, and SMV)

20. PA, PA axial, and parietoacanthial projections will demonstrate a possible bony nasal septal deviation.

PART IV: LEARNING EXERCISES

Review Exercise A: Critique Radiographs of the Cranium

A. Lateral skull: 4-year-old (Fig. 11.28)
1. Foreign bodies (earrings) obscuring essential anatomic structures
2. Correct part positioning, but patient's hand seen supporting mandible; can use positioning sponge if needed to support skull
3. No evidence of collimation; correct central ray and IR placement
4. Appears underexposed on this printed copy (may be a repeatable error if actual radiograph also appears similarly underexposed)
5. No evidence of anatomic side marker
Repeatable errors: 1 (anatomy demonstrated) and possibly 4 (slightly underexposed)

B. Lateral skull: 54-year-old, posttraumatic injury (Fig. 11.29)
1. Vertex of the skull just slightly cut off (may be repeatable error because of proximity to the site of trauma)
2. Tilted and rotated skull (separation of the orbital plates from the tilt; separation of the greater wings of the sphenoid, the rami of the mandible, and the EAMs—all indicating rotation)
3. No evidence of collimation; slightly high central ray centering if the photo borders are also the collimation borders, which would add to the tilt appearance
4. Acceptable exposure factors
5. No evidence of anatomic side marker
Repeatable errors: 1 (anatomy demonstrated) and 2 (part positioning)

C. AP axial skull (Towne) (Fig. 11.30)
1. Entire occipital bone and foramen magnum demonstrated
2. Correct part positioning
3. No evidence of collimation; overangled central ray; anterior arch of C1 projected into the foramen magnum rather than the dorsum sellae

4. Acceptable but slightly underexposed exposure factors
5. No evidence of anatomic side marker
Repeatable errors: 3 (part positioning)

D. AP or PA skull (Fig. 11.31) AP 15-degree cephalad projection, as indicated by the large size of the orbits, which was caused by magnification from increased OID (can compare with radiograph that follows)
1. All pertinent anatomic structures demonstrated but with some foreshortening of frontal bone
2. Petrous ridges not in the lower third of orbits; position requires more flexion or less central ray angle as an AP; skull slightly rotated (note distance between orbits and lateral margins of skull)
3. No evidence of collimation; less central ray angle needed (can also compare with correctly angled central ray on PA radiograph in Fig. 11.32)
4. Acceptable exposure factors
5. No evidence of anatomic side marker
Repeatable errors: 2 (part positioning) and 3 (collimation and CR angle)

E. AP or PA skull (Fig. 11.32) PA 15-degree Caldwell projection
1. All pertinent anatomic structures not demonstrated; patient ID marker and side marker obscuring skull
2. Correct part positioning
3. Evidence of collimation (circular cone); size of IR too small for the skull; correct central ray placement and angle (petrous ridges in lower third of orbit)
4. Acceptable exposure factors
5. Evidence of anatomic side marker, but placed over skull; patient ID marker over upper right cranium—both repeatable errors
Repeatable errors: 1 (anatomy demonstrated) and 5 (incorrect placement of ID marker)

536

Answers to Review Questions

Copyright © 2025 by Elsevier Inc.
All rights reserved, including those for text and data mining, AI training, and similar technologies.

Review Exercise B: Critique Radiographs of the Facial Bones

A. Parietoacanthial (Waters) projection (Fig. 11.33)
1. Petrous ridges are projected into maxillary sinuses which could obscure pathology in this region.
2. Skull is underextended. This led to the petrous ridges being projected into the lower maxillary sinuses. Also, skull appears to be rotated.
3. Collimation is not evident. CR and image receptor appears correct.
4. Acceptable exposure factors
5. Anatomic side marker is not evident.
   Repeatable error(s): 2 (part positioning)
B. SMV mandible (Fig. 11.34)
1. Pertinent anatomy is included but is not well demonstrated because of positioning error.
2. Skull is underextended. (IOML was not parallel to IR and not perpendicular to CR.) Mandible is foreshortened and rami projected into temporal bone.
3. Collimation is not evident. CR centering and IR placement are correct.
4. Image appears to be slightly underexposed.
5. Anatomic side marker is not evident.
   Repeatable error(s): 2 (part positioning) (possibly 4—underexposed)
C. Optic foramina, parieto-orbital oblique Rhese method (Fig. 11.35)
1. Optic foramen is included but is slightly distorted.
2. Skull is rotated excessively toward a PA. (The skull is rotated >53 degrees from the lateral position. This led to the optic foramen being projected into the middle lower aspect of the orbit.)
3. Collimation is not evident. CR and IR placement are correct.
4. Exposure factors are acceptable.
5. Anatomic side marker is not evident.

   Repeatable error(s): 2 (The foramen is demonstrated; therefore, this may not be a repeatable error.)
D. Optic foramina, parieto-orbital oblique Rhese method (Fig. 11.36)
1. Optic foramen is distorted and totally obscured.
2. Skull appears to be overextended. (The AML was not perpendicular.) This projects the optic foramina into the infraorbital rim structure. Skull also appears to be under-rotated toward a lateral position. (If the skull is rotated <53 degrees from the lateral position, the optic foramen will be projected into the lateral margin of the orbit.)
3. Collimation is evident and appears satisfactory. CR and IR placement are correct.
4. Exposure factors are acceptable.
5. Anatomic side marker is not evident.
   Repeatable error(s): 1 (anatomy demonstrated) and 2 (part positioning)
E. Lateral facial bones (Fig. 11.37)
1. Very distal end of mandible is cut off. Probably would not justify repeat exposure unless this was a specific area of interest.
2. Skull is rotated. (Note the separation of rami of mandible, greater wings of sphenoid, and orbits.)
3. Collimation is evident and acceptable (except for cutoff of lower tip of mandible). CR and IR placement are acceptable.
4. Exposure factors appear to be satisfactory.
5. Anatomic side marker is not evident.
   Repeatable error(s): 2 (part positioning) (possibly 1—anatomy demonstrated)

Review Exercise C: Critique Radiographs of the Paranasal Sinuses

A. Parietoacanthial transoral (open-mouth Waters method) (Fig. 11.38)

1. Sphenoid and maxillary sinuses not well demonstrated. Petrous ridges are projected into lower aspect of maxillary sinuses. The base of the skull is superimposed over the sphenoid sinus.
2. Skull is underextended leading to errors previously described. (Chin is not elevated sufficiently.)
3. Collimation is not centered to image receptor. CR is centered too low (inferior) according to circular collimation on top, but this is not a repeatable error by itself.
4. Exposure factors are acceptable.
5. Anatomic side marker is not evident.
   Repeatable errors: 1 (anatomy demonstrated) and 2 (part positioning)
B. Parietoacanthial (Waters) (Fig. 11.39)
1. Maxillary sinuses not well demonstrated. Petrous ridges are projected into lower aspect of maxillary sinuses. Artifacts appear to be either surgical clips and devices or external hairpins or clips.
2. Skull is underextended and severely rotated.
3. Collimation is not evident. CR centering and film placement are slightly low.
4. Exposure factors are acceptable.
5. Anatomic side marker is not evident.
   Repeatable errors: 1 (anatomy demonstrated) and 2 (part positioning)
C. Submentovertical (SMV)-Paranasal Sinuses (Fig. 11.40)
1. Maxillary and ethmoid sinuses not well demonstrated and partially cut off. Mandible is superimposed over sinuses.
2. Skull is grossly underextended and tilted. (Also, slight rotation.)
3. Collimation would have been satisfactory if centering had

been correct. CR centering is off laterally. This led to cut-off of the anatomy.
   4. Exposure factors are acceptable.
   5. Anatomic side marker is not evident.
      Repeatable errors: 1 (anatomy demonstrated), 2 (part positioning), and 3 (CR centering)
D. Lateral projection—Paranasal sinuses (Fig. 11.41)
   1. Aspect of ethmoid and maxillary sinuses not well demonstrated because of superimposed mandible.
   2. Slight rotation with considerable tilt evident by poor superimposition of orbital plates.
   3. Collimation is acceptable. CR centering and film placement are acceptable but slightly anterior.
   4. Exposure factors are acceptable for the sphenoid/ethmoid sinuses.
   5. Anatomic side marker is evident.
      Repeatable errors: 1 (anatomy demonstrated) and 2 (part positioning)

CHAPTER 12

Review Exercise A: Radiographic Anatomy and Clinical Indications of the Pathology of the Gallbladder and Biliary System

1. 3–4 pounds (1.5–2 kg), or 1/36 of total body weight
2. Right upper quadrant (RUQ)
3. Falciform ligament
4. Right
5. A. Quadrate
   B. Caudate
6. True
7. False (1 quart, or 800–1000 mL)
8. A. Store bile
   B. Concentrate bile
   C. Contracts to release bile into duodenum
9. True
10. Duodenal papilla
11. True
12. False (duct of Wirsung)
13. Anteriorly
14. 1. C

   2. A
   3. C
   4. C
15. A. Left hepatic duct
    B. Common hepatic duct
    C. Common bile duct
    D. Pancreatic duct (duct of Wirsung)
    E. Hepatopancreatic ampulla (ampulla of Vater)
    F. Duodenal papilla (papilla of Vater)
    G. Duodenum
    H. Fundus of gallbladder
    I. Body of gallbladder
    J. Neck of gallbladder
    K. Cystic duct
    L. Right hepatic duct
16. A. No ionizing radiation
    B. Better detection of small calculi
    C. No contrast media required
    D. Less patient preparation
17. Study of both the gallbladder and the biliary ducts
18. D. Nuclear medicine (NM)
19. True
20. 1. C
    2. D
    3. F
    4. A
    5. E
    6. B

Review Exercise B: Specific Anatomy of the Upper Gastrointestinal System

1. A. Mouth
   B. Pharynx
   C. Esophagus
   D. Stomach
   E. Small intestine
   F. Large intestine
   G. Anus
2. A. Salivary glands
   B. Pancreas
   C. Liver
   D. Gallbladder
3. A. Intake and digestion of food
   B. Absorption of digested food particles
   C. Elimination of solid waste products
4. Esophagography or barium swallow
5. Upper gastrointestinal (UGI) series or upper GI
6. A. Parotid

   B. Sublingual
   C. Submandibular
7. Deglutition
8. A. Nasopharynx
   B. Oropharynx
   C. Laryngopharynx
9. A. Aortic arch
   B. Left primary bronchus
10. A. Esophagus
    B. Inferior vena cava
    C. Aorta
11. Duodenal bulb or cap
12. Duodenojejunal flexure (suspensory muscle of the duodenum or ligament of Treitz)
13. Retroperitoneal (or "behind peritoneum")
14. A. Tongue
    B. Oral cavity (mouth)
    C. Hard palate
    D. Soft palate
    E. Uvula
    F. Nasopharynx
    G. Oropharynx
    H. Epiglottis
    I. Laryngopharynx
    J. Larynx
    K. Esophagus
    L. Trachea
15. False (inferiorly and anteriorly)
16. A. Fundus
    B. Greater curvature
    C. Body
    D. Gastric canal
    E. Pyloric portion (pylorus)
    F. Pyloric orifice (or just pylorus)
    G. Angular notch (incisura angularis)
    H. Lesser curvature
    I. Esophagogastric junction (cardiac orifice)
    J. Cardiac antrum
    K. Cardiac notch (incisura cardiaca)
17. A. Fundus (labeled A on Fig. 12.3)
    B. Body (labeled C)
    C. Pylorus (labeled E)
18. Pyloric antrum and pyloric canal
19. Rugae
20. A. Supine
    B. Prone
    C. Erect
21. A. Pylorus (pyloric sphincter)
    B. Bulb or cap of duodenum

C. First (superior) portion of duodenum

D. Second (descending) portion of duodenum

E. Third (horizontal) portion of duodenum

F. Fourth (ascending) portion of duodenum

G. Head of pancreas

H. Duodenojejunal flexure

22. A. Head of pancreas
    B. C-loop of duodenum

23. A. Distal esophagus
    B. Area of esophagogastric junction (Cardiac orifice)
    C. Lesser curvature of stomach
    D. Angular notch (incisura angularis)
    E. Pyloric region of stomach
    F. Pyloric orifice (pyloric sphincter)
    G. Duodenal bulb
    H. Second (descending) portion of duodenum
    I. Body of stomach
    J. Greater curvature of stomach
    K. Mucosal folds or rugae of stomach
    L. Fundus of stomach

Review Exercise C: Mechanical and Chemical Digestion and Body Habitus

1. True
2. A. Pharynx
3. Chyme
4. Rhythmic segmentation
5. A. Carbohydrates
   B. Proteins
   C. Lipids (fats)
6. Enzymes
7. A. Simple sugars
   B. Fatty acids and glycerol
   C. Amino acids
8. Bile
9. Large fat droplets are broken down to small fat droplets, which have greater surface area (to volume) and give enzymes greater access for the breakdown of lipids.
10. A. Small intestine
    B. Stomach
11. Carbohydrates
12. Large intestine
13. Mechanical
14. Chyme
15. A. Hypersthenic
16. C. Hyposthenic/asthenic

17. 1–2 inches (2.5–5 cm)
18. A. Stomach
    B. Gallbladder
19. Inferior, because of its proximity to the diaphragm
20. 1. A, B
    2. B
    3. B, C
    4. C, D
    5. C, E

Review Exercise D: Contrast Media, Fluoroscopy, and Clinical Indications and Contraindications for Upper Gastrointestinal Studies

1. True
2. Radiolucent contrast medium
3. Calcium or magnesium citrate
4. Barium sulfate
5. Suspension (colloidal)
6. True
7. True
8. One part water to one part barium sulfate (1 : 1 ratio)
9. $BaSO_4$
10. When the mixture may escape into the peritoneal cavity
11. Sensitivity to iodine
12. Better coating and visibility of the mucosa. Polyps, diverticula, and ulcers are better demonstrated.
13. Motility
14. It forces the barium sulfate against the mucosa for better coating.
15. C. CCD (charge-coupled device)
16. C. Bucky slot shield
17. By moving the Bucky tray all the way to the end of the table
18. B. 0.5 mm Pb/Eq apron
19. C. Reduces exposure to arms and hands of the fluoroscopist
20. Leaded glove
21. A. Time
    B. Distance
    C. Shielding
22. Distance
23. A. Optional postfluoroscopy overhead images
    B. Multiple frames formatting and multiple original images
    C. Cine loop capability
    D. Image enhancement and manipulation
24. Cine loop capability
25. A. 7
    B. 5
    C. 6

D. 3
E. 2
F. 1
G. 4

26. A. 4
    B. 5
    C. 8
    D. 3
    E. 7
    F. 1
    G. 6
    H. 2

27. A. 5
    B. 6
    C. 7
    D. 3
    E. 2
    F. 8
    G. 4
    H. 1

28. Endoscopy
29. Antral muscle at the orifice of the pylorus
30. Diagnostic medical sonography (DMS)

Review Exercise E: Patient Preparation and Positioning for Esophagography and Upper Gastrointestinal Study

1. Literally stands for *non per os*, a Latin phrase meaning "nothing by mouth"
2. False (8 hours NPO for an upper GI but not for esophagography)
3. True
4. Barium-soaked cotton balls, barium pills, or marshmallows followed by thin barium
5. A. Breathing exercises
   B. Water test
   C. Compression (paddle) technique
   D. Toe-touch maneuver
6. Valsalva maneuver
7. LPO (slight)
8. Esophagogastric junction
9. Oral, water-soluble iodinated contrast media
10. 8 hours
11. Both activities tend to increase gastric secretions
12. D. All of the above
13. Left hand
14. Newborn to 1 year: 2–4 ounces
    1–3 years: 4–6 ounces
    3–10 years: 6–12 ounces
    >10 years: 12–16 ounces

539

15. Pulsed, grid-controlled fluor-oscopy (to reduce dose for all patients, but especially for children)
16. D. Endoscopy
17. B. Radionuclides
18. Places the esophagus between the vertebral column and heart
19. 35–40 degrees
20. Optional cervicothoracic (Swimmer's) lateral
21. A. RAO
    B. Left lateral
    C. AP
22. B. Pylorus of stomach and C-loop
23. C. 40–70 degrees
24. 110 to 125 kVp
25. Body and pylorus of stomach and duodenal bulb
26. To prevent superimposition of the pylorus over the duodenal bulb, and to visualize better the lesser and greater curvatures of the stomach
27. C. 35–45 degrees cephalad
28. B. Lateral
29. 90–100 kVp range
30. Upright (erect)
31. A. RAO
    B. PA
    C. Right lateral
    D. LPO
    E. AP
32. Left upper quadrant (LUQ)
33. Right
34. False (expiration)

Review Exercise F: Problem Solving for Technical and Positioning Errors

1. When using thin barium, have the patient drink continuously during the exposure. With thick barium, have the patient hold two or three spoonful in the mouth and make the exposure immediately after swallowing.
2. When using barium sulfate as a contrast medium, 100–125 kVp should be used to ensure proper penetration of the contrast-filled stomach and to visualize the mucosa; 90–100 kVp would be adequate for a double-contrast study.
3. AP. Because the fundus is more posterior than the body or pylorus, it will fill with barium

when the patient is in a supine (AP) position.
4. With a hypersthenic patient, more rotation (≤70 degrees) may be required to profile the duodenal bulb better. (Note: The radiologist under fluoroscopic guidance will frequently move the patient as needed for the overhead oblique to best profile the duodenal region. Observe the degree of rotation of the body required to profile the stomach during fluoroscopy.)
5. The LPO position (recumbent) produces an image in which the fundus and body are filled with barium but the duodenal bulb is air filled.
6. Upper GI series
7. Oral, water-soluble contrast media should be used for an upper GI when a ruptured viscus or bowel is suspected (not barium sulfate, which is not water soluble).
8. With radiolucent foreign bodies in the esophagus, shredded cotton soaked in barium sulfate may be used to help locate them. But today, most foreign body studies of the esophagus are located and removed through endoscopy.
9. Would center these lower than usual, to the mid-L3 to L4 region, or about 1½–2 inches (4–5 cm) above the level of the iliac crest
10. A mass of undigested material that gets trapped in the stomach; a rare condition that can be diagnosed with an upper GI study
11. Underrotation of the body into the RAO position led to the esophagus being superimposed over the vertebral column. An increase in rotation of the body during the repeat exposure will separate the esophagus from the spine.
12. Angle the CR 20–25 degrees cephalad to open up the body and pylorus of the stomach.
13. The lateral position best demonstrates a gastric diverticulum located in the posterior region of the stomach.

14. Nuclear medicine is an effective modality in detecting Barrett esophagus.
15. Hemochromatosis is a condition of abnormal iron deposits in the liver parenchyma. MR is an effective imaging modality in diagnosing this condition.

CHAPTER 13

Review Exercise A: Radiographic Anatomy of the Lower Gastrointestinal System

1. A. 23 feet, or 7 m
   B. 15–18 feet, or 4.5–5.5 m
   C. 5 feet, or 1.5 m
2. A. Duodenum
   B. Jejunum
   C. Ileum
3. Duodenum
4. LUQ and LLQ
5. Jejunum
6. Ileum
7. Cecum and rectum
8. Four sections; two flexures
9. A. Prevents contents of the ileum from passing too quickly into cecum
   B. Prevents reflux back into the ileum
10. Vermiform appendix
11. 1. H
    2. F
    3. D
    4. B
    5. C
    6. I
    7. E
    8. A
    9. G
12. A. *Taeniae coli*
    B. Haustra
13. Plicae circulares
14. A. Vermiform appendix (appendix)
    B. Cecum
    C. Ileocecal valve (sphincter)
    D. Ascending colon
    E. Right colic (hepatic) flexure
    F. Transverse colon
    G. Left colic (splenic) flexure
    H. Descending colon
    I. Sigmoid colon
    J. Rectum
    K. Anal canal
    L. Anus
    M. Sacrum
    N. Coccyx

O. Anal canal
P. Anus
Q. Rectal ampulla
R. Rectum
15. Jejunum
16. Ileum
17. Ileum
18. Duodenojejunal flexure
19. Right lower quadrant (RLQ)
20. Suspensory muscle of the duodenum or ligament of Treitz (This site is a reference point for certain small bowel exams because it remains in a relatively fixed position.)
21. Cecum
22. Left colic (splenic)
23. Appendicitis
24. B. Transverse colon
    D. Sigmoid colon
25. A. Small intestine
26. C. Large intestine
27. A. Peristalsis
28. A. Duodenum
    B. Region of suspensory ligament (Ligament of Treitz) of duodenum/duodenojejunal flexure
    C. Jejunum
    D. Ileum
    E. Region of ileocecal sphincter (valve)
29. A. Cecum
    B. Ascending colon
    C. Right colic (hepatic) flexure
    D. Transverse colon
    E. Left colic (splenic) flexure
    F. Descending colon
    G. Sigmoid colon
    H. Rectum
30. 1. A
    2. B
    3. A
    4. B
    5. A
    6. B
    7. C
    8. B
    9. A
    10. A

Review Exercise B: Clinical Indications and Radiographic Procedures for the Small Bowel Series and Barium Enema

1. D. All of the above
2. A. Possible perforated hollow viscus
   B. Large bowel obstruction
3. Young and dehydrated

4. A. 3
   B. 8
   C. 1
   D. 4
   E. 2
   F. 6
   G. 5
   H. 7
5. A. 3
   B. 5
   C. 1
   D. 4
   E. 2
   F. 6
6. D. All of the above
7. D. Nuclear medicine
8. B. Proximal small intestine
9. 2 cups or 16 ounces
10. When the contrast medium passes through the ileocecal valve
11. 2 hours
12. 15–30 minutes after ingesting the contrast medium
13. True
14. Double-contrast method
15. High-density barium sulfate and air or methylcellulose
16. Regional enteritis (Crohn disease) and malabsorption syndromes
17. False (24 hours)
18. A. Duodenojejunal flexure (suspensory ligament)
19. It dilates the intestinal lumen to produce a more diagnostic study.
20. C. Therapeutic intubation
21. NPO for at least 8 hours before procedure; no smoking or gum chewing
22. Prone. To separate the loops of intestine
23. A. 4
    B. 2
    C. 6
    D. 5
    E. 3
    F. 1
24. Infant (<2 years of age)
25. Diverticulosis
26. C. Volvulus
27. A. Ulcerative colitis
28. C. Adenocarcinoma
29. False
30. True
31. False
32. True
33. A. Gross bleeding
    B. Severe diarrhea

C. Obstruction
   D. Inflammatory lesions
34. False (castor oil is an irritant cathartic)
35. A. Plastic disposable
    B. Rectal retention
    C. Air-contrast retention
36. True
37. Warm temperature (85°F–90°F; 29°C–32°C)
38. B. Lidocaine
39. Left lateral recumbent position
40. C. Umbilicus
41. B. Double-contrast barium enema
42. C. Anorectal angle
43. C. Rectal prolapse
44. C. Evacuative proctogram
45. D. Lateral
46. True
47. False (not more than 24 inches (60 cm) above tabletop when beginning the procedure)
48. True
49. True
50. False
51. B. 0.1% barium sulfate suspension is often instilled before the procedure
52. Virtual colonoscopy
53. False
54. C. To mark or "tag" fecal matter
55. A. Cannot remove polyps discovered during CTC

Review Exercise C: Positioning of the Lower Gastrointestinal System

1. False
2. D. Prone posteroanterior (PA)
3. True
4. Every 20–30 minutes
5. False (generally should not be removed until after overhead projections are completed unless directed to do so by the radiologist)
6. Ventral decubitus
7. 110–125 kVp
8. C. 2 inches (5 cm) above iliac crest
9. Make exposure on expiration
10. Ileocecal valve—large intestine
11. A. Hypersthenic
12. RAO or LPO
13. 35–45 degrees
14. RPO
15. Left lateral decubitus
16. Level of ASIS at the midcoronal plane

541

17. Right lateral decubitus (left side up)
18. Rectosigmoid region
19. Creates less superimposition of the rectosigmoid segments
20. A. Butterfly projections
    B. AP: CR angled 30–40 degrees cephalad
    C. PA: CR 30–40 degrees caudad
21. A. PA prone
22. 90–100 kVp
23. A. 110–125 kVp
    B. 90–100 kVp
24. Glucagon (review patient history before administration to ensure patient is not diabetic)

Review Exercise D: Problem Solving for Technical and Positioning Errors

1. PA prone. Because the transverse colon is an intraperitoneal aspect of the large intestine located more anteriorly, it will fill with barium in the PA prone position.
2. Even with the use of a wedge compensating filter, a reduction in kVp is required. Because less barium sulfate is used during an air-contrast procedure, the kVp range should be 90–100.
3. The CR was angled in the wrong direction. The AP axial projection requires a 30- to 40-degree cephalad angle.
4. Use two field sizes of 14 × 17 inches (35 × 43 cm) in landscape for the AP/PA and oblique projections, one centered higher and one lower. Because hypersthenic patients have a wider distribution of the large intestine, two landscape-placed cassettes will ensure that all of the pertinent anatomy is demonstrated.
5. Retention catheters should be fully inflated only by the radiologist under fluoroscopic guidance.
6. Lie on left side and flex head and upper body forward, drawing the right leg up above the partially flexed left leg.
7. Enteroclysis, which is a double-contrast small bowel procedure. A routine small bowel series may also demonstrate this condition, but the enteroclysis with double contrast is more effective in demonstrating mucosal

changes. A CT enteroclysis may provide further evidence of obstruction or narrowing of the small intestine.
8. Because the patient is having surgery soon after the small bowel series, a water-soluble, iodinated contrast medium should be used. Barium sulfate should not be administered to presurgical patients.
9. A diagnostic intubation small bowel series is preferred. A nasogastric tube is passed into the small intestine, allowing the contrast medium to be instilled. This procedure is effective for patients who cannot swallow.
10. A barium enema or air enema often leads to re-expansion of the telescoped aspect of the large intestine.
11. Inform the radiologist and have him or her insert the tip under fluoroscopic guidance.
12. RAO or LPO projections
13. A small bowel series (Enteritis is an inflammation or infection of the small intestine.)
14. A small bowel series (Giardiasis is a parasitic infection of the small intestine.)
15. The patient should undergo a cleansing bowel preparation. The morning of the procedure, food intake should be limited to clear liquids. The patient should wear loose-fitting clothing without any metal snaps or clips.

CHAPTER 14

Review Exercise A: Radiographic Anatomy of the Urinary System

1. D. Retroperitoneal
2. Suprarenal (adrenal) glands
3. Psoas major muscles
4. Perirenal fat or adipose capsule
5. 30 degrees
6. Xiphoid process and iliac crest
7. Nephroptosis
8. A. Remove nitrogenous waste
   B. Regulate water levels
   C. Regulate acid-base balance and electrolyte levels in the blood
9. B. Uremia
10. Hilum
11. Cortex

12. Renal parenchyma
13. Nephron
14. False (afferent)
15. Bowman capsule
16. False (located in the cortex)
17. Renal pyramids
18. A. Renal pelvis
    B. Major calyx
    C. Minor calyx
    D. Renal sinuses
    E. Cortex
    F. Medulla
    G. Ureter
19. A. Loop of Henle, medulla
    B. Distal convoluted tubule, cortex
    C. Afferent arteriole, cortex
    D. Efferent arteriole, cortex
    E. Glomerular capsule, cortex
    F. Proximal convoluted tubule, cortex
    G. Descending limb, medulla
    H. Ascending limb, medulla
    I. Collecting tubule, medulla
20. A. Peristalsis
    B. Gravity
21. C. Urinary bladder
22. Ureterovesical junction (UVJ)
23. Trigone
24. Prostate gland
25. C. 350 to 500 mL
26. D. Kidneys
27. A. Minor calyces
    B. Major calyces
    C. Renal pelvis
    D. Ureteropelvic junction (UPJ)
    E. Proximal ureter
    F. Distal ureter
    G. Urinary bladder

Review Exercise B: Venipuncture

1. A. Bolus by hand injection, bolus by power injector
   B. Drip infusion
2. True
3. D. Antecubital fossa
4. C. 18–22 gauge
5. Butterfly and over-the-needle catheter
6. 1. Wash hands and put on gloves.
   2. Select site, apply tourniquet, and cleanse the site.
   3. Initiate puncture.
   4. Confirm entry and secure needle.
   5. Prepare and proceed with injection.
   6. Remove needle or catheter.

542

Answers to Review Questions

Copyright © 2025 by Elsevier Inc.
All rights are reserved, including those for text and data mining, AI training, and similar technologies.

7. False (facing upward)
8. False (The needle should be withdrawn and pressure applied.)
9. True
10. False (The technologist or person performing the venipuncture is responsible.)

Review Exercise C: Contrast Media and Urography

1. A. N
   B. N
   C. I
   D. I
   E. I
   F. N
   G. N
   H. I
   I. N
   J. I
2. A. Diatrizoate or iothalamate
3. D. Chemotoxic theory
4. 60 mL/min or greater
5. 0.6 and 1.5 mg/dL
6. 8 and 25 mg/100 mL
7. A. Diabetes mellitus
   B. 48 hours
8. Extravasation (infiltration)
9. A. Local
   B. Systemic
10. Anaphylactic reaction
11. Vasovagal reaction
12. False
13. A. 3
    B. 2
    C. 2
    D. 1
    E. 3
    F. 3
    G. 3
    H. 3
    I. 1
14. True
15. False (the term for hives)
16. C. Severe
17. A. 4
    B. 1
    C. 3
    D. 4
    E. 2
    F. 2
    G. 1
    H. 4
    I. 4
    J. 5
    K. 3
18. Call for medical assistance
19. To reduce the severity of contrast media reactions

20. C. Combination of Benadryl and prednisone
21. B. Asthmatic patient
22. Elevate the affected extremity or use a cold compress followed by a warm compress
23. False—peaks 24–48 hours after extravasation
24. True
25. A. Hypersensitivity to iodinated contrast media
    B. Anuria
    C. Multiple myeloma
    D. Diabetes mellitus
    E. Severe hepatic or renal disease
    F. Congestive heart failure
    G. Pheochromocytoma
    H. Sickle cell anemia
    I. Patients taking metformin or similar medication
    J. Renal failure, acute or chronic

Review Exercise D: Radiographic Procedures, Pathologic Terms, and Clinical Indications

1. Lasix (Furosemide)
2. A. An IVP (intravenous pyelogram) is a study of the renal pelvis (hence, *pyelo-*).
   B. Intravenous urogram (IVU)
3. The collecting system of the kidney (minor and major calyces, renal pelvis, and proximal ureters)
4. C. Hematuria
5. A. Pheochromocytoma
6. A. 5
   B. 8
   C. 3
   D. 10
   E. 1
   F. 11
   G. 12
   H. 4
   I. 2
   J. 7
   K. 9
   L. 6
7. A. 7
   B. 4
   C. 8
   D. 1
   E. 5
   F. 2
   G. 3
   H. 6
8. A. 5
   B. 7

   C. 8
   D. 3
   E. 2
   F. 1
   G. 4
   H. 6
9. Angioedema
10. Bronchospasm
11. Syncope
12. Urticaria
13. Staghorn calculi
14. True
15. To enhance filling of the renal pelvic-calyceal system and proximal ureters with contrast media
16. A. Possible ureteric stones
    B. Abdominal mass
    C. Abdominal aortic aneurysm
    D. Recent abdominal surgery
    E. Severe abdominal pain
    F. Acute abdominal trauma
17. At the start of the injection of contrast media
18. A. 1-minute nephrogram
    B. 5-minute full KUB
    C. 10- to 15-minute full KUB
    D. 20-minute posterior R and L oblique positions
    E. Postvoid (prone PA or erect AP)
19. An IVU introduces contrast via venipuncture whereas a retrograde urography introduces contrast directly into the pelvicalyceal system via a catheter.
20. Surgery (inpatient or outpatient facility)
21. False (nonfunctional exam)
22. False (used for males only)
23. D. All of the above
24. C. Magnetic resonance imaging (MR)
25. True
26. True
27. Height and weight
28. True
29. A. MR
30. True

Review Exercise E: Radiographic Positioning of the Urinary System

1. The prostate gland will indent the floor of the bladder.
2. Just medial to the ASIS and lateral to the spine (placed over the outer pelvic brim)
3. Place the patient in a 15-degree Trendelenburg position.

4. Renal pelvis, major and minor calyces of the kidneys
5. A. Verify patient preparation
   B. Determine whether exposure factors are acceptable
   C. Verify positioning
   D. Detect any abnormal calcifications
6. A. Primarily the ureters
7. 30-degree RPO
8. 80–85 kVp
9. False (both an AP erect and a supine IVU image have a recommended 40-inch SID)
10. False (the CR is at the iliac crest)
11. Symmetry of iliac wings and rib cage
12. True. The recommended collimation field size for a nephrogram is 10 × 12 inches (24 × 30 cm) and an AP scout is 14 × 17 inches (35 × 43 cm)
13. D. Within 1 minute after injection
14. B. Midway between the xiphoid process and the iliac crest
15. RPO
16. 30 degrees
17. Erect position
18. C. 10–15 degrees caudad
19. True

Review Exercise F: Problem Solving for Technical and Positioning Errors

1. A second projection of the bladder should be taken, using a smaller field size placed in landscape orientation to include this region. The larger field size should be centered 1 or 2 inches (2–5 cm) higher to include the upper abdomen.
2. Too long a delay between the injection of contrast media and the imaging of the nephrogram. The nephrogram needs to be taken ≤60 seconds after injection.
3. Decrease the obliquity of the RPO to ≤30 degrees.
4. Place the pneumatic paddles just medial to the ASIS to allow for compression of the distal ureters against the pelvic brim.
5. Increase caudad angulation of the central ray to project the symphysis pubis below the bladder. The typical CR angle is 10–15 degrees caudad.

6. Decrease the time span between projections to capture all phases of the urinary system. (Take images at 1, 2, and 3 minutes rather than at 1, 5, and 15 minutes.)
7. The technologist should not perform the compression phase of the study. Ureteric compression is contraindicated when an abdominal aortic aneurysm is suspected. (The technologist should consult with the radiologist or physician.)
8. The erect prevoid AP projection will best demonstrate an enlarged prostate gland.
9. Ultrasound, CT, or nuclear medicine scan
10. CT is preferred, but a nuclear medicine procedure could also be performed.
11. The patient should be asked whether he is taking metformin or similar medication to control diabetes. If the response is yes, document and inform the radiologist of the patient's condition and medication history before injection. The referring physician may be asked to check kidney function before the patient resumes this medication.
12. These are expected side effects, and the technologist should reassure the patient. No medical treatment is required.
13. Although the technologist should inform the radiologist or injecting technologist of the blood chemistry levels, both BUN, creatinine, and eGFR levels are within the normal range.

CHAPTER 15

Review Exercise A: Mobile X-Ray Equipment and Radiation Protection

1. A. Battery operated, battery-driven type
   B. Standard AC power source, nonmotor drive
2. True
3. 8 hours
4. Standard power source, nonmotor drive
5. C-arm

6. A. X-ray tube
   B. Image intensifier
7. Because it results in a significant increase in exposure to the head, eyes, and neck region of the operator, and increases the OID, resulting in decreased image resolution and increased scatter.
8. A. Intensifier side
   B. The radiation field pattern extends out farther on the x-ray tube side.
9. Left monitor
10. True
11. True
12. Four
13. False (can be used)
14. Roadmapping
15. C. 50–100 mR/h
16. A. 5 mR (60 mR ÷ 60 minutes = 1 mR × 5 minutes = 5)
17. B. 25 mR/h
18. 67 mR (400 ÷ 60 × 10 = 67)
19. C. 100–300 mR/h
20. False (reduces exposure to patient)

Review Exercise B: Skeletal Trauma and Fracture Terminology

1. Adaptation
2. Move the CR and IR around the patient to produce similar projections rather than moving the patient.
3. Two. Two projections should be taken 90 degrees to each other.
4. Two. Both joints must be included on the initial study.
5. False (must include at least one joint nearest injury)
6. True
7. True
8. False (It is important to rotate the x-ray tube and image receptor around patients if they are unable to move.)
9. Dislocation
10. A. Shoulder
    B. Fingers or thumb
    C. Patella
    D. Hip
11. Subluxation
12. Sprain
13. Contusion
14. Alignment
15. Bayonet apposition
16. A. Varus (deformity) angulation
    B. A lateral apex

17. A simple fracture does not break through the skin, but a compound fracture protrudes through the skin.
18. A. Torus fracture
    B. Greenstick fracture (hickory or willow stick fracture)
19. Butterfly fracture
20. Impacted fracture
21. A. Chauffeur's
    B. Mallet
    C. Open
    D. Ping-pong
    E. Closed
22. False. (A chip fracture involves an isolated fracture not associated with a tendon or ligament.)
23. Closed reduction
24. 1. G
    2. H
    3. A
    4. I
    5. D
    6. J
    7. B
    8. M
    9. L
    10. N
    11. F
    12. O
    13. E
    14. K
    15. C
25. A. Colles fracture
    B. Distal radius, posterior displacement of distal fragment
    C. Fall on outstretched arm
26. A. Pott fracture
    B. Distal fibula and occasionally the distal tibia or medial malleolus

Review Exercise C: Trauma and Mobile Positioning and Procedures

1. Centered 3–4 inches (8–10 cm) below jugular notch, angled caudad so as to be perpendicular to sternum
2. A. Landscape
   B. To prevent cutoff of the right or left lateral margins of the chest. More important with portable chests because of increased divergence of x-ray beam at the shorter SID.
3. False (not recommended because of probable grid cutoff)

4. 15- to 20-degree LPO
5. Landscape
6. 30- to 40-degree cross-angled mediolateral projection (Note: This results in image distortion and should be done as a last resort.)
7. A. Left lateral decubitus
8. D. Dorsal decubitus
9. Increased OID of the thumb (increases distortion of the CMC joint)
10. PA and lateral projections
11. True
12. True
13. AP and horizontal beam, transthoracic lateral or AP oblique (scapular Y) projection
14. A horizontal beam transthoracic lateral or an AP oblique (Scapular Y) projection
15. A. 25–30
16. B. 15 degrees
17. C. 10 degrees posteriorly from perpendicular to the plantar surface (Note: This would also be 10 degrees posteriorly from the plane of IR.)
18. Angle the CR 15–20 degrees lateromedially to the long axis of the foot. (perpendicular to the intermalleolar plane)
19. AP and horizontal beam lateral with no flexion of the knee
20. 45-degree lateromedial cross-angle AP projection of the knee and proximal tibia/fibula
21. A. Danelius-Miller (inferosuperior, axiolateral) method
22. Direct horizontal CR perpendicular to the femoral neck and to the plane of the IR
23. D. Fuchs method (Review Chapter 8 for details)
24. Cervicothoracic projection (Swimmer's lateral) using a horizontal beam CR
25. D. 35- to 40-degree cephalad axial projection (CR parallel to MML)
26. AP axial trauma oblique projections
27. A. 45 degrees lateromedial
    B. 15 degrees cephalad
28. False. A grid cannot be used for this projection because of the double angulation.
29. C. Horizontal beam lateral skull

30. C. AP axial, CR 15 degrees cephalad to OML
31. False (should not exceed 45 degrees)
32. True
33. Parallel to the mentomeatal line, centered to acanthion
34. 25–30 degrees cephalad and possibly 5–10 degrees posterior to clear the shoulder
35. D. PA or AP and horizontal beam lateral forearm
36. A. Pediatric
37. A. AP and horizontal beam lateral lower leg
38. C. Stellate fracture

Review Exercise D: Surgical Radiography

1. A. Confidence
   B. Mastery
   C. Problem-solving skills
   D. Communication
2. 1. E
   2. A
   3. B
   4. D
   5. F
   6. C
3. False
4. False (The technologist is responsible to ensure radiation safety in the OR.)
5. True
6. False. Only sterile items are permitted to be on a sterile field.
7. D. Surgical asepsis
8. C. The shoulders to the level of the sterile field, as well as the sleeve from the cuff to just above the elbow
9. False
10. A. Drape the image intensifier, x-ray tube, and C-arm using a sterile cloth and/or bag.
    B. Drape the patient or surgery site with an additional sterile cloth before the undraped C-arm is positioned over the anatomy.
    C. Maintain the sterile area by using a "shower curtain."
11. False
12. True
13. True
14. False
15. Aerosol
16. Can add to patient dose and to the surrounding surgical team

545

17. Brighter image
18. Distance
19. A. Time
    B. Distance
    C. Shielding
20. C. Use intermittent or "foot-tap-ping" fluoroscopy
21. Biliary ductal system
22. "Pizza pan"
23. Landscape orientation to prevent grid cutoff
24. 6–8 mL
25. A. Can be performed as an out-patient procedure
    B. Less-invasive procedure
    C. Reduced hospital time and cost
26. A. Right hepatic duct
    B. Left hepatic duct
    C. Common hepatic duct
    D. Common bile duct
    E. Duodenum
27. D. Retrograde pyelogram
28. B. Modified lithotomy position
29. C. Closed reduction
30. D. Ilizarov device
31. A. Cannulated screw assembly
32. A. Intramedullary nail
33. Modular bipolar hip prostheses
34. Laminectomy
35. Interbody fusion cages
36. Supine
37. A. Harrington rods
    B. Luque rods
38. A. 4
    B. 5
    C. 3
    D. 8
    E. 9
    F. 10
    G. 7
    H. 2
    I. 1
    J. 6
39. A. Compression fracture of the vertebral body

CHAPTER 16

Review Exercise A: Immobilization, Ossification, Radiation Protection, Pre-Exam Preparation, and Clinical Indications

1. A. Technologist's attitude and approach to a child
   B. Technical preparation of the room
2. A. Serve as an observer in the room to lend support and comfort to the child.
   B. Serve as a participator to assist with immobilization.
   C. Remain in the waiting room, and do not accompany the child into the room.
3. False (may be permissible with proper lead shielding if not pregnant)
4. True
5. True
6. Pigg-O-Stat
7. Erect chest and abdomen studies
8. It can damage the skin.
9. A. Twisting the tape so that the adhesive surface is not against the skin
   B. Placing a gauze pad between the tape and the skin
10. 1. Place the sheet on the table folded in half or thirds portrait.
    2. Place patient in middle of sheet with the right arm down to the side. Fold sheet across the patient's body and pull sheet across the body, keeping the arm against the body.
    3. Place the patient's left arm along the side of the body and on top of the sheet. Bring the free sheet over the left arm to the right side of the body. Wrap the sheet around the body as needed.
    4. Pull the sheet tightly so that the patient cannot free arms.
11. Diaphysis
12. Epiphyses
13. Metaphysis
14. 1. Forensic
    2. Pathology
    3. Determine future growth potential
15. Single PA; Left hand or wrist
16. B. 3–14 months
17. 1. Greulich-Pyle (GP)
    2. Tanner-Whitehouse (TW)
18. 1. Neglect
    2. Physical abuse
    3. Sexual abuse
    4. Psychological maltreatment
    5. Medical neglect
19. Multiple and posterior fractures are an indication of a child being held up under the axillae and shaken.
20. A. Proper immobilization
    B. Short exposure times
    C. Accurate manual technique charts
21. A. Close collimation
    B. Low-dosage techniques
    C. Minimum number of exposures
22. 1. B
    2. A
    3. B
    4. A
    5. B
    6. A
23. False (These items may cause artifacts and should be removed.)
24. False
25. 4–4 ½ inches (10–12 cm), unless using virtual grid software
26. True
27. A. Diagnostic medical sono-graphy (DMS)
28. A. Diagnostic medical sono-graphy (DMS)
29. C. Hydrocephalus
30. A. 4
    B. 2
    C. 7
    D. 1
    E. 3
    F. 5
    G. 6
31. A. 6
    B. 7
    C. 4
    D. 8
    E. 2
    F. 1
    G. 3
    H. 5
32. A. 5
    B. 1
    C. 6
    D. 3
    E. 7
    F. 2
    G. 4
33. A. (-)
    B. (-)
    C. (-)
34. C. Dark green secretion of the liver and intestinal glands mixed with amniotic fluid
35. True

Answers to Review Questions

Copyright © 2025 by Elsevier Inc.
All rights are reserved, including those for text and data mining, AI training, and similar technologies.

Review Exercise B: Pediatric Positioning of the Chest, Skeletal System, and Skull

1. True
2. A. Nongrid
   B. 75–85 kVp
   C. Landscape
   D. 50–60 inches (125–150 cm)
   E. 72 inches (180 cm)
3. 80–85 kVp
4. No
5. 2–4
6. As the child fully inhales and holds his or her breath
7. The sternoclavicular joints and lateral rib margins should be equidistant from the vertebral column.
8. Horizontally
9. False (9–10)
10. True
11. True
12. A. 1
    B. 2
    C. 1
    D. 2
    E. 1
13. Bilateral frog-leg
14. AP and lateral feet, Kite method
15. False (Take two projections 90 degrees from each other.)
16. False
17. Base selection on the size of the anatomy (10 × 12 inches or 24 × 30 cm, if the skull is near adult size)
18. A. 15 degrees cephalad to OML
19. C. Craniosynostosis
20. B. OML
21. False
22. True
23. A. Mammillary (nipple) line
    B. 1 inch (2.5 cm) above umbilicus
    C. At level of iliac crest
    D. Glabella

Review Exercise C: Positioning of the Pediatric Abdomen and Contrast Media Procedures

1. Vesicoureteral reflux
2. False (Retention tips should not be used on small children.)
3. Air for the pneumatic reduction of intussusception
4. 24 inches (60 cm) (for pediatric patients unless otherwise directed by the radiologist)
5. True

6. False (Most bony landmarks are nonexistent in infants.)
7. True
8. False (Contrast is low)
9. A. 4 hours
   B. 3 hours
   C. No prep required
   D. 4 hours (solid food)
10. A. Hirschsprung disease
    B. Extensive diarrhea
    C. Appendicitis
    D. Obstruction
    E. Dehydration (patients who cannot withstand fluid loss)
11. The following indicators apply: B, C, D, F, G
12. 1 inch (2.5 cm) above the umbilicus
13. A. 60–75 kVp
    B. 4–4 ½ inches (10–12 cm), unless using virtual grid software
14. C. Dorsal decubitus abdomen
15. A. Wilms tumor
16. Urinary tract infection (UTI)
17. A. NEC
18. D. Acute abdomen series
19. True
20. A. Infants: 30–75 mL
    B. Adolescents: 480 mL
21. Insert a nasogastric tube into the stomach.
22. False (usually 1 hour)
23. False (Latex tips should not be used because of possible allergic response to latex.)
24. AP and oblique positions (LPO and RPO)
25. True

Review Exercise D: Problem Solving and Analysis

1. C. Have another (nonradiology) health professional hold the child and have the guardian wait outside the room.
2. B. Pigg-O-Stat
3. A. AP and lateral upper airway
4. D. Chest
5. C. AP and lateral hip
6. A. Foot
7. C. AP and lateral foot—Kite method
8. D. Barium enema
9. D. Upper GI
10. A. Functional MRI (fMRI)

CHAPTER 17

Review Exercise A: Radiographic Anatomy

1. A. Cardiovascular
   B. Lymphatic
2. A. Heart
   B. Blood vessels
   C. Heart to lungs
   D. Throughout the body
3. A. Transportation of oxygen, nutrients, hormones, and chemicals
   B. Removal of waste products
   C. Maintenance of body temperature, water, and electrolyte balance
4. A. Heart
   B. Artery
   C. Arteriole
   D. Capillary
   E. Venule
   F. Vein
5. B. (artery) and C. (arteriole)
6. E. (venule) and F. (vein)
7. 1. A. Red blood cells
      B. Transports oxygen
   2. A. White blood cells
      B. Defends against infection and disease
   3. A. (no other term given)
      B. Repairs tears in blood vessels and promotes blood clotting
8. A. 92%
   B. 7%
9. A. Right ventricle
   B. Left ventricle
   C. Left atrium
   D. Capillaries of left lung
   E. Pulmonary arteries
   F. Aorta (arch)
   G. Superior vena cava
   H. Capillaries of right lung
   I. Pulmonary veins
   J. Right atrium
   K. Inferior vena cava
10. A. Pulmonary arteries
    B. Pulmonary veins
11. A. Superior vena cava
    B. Inferior vena cava
    C. Right atrium
12. A. Tricuspid (right atrioventricular) valve
    B. Pulmonary (pulmonary semilunar) valve

547

C. Bicuspid (left atrioventricular or mitral) valve
   D. Aortic (aortic semilunar) valve
13. A. Right and left coronary arteries
   B. Aortic bulb (root)
14. A. Great cardiac vein
   B. Middle cardiac vein
   C. Small cardiac vein
15. A. Left subclavian
   B. Left common carotid
   C. Left vertebra
   D. Left internal carotid
   E. Right and left external carotid
   F. Right internal carotid
   G. Right vertebra
   H. Right common carotid
   I. Right subclavian
   J. Brachiocephalic
16. A. Right common carotid artery
   B. Left common carotid artery
   C. Right vertebral artery
   D. Left vertebral artery
17. A. Brachiocephalic artery
   B. Left common carotid artery
   C. Left subclavian artery
18. False (right common carotid and right subclavian)
19. True
20. Internal and external carotid
21. D. Carotid siphon
22. A. Anterior cerebral artery
   B. Middle cerebral artery
23. Anterior cerebral
24. Vertebrobasilar arteries
25. Basilar
26. Middle cerebral arteries
27. Lateral
28. A. Anterior cerebral artery
   B. Middle cerebral artery
   C. Internal cerebral artery
29. 1. Posterior cerebral arteries
   2. Posterior communicating arteries
   3. Middle cerebral arteries
   4. Anterior cerebral arteries
   5. Anterior communicating arteries
   6. A. Hypophysis (pituitary) gland
      B. Vertebral arteries
      C. Basilar
30. A. Right and left internal jugular veins
   B. Right and left external jugular veins
   C. Right and left vertebral veins

31. A. Brachiocephalic
   B. Superior vena cava; right atrium
32. True
33. A. Superior sagittal sinus
   B. Inferior sagittal sinus
   C. Straight sinus
   D. Transverse sinus
   E. Confluence of sinuses
   F. Occipital sinus
   G. Sigmoid sinus

Review Exercise B: Anatomy of Thoracic and Abdominal Arteries and Veins, Portal System, and Upper and Lower Arteries and Veins

1. A. Aortic bulb (root)
   B. Ascending aorta
   C. Aortic arch
   D. Descending aorta
2. A. Left circumflex
   B. Inverse aorta
   C. Pseudocoarctation
3. B. Azygos vein
4. 1. Celiac artery
   2. Superior mesenteric arteries
   3. Right renal arteries
   4. Left renal artery
   5. Inferior mesenteric artery
5. B. T12
6. A. Liver
   B. Spleen
   C. Stomach
   D. Left common iliac artery
   E. Left external iliac artery
   F. Left internal iliac artery
7. L4
8. A. Left external iliac vein
   B. Left internal iliac vein
   C. Inferior mesenteric vein
   D. Splenic vein
   E. (Inferior vena cava)
   F. Hepatic vein
   G. Hepatic portal vein
   H. Right renal vein
   I. Superior mesenteric vein
   J. Right common iliac vein
9. A. Superior mesenteric vein
   B. Splenic vein
   C. Hepatic portal vein
   D. Hepatic veins
   E. Inferior vena cava
10. A. Brachiocephalic
   B. Subclavian
   C. Axillary
   D. Brachial
   E. Radial
   F. Ulnar

11. A. Superficial palmar arch vein
   B. Deep palmar arch vein
   C. Median cubital
   D. Brachial
   E. Superior vena cava
   F. Subclavian
   G. Cephalic
12. Median cubital vein
13. A. External iliac
   B. Femoral
   C. Deep artery of thigh (profunda femoris)
   D. Lateral circumflex femoral
   E. Popliteal
   F. Dorsalis pedis
14. A. Dorsalis pedis (dorsal venous arch)
   B. Anterior tibial
   C. Great (long) saphenous
   D. Deep femoral (profunda femoris)
   E. Femoral
   F. External iliac
   G. Internal iliac
   H. Inferior vena cava
15. Great (long) saphenous vein

Review Exercise C: Angiographic Procedures, Equipment, and Supplies

1. B. Respiratory therapist
2. A. Vascular interventional (VI)
   B. Cardiac interventional (CI)
3. True
4. Seldinger technique
5. A. Insertion of compound (Seldinger) needle
   B. Placement of needle in lumen of vessel
   C. Insertion of guide wire
   D. Removal of needle
   E. Threading of catheter to area of interest
   F. Removal of guide wire
6. A. Femoral artery
7. C. Help the patient relax
8. Water-soluble, nonionic contrast media
9. 1. Bleeding at the puncture site
   2. Thrombus formation
   3. Embolus formation
   4. Dissection of a vessel
   5. Infection of puncture site
   6. Contrast media reaction
10. B. Just inferior to the inguinal ligament
11. C. 4 hours
12. D. 30 degrees
13. True

14. 1. Wrap-around lead aprons
    2. Thyroid shields
    3. Lead glasses
15. Oxygen and suction
16. A. Single
    B. Biplane
17. False (An island-type table is needed)
18. Overlying anatomic structures
19. A. Pixel-shifting or remasking
    B. Magnified or zooming
    C. Quantitative analysis of image to measure distances and to calculate stenosis
20. Length and diameter
21. A. To maintain temperature of contrast media at body temperature
    B. To reduce viscosity of the contrast media
22. True
23. False (does require iodinated contrast media)
24. True
25. False
26. True
27. False (does not require contrast media)
28. False (up to 180 degrees)
29. False
30. False

Review Exercise D: Interventional Imaging Procedures

1. A. Vascular stenosis and occlusions
   B. Aneurysms
   C. Trauma
   D. Arteriovenous malformations
   E. Neoplastic disease
2. Lateral
3. A. Common carotid arteries
   B. Internal carotid arteries
   C. External carotid arteries
   D. Vertebral arteries
4. A. Arterial
   B. Capillary
   C. Venous
5. A. Aneurysm
   B. Congenital abnormalities
   C. Vessel stenosis
   D. Embolus
   E. Trauma
6. False (CT has become the modality of choice for pulmonary emboli.)
7. A. Femoral vein
8. D. Femoral artery
9. A. Femoral vein

10. D. 30–50 mL
11. C. 45 degrees
12. A. Coronary arteries
13. Femoral vein
14. C. 15–30 frames per second
15. A. Ejection fraction
16. Venacavography
17. A. Aneurysm
    B. Congenital abnormality
    C. GI bleed
    D. Stenosis or occlusion
    E. Trauma
18. Femoral artery
19. A. Renal arteries
    B. Celiac artery
    C. Superior and inferior mesenteric arteries
20. True
21. D. Left subclavian artery
22. True
23. Radiologic procedures that intervene in disease process, providing a therapeutic outcome
24. B. Shorter hospital stays
25. False (primarily for treatment of disease)
26. False (performed primarily in angiographic/interventional suite)
27. Embolization of the uterine artery can shrink fibroids and eliminate associated pain and bleeding.
28. 1. A
    2. A
    3. B
    4. B
    5. A
    6. A
    7. B
    8. B
    9. A
    10. B
    11. B
    12. A
29. Through the right jugular vein
30. Vasoconstrictor
31. Endovascular retrieval devices (snare wire loop) snare
32. Kyphoplasty or vertebroplasty
33. Kyphoplasty balloon
34. Transluminal balloon catheter
35. Thrombolysis
36. D. Unresectable malignant disease
37. False (>80%)
38. True
39. D. Frictional heating

CHAPTER 18

Review Exercise A: Basic Principles of Computed Tomography

1. False. While it may still be commonly heard, it is not an accurate name.
2. Movement of the x-ray tube; design and construction of detectors.
3. A. Slip rings
4. True
5. False (multiple rotations possible)
6. True
7. D. Low-cost system to operate
8. C. Multiplanar reconstruction
9. B. Dual-source CT
10. A. Gantry
    B. Operator control console
    C. Computer
11. Gantry
12. Aperture
13. Cadmium tungstate or rare earth oxide ceramic crystals
14. A. Size of detector row
15. D. 262,144
16. A. Picture archiving and communication system
17. Attenuation of radiation by a given tissue
18. Volume element
19. Three, two
20. A. Slice thickness
21. B. Isotropic
22. Lower
23. Attenuation (Linear attenuation coefficient)
24. A. Cortical bone: +1000
    B. White brain matter: +45
    C. Blood: +20
    D. Fat: -100
    E. Lung tissue: –200
    F. Air: –1000
    G. Water: 0
25. Water
26. A. 1
    B. 2
    C. 3
    D. 1
27. B. Displayed image contrast
28. A. Image brightness
29. Amount of anatomy examined during a particular scan
30. Table speed and slice thickness
31. 2:1 pitch
32. A. Undersampling

33. C. 10-mm couch movement and 20-mm slice thickness
34. A. ≤1%
35. True
36. B. Power injector
37. False. A lower pitch results in a higher patient dose

Review Exercise B: Clinical Applications of Computed Tomography

1. A. Visualization of anatomic structures with no superimposition
   B. Increased contrast resolution between various types of soft tissue
   C. MPR (multiplanar reconstruction)
   D. Manipulation of attenuation data
2. B. Scout view
3. 50%–90%
4. False (4 minutes)
5. False (not able to pass through)
6. True
7. A. Proteins
8. True
9. False (lower pitch ratio leads to a higher dose)
10. D. Dose modulation
11. To strive to reduce dose to children during CT procedures through the application of accepted protocols, safety measures, and open dialogue with patients and the health care team.
12. True

Review Exercise C: Cranial Anatomy and Head CT Procedures

1. A. Brain
   B. Spinal cord
2. A. L1
   B. Conus medullaris
3. A needle can enter the subarachnoid space without damaging the spinal cord.
4. A. Dura mater
   B. Arachnoid mater
   C. Pia mater
   D. Epidural space
   E. Subdural space
   F. Subarachnoid space
5. Venous sinuses
6. A. Midbrain
   B. Pons
   C. Medulla

7. A. Tracts of myelinated axons of nerve cells
   B. Primarily dendrites and cell bodies
8. A. Gray
   B. White
9. A. Frontal lobe
   B. Parietal lobe
   C. Occipital lobe
   D. Temporal lobe
   E. Insula or central lobe
10. A. Cerebrum
    B. Thalamus
    C. Hypothalamus
    D. Cerebellum
    E. Pons
    F. Medulla (medulla oblongata)
11. A. Occipital lobe
    B. Parietal lobe
    C. Frontal lobe
    D. Longitudinal fissure
12. E. Anterior (precentral) central gyrus
    F. Central sulcus
    G. Posterior (postcentral) central gyrus
13. D. Corpus callosum
14. B. Longitudinal fissure
15. C. Choroid plexus
16. A. Cisterns
    B. Cistern cerebellomedullaris (Cisterna magna)
17. Brainstem
18. C. Thalamus
19. Hypothalamus
20. C. Pituitary
21. Infundibulum
22. B. Cerebellum
23. D. Hypothalamus
24. B. Pituitary gland
25. A. Caudate nucleus
    B. Lentiform nucleus
    C. Claustrum
    D. Amygdaloid nucleus
26. A. Lateral
    B. Third
    C. Fourth
    1. Posterior horn
    2. Body
    3. Anterior horn
    4. Interventricular foramen
    5. Cerebral aqueduct
    6. Inferior horn
    7. Lateral recess
    8. Pineal gland
27. A. Olfactory
    B. Optic
    C. Oculomotor
    D. Trochlear

E. Trigeminal
F. Abducens
G. Facial
H. Acoustic (Vestibulocochlear)
I. Glossopharyngeal
J. Vagus
K. Spinal accessory
L. Hypoglossal
28. A. Narrow window (soft tissue and brain tissue visualized)
    B. Wide window (bony detail visualized)
29. Rotation, tilt
30. Subdural hematoma
31. A. Anterior corpus callosum-genu
    B. Anterior horn of left lateral ventricle
    C. Head of caudate nucleus
    D. Region of thalamus
    E. Third ventricle
    F. Superior sagittal sinus
    G. Posterior horn of left lateral ventricle
32. A. Anterior corpus callosum-genu
    B. Anterior horn of left lateral ventricle
    C. Third ventricle
    D. Region of pineal gland
    E. Internal occipital protuberance

Review Exercise D: Additional and Specialized Computed Tomography Procedures and Computed Tomography Terminology

1. A. 2–3 mm
2. True
3. C. Spinal cord deformity
4. C. Both bone and soft tissue window settings
5. False
6. True
7. Air
8. Carbon dioxide
9. False
10. D. Up to 2000 mL
11. To ensure that the heart is scanned only during the times of the least motion in the cardiac cycle
12. True
13. True
14. C. 8–12 images per second
15. D. Biopsies
16. D. Special needle holders
17. True

18. D. 85%
19. Gantry
20. Matrix
21. Scanogram, topogram, or scout
22. Slip rings
23. Window level (WL)
24. Window width (WW)
25. Maximum intensity projection (MIP)

CHAPTER 19

Review Exercise A: Arthrography

1. Synovial joints
2. Magnetic resonance imaging (MR) or computed tomography (CT)
3. A. Tears of the joint capsule
   B. Tears of the menisci
   C. Tears of ligaments
4. Baker cyst
5. Allergic reactions to iodine-based contrast media and allergic reactions to local anesthetics
6. True
7. False (needs to be flexed to distribute contrast media)
8. Clear and tinged yellow
9. A. Positive or radiopaque media such as iodinated, water-soluble contrast agent
   B. Negative or radiolucent contrast agents, such as room air, oxygen, or carbon dioxide
10. A. AP
    B. Lateral
11. A. Nine images per meniscus
    B. 20 degrees
12. A. Joint capsule
    B. Rotator cuff
    C. Long tendon of biceps muscle
    D. Articular cartilage
13. Rotator cuff
14. 2¾- to 3½-inch spinal needle
15. A. Chronic pain
    B. General weakness
    C. Suspected tear in the rotator cuff
16. A. AP scout
    B. AP internal rotation
    C. AP external rotation
    D. Glenoid fossa AP oblique (Grashey method) projection
    E. Transaxillary (inferosuperior axial) projection
    F. Intertubercular (bicipital) sulcus projection

Review Exercise B: Biliary Duct Procedures

1. B. Biliary stones
2. False
3. A. BUN
   B. Creatinine
4. Contrast media that are too concentrated may obscure small stones in the biliary ducts
5. False
6. RPO position
7. In the radiology department
8. C. Removal of a biliary stone
9. A. Endoscopic retrograde cholangiopancreatogram
   B. ERCP
   C. Duodenoscope or video endoscope
   D. Gastroenterologist
   E. To prevent aspiration of food or liquid into the lungs
10. Pseudocyst

Review Exercise C: Hysterosalpingography

1. Uterus and uterine tubes
2. Rectosigmoid colon, urinary bladder
3. A. Fundus
   B. Corpus (or body)
   C. Isthmus
   D. Cervix
4. Corpus (or body)
5. Cervix
6. A. Endometrium
   B. Myometrium
   C. Serosa
7. A. Cornu
8. True
9. True
10. B. Patency
11. Assessment of female infertility
12. A. Demonstration of intrauterine pathology
    B. Evaluation of the uterine tubes after tubal ligation or reconstructive surgery
13. A. Endometrial polyps
    B. Uterine fibroids
    C. Intrauterine adhesions
14. A. Water-soluble, iodinated
15. Tenaculum
16. Slight Trendelenburg
17. A. LPO
    B. RPO
18. D. 2 inches (5 cm) superior to the symphysis pubis

Review Exercise D: Myelography

1. A. Spinal cord
   B. Nerve root branches
2. A. Herniated nucleus pulposus (HNP)
   B. Cancerous or benign tumors
   C. Cysts
   D. Possible bone fragments (in the case of trauma)
3. Herniated nucleus pulposus (HNP)
4. False (Most common are cervical and lumbar regions.)
5. A. Blood in the cerebrospinal fluid
   B. Arachnoiditis
   C. Increased intracranial pressure
   D. Recent lumbar puncture (within 2 weeks)
6. 1 hour
7. 90/45-degree or 90/90-degree tilting table
8. Subarachnoid space
9. A. Lumbar (L3–L4)
   B. Cervical (C1–C2)
10. Lumbar (L3–L4)
11. A. Prone or left lateral
    B. Erect or prone
12. For spinal flexion to widen the interspinous spaces to facilitate needle placement
13. Nonionic, water-soluble, iodine-based
14. C. 1 hour
15. C. 9–15 mL
16. A. 4
    B. 5
    C. 8
    D. 1
    E. 6
    F. 2
    G. 7
    H. 3
17. Cervicothoracic (Swimmer's) lateral with a horizontal x-ray beam
18. To keep the contrast media from entering the cranial subarachnoid space
19. True (Right and left lateral decubitus positions are taken.)
20. 1. A. Horizontal beam lateral (prone), C5
       B. Horizontal beam cervicothoracic lateral (Swimmer's), C7
    2. A. R lateral decubitus (AP or PA), T7

551

B. L lateral decubitus (AP or PA), T7
C. R or L lateral, vertical beam, T7
3. A. Semierect horizontal beam lateral (prone), L3
21. True
22. Excreted by kidneys

Review Exercise E: Hip-to-Ankle Long Bone Measurement

1. To determine limb length discrepancies and lower limb extremity alignment.
2. To determine hardware needs and prothesis or appliance placement.
3. 120 inches (300 cm)
4. A wedge filter or the anode-heel effect.
5. 8 inches (20 cm)
6. Perpendicular to the knee joint

Review Exercise F: Radiographic Skeletal Survey (Bone Survey)

1. Radiographic images that encompass the entire skeleton or those regions appropriate for the clinical indications.
2. To accurately identify the focal and diffuse abnormalities of the skeleton such as, evaluation of fractures, bone lesions, metabolic bone disease, skeletal dysplasia, developmental changes, or anatomic variants.
3. B. Thorax
4. D. Lumbosacral spine
5. True (Radiographic skeletal surveys may be performed as the initial imaging procedure based on the findings or no findings from other modalities.)
6. True (A skeletal survey may be requested following a positive radionuclide bone scan to further evaluate the structure.)

Review Exercise G: Digital Tomosynthesis

1. B. Gastric
2. False. DTS often delivers lower dose and is less expensive that CT
3. Multiple very low-dose x-ray projection images acquired from different angles during a single linear sweep of the x-ray tube across a stationary detector
4. The structures in each plane are more clearly visible without the interference of tissue in front or in back of the plane of interest.
5. True
6. Parallax
7. Superimposition or overlapping structures

CHAPTER 20

Review Exercise A: Nuclear Medicine and PET

1. Radiopharmaceuticals
2. True
3. D. All of the above
4. C. Technetium 99 m (Tc-99m)
5. D. 48 hours
6. Planar (static); dynamic
7. Single-photon emission computed tomography
8. 200 microcuries (μCi) and 30 millicuries (mCi)
9. 2 years
10. A. Kidney transplants
11. B. Gastric emptying
12. B. Myocardial perfusion Imaging (stress/rest cardiac imaging)
13. C. Sodium iodide 123 (^{123}I)
14. A. 1
    B. 3
    C. 1
    D. 1
    E. 2
    F. 3
    G. 2
    H. 4
    I. 3
    J. 1
15. A. 3
    B. 6
    C. 2
    D. 8
    E. 1
    F. 5
    G. 4
    H. 7
16. Positron emission tomography
17. C. Metabolic and biochemical changes in tissue
18. False (The PET scanner itself does not produce radiation.)
19. B. Positrons
20. Annihilation radiation
21. A. Emitted photons
22. Fused or coregistered
23. D. Carbon and fluorine
24. C. Cellular reproduction
25. A. 2
    B. 1
    C. 4
    D. 3
26. Cyclotron
27. A. 120 seconds to 110 minutes
28. False
29. True
30. C. Staging
31. False
32. True
33. A. 82Rbn chloride
34. True
35. True
36. D. Identify the location of key motor and sensory regions of the brain
37. Decreased
38. D. Fusion technology
39. Electroencephalography
40. True

Review Exercise B: Radiation Oncology (Therapy)

1. True
2. Simulation
3. A. 3D imaging
    B. 4D imaging
4. Brachytherapy
5. A. CT
    B. MR
6. Gamma knife
7. D. Bragg peak
8. Respiratory and cardiac
9. Stereotactic body radiation therapy
10. Intensity modulated radiation therapy (IMRT)
11. MR based linear accelerator
12. Short-distance therapy

Review Exercise C: Diagnostic Medical Sonography (Sonography)

1. A. Sonography
    B. Ultrasonography
    C. Echosonography
    D. Ultrasound
2. 2 and 20 MHz
3. Converts electrical energy to waves of (sound) energy
4. True
5. True
6. A. General
    B. Echocardiography
    C. Vascular
7. False
8. No ionizing radiation
9. True
10. World War II

11. Echo location
12. C. Computers
13. B. B-mode (brightness mode)
14. D. Doppler
15. D. The stiffness of normal versus abnormal tissues
16. True
17. False
18. False
19. True
20. Lowest MI and TI settings
21. True
22. False
23. True
24. B. Stomach
25. True
26. True
27. C. Gel
28. True
29. A. 8
    B. 3
    C. 9
    D. 1
    E. 7
    F. 5
    G. 10
    H. 4
    I. 2
    J. 6
30. B. Heterogeneous

MAMMOGRAPHY

Review Exercise A: Breast Cancer, Mammography Quality Standards Act, Anatomy of the Breast, and Breast Classifications

1. Mammography
2. B. 40
3. C. 1994
4. 2.26 million
5. 1%–2%
6. 2 cm
7. B. 15%
8. Canadian Association of Radiologists
9. B. VA facilities
10. Inframammary fold
11. Areola
12. Axillary prolongation
13. Mediolateral
14. Lower inner quadrant (LIQ)
15. 10 o'clock
16. Pectoralis major muscle
17. Retromammary
18. Lactation or secretion of milk

19. A. Glandular
    B. Fibrous or connective
    C. Adipose (fatty)
20. Trabeculae
21. Cooper (suspensory) ligaments
22. 1. FG
    2. FG
    3. FF
    4. FG
    5. F
    6. F
    7. FG
    8. F
23. Adipose
24. Fig. 20.1
    A. Skin
    B. Pectoralis major muscle
    C. Retromammary space
    D. Adipose (fatty) tissue
    E. Glandular tissue
    F. Nipple
    G. Inframammary crease
    H. Sixth rib (lower breast margin—varies among individuals)
    I. Second rib (upper breast margin)
    J. Clavicle
25. Fig. 20.2
    A. Areola
    B. Nipple
    C. Ampulla
    D. Ducts
    E. Alveoli
    F. Mammary fat
    G. Lobe
    H. Cooper ligament
26. 15–20
27. Base
28. Apex
29. A. Compressed breast thickness
    B. Tissue density
30. Breast density

Review Exercise B: Mammography: Patient Preparation, Technical Considerations, Alternative Modalities, and Radiographic Positioning

1. Talcum powder and antiperspirant deodorant
2. True
3. A. Number of pregnancies? Are you currently pregnant?
    B. Is there a family history of cancer, including breast cancer?

C. Medications currently taking?
    D. Previous breast surgery?
    E. Had previous mammogram? When and where?
    F. Reason for current examination? Screening mammogram? Any changes in breast, including lumps, pain, or discharge?
4. False
5. Base
6. 0.1 and 0.3 mm
7. 15–30 pounds (40 lb maximum)
8. A. Decreases the thickness of the breast
    B. Brings the breast structures as close to the IR as possible
    C. Decreases dose and scattered radiation
    D. Decreases motion and geometric unsharpness
    E. Increases radiographic contrast
    F. Separates breast structure
9. A. Reduces scatter radiation
    B. Separation of superimposed structures in breast
10. B. Magnify specific regions of interest
11. A. The characteristics of the equipment being used.
    B. The technique factors selected for the examination.
    C. The size and density of the patient's breast.
12. False
13. B. 5%
14. True
15. A. Fine detail (high resolution)
    B. Edge sharpness
    C. Soft tissue visibility
16. C. Overall spatial resolution is higher (Analog imaging is higher)
17. A. Algorithms
18. D. Iodinated
19. Flat panel detector (also termed thin film transistor [FPD-TFT] technology in Chapter 1)
20. False
21. B. 15%
22. Distinguishing a cyst from a solid mass
23. True
24. True
25. D. Technetium-99m-sestamibi

26. B. Detect metastasis to a lymph node surrounding the breast
27. A. Sulfur colloid
28. C. Glucose (sugar) metabolism
29. Gamma camera is much smaller, therefore in closer proximity to the patient's breast
30. A. Higher cost
    B. Radiation exposure to the patient
31. False
32. A. High false-positive rate
    B. Higher cost
    C. Length of the exam time
33. B. Digital breast tomosynthesis
34. A. Fibroadenoma
35. C. Infiltrating (invasive) ductal carcinoma
36. C. Fibroadenoma
37. True
38. A. Craniocaudal (CC)
    B. Mediolateral oblique (MLO)
39. Inframammary fold
40. Axillary
41. Nipple
42. Away from
43. Mediolateral oblique (MLO)
44. 45 degrees from vertical (Note: CR is perpendicular to the patient's pectoral muscle.)
45. False
46. B. Forward, toward the front of the body
47. Exaggerated craniocaudal (lateral), or XCCL
48. Base
49. Exaggerated craniocaudal (lateral), or XCCL
50. Exaggerated craniocaudal (lateral), or XCCL
51. 90 degrees from vertical
52. A. True
    B. False
    C. False
    D. True
    E. False
    F. False (overexposed image)
    G. True
    H. True
    I. False
    J. True
53. Eklund method
54. The breast implant needs to be "pinched" or carefully pushed posterior toward the chest wall out of the exposure field.
55. D. Axillary tail

56. A. Mediolateral oblique
    B. Superolateral-inferomedial oblique
    C. Axillary tail
    D. Craniocaudal
    E. Rolled lateral
    F. Lateromedial
    G. Exaggerated craniocaudal (laterally)
    H. Lateromedial oblique
    I. Implant displaced

Review Exercise C: Critique Radiographs of the Breast

A. CC projection (Fig. 20.3)
   1. Folds of fatty tissue superimpose breast tissue.
   2. Breast is not pulled away from chest wall; folds of tissue are not pulled back.
   3. Collimation is not applicable for mammography. CR centering is acceptable.
   4. Exposure factors are acceptable.
   5. Anatomic side marker is visible.
      Repeatable error(s): 1 (anatomy demonstrated) and 2 (part positioning)
B. MLO projection (Fig. 20.4)
   1. Pertinent muscle is not seen to nipple level, and outer tissue is not compressed.
   2. Lower part of breast not pulled away from chest wall onto IR sufficiently.
   3. Collimation not applicable for mammography. CR centering is acceptable.
   4. Exposure factors are acceptable.
   5. Anatomic side marker is visible.
      Repeatable error(s): 1 (anatomy demonstrated) and 2 (part positioning)
C. CC projection (Fig. 20.5)
   1. Part of lateral posterior breast is cut off.
   2. Medial posterior breast is not included, and shoulder is superimposed over the lateral posterior tissue.
   3. Collimation is not applicable for mammography. CR centering is acceptable.

   4. Exposure factors are acceptable
   5. Anatomic side marker is visible.
      Repeatable error(s): 1 (anatomy demonstrated) and 2 (part positioning)
D. MLO projection (Fig. 20.6)
   1. Posterior medial breast is cut off; no pectoral muscle is visible. (White specks are calcifications; they are not dust artifacts.)
   2. Breast is not pulled out away from chest wall.
   3. Collimation is not applicable for mammography. CR centering is acceptable.
   4. Exposure factors are acceptable.
   5. Anatomic side marker is visible.
      Repeatable error(s): 1 (anatomy demonstrated) and 2 (part positioning)
E. CC projection (Fig. 20.7)
   1. Motion is present, which obliterates all detail.
   2. Acceptable—dark half-circle indicates posterior breast is included.
   3. Collimation is not applicable for mammography. CR centering is acceptable.
   4. Exposure factors are acceptable.
   5. Anatomic side marker is visible.
      Repeatable error(s): 1 (anatomy demonstrated)
F. CC projection (Fig. 20.8)
   1. Hair artifacts are evident on posterior breast tissue, obscuring breast tissue detail.
   2. Acceptable.
   3. Collimation is not applicable for mammography. CR is slightly off-centered toward medial side.
   4. Exposure factors are acceptable.
   5. Anatomic side marker is visible.
      Repeatable error(s): 1 (anatomy demonstrated)
      Review Exercise: Bone densitometry

1. 72.2 million
2. A. Bone density
   B. Bone quality
3. 30%–50%
4. Osteoblasts, osteoclasts
5. 35 years
6. 90% collagen and 10% other proteins
7. Bone mineral content (BMC)
8. D. All of the above
9. D. Polycystic kidney disease
10. True
11. B, C, G, I
12. False (less risk)
13. True
14. True
15. D. 2.5 standard deviations below the average for the young normal population
16. The number of standard deviations an individual's BMD is from the mean BMD of an average, young individual of the same sex and ethnicity.
17. A. Normal bone
18. Z-scores
19. B. Parathyroid hormone analog (PTH I-34)
20. True
21. A. Dual-energy x-ray absorptiometry (DXA)
    B. Quantitative computed tomography (QCT)
    C. Quantitative ultrasound (QUS)
22. B. Dual-energy x-ray absorptiometry (DXA)
23. False (Fan-beam)
24. Micro-Sieverts (µSv)
25. <5 µSv
26. B. An average individual of the same sex and age
27. C. T12–L5
28. True
29. False
30. Trabecular and cortical
31. 30 µSv
32. C. Calcaneus (Os calcis)
33. C. QUS
34. A. Lumbar spine
    B. Hip (proximal femur)
35. True
36. True
37. True
38. False
39. False
40. B. Reproducibility
41. A. Patient positioning
42. 10%
43. 70 years
44. A. Thoracolumbar spine
45. B. Femoral neck or total hip
46. False

MAGNETIC RESONANCE IMAGING

Review Exercise A: Physical Principles of MR and MR Magnets

1. Magnetic fields, radiofrequency pulses, and a computer system
2. False. MR does not use ionizing radiation.
3. A. T1
4. Fourier Transform (FT)
5. A. Hydrogen (single-proton nucleus)
   B. The large amount of hydrogen present in any organism. (Hydrogen atoms are present in each water molecule, and the body is roughly 85% water.)
6. Proton
7. It is similar to the wobble of a slowly spinning top
8. Increases
9. A. Larmor frequency
   B. Resonance frequency
10. Net magnetization (NM)
11. True
12. Resonance
13. False. Only hydrogen protons will resonate
14. A. Forces precessing protons into the transverse plane away from the static magnetic field (B0).
    B. Forces the protons to process in phase (same direction).
15. T1 relaxation and T2 relaxation
16. Longitudinal
17. Transverse
18. Spin (or proton) density
19. A. Permanent
    B. Resistive
    C. Superconductive Superconductive
20. C. Tesla
21. D. 0005 (1 T = 10,000 G)
22. C. Superconducting

Review Exercise B: Patient Aspects: Contraindications, Preparation, Anxiety, and Monitoring MR Safety, and Pulse Sequences

1. D. Any of the above
2. False. Some contraindicated devices may be MR conditional and examinations are possible.
3. A. Thorough medical history
4. C. MR technologist
5. D. All of the above
6. C. Use restraints
7. C. Xanax
8. A. 2 (Zone II)
   B. 4 (Zone IV)
   C. 1 (Zone I)
   D. 3 (Zone III)
9. C. Level 2
10. D. MR medical director
11. Missile effect
12. False
13. A. Translational force
    B. Torque
14. D. A or B
15. Specific absorption rate (SAR)
16. C. Watts per kilogram
17. A. Normal
18. B. SED (Specific energy dose)
19. True
20. True
21. C. Gadolinium
22. C. Within 1 hour
23. C. eGFR
24. A. T1
    B. T2
    C. Proton density (PD)
25. A. Spin echo (SE)
    B. Gradient echo (GRE)
    C. Echo planar imaging (EPI)

Review Exercise C: MR Examinations

1. A. T1
   B. T2
   C. PD
2. D. Intervertebral disc
3. FLAIR
4. A. T1
5. B. Pons
6. Magnetic resonance angiography (MRA)
7. Magnetic resonance venogram (MRV)
8. C. Circle of Willis
9. A. Soft tissue

555

B. Ligaments
C. Tendons
D. Cartilage
E. Bone
10. D. Any of the above
11. False
12. A. Rotator cuff tear (Shoulder)
13. True
14. C. 7–14 days from the start of menstruation
15. Anatomic structures and function
16. Water molecules
17. False

18. White matter fiber tracks
19. A. Functional Magnetic Resonance Imaging (fMRI)
    B. Blood oxygenation level dependent (BOLD)
20. A. (9) Larmor frequency
    B. (7) Gating
    C. (4) Flip angle
    D. (2) Coil
    E. (6) Fringe field
    F. (10) MR conditional
    G. (1) B0
    H. (5) Fourier transform

I. (3) Echo time
J. (8) Gradient coils
21. A. (3) Relaxation time (TR)
    B. (9) Tesla
    C. (7) T1 relaxation
    D. (1) Precession
    E. (6) Specific absorption rate
    F. (2) Pulse sequence
    G. (5) Spatial resolution
    H. (8) T2 relaxation
    I. (10) Torque
    J. (4) Resonance